D0875777

Immunochemistry:
An Advanced Textbook

Immunochemistry: An Advanced Textbook

Edited by

L. E. Glynn and M. W. Steward

Kennedy Institute of Rheumatology,
and
London School of Hygiene and Tropical Medicine
London

A Wiley–Interscience Publication

JOHN WILEY & SONS

CHICHESTER · NEW YORK · BRISBANE · TORONTO

Library of Congress Cataloging in Publication Data:
Main entry under title:

Immunochemistry: An Advanced Textbook

    'A Wiley–Interscience publication.'
    Includes bibliographical references and indexes.
    1. Immunochemistry.   I. Glynn, Leonard Eleazer.
II. Steward, Michael W.
QR182.I46   612′.11822   77-1630
ISBN 0 471 99508 8

Printed by William Clowes & Sons, Limited, London, Beccles and Colchester.

Contributors

R. ARNON — *Department of Chemical Immunology, The Weizmann Institute of Science, Rehovot, Israel*

K. F. AUSTEN — *Robert B. Brigham Hospital, Boston, Massachusetts, U.S.A.*

D. BEALE — *Agricultural Research Council, Institute of Animal Physiology, Babraham, Cambridge CB2 4AT, U.K.*

H. K. BEARD — *Medical Research Council Rheumatism Research Unit, Canadian Red Cross Hospital, Taplow, Berkshire, U.K.*

L. CONOCHIE — *Medical Research Council Rheumatism Research Unit, Canadian Red Cross Hospital, Taplow, Berkshire, U.K.*

D. W. DRESSER — *National Institute for Medical Research, Mill Hill, London NW7 1AA, U.K.*

D. T. FEARON — *Robert B. Brigham Hospital, Boston, Massachusetts, U.S.A.*

A. FEINSTEIN — *Agricultural Research Council, Institute of Animal Physiology, Babraham, Cambridge CB2 4AT, U.K.*

J. GAFNI — *Tel-Aviv University School of Medicine, Israel*

B. GEIGER — *Department of Chemical Immunology, The Weizmann Institute of Science, Rehovot, Israel*

L. E. GLYNN — *The Kennedy Institute of Rheumatology, London W6 7DW, U.K.*

T. J. KINDT — *The Rockefeller University, New York, New York 10021, U.S.A.*

W. H. KONIGSBERG — *Yale University School of Medicine, New Haven, Connecticut 16510, U.S.A.*

W. PAGE-FAULK — *Medical Research Council Rheumatism Research Unit, Canadian Red Cross Hospital, Taplow, Berkshire, U.K.*

D. PARKER — *Department of Pathology, Royal College of Surgeons of England, London WC2A 3PN, U.K.*

R. M. E. PARKHOUSE — *National Institute for Medical Research, Mill Hill, London NW7 1AA, U.K.*

M. PRAS — *Department of Internal Medicine and Heller Institute of Medical Research, Sheba Medical Centre at Tel-Hashomer, Israel*

F. F. RICHARDS — *Yale University School of Medicine, New Haven, Connecticut 16510, U.S.A.*

R. W. ROSENSTEIN — *Yale University School of Medicine, New Haven, Connecticut 16510, U.S.A.*

J. A. SOGN — *The Rockefeller University, New York, New York 10021, U.S.A.*

N. A. STAINES — *Searle Research Laboratories, High Wycombe, Buckinghamshire HP12 4H2, U.K. Now at: Kennedy Institute of Rheumatology, London W6 7DW*

D. R. STANWORTH — *Department of Experimental Pathology, The University of Birmingham, Birmingham B15 2TJ, U.K.*

M. W. STEWARD — *Division of Immunology, Kennedy Institute of Rheumatology, London W6 7DW, U.K. Now at: London School of Hygiene, Keppel Street, London WC1E 7HT, U.K.*

I. W. SUTHERLAND — *Department of Microbiology, University of Edinburgh, Edinburgh EH9 3JG, U.K.*

J. L. TURK — *Department of Pathology, Royal College of Surgeons of England, London WC2A 3PN, U.K.*

M. W. TURNER — *Department of Immunology, Institute of Child Health, Guilford Street, London WC1N 1EH, U.K.*

J. M. VARGA — *Yale University School of Medicine, New Haven, Connecticut 16510, U.S.A.*

M. W. WHITEHOUSE — *Department of Experimental Pathology, John Curtin School of Medical Research, The Australian National University, Canberra ACT 2601, Australia*

A. R. WILLIAMSON — *Department of Biochemistry, University of Glasgow, Glasgow G12 8QQ, U.K.*

Contents

Preface

The subject of Immunochemistry owes much to the pioneering work of Paul Ehrlich, but it was the physical chemist Arrhenius who, in 1907 first coined the word Immunochemistry to describe:

> *the chemical reactions of substances that are produced by the injection of foreign substances into the blood of animals (i.e. by immunization) and that the substances with which these products react as proteins and ferments are to be considered with respect to their chemical properties.*

The field of modern immunochemistry still has as its central theme the study of the chemistry of antibodies and antigens and of their interaction, but in addition, research interests within this discipline have broadened to include investigations of the nature of other substances of immunological importance, for example components of the complement system.

In the compilation of this book, we have taken into account the fact that although there are many specialized texts and reviews of aspects of this topical area of biomedical research, no single volume exists which gives an up-to-date and comprehensive coverage of the broad field of immunochemistry. We feel that this book meets such a need and will be of particular value for final-year undergraduates in both science and medical faculties who are interested in these exciting areas of modern immunology; for postgraduates in both scientific and medical disciplines and for research workers in immunochemistry and other areas of immunology who wish to be acquainted with the current state of knowledge in fields other than their own.

The book is an 'advanced textbook' in that the authors have assumed, in the preparation of their chapters, that readers will have a general background knowledge of immunology, biochemistry, and biology. All the authors have gained international recognition for their contributions to their respective fields of research, and the chapters have been carefully selected to ensure that all the areas attracting the current attention of immunochemists are discussed. These include the structure, function and genetics of immunoglobulins and antibodies; the immunochemistry of a wide variety of antigens; the immunochemistry of complement and the immunology of cell antigens; a discussion of the current understanding of adjuvant substances; and two clinically important subjects— the immunoglobulinopathies and the nature of amyloid.

It is our hope that this book will acquaint its readers with the achievements, failures, and future hopes of research in this challenging field of biomedical research.

L.E.G.
M.W.S.
London, 1977.

CHAPTER 1

Structure and Function of Immunoglobulins

M. W. Turner

1 GENERAL INTRODUCTION

Immunoglobulins are a family of structurally related proteins which mediate circulating antibody responses. There are five major classes of protein in most

1

Table 1 Human immunoglobulins

Present nomenclature	Abbreviation	Previous nomenclature
Immunoglobulin G	IgG	γ-G globulin, 7 S γ-globulin
Immunoglobulin A	IgA	γ-A globulin, β_2A-globulin
Immunoglobulin M	IgM	γ-M globulin, 19 S γ-globulin
Immunoglobulin D	IgD	—
Immunoglobulin E	IgE	reagin, IgND

higher mammals although when the name immunoglobulin (Ig) was proposed by Heremans (1959) only three classes were known, namely IgG, IgA, and IgM. To these have now been added the classes IgD and IgE. Table 1 gives the present nomenclature recommended by WHO*.

Immunoglobulins are the products of lymphoid cells, particularly plasma cells, which synthesize large quantities of these proteins (see Chapter 4). Most immunoglobulin molecules produced by these cells are found in the serum and secretions of the body and are responsible for the humoral immune response. In addition, a small proportion of immunoglobulin molecules become firmly bound to the surface membranes of lymphocytes and macrophages and may function as antigen receptors, thus playing a role in implementing cell-mediated immunity.

The physicochemical heterogeneity of antibodies has been recognized for nearly 40 years and was a major problem in early structural investigations. However, in the mouse, rat, and man, pathological proteins occur known as myeloma proteins which are structurally homogeneous immunoglobulins produced by neoplastic plasma cells. Each of these proteins is thought to represent an overproduction of a single 'normal' immunoglobulin molecule, and in many cases sufficient protein has been isolated from serum to permit full immunochemical characterization. In the absence of myeloma proteins, such investigations would be almost impossible for the quantitatively unimportant IgD and IgE classes.

This chapter will attempt to provide a selective review of our present knowledge of the immunoglobulins. The emphasis will be largely on the human system but some information for other species will be included also, especially when notable differences occur. For convenience, the chapter is divided into a section dealing with general aspects of structure and a section devoted to the structural basis for effector or adjunctive functions such as complement fixation and interactions with membranes. The close relationships between primary structure and conformation are covered in Chapter 8 which should be considered conjointly with the present review.

* This and other aspects of immunoglobulin nomenclature have been published by various Committees on Nomenclature for Human Immunoglobulins. *Bull. Wld Hlth Org.*, (1964) **30**, 447; (1965) **33**, 721; (1966) **35**, 953; (1968) **38**, 151; (1969) **41**, 975.

2 STRUCTURE OF IMMUNOGLOBULINS

2.1 Introduction and General Considerations

Although myeloma proteins have made a major contribution to our knowledge of immunoglobulin structure, it was work on pooled rabbit IgG which provided the basis for many present-day concepts. In 1959, Porter showed that rabbit IgG antibodies could be split by the plant protease papain into three large fragments and, furthermore, that these fragments could be separated by ion-exchange chromatography. Two of these fragments were identical and retained univalent antigen-binding capacity (now known as Fab—Fragment antigen binding), whereas the third fragment could be crystallized (now called Fc—Fragment crystalline). The latter fragment has been shown subsequently to be associated with various effector or adjunctive functions of the antibody molecule. Examples of such functions are the binding of the complement protein C1q, macrophage binding, and membrane transmission. The effector functions of immunoglobulins are discussed in detail in Section 3 of this chapter.

Chemical methods of separating the constituent peptide chains of immunoglobulins were described by Edelman and Poulik (1961), and by Fleischman *et*

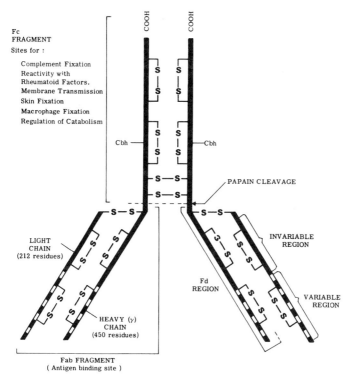

Figure 1 Schematic representation of the four-chain structure of human IgG1 showing inter and intra-chain disulphide bridges, papain fragments, and location of effector functions

al. (1961) and shortly afterwards Porter (1962) proposed a four-chain model for immunoglobulin molecules based on two distinct types of polypeptide chain. This basic four-chain model, which is illustrated in Figure 1, appears to occur throughout the vertebrate kingdom and comprises two small (light) polypeptide chains (molecular weight 22 000) and two larger (heavy) polypeptide chains (molecular weight 50 000–77 000). The heavy chains are invariably covalently bound through disulphide bridges, and usually each heavy chain is bound similarly to a light chain. Occasionally, however, the disulphide bridges between heavy and light chains are absent, and instead the light chains are linked covalently. This is the case with certain IgA molecules in man and the mouse. In all cases, noncovalent forces also help to maintain overall molecular stability.

The light chains are common to all classes of immunoglobulin whereas the heavy chains have the antigenic, immunological, and chemical characteristics of only one of the five classes. The heavy chains characteristic of immunoglobulin chains are designated by appropriate Greek letters—γ chains for IgG, α for IgA, μ for IgM, δ for IgD, and ε for IgE. The light chains of most vertebrates have been shown to exist in two antigenically distinct forms called Kappa (κ type) and lambda (λ type). In any one molecule, both light chains are of the same type and hybrid molecules have never been observed. Both types are present usually in any one individual but the $\kappa : \lambda$ ratio differs from species to species, from class to class, and from subclass to subclass. Thus for human immunoglobulins, the overall ratio is $6:4$ but for circulating human IgD it is $2:8$. The ratio of light chain types in each of the four subclasses of human IgG is shown in Table 2. In the serum of other animals, the proportions of κ and λ chains range from more than 95 per cent λ chains in the horse to more than 95 per cent κ chains in the mouse. There is evidence that the relative proportions of κ and λ chains change during immunization. This is presumably a reflection of the particular classes and subclasses involved at different stages of the immune response.

Table 2 κ and λ-light chains in human IgG subclasses

Human subclass	$\kappa : \lambda$ ratio	
	a	*b*
IgG1	2·41	1·42
IgG2	1·10	0·96
IgG3	1·12	1·25
IgG4	5·0	7·0

a data from Terry *et al.* (1965)
b data from Schur (1972)

The realization that serum myeloma proteins and urinary Bence–Jones proteins represent pathological counterparts of normal intact immunoglobulins and free light chains, respectively (Edelman and Gally, 1962), initiated the application of protein-sequencing techniques to these proteins, and many sequences for several species are now available. Only selected sequences are

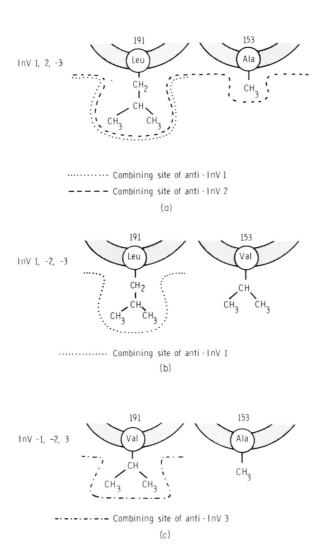

Figure 2 InV (or Km) antigens and amino acid sequence. Antisera that detect the InV1 (Km (1)) antigen probably interact with a leucine residue at position 191, but do not encompass residue 153. In contrast, antisera to InV2 (Km (2)) recognize the leucine residue at position 191, but also encompass an alanine residue at position 153 (*a*). If the alanine residue is replaced by valine the anti-InV2 (Km (2)) reagent is no longer able to recognize the complete antigenic determinant, possibly because of steric hindrance by the larger valine residue (*b*). The third InV allotype (InV3 or Km (3)) is expressed when a valine residue occurs at position 191 and appears to be independent of residue 153, although this is uncertain (*c*)

6

included in this review but the interested reader can obtain information from the annually updated *Atlas of Protein Structure* (Dayhoff, M. O., ed.), National Biomedical Research Foundation, Silver Spring, Maryland, U.S.A.

The work of Hilschmann and Craig (1965), Baglioni *et al.* (1966), Milstein (1966), and Putnam *et al.* (1966) established the important principle that when light chains of the same type (and from the same species) are sequenced they are seen to comprise two distinct regions. The C-terminal half of the chain (approximately 107 amino acid residues) does not vary except for certain minor differences which reflect either allotypic or isotypic variations. In human κ-chains, for example, alternative amino acid residues may occur at positions 191 and 153 of the peptide chain. These alternative residues correlate with the allotypic antigens InV1, InV2, and InV3 (now called Km(1), Km(2), and Km(3)) as illustrated schematically in Figure 2.

In the case of human λ chains, amino acid differences have been noted at positions 190 and 152, and these correlate with the so-called Oz and Kern

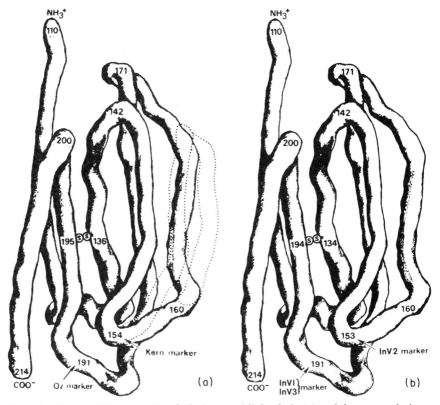

Figure 3 Model of C-terminal half of a human λ light chain (*a*) and, by extrapolation, a similar model for human κ light chain (*b*) showing the basic 'immunoglobulin fold' in both. The approximate location of residues which determine Oz and Kern isotypes and the InV (or Km) allotypes are indicated. The dotted line indicates the position of the extra loop in the V_L region. Modified, with permission, from Poljak (1975)

markers. Unlike the InV (or Km) markers, however, these are both isotypic antigens, that is, all normal individuals have both Oz(+) and Oz(−), and Kern(+) and Kern(−) λ chains.

Recent X-ray crystallographic analyses indicate that each of these amino acid residues is located at the surface and available to the external environment (see Figure 3, and Chapter 7).

In contrast to the C-terminal half of the light polypetide chain the N-terminal region shows much sequence variability. However, the variability observed is not distributed evenly throughout the length of the region. Some positions in the sequence show exceptional variability, and in both κ and λ light chains such hypervariable regions are located near positions 30, 50, 95, and 106 (see Figure 4). It is now generally accepted that such hypervariable residues are involved directly in the formation of the antigen binding site. A feature associated with hypervariable regions is the presence of adjacent constant residues, particularly cysteine, glycine, and tryptophan. These residues are sometimes called 'framework' residues and are thought to create the necessary rigid framework near which apparently unrestricted amino acid variability can occur.

In addition to the hypervariable residues, the N–terminal half of light chains is composed of residues showing a more restricted variation in different proteins. Indeed when sequences are examined for evidence of homology, it is found that the variable regions of both κ and λ chains are divisible into subgroups. In man, κ

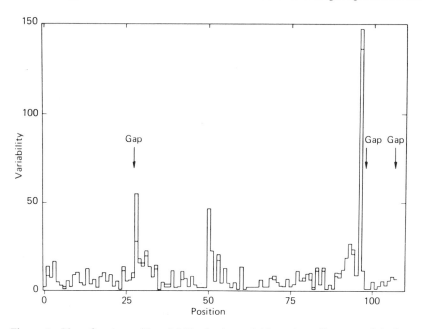

Figure 4   Plot of amino acid variability in the variable region of immunoglobulin light chains according to sequence number. Extra amino acids occur in some sequences and to enhance the comparison these have been excluded as indicated by the arrows. Reproduced from Wu and Kabat (1970), with permission

Table 3 Prototype N-terminal sequences of the subgroups of human κ and λ-light chains

Subgroups	Sequence
κ chains	
$V_\kappa I$	Asp-Ile -Gln-Met-Thr-Gln-Ser -Pro-Ser -Ser -Leu-Ser -Ala-Ser -Val -Gly-Asp-Arg-Val -Thr
$V_\kappa II$	Glu-Ile -Val -Leu-Thr-Gln-Ser -Pro-Gly-Thr-Leu-Ser -Leu-Ser -Pro-Gly-Glu-Arg-Ala -Thr
$V_\kappa III$	Asp-Ile -Val -Met-Thr-Gln-Ser -Pro-Leu-Ser -Leu-Pro-Val -Thr-Pro-Gly-Glu-Pro-Ala-Ser
λ chains	
$V_\lambda I$	*Glp-Ser -Val -Leu-Thr-Gln-Pro-Pro-( )-Ser -Val -Ser -Gly-Ala-Pro-Gly-Gln-Arg-Val -Thr
$V_\lambda II$	*Glp-Ser -Ala -Leu-Thr-Gln-Pro-Ala-( )-Ser -Val -Ser -Gly-Ser -Pro-Gly-Gln-Ser -Ile -Thr
$V_\lambda III$	( )-Tyr-Val -Leu-Thr-Gln-Pro-Pro-( )-Ser -Val -Ser -Val -Ser -Pro-Gly-Gln-Thr-Ala-Ser
$V_\lambda IV$	*Glp-Ser -Ala -Leu-Thr-Gln-Pro-Pro-( )-Ser -Ala-Ser -Gly-Ser -Pro-Gly-Gln-Ser -Val -Thr
$V_\lambda V$	( )-Ser -Glu-Leu-Thr-Gln-Pro-Pro-( )-Ala -Val -Ser -Val -Ala-Leu-Gly-Gln-Thr-Val -Arg

* Residue derived from pyrrolid-2-one-5-carboxylic acid

chains fall into three subgroups and λ chains into five. Prototype sequences of the first 20 residues of such subgroups are illustrated in Table 3.

Sequence studies on heavy chains of monoclonal human immunoglobulins have revealed that, in common with the light chains, there is a V region at the N-terminus of the peptide chain. Generally, V_H regions are slightly longer than V_L regions, comprising 118–124 amino acid residues and having four regions of hypervariability between residues 31–37, 51–68, 84–91, and 101–110. A point of major interest is that V_H-region sequences seem to be shared by all classes. Three V_H subgroups ($V_H I$, $V_H II$, and $V_H III$), have been recognized and within a subgroup sequence homology is of the order of 80–95 per cent (hypervariable regions excluded). The concentration of the heavy chains of the $V_H III$ subgroup in normal immunoglobulin (20 per cent of all heavy chains) is close to the frequency of myeloma proteins of the $V_H III$ subgroup. However, a high proportion of IgA proteins studied (75 per cent) seem to belong to the $V_H III$ subgroup, suggesting that the association between a V-region subgroup and the class-specific C region is not entirely random.

A suggestion by Dreyer and Bennett (1965), that two genes control the synthesis of each immunoglobulin chain is now generally accepted, although genetically unorthodox. According to this view, one gene codes for the constant part of the chain and another for the variable portion. The genes are then brought together by an unknown mechanism and, thereafter, function as a single unit. Studies in several species suggest that there are three distinct linkage groups of immunoglobulin structural genes. These determine the primary structure of κ, λ, and heavy chains (see Figure 5). Within any linkage group any V-region subgroup gene can associate with any C-region gene (Kohler *et al.*, 1970), although some associations may be preferred (for example, IgA–V_HIII).

Recently, it has been suggested that three, rather than two, structural genes may interact to produce each immunoglobulin peptide chain (Capra and Kindt, 1975). According to this hypothesis a limited number of *group one* genes would code for the relatively invariant portions of the V region (perhaps one for each subgroup), a larger number of *group two* genes would encode hypervariable regions, and a small number of *group three* genes would code for the C regions. This hypothesis is elaborated in more detail by one of the authors elsewhere in this volume (see Sogn and Kindt, Chapter 4).

As shown in Figure 1 there are two intra-chain disulphide bridges in the light chain—one in the variable and one in the constant region. Similarly, there are four such bridges in the heavy (γ) chain, which is twice the length of a light chain. Each bridge encloses a peptide loop of 60–70 amino acid residues and if the amino

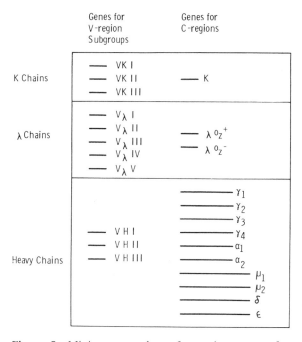

Figure 5 Minimum number of genetic systems for human immunoglobulin synthesis. Each box encloses a set of genes (represented by bars) which are probably linked. One V-region gene and one C-region gene contribute to each immunoglobulin chain, and other genes (not shown) may contribute to hypervariability. The heavy, κ, and λ-chain systems appear to be three unlinked systems. In the figure, genes are labelled by the name of their protein product

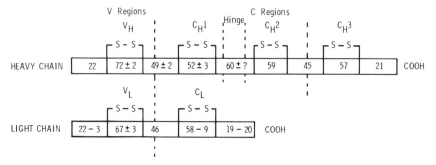

Figure 6 Schematic diagram of human IgG homology regions showing number of amino acid residues enclosed by each disulphide bridge (range for four subclasses shown). Modified from Milstein and Svasti (1971)

acid sequences of these loops are compared within a given heavy chain a striking degree of homology is revealed. Each loop represents the central portion of a so-called homology region or 'domain' which comprises some 110 amino acid residues. In the light chain, these regions are called V_L and C_L, respectively, for the variable and constant regions. In the heavy chain, the N-terminal homology region is called the V_H region and there are at least three homology regions in the constant part of the chain called C_H1, C_H2, and C_H3 (see Figure 6). There are known to be three constant homology regions in γ and α heavy chains and four such regions in μ and ε chains. There are probably four in δ chains also. A specific nomenclature may be used to describe the homology regions of different classes, for example $C_\gamma1$, $C_\gamma2$, and $C_\gamma3$ for IgG, and $C_\mu1$, $C_\mu2$, $C_\mu3$, and $C_\mu4$ for IgM. The variation in size of the homology regions of human IgG subclasses is indicated in Figure 6. This shows that the V_H and V_L disulphide-bridged loops are larger than the C-region loops of these chains. Furthermore the regions between loops are of comparable size except that between the C_H1 and C_H2 loops which is longer (especially in IgG3). The latter feature (sometimes called the 'hinge' region) is common to the four-domain IgG and IgA molecules, but is not shared apparently with the five-domain IgM and IgE molecules. In IgG and IgA, the hinge region shows no sequence homology with any other part of the polypeptide structure and appears to have evolved independently. An intriguing possibility proposed recently by Bennich (personal communication) is that the hinge regions of IgG and IgA represent 'collapsed' domains, thus these regions are the equivalent of $C_\varepsilon2$ and $C_\mu2$ domains.

Edelman and Gall (1969) proposed that each homology region is folded into a compact globular structure and linked to neighbouring domains by more loosely folded portions of peptide chain. Furthermore, it was suggested by Edelman (1970) that each homology region has evolved to fulfil a specific function, for example, antigen binding would be the major function of the V_L and V_H domains. There is much evidence to support this concept. This will be discussed in Section 3.

In the last five years, the three-dimensional structure of immunoglobulins has been under active investigation and high resolution data are now available for the

Fab regions of human IgG1 (Amzel *et al.*, 1974) and mouse IgA (Segal *et al.*, 1974), as well as human λ Bence–Jones dimer (Edmundson *et al.*, 1974). Much of this work is reviewed elsewhere in this volume (Richards *et al.*, Chapter 2), but the major conclusions of this work are summarized here.

Within each homology region two roughly parallel β-pleated sheets surround a tightly coiled internal structure of hydrophobic side chains. The two β sheets are linked covalently by the intra-chain disulphide bridge, and there appears not to be any α-helical structure present. Many of the 'framework' residues of the two variable regions (V_H and V_L) occur at hairpin bends, or contribute to the intra- and inter-subunit bonds thereby enhancing the overall structural stability. At such positions, only specific amino acids are compatible with the requirements for a constant three-dimensional structure for all homology subunits. On the other hand, the hypervariable portions of the V_L and V_H regions come together at the N-terminal surface of the molecule and appear not to be subject to structural constraints. These combined hypervariable regions are thought to constitute the 'contact residues' of the antigen binding site (see also Feinstein and Beale Chapter 8).

Subclasses of human IgG and IgA exist and probably also of IgM and IgD. Most mammals, with the exception of the rabbit, appear to have two or more subclasses of IgG but there are no clear relationships between species suggesting that the subclasses are relatively recent evolutionary events which have arisen independently in each species. All healthy individuals have the subclass variants of IgG and IgA in their serum and the antigenic markers of these proteins are termed isotypic markers. Certain genetic markers are also identifiable. These are inherited as autosomal codominant factors called allotypic markers and are found on γ chains (Gm antigens), α chains (Am antigens) and κ light chains (Km antigens).

Table 4 Physicochemical properties of human immunoglobulins

Immuno-globulin	Heavy chain	Sedimen-tation constant (S)	Total molecular weight	Molecular weight of heavy chain	Number of heavy chain domains	Carbo-hydrate (per cent)
IgG1	γ_1	7	146 000	51 000	4	2–3
IgG2	γ_2	7	146 000	51 000	4	2–3
IgG3	γ_3	7	170 000	60 000	4*	2–3
IgG4	γ_4	7	146 000	51 000	4	2–3
IgM	μ	19	970 000	65 000	5	12
IgA1	α_1	7	160 000	56 000	4	7–11
IgA2	α_2	7	160 000	52 000	4	7–11
sIgA†	α_1 or α_2	11	385 000	52 000–56 000	4	7–11
IgD	δ	7	184 000	69 700	5	9–14
IgE	ε	8	188 000	72 500	5	12

* The hinge region of IgG3 may incorporate an intra-chain disulphide bridge but this would not constitute a domain of 110 residues
† secretory IgA

12

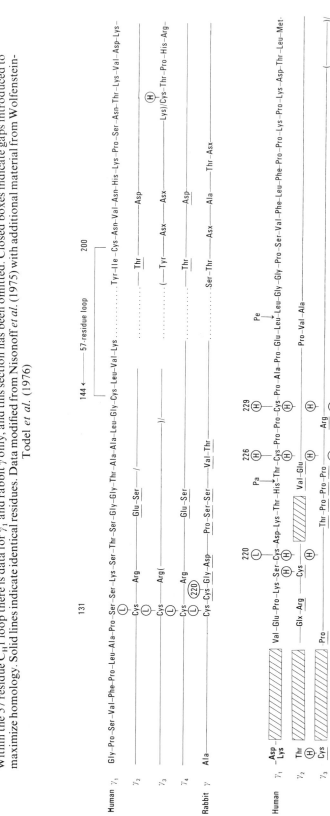

Figure 7 Partial sequences of the three C$_H$ regions of four subclasses of human γ chains and the rabbit γ chain. The symbols L or H adjacent to a Cys residue indicate a disulphide bond linking that Cys to a light or heavy chain, respectively. Other Cys residues form intra-chain disulphide bridges. Carbohydrate (CBH) is attached to an asparagine residue (no. 297). Residue numbering according to the Eu sequence of Edelman *et al.* (1969). Pa and Pe indicate cleavage points of papain and pepsin, respectively. Allotype related substitutions are indicated by alternative residues. Within the 57 residue C$_H$1 loop there is data for γ$_1$ and rabbit γ only, and this section has been omitted. Closed boxes indicate gaps introduced to maximize homology. Solid lines indicate identical residues. Data modified from Nisonoff *et al.* (1975) with additional material from Wolfenstein-Todel *et al.* (1976)

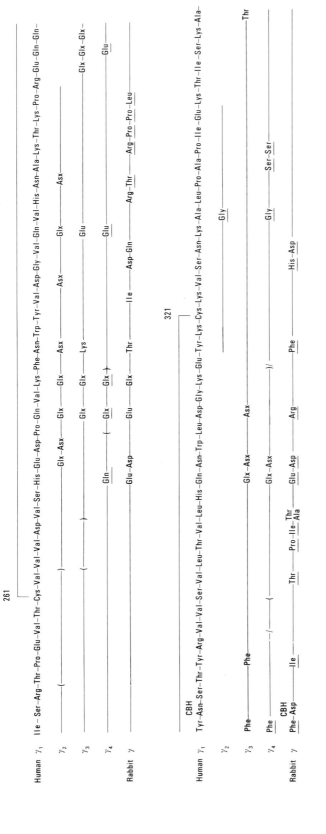

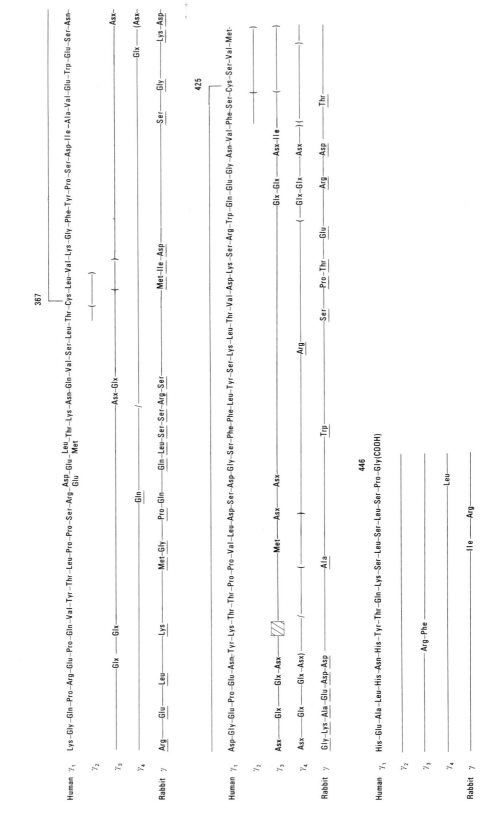

The major physicochemical properties of the classes and subclasses of human immunoglobulin are shown in Table 4. The structural characteristics of each class will now be considered in greater detail.

2.2 Structure of Immunoglobulin G

2.2.1 Human Immunoglobulin G

IgG is the major immunoglobulin in normal human serum accounting for 70–75 per cent of the total immunoglobulin pool. Isolated pooled IgG is a monomeric protein with a sedimentation coefficient (s_{20°, w) of 6·6 S and a molecular weight of 146 000. However, studies of subclass proteins have indicated that IgG3 proteins are slightly larger than the other subclasses (see Table 4). Following electrophoresis IgG shows a broad range of mobilities from slow γ to α_2. This range of net charge (partly a reflection of the subclass content) is also seen on isoelectric focusing and ion-exchange chromatography.

Four subclasses of human IgG (IgG1, IgG2, IgG3, and IgG4) have been recognized and occur in the approximate proportions of 66, 23, 7, and 4 per cent, respectively. These subclasses cross-react antigenically but also possess subclass-specific antigenic determinants in the C_H regions. These antigenic differences are, of course, reflected in the amino acid sequences of heavy chains from myeloma proteins of different subclasses. The first human γ chain to be sequenced completely was the γ_1 chain of the Eu protein (Edelman et al., 1969), and the numbering system for this chain is used frequently as a basis for comparisons between γ-chain sequences. Partial C-region sequences of human $\gamma_1, \gamma_2, \gamma_3$, and γ_4 chains and rabbit γ chain are shown in Figure 7. Inspection of these sequences shows that each protein has three homology regions or domains. Each of these domains encompasses a disulphide-bridged loop of 52–59 residues (see Figure 6). More variable than the number of residues within the loops is the number *between* the loops. For example in IgG1, IgG2, and IgG4 there are 10–15 more residues between the C_H1 and C_H2 disulphide loops than between the C_H2 and C_H3 loops. These extra residues occur in what has become known as the hinge or bridge region, and it is here that structural and sequential differences between subclasses are greatest. Two amino acid residues are especially frequent in this region, namely half-cystine and proline. Although in IgG1 the half-cystine at residue 220 contributes to the light–heavy chain bridge, most of the half-cystine residues in the hinge region are those involved in inter-heavy chain disulphide bridges. There are two inter-chain disulphide bonds between both γ_1 and γ_4 chains, and four between γ_2 chains. The number of such bonds in IgG3 is still controversial; estimates range from five (Frangione and Milstein, 1968) to 15 (Michaelsen, 1973). It is possible that the hinge-region peptide of IgG3 originally sequenced by Frangione and Milstein (1968), and containing five half-cystines, is triplicated to give the 15 half-cystines suggested subsequently. This is consistent with the presence of approximately 95 extra amino acid residues in the γ_3 chain and would account for its higher molecular weight of 60 000 (see Table 4). The disulphide-bridge patterns of the human IgG subclasses are illustrated in Figure 8.

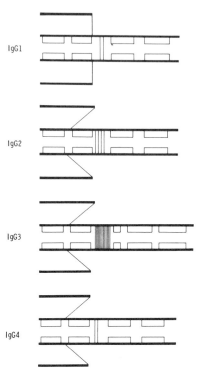

Figure 8 Gross structure of human IgG subclasses showing heavy and light polypeptide chains (long and short thick lines) and both inter and intra-chain disulphide bridges (thin lines). The positions of the bridges are based on comparisons with homologous sequences in human IgG1 molecules. Data for IgG3 are tentative

The hinge regions of the γ chains are also rich in proline (see Figure 7), and it has been suggested by Welscher (1970) that this amino acid stabilizes the structure of the hinge. Whether or not this is the case, there is evidence that the peptide structure is exposed and particularly susceptible to proteolysis in this region. A wide range of proteolytic enzymes cleave IgG molecules in the hinge region but the most extensively used enzymes have been papain and pepsin. Using papain, Fc and Fab fragments can be obtained from all four IgG subclasses, although there are marked differences in susceptibility to the enzyme; IgG3 is the most susceptible followed by IgG1, IgG4, and IgG2. The enzyme cleaves the γ chains of each subclass on the N-terminal side of the inter-heavy chain disulphide bonds but can also cleave at other points. For example, a fragment derived from the C_H3 domain and called Fc′ is detected frequently after

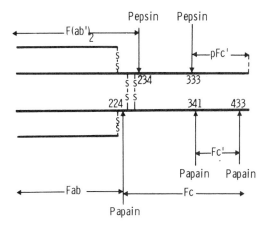

Figure 9 Pepsin and papain cleavage points of human IgG1. Numbers refer to the amino acid on the N-terminal side of the bond cleaved and are based on the Eu sequence of Edelman *et al.* (1969). Reproduced, with permission, from Stanworth and Turner (1973)

prolonged papain digestion (Turner and Bennich, 1968). The major papain cleavage points of human IgG1 are illustrated in Figure 9.

Pepsin at pH 4·0–4·5 can cleave γ chains also in the hinge region, but in this case the susceptible bond is on the C-terminal side of the inter-heavy chain disulphide bridges (see Figure 9 for cleavage point of IgG1). This yields a divalent fragment called F(ab')₂ which essentially consists of the two Fab regions held together by the hinge region. At pH 4·0, the rest of the Fc region is destroyed, but at pH 4·5 a fragment corresponding closely to the C_H3 domain of each subclass (pFc') is readily obtained (Turner *et al.*, 1970).

The generation of Fc' and pFc' by cleavage of peptide bonds between the C_H2 and C_H3 regions suggests that controlled enzymic cleavage between other domains may permit their isolation for structural and biological studies. Such indeed appears to be the case and methods for isolating the C_H2 domain using brief exposure to trypsin (Yasmeen *et al.*, 1973) or treatment with pepsin at a high temperature (70°, pH 4·5, 50 minutes incubation, enzyme:substrate ratio 1:100) have been reported (Seon and Pressman, 1975).

An apparently large structural difference between human IgG1 and the other IgG subclasses is the location of the heavy chain half-cystine which links to the light chain half-cystine. This is residue 220 in IgG1 but a residue homologous to position 131 in the other subclasses (and indeed in most other immunoglobulin classes). X-Ray crystallographic analysis of the human IgG1 protein (NEW) to a resolution of 0·2 nm (Amzel *et al.*, 1974) has, however, shown that positions 131 and 220 of the γ_1 chain in fact are spatially very close and that the overall three-

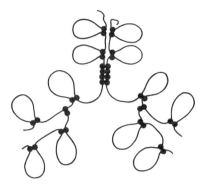

Figure 10 Schematic diagram of human IgG2 showing both intra and inter-chain disulphide bridges between $\frac{1}{2}$-cystine residues (●●). Note the proximity of the C-terminus of the light chain to both the N-terminal and C-terminal sides of the C_H1 loop

dimensional structure of the molecule is not influenced greatly whichever alternative operates. This point is illustrated diagrammatically in Figure 10.

All subclasses of IgG contain carbohydrate and it is probable that this is located on the outside of the C_H2 domain and (by extrapolation from studies on IgG1) attached to an asparagine at residue 297 of each heavy chain (see Figure 7). The obligatory triplet sequence Asn–X–Ser/Thr occurs at positions 297–299 of both γ_1 and γ_4 chains (Edelman *et al.*, 1969; Pink *et al.*, 1970), but not elsewhere in the C regions of these proteins. Although there is a wide variation in the sugar groups associated with IgG myeloma proteins, there is no evidence that this variation is linked in a specific way to the subclasses.

The ease with which papain cleaves the IgG molecule into two Fab fragments and one Fc fragment suggests that the molecule has a natural tripartite structure. This is confirmed apparently by the electron micrographs obtained by Valentine and Green (1967). These workers used a rabbit antibody with specificity for a DNP hapten. When the antibody was mixed with the bivalent hapten DNP-NH-$(CH_2)_n$-NH-DNP (where n was 8 or more), a number of closed structures including cyclic dimers, trimers, tetramers, and pentamers was visualized readily in the electron microscope (see Fearon and Beale, chapter 8). These micrographs suggest that IgG is a Y-shaped molecule in which the three limbs represent the Fc and the two Fab regions. The angle between the Fab limbs in these complexes varies between 10° and 180°. These results confirm earlier work by Feinstein and Rowe (1965) which suggested a highly flexible structure.

A large number of allotypic antigens (Gm markers) has now been described for human γ chains. These are listed in Table 5 together with the subclass to which the antigen is restricted. A feature of the Gm system, which has not yet been described in any other animal allotype system, is the association of so-called 'iso-allotypes' with many Gm antigens. Such antigens are shared by two or more

Table 5 Established Gm allotypes of human immunoglobulin G

Original nomenclature	New nomenclature	IgG subclass
a	G1m(a)	IgG1
x	G1m(x)	IgG1
f	G1m(f)	IgG1
z	G1m(z)	IgG1
n	G2m(n)	IgG2
g	G3m(g)	IgG3
b^0	G3m(b^0)	IgG3
b^1	G3m(b^1)	IgG3
b^3	G3m(b^3)	IgG3
b^4	G3m(b^4)	IgG3
b^5	G3m(b^5)	IgG3
c^3	G3m(c^3)	IgG3
c^5	G3m(c^5)	IgG3
s	G3m(s)	IgG3
t	G3m(t)	IgG3

subclasses and are structurally antithetic to a Gm marker in one subclass only. The most widely studied example is nG1m(a), an antigen present on all IgG2 and IgG3 proteins but only on IgG1 molecules lacking the Gm(a) antigen. A plausible explanation for the existence of both classical allotypic antigens and antithetic antigens is that Gm antigens have arisen following a mutation in a portion of the C-region gene controlling a subclass-specific segment of the γ polypeptide chain. G1m(z) and G1m(f) at residue number 214 of the γ_1 chain are examples of such classical allelic antigens. In contrast, mutations in a part of the gene controlling

Table 6 Probable structural location of some human γ-chain allotypes and iso-allotypes

Allotype or Iso-allotype	Chain	Homology region	Sequence	Amino acid
G1m(a)	γ_1	$C_\gamma 3$	355–358	Arg-*Asp*-Glu-*Leu*
nG1m(a)	$\gamma_1, \gamma_2, \gamma_3$	$C_\gamma 3$	355–358	Arg-Glu-Glu-Met
G1m(f)	γ_1	$C_\gamma 1$	214	Arg
G1m(z)	γ_1	$C_\gamma 1$	214	Lys
nG4m(a)	$\gamma_1, \gamma_3, \gamma_4$	$C_\gamma 2$	309	Val-Leu-His
nG4m(b)	γ_2, γ_4	$C_\gamma 2$	309	Val-His
G3m(g)	γ_3	$C_\gamma 2$	296*	Tyr
nG3m(g)	γ_2, γ_3	$C_\gamma 2$	296*	Phe
G3m(b^0)	γ_3	$C_\gamma 3$	436**	Phe
nG3m(b^0)	$\gamma_1, \gamma_2, \gamma_3$	$C_\gamma 3$	436**	Tyr

* and ** Correlative sequence differences observed in incompletely sequenced chains.

regions common to other subclasses may give rise to a genetic marker in one subclass—for example G1m(a)—but the antithetic marker (nG1m(a)) is shared with two other subclasses (IgG2 and IgG3).

A combination of peptide mapping, mild proteolytic fragmentation, and amino acid analysis has permitted the partial structural localization of several Gm and antithetic antigens. Some of these data are summarized in Table 6.

Extrapolation of the X-ray crystallographic data on the constant (C_H1) homology region of Fab fragments suggests that if a similar folding of the γ-polypeptide chain exists in the C_H2 and C_H3 regions then all of the antigens listed in Table 6 will occupy surface positions, usually near bends and corners (see also Fearon and Beale, Chapter 8).

The structural localization of effector sites in the IgG molecule is still in its infancy but there has been limited progress in the case of both the complement-fixing site and the macrophage/monocyte-binding site. These data are considered in more detail in Section 3.

2.2.2 Immunoglobulin G from Other Species

The IgG class of several mammalian species has now been studied in some detail. This section will deal briefly with some of the points of major interest; readers requiring a more detailed review are recommended to consult Nisonoff *et al.* (1975).

The known subclasses and overall structure of IgG from rabbit, mouse, guinea-pig, and goat are shown in Figure 11. The rabbit is unusual in that its IgG exists as a single major subclass. The protein has a single inter-heavy chain disulphide bond, two intra-chain disulphide loops in the C_1 region and a light–heavy bond which joins the heavy chain near the V–C junction. Much of the early elucidation of immunoglobulin structure was performed on rabbit IgG (see Porter, 1959; Hill *et al.*, 1966).

Four subclasses of IgG have been described in the mouse (IgG1, IgG2a, IgG2b, and IgG3). The availability of myeloma proteins representative of each of these subclasses has permitted extensive structural work to be carried out. IgG2a (quantitatively the most important) and IgG2b are structurally similar and are difficult to isolate from each other. Mouse IgG3 is present at low concentrations and is the least studied of the four subclasses. All four subclasses are cleaved readily by papain to give Fc and Fab fragments.

Two major subclasses of guinea-pig IgG (called IgG1 and IgG2) have been described, and a third minor subclass is suggested by the work of Parish (1970). IgG1 and IgG2 of guinea-pig differ extensively in the structure of the Fc regions and also in their biological effector functions. Both subclasses may be digested readily with papain to give Fc and Fab fragments.

Studies on the inter-chain disulphide bridges of goat IgG (Strausbauch *et al.*, 1971) show that it is similar to rabbit IgG with a single bond between the heavy chains and light–heavy bonds to residue 131 of the heavy chains (see Figure 11).

Recent work from the laboratory of Marchalonis (Atwell and Marchalonis,

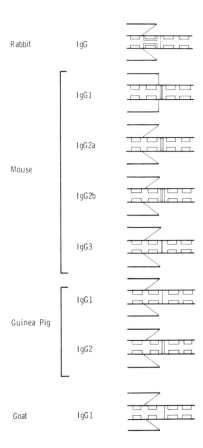

Figure 11 Gross structure of IgG subclasses from rabbit, mouse, guinea pig, and goat. Heavy and light polypeptide chains are indicated by the long and short thick lines, respectively, and inter and intra-chain disulphide bridges by thin lines. Data from De Préval *et al.* (1970); O'Donnell *et al.* (1970); Grey *et al.* (1971); Oliveira and Lamm (1971); Svasti and Milstein (1972)

1975, 1976) suggests that the low molecular weight non-IgM antibodies of lower vertebrates, including amphibians, reptiles, and birds, are distinct from the IgG class of mammals. The protein present in the serum of lower vertebrates has light chains which are of normal molecular weight (23 000) but the heavy chains are larger than the mammalian ones with a molecular weight of 61 400 in the case of the marine toad *Bufo marinus*. This gives a total molecular weight of 168 000 for the intact four-chain molecule which is close to that of the human IgG3. It is possible that the human subclass has a close phylogenetic relationship with the low

		1						10						20						30			
κ	C1							Ala	Val		Phe	Ile	Phe	Pro	Pro	Ser	Ser		Glu	Gly	Ser	Lys	Thr
λ	C2							Ala	Ala	Thr	Thr	Leu	Phe	Pro	Pro	Ser				Asn	Ala		Lys
γ₁	C3	Gly	Val	Gln		Ala		Ala		Phe		Phe	Leu	Pro	Pro	Lys	Pro		Lys	Ser	Gly	Ser		Thr
μ	C1	Val		Ser	Ala	Pro	Thr	Ala	Gly		Pro	Thr	Pro	Ser	Val	Phe	Leu	Thr		Ile	Ser	Arg		Thr
	C2	Val		Gln	Ala	Pro		Gly		Phe	Ser	Tyr	Phe	Val	Leu	Ser	Val		Arg	Glu	Gln	Arg		Ser
	C3			Ser	Lys	Arg	Ser	Thr		Thr	Pro	Phe	Val	Ala	Ser			Glu		Gln	Thr	Ala		Ser
	C4			Glx	Asp		Ala	His		Ser	Tyr	Leu	Ser	Asp	Ala	Asp		Arg		Glu	Thr	His		Ser
α₁	C1				Ser	Arg					Thr	Phe	Pro	Pro	Pro			Glx		Glx	Gln	Ala		Gln
	C2	Gly	Ser		Leu	Ser	Arg		His	His	Ala	Arg	Thr	Ser	Ser	Gly		Ala	Leu	Ser	Ala	His		Arg
	C3	Val	Ala		Asn	Thr	Leu		Thr	Thr	Pro	Phe	Pro	Leu	Thr	Ser	Pro	Arg		Lys	Ser	Arg		Arg
ε	C1	Val	Asp		Asx	Thr	Pro	Asx		Gly			Glx	Ile	Leu	Ser	Ser	Phe	Thr		Gln	His	Ala	
	C2			Ser					Phe		Ala	Met		Pro	Pro	Pro			Phe	Asp	Glu	Arg		Lys
	C3			Ser	Asp		Pro					Trp			Gly	Ser		Pro			Ala	Ala	Pro	

				40									50							60				
κ	C1	Ser	Leu	Asn		Asn	Phe	Ile	Phe	Val	Pro	Pro	Ser	Ser	Leu	Gln	Lys	Leu	Gln	Val	Gly
λ	C2	Thr	Ile	Ser		Asp	Thr	Leu	Pro	Ala	Pro	Pro	Ser	Ala	Met	Glu	Asp	Glu	Ser	Ala	Asn
γ₁	C3	Ala	Val	Lys		Asp	Val	Leu	Leu	Val	Pro	Pro	Asp	Ser	Pro	Ser	Asp	Ser	Gly	Asx	Leu
μ	C1	Val	Val	Lys		Gly	Val	Thr	Phe	Ser	His	Pro	Ser	Tyr	Phe	Arg	Leu	Glx	Pro	Ala	Ser
	C2	Leu	Ala	Gln	Thr	Asp	Pro	Leu	Tyr	Asp		Pro	Ser	Tyr	Met	Gln	Asp	Ser	Asp	Asn	Glu
	C3	Glu	Ala	Thr	Ala	Thr	Tyr	Leu	Phe	Pro	Arg	Arg	Ser	Thr	Gln	Thr	Thr	Gly	Arg	Leu	Glu
	C4	Asn	Leu	Leu	Ala	Asp	Leu	Ala	Phe	Asp	Phe	Phe	Thr	Arg	Thr	Ser	Ala	Glx	Thr	Leu	Asn

						70						80					90				95			
κ	C1	Gln	Ser	Val	Ala	Cys	Leu	Ser	Glu	Val	Thr	Asp	Lys	Trp	Glu	Ile	Gln	Gly	Ser	Leu	Ser
λ	C2	Lys	Ala	Val	Thr	Cys	Leu	Asn	Lys	Thr	Pro	Asn	Asp	Trp	Ser	Asn	Ser	Tyr	Ala	Val
γ₁	C3	Asp	Gly	Val	Thr	Cys	Val	Val	Pro	Ser	Pro	Ser	Tyr	Trp	Gly	Gly	Ser	Tyr	Arg	Leu
μ	C1	Glu	Asp	Glu	Thr	Cys	Lys	Phe	Lys	Thr	Pro	Ile	Trp	Gly	Cys	Leu	Val	Phe	Thr	Thr
	C2	Leu	Asn	Thr	Thr	Cys	Leu	Glx	Phe	Gly	Thr	Pro	Leu	Trp	Glu	Gln	Tyr	Thr	Ala
	C3	Thr	Pro	Asx	Cys	Leu	Pro	Met	Gln	Asx	Gly	Gly	Ser	Thr	His	Ser	Ala
α₁	C1	Arg	Glu	Arg	Gln	Thr	Leu	His	Ser	Gly	Leu	Leu	Glu	Leu	Ala
	C2	Thr	His	Glu	Pro	Thr	Cys	Gly	Ala	Val	Leu	Gix	Leu	Gln
ε	C3	Ser	Leu	Thr	Glu	Gly	Glu	Cys	Gly	Glu	Leu	Leu	Thr	Thr

					100										110										120								
κ		Ser	Thr	Leu	Thr	Leu	Ser	—	Lys	Ala	—	Asp	Tyr	—	Glu	Lys	His	Lys	Val	Tyr	Ala	—	Cys	Glu	Val	Thr	His	Gln	Gly	—	Leu	Ser	Ser
λ		Ser	Tyr	Leu	Ser	Leu	Thr	Pro	—	—	Glu	Gln	Trp	Lys	Ser	—	His	Arg	Ser	Tyr	Ser	—	Cys	Gln	Val	Thr	His	Glu	Gly	—	—	Ser	Thr
γ_1	C1	Ser	Val	Val	Thr	Val	Pro	Ser	—	Ser	—	—	Ser	Leu	—	Gly	Thr	Gln	Thr	Tyr	Ile	—	Cys	Asn	Val	Asn	His	Lys	Pro	—	Ser	Asn	Thr
	C2	Ser	Val	Leu	Thr	Val	Leu	—	—	His	Gln	Asp	Trp	Leu	Asp	Gly	—	Lys	Glu	Tyr	Lys	—	Cys	Lys	Val	Ser	Asn	Lys	Ala	—	Leu	Pro	Ala
	C3	Ser	Lys	Leu	Thr	Val	Asp	—	Lys	Ser	—	Arg	Trp	Gln	Gln	Gly	—	Asn	Val	Phe	Ser	—	Cys	Ser	Val	Met	His	Glu	Ala	—	Leu	His	Asn
μ	C1	Ser	Gln	Val	Leu	Leu	Pro	Ser	Lys	—	—	Asp	Val	Met	Gln	Gly	Thr	Asn	Glu	His	Val	Val	Cys	Lys	Val	Glx	His	Pro	—	—	Asx	Gly	Asx
	C2	Ser	Thr	Leu	Thr	Ile	Lys	Glu	—	Ser	—	Asx	Trp	Leu	Ser	Gln	—	Ser	Met	Phe	Thr	—	Cys	Arg	Val	Asp	His	Arg	Gly	—	Leu	—	Thr
	C3	—	—	—	—	—	—	—	—	Glu	Asx	Asx	Trp	Asn	Ser	Gly	—	Glu	Arg	Phe	Thr	—	Cys	Thr	Val	Thr	His	Thr	Asp	—	Leu	Pro	Ser
	C4	Ser	Ile	Leu	Thr	Val	Ser	—	—	Glu	Glu	Glu	Trp	Asn	Thr	Gly	—	Glu	Thr	Tyr	Thr	—	Cys	Val	Val	Ala	His	Glu	Ala	—	Leu	Pro	Asn
α_1	C1	Ser	Gln	Leu	Thr	Leu	Pro	—	—	Ala	Thr	Glx	Cys	Leu	Ala	Gly	—	Lys	Ser	Val	Thr	—	Cys	His	Val	Lys	His	Tyr	Thr	—	Asx	Pro	Ser
	C2	Ser	Val	Leu	Ser	Gly	Cys	—	—	Ala	Gln	Pro	Trp	Asp	His	Gly	—	Lys	Thr	Phe	Thr	—	Cys	Thr	Ala	Ala	Tyr	Pro	Glu	—	Ser	Lys	Thr
	C3	Ser	Ile	Leu	Arg	Val	Ala	—	—	Ala	Glx	Asx	Trp	Lys	Lys	Gly	—	Asp	Thr	Phe	Ser	—	Cys	Met	Val	Gly	His	Glu	Ala	—	Leu	Pro	Leu
ε	C1	Ser	Leu	Leu	Thr	Val	Ser	Gly	—	Ala	—	—	Trp	Ala	Lys	—	—	Gln	Met	Phe	Thr	—	Cys	Arg	Val	Ala	His	Thr	Pro	—	Ser	Ser	Thr
	C2	Ser	Glu	Leu	Thr	Leu	Ser	Gln	Lys	His	—	—	Trp	Leu	Ser	Asp	—	Arg	Thr	Tyr	Thr	—	Cys	Glu	Val	Thr	Tyr	Glx	Gly	—	—	His	Thr
	C3	Ser	Thr	Leu	Pro	Val	Gly	Thr	Arg	—	—	Asx	Trp	Ile	Glu	Gly	—	Glu	Thr	Tyr	Glx	—	Cys	Arg	Val	Thr	His	Pro	His	—	Leu	Pro	Arg
	C4	Ser	Arg	Leu	Glu	Val	—	Thr	Arg	Ala	Glu	—	Trp	Gln	Glu	Lys	—	Asp	Glu	Phe	Ile	—	Cys	Arg	Ala	Val	His	Glu	Ala	Ala	Ser	Pro	Ser

			130										140											150								159
κ		Pro	Val	Thr	—	Lys	Ser	Phe	Asn	Arg	Gly	Glu	Cys	—																		
λ		—	Val	—	Glu	Lys	Thr	Val	Ala	Pro	Thr	Glu	Cys	Ser																		
γ_1	C1	Lys	Val	—	Asp	Lys	Lys	Val	Glu	Pro	Lys	Ser	Cys	Asp	Lys	Thr	His	Thr	Cys	Pro	Pro	Cys	Pro	Ala	Pro							
	C2	Pro	Ile	—	Glu	Lys	Thr	Ile	Ser	Lys	Ala	Lys	Gly	—																		
	C3	His	Tyr	Thr	Gln	Lys	Ser	Leu	Ser	Leu	Ser	Pro	Gly	—																		
μ	C1	Lys	—	—	Glu	Lys	Asp	Val	—	Pro	Leu	Pro	—	—																		
	C2	Phe	Gln	—	Gln	Asx	—	—	Ala	Ser	Ser	Met	Cys	—																		
	C3	Pro	Leu	Lys	Gln	—	Thr	Ile	Ser	Arg	Pro	Lys	Gly	—																		
	C4	Arg	Val	Thr	Glu	Arg	Thr	Val	Asp	Lys	Ser	Thr	Gly	Lys	Pro	Thr	Leu	Tyr	Asx	Val	Ser	Leu	Val	Met	Ser	Asx	Thr	Ala	Gly	Thr	Cys	Tyr
α_1	C1	—	—	—	Glx	Asx	—	Val	Thr	—	Val	Pro	Cys	—	Pro	Val	Pro	Ser	Thr	Pro	Pro	Thr	Pro	Ser	Pro							
																		Ser	Thr	Pro	Pro	Thr	Pro	Ser	Pro	—	—	—	—	Ser	Cys	Cys
	C2	Pro	Leu	Thr	Ala	—	Thr	Leu	Ser	Lys	—	Ser	Gly	—																		
	C3	Ala	Phe	Thr	Gln	Lys	Thr	Ile	Asp	Arg	Leu	Ala	Gly	Lys	Pro	Thr	His	Val	Asx	Val	Ser	Val	Val	Met	Ala	Glu	Val	Asp	Gly	Thr	Cys	Tyr
ε	C1	Asx	Asn	—	Val	Lys	Thr	Phe	Ser	Val	—	—	Cys	Ser																		
	C2	Phe	—	—	Glx	Asx	Ser	—	Thr	Lys	—	Lys	Cys	Ala																		
	C3	Ala	Leu	—	Met	Arg	Ser	Thr	Thr	Lys	Thr	Ser	Gly	—																		
	C4	Gln	Thr	Val	Gln	Arg	Ala	Val	Ser	Val	Asn	Pro	Gly	Lys																		

Figure 12 Primary amino acids sequence of the constant regions of κ, λ, γ_1, μ, α_1, and ε chains. Gaps have been introduced to maximize homology. Adapted, from Kratzin *et al.* (1975). Reproduced by permission of authors and publishers

molecular weight immunoglobulins of lower vertebrates. However, more detailed structural studies, particularly of the hinge region, are required to establish such a possibility.

2.3 Structure of Immunoglobulin A

2.3.1 Serum Immunoglobulin A

IgA was first identified as β_x-globulin by immunoelectrophoresis of human serum (Graber and Williams, 1953), where it accounts for about 15–20 per cent of the total immunoglobulin pool. In man, more than 80 per cent of IgA occurs as 7 S four-chain monomers ($\alpha_2 L_2$) with the remainder as polymers having sedimentation coefficients of 10, 13, and 15 S. In most mammals, the IgA in serum is predominantly 10 S. IgA polymers may be reduced to four-chain monomers by thiol treatment and are stabilized presumably by inter-monomer disulphide bonds. Monomeric IgA has a molecular weight of 160 000, while the isolated α chains have a molecular weight of 52 000–56 000. This is similar to γ chains which also have four domains per chain.

Two subclasses of IgA—IgA1 and IgA2—have been identified in normal human serum using antisera raised in other species (Feinstein and Franklin, 1966; Kunkel and Prendergast, 1966; Vaerman and Heremans, 1966). In serum, IgA1 is the predominant subclass (80–90 per cent), but in seromucous secretions the α_1 and α_2 chains are present in secretory IgA in approximately equal proportions (Grey et al., 1968). The α_1 and α_2 chains have been reported by Montgomery et al. (1969) and by Dorrington and Rockey (1970) to have slightly different molecular weights (52 000 and 56 000, respectively), although it is not known where the additional residues in the α_2 chain are located.

Recently, the primary structure of a monoclonal human IgA1 protein has been determined in Hilschmann's laboratory (Kratzin et al., 1975; Scholz and Hilschmann, 1975). The α_1 chain of this protein comprises 472 amino acid residues with a V region extending from residue 1 to 119. The C region of the α chain consists of three homology regions each showing sequence homology with the C regions of light chains and other immunoglobulin heavy chains (see Figure 12). A feature shared with IgM is the presence of an additional C-terminal octadecapeptide with a penultimate cysteine which is able to bind covalently to the J chain in polymeric molecules. The $C_\alpha 1$ and $C_\alpha 2$ homology regions are each distinguished by the presence of an additional intra-chain disulphide bridge and in each $C_\alpha 2$ homology region there are two cysteine residues of unknown function. It is possible that these are the residues involved in covalent binding to the secretory component but as yet there is no direct evidence for this. A schematic structure for human serum IgA1 based on the work of Kratzin et al. (1975) is shown in Figure 13. It is in the hinge region that the greatest differences between IgA1 and IgA2 molecules are seen, for example, α_2 chains lack 12 amino acid residues and the two galactosamine-rich carbohydrate moieties which are present in the hinge of α_1 chains (Frangione and Wolfenstein-Todel, 1972).

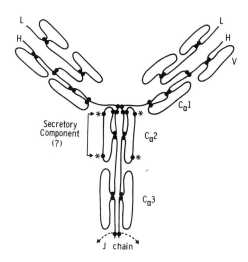

Figure 13 Polypeptide structure of human IgA1 showing intra and inter-chain disulphide bridges between $\frac{1}{2}$-cystine residues ($\bullet\bullet$). The secretory-component binding role of the cysteine residues in the $C_\alpha 2$ region is speculative

Furthermore, there is a duplicated sequence of seven amino acid residues in the α_1 hinge which does not occur in the α_2 hinge (see Figure 14).

IgA2 molecules exist in two allotypic forms—$A_2m(1)$ and $A_2m(2)$. The $A_2m(1)$ molecules have been shown to possess an unusual molecular structure. The light chains are disulphide bonded to each other but not to the α chains (Grey *et al.* 1968). There are, however, strong non-covalent forces between the light and heavy chains. A second Am allotype, which appears to be located in the Fd region of IgA2 molecules, has been described by Wang *et al.* (1973).

Treatment of IgA with proteolytic enzymes has been relatively unproductive. Digestion with papain was found by Bernier *et al.* (1965) to yield Fab-like fragments and, recently, treatment with a streptococcal IgA protease has been reported to produce both Fab and Fc-like fragments from IgA1 but not from IgA2 proteins (Plaut *et al.*, 1974).

2.3.2 Secretory Immunoglobulin A

In 1963, Chodirker and Tomasi reported that IgA is the predominant immunoglobulin in seromucous secretions. Such secretory IgA is found only in external secretions such as saliva, tracheobronchial secretions, colostrum, milk, and genitourinary secretions. In these secretions, the IgG:IgA ratio is always less than one, whereas in internal secretions such as synovial, amniotic, pleural, and cerebrospinal fluids, and in the aqueous humour of the eye the IgA is not of the secretory type and the IgG:IgA ratio is similar to plasma, that is approximately 5:1.

26

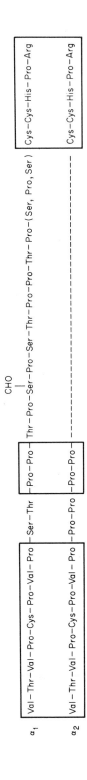

Figure 14 Primary amino acid sequence of human IgA α_1 and α_2 chains in the hinge region of the molecule according to Frangione and Wolfenstein-Todel (1972)

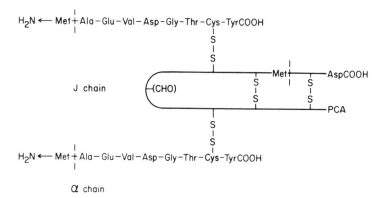

Figure 15 Suggested model for attachment of J chain to α chain in polymeric human IgA. Reproduced from Mestecky *et al.* (1974), with permission

Secretory IgA exists mainly in the 11 S form and has a molecular weight of 380 000. The complete molecule is made up of two four-chain units of IgA, one secretory component (molecular weight 70 000) and one J chain (molecular weight 15 000). It is not at present clear how the various peptide chains are linked

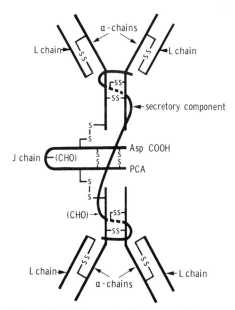

Figure 16 Schematic diagram of human secretory IgA showing possible arrangement of IgA monomers, secretory component, and J chain

together. It is known, however, that the J chain is a product of the plasma cells which synthesize the IgA molecule and that it is added just before secretion. It is also known that the J chain is attached to the penultimate half-cystine of the α chain (Figure 15) and that one or two half-cystines join the J chain to an α chain (Mestecky et al., 1974). As in the case of polymeric IgM (see p. 29), it is not yet clear whether the J chain is linked to two four-chain units of IgA or to one or both heavy chains of a single IgA subunit.

In contrast to the J chain, the secretory component is not synthesized by plasma cells but probably by epithelial cells. Poger and Lamm (1974) have suggested that assembly of the secretory component and IgA probably occurs in the golgi apparatus or in the adjacent apical cytoplasm of epithelial cells. The secretory component is a single polypeptide chain containing carbohydrate (approximately 9 per cent) which becomes covalently bound to α chains in the Fc region of 80 per cent of secretory IgA molecules. Strong non-covalent interactions also help to stabilize the molecule. A schematic diagram of the secretory IgA molecule is shown in Figure 16. Both IgA1 and IgA2 are able to bind the secretory component, and there is no evidence of any structural difference between bound and free forms of the secretory component. The secretions of patients lacking IgA have been shown by South et al. (1966) to contain free secretory component in increased amounts. Such patients frequently have detectable secretory IgM instead of secretory IgA (Thompson, 1970).

2.4 Structure of Immunoglobulin M

2.4.1 Human Immunoglobulin M

IgM, also known as 19 S γ-globulin or γ-macroglobulin, occurs pre-dominantly in man as a pentamer $(\mu_2 L_2)_5$ with a molecular weight of 950 000–1 000 000. However, both larger polymers and monomeric forms of IgM have been reported. The low molecular weight form (7 S IgM) is present at low concentrations in normal human serum, but at higher concentrations in patients with various immunological disorders (especially Waldenström's macroglobu-linaemia, systemic lupus erythematosus, and ataxia telangiectasia).

The complete amino acid sequences of the μ chains from two Waldenström macroglobulins (Gal and Ou) have been reported (Watanabe et al., 1973; Putnam et al., 1973a, b) (see Figure 12), and the overall arrangement of polypeptide chains and disulphide bonds is illustrated in Figure 17. The macroglobulin is a pentamer of four-chain subunits, thus consisting of a total of ten light chains and ten heavy chains, plus one J chain. The μ chain has five intra-chain disulphide loops or domains, each of similar size to the γ-chain domains. An allotypic marker on human IgM, designated Mm1, has been described by Wells et al. (1973), but little is known about its structural location. The μ chain is rich in carbohydrate having five oligosaccharide groups per chain (see Figure 17). These oligosaccharides are either simple or complex, but all contain glucosamine and are attached to asparagine residues in the obligatory sequence Asn–X–Ser/Thr. The function of these oligosaccharides has yet to be established

POLYPEPTIDE STRUCTURE OF HUMAN IgM

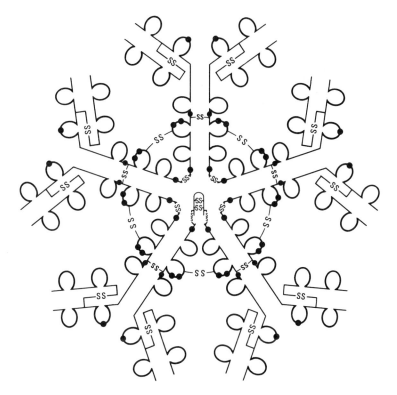

Figure 17 Schematic diagram of human IgM showing homology regions, carbohydrate side chains (●), and possible location of J chain (centre)

although it is known that they increase the solubility of the molecule and influence its conformation.

A single J chain occurs in each pentameric IgM molecule (Chapuis and Koshland, 1974) but the exact method of attachment remains open to discussion. Two different models of J-chain linkage have been proposed. In one the IgM monomer subunits are all disulphide-linked to the J chain which is held in a circular configuration by an intra-chain disulphide bridge. An alternative model envisages the J chain joined by disulphide bonds to two IgM monomers (a dimer clasp) or possibly disulphide bonded to one or both μ chains of a single monomer (a monomer clasp). The first (bracelet) model is now thought unlikely since recent evidence suggests that a single J chain is linked by disulphide bonds to the penultimate half-cystine residue of one or two μ chains only (Inman and Ricardo, 1974; Mestecky *et al.*, 1974). If this is so the J chain constitutes an asymmetric feature of polymeric IgM (see Figure 17) and it is suggested that the pentameric structure is stabilized through inter-subunit disulphide bridges between adjacent $C_\mu 3$ domains (Putnam *et al.*, 1973a).

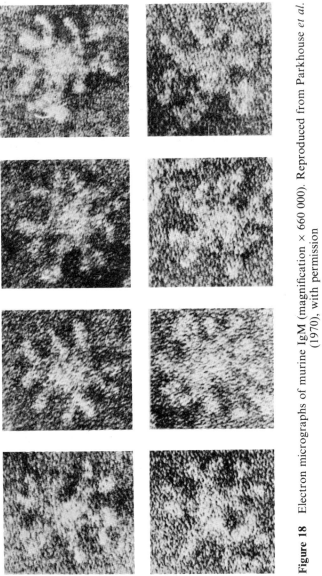

Figure 18 Electron micrographs of murine IgM (magnification × 660 000). Reproduced from Parkhouse *et al.* (1970), with permission

The IgM molecule has been a rewarding molecule for the electron microscopist. It has been shown that all the mammalian proteins studied have a characteristic stellate structure in which the individual Fab arms of the five subunits may sometimes be observed (see Figure 18).

The pentameric IgM molecule can be readily broken down to 7 S subunits by mild reduction using, for example 0·015 M 2-mercaptoethylamine at neutral pH (Morris and Inman, 1968). The 7 S subunits ($\mu_2 L_2$) are designated IgMs (where s indicates subunit) and the ease with which they are obtained, in the absence of

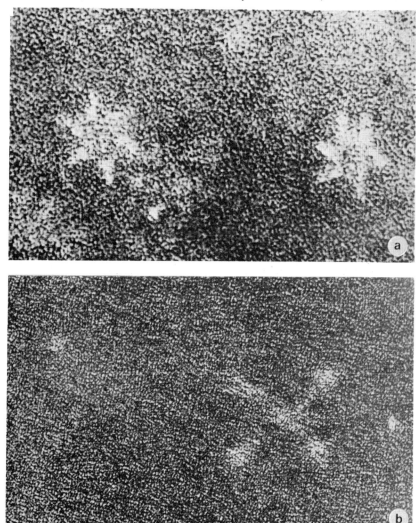

Figure 19 Electron micrographs of tetrameric IgM-like protein from the carp (*a*) and hexameric IgM-like protein from the toad *Xenopus levi* (*b*). Micrographs by Dr. E. Shelton and Dr. R. M. E. Parkhouse, respectively, and reproduced, with permission, from Metzger (1970)

any dissociating agent, suggests that the stabilization of the pentamer is mainly through disulphide bridges. When $0\cdot1-0\cdot2$ M 2-mercaptoethanol is used for dissociation, half-molecules (μL) sedimenting at 5 S may be obtained and these may then be used to prepare hybrid molecules (Frank and Humphrey, 1969; Solheim and Harboe, 1972). IgM can also be separated into its constituent heavy and light chains by conventional reduction procedures followed by alkylation and gel filtration in dissociating solvents (Cohen, 1963). Such procedures also release J chain and the separation of J and L chains requires an additional electrophoretic step.

Fragments of IgM analogous to the Fc, Fab, and $F(ab')_2$ of IgG may be produced by proteolytic cleavage with enzymes such as trypsin, papain, pepsin, and chymotrypsin—as reviewed by Metzger (1970). Treatment of the IgMs subunit with trypsin at $25°$ yields a Fab fragment (molecular weight 47 000), while treatment of the pentameric IgM with trypsin gives a $F(ab')_2$ fragment (molecular weight 114 000). Digestion of IgM with papain in the absence of thiols (Onoue *et al.*, 1968) or with trypsin at $60°$ (Plaut and Tomasi, 1970) yields a pentameric $(Fc)_5\mu$ fragment (320 000–340 000) comprising the $C_\mu 3$ and $C_\mu 4$ domains of the μ chains.

2.4.2 Immunoglobulin M from Other Species

An IgM-like protein is present in the serum of nearly all vertebrates but its structure is variable. Whereas the molecule occurs in a pentameric form in mammals, birds, and reptiles, it exists as a hexamer in most amphibia, and as a tetramer in most teleosts (Figure 19). Marchalonis (1972) has shown that there are very few differences in amino acid composition between the high molecular weight immunoglobulins of lower vertebrates and the IgM of mammals. Moreover, the primitive IgM-like proteins resemble human IgM more closely than do human IgG or IgA.

Recent studies by Milstein *et al.* (1975) have shown that murine IgM has a subunit structure which closely resembles human IgM with the exception of the inter-subunit bonds in the two species. There is no disulphide bridge between adjacent $C_\mu 3$ domains in the mouse as in human IgM. The polymer appears to be bonded covalently solely through the penultimate cysteines of the $C_\mu 4$ domain (Figure 20).

2.5 Structure of Immunoglobulin D

IgD was first described by Rowe and Fahey (1965a, b) following investigations of an unusual myeloma protein. In normal human serum, the protein accounts for less than 1 per cent of the total plasma immunoglobulin and correspondingly only 1–3 per cent of cases of multiple myeloma involve this class.

Molecular weight studies of three IgD myeloma proteins (Leslie *et al.*, 1971) indicate an average molecular weight of 69 000 for the δ chain and a molecular weight of 184 000 for the intact IgD molecule. This suggests that there may be five domains in the δ chain but this still has to be confirmed by sequence analysis.

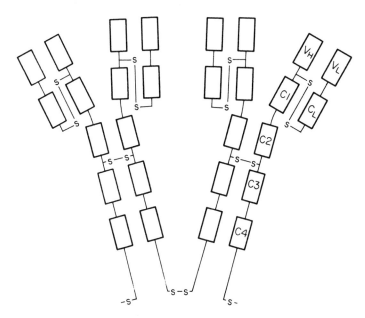

Figure 20 Possible arrangement of disulphide bridges in murine IgM. Reproduced from Milstein *et al.* (1975), with permission

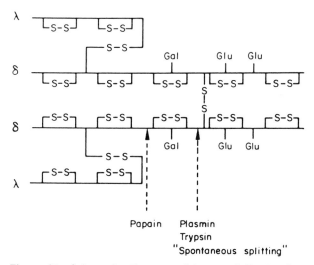

Figure 21 Schematic diagram of human IgD showing possible location of oligosaccharide units and the single inter-heavy chain disulphide bond. Reproduced from Stanworth and Turner (1973) with permission

Structural studies of IgD by Spiegelberg *et al.* (1970) have shown that the protein is unique among the human immunoglobulins in having only a single disulphide bridge between the two heavy chains (Figure 21). This immunoglobulin is rich in carbohydrate; the total amount present has been reported to range from 9 to 18 per cent. A striking finding is the presence of *N*-acetylgalactosamine (Jefferis *et al.*, 1975) which occurs also in IgA1 but no other immunoglobulin.

IgD is difficult to isolate from normal serum because it is present in low concentration. It is also liable to undergo spontaneous proteolysis by plasmin if ε-aminocaproate is not added to serum as an enzyme inhibitor. Spiegelberg *et al.* (1970) found that the protein is more susceptible to proteolysis than IgG1, IgG2, IgA, or IgM. Papain and trypsin both cleave the δ chains on the N-terminal side of the inter-heavy chain disulphide bridge, but trypsin cleaves at a point nearer to this bond to yield a larger Fab fragment (see Figure 21). Cleavage of the Fc_δ fragment with trypsin results in the loss of a hinge-region peptide (Spiegelberg *et al.*, 1970). Jefferis *et al.* (1975) have shown that, whereas the Fc_δ fragment contains all the carbohydrate of the intact molecule, the tFc_δ fragment lacks all the *N*-acetylgalactosamine and some ten residues of galactose. This suggests that the hinge region of IgD may be structurally similar to the hinge region of IgA1 (see p. 24).

2.6 Structure of Immunoglobulin E

Ishizaka *et al.* (1966) provided evidence for a fifth class of immunoglobulin having all the characteristics of homocytotropic or reaginic antibody. The concentration of the protein in normal serum is exceedingly low and further work on this immunoglobulin has been facilitated greatly by the identification of IgE myeloma proteins. A total of seven such proteins has now been described and studies on two of these (ND and PS) have provided most of the structural information about this class. Several aspects of this work have been reviewed by Bennich and Johansson (1971).

Electrophoretically IgE migrates in the fast γ region and is sedimented in the 8·0 S fraction following ultracentrifugation. The molecular weight of the whole molecule is about 188 000 and that of the isolated ε chain is about 72 500. The molecule exists as a four-chain unit with two light chains and two ε chains. The molecular weight of the ε chain without carbohydrate is about 61 000 which suggests that there are five structural domains in the molecule. Sequential analysis by Bennich and Bahr-Lindström has confirmed this.

When IgE is digested with papain, a 5 S Fc fragment with a molecular weight of 98 000 is released (Figure 22). This fragment which contains many of the IgE-specific determinants of the whole molecule and binds to the mast cell surface (see p. 000) also shares antigenic determinants (D1) with the $F(ab')_2$ fragment produced by pepsin (Bennich and Johansson, 1971). A fragment corresponding to the region of overlap has also been isolated and called Fc".

The complete amino acid sequence of the ε chain of IgE (ND) was published by Bennich and Bahr-Lindström in 1974, and partial sequences of IgE (PS) are also

POLYPEPTIDE STRUCTURE OF HUMAN IgE

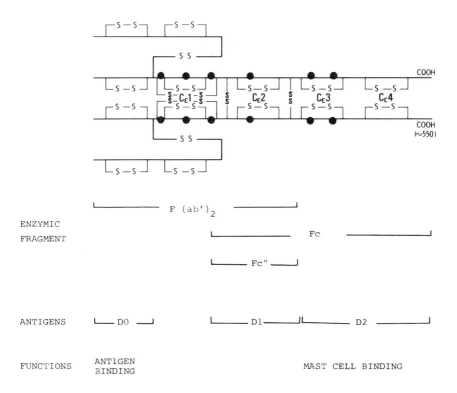

Figure 22 Schematic diagram of human IgE showing position of oligosaccharides (●). The location of various enzymic fragments, antigenic determinants, and biological activities are indicated. Data from Bennich and von Bahr-Lindström (1974)

available. Comparison of the C-region sequences from μ, γ, and α chains (see Figure 12) with the ε-chain sequence suggests that IgE has greatest homology with IgG (33 per cent).

IgE is unusual in having two inter-heavy chain disulphide bridges separated by a complete domain, that is, an inter-chain disulphide bridge between $C_\varepsilon 1$ and $C_\varepsilon 2$, and also between $C_\varepsilon 2$ and $C_\varepsilon 3$. Another feature which has been reported previously for rabbit IgG is the presence of an extra intra-chain disulphide bridge in the $C_\varepsilon 1$ homology region.

Since few human monoclonal IgE proteins have been described there is no evidence at present for the existence of any subclasses of IgE with possibly differing effector functions, nor is there any data on the structure of IgE from non-human species. However, the availability of monoclonal rat IgE will now make such studies feasible in this species (Bazin *et al.*, 1974).

3 RELATIONSHIP BETWEEN STRUCTURE AND EFFECTOR FUNCTIONS OF IMMUNOGLOBULINS

3.1 Introduction

The primary function of immunoglobulins is, of course, to bind to antigen and the structure–activity relationships of the antigen-binding site are the subject of a separate chapter in this volume (Richards *et al.*, Chapter 2). This section will deal only briefly with this primary function and will consider solely the spectrum of antibody responses observed in immunoglobulin classes and subclasses. The remainder of Section 3 is concerned with the so-called 'secondary' manifestations of antigen–antibody interactions and the structural basis for such phenomena. The effector functions of the various proteins that constitute the human immunoglobulin system are summarized in Table 7.

Table 7 Major effector functions of human immunoglobulins

Immuno-globulin	Mean serum concen-tration (mg/ml)	Classical complement fixation	Alternate pathway comple-ment activation	Placental transfer	Binding to mono-nuclear cells	Binding to mast cells and basophils	Reactivity with staphy-lococcal protein A
IgG1	9	+ +	−	+	+	−	+
IgG2	3	+	−	+	−	−	+
IgG3	1	+ + +	−	+	+	−	−
IgG4	0·5	−	− *	+	−	(?)	+
IgM	1·5	+ + +	−	−	−	−	−
IgA1	3·0	−	+	−	−	−	−
IgA2	0·5	−	+	−	−	−	−
sIgA	0·05	−	−	−	−	−	−
IgD	0·03	−	−	−	−	−	−
IgE	0·00005	−	− *	−	− †	+ + +	−

* Aggregated molecules may activate complement by alternate pathway
† Human IgE has been reported to bind to macrophages

3.2 Antibody Populations and Immunoglobulin Classes

The nature of antibody populations is surprisingly variable and can range from essentially monoclonal responses (Braun *et al.*, 1969) to the widest possible heterogeneity involving all classes and subclasses. Many antibody responses, however, share certain common features such as an early IgM response (usually of low binding affinity) and a later, mainly IgG, response (usually of high binding affinity). In studies of human antibody responses to injected protein antigens, such as tetanus toxoid, diphtheria toxoid, and thyroglobulin, it has been shown that antibody activity is present in all four IgG subclasses in approximately the same proportions as the subclass proteins themselves (Carrel *et al.*, 1972; Hay and Torrigiani, 1973; Spiegelberg, 1974). In contrast, some carbohydrate antigens give rise to a more restricted antibody response. For example, human antibody responses to injected dextrans and levans seem to be largely restricted to the IgG2 subclass (Yount *et al.*, 1968) and antibodies to the coagulation Factor VIII are found primarily in the IgG4 subclass (Anderson and Terry, 1968; Robboy *et al.*, 1970). In studies of IgG antibodies formed by grass pollen-allergic patients during immunotherapy, van der Giessen (1975) found that a relatively high proportion of grass pollen-specific antibodies belong to the IgG4 subclass. Other antibody responses appear to be restricted to two of the four subclasses. For example, anti-Rh antibodies (Natvig and Kunkel, 1973) are found in the IgG1 and IgG3 subclasses. Each of these restrictions may indicate that combinations between V and C-region genes are not totally random.

Injection is not, of course, the natural route of entry of an antigen. In studies of local responses to antigens introduced orally (polio virus—Ogra and Karzon, 1969) or intranasally (tetanus toxoid—Butcher *et al.*, 1975), it has been shown consistently that IgA is the predominant antibody class present in the local secretion, although in the case of a replicating antigen a specific antibody response also is elicited in all the major serum immunoglobulin fractions.

IgM antibody responses appear to be associated strongly with micro-organisms having a blood phase. This applies both to bacterial infections and protozoal parasites such as malaria and trypanosomiasis. The combined characteristics of good complement fixation, efficient agglutination, and pre-dominantly intravascular location suggests that IgM plays a special role in eliminating micro-organisms from the blood stream. High levels of serum IgM in the newborn usually indicate an intrauterine infection such as rubella, syphilis, toxoplasmosis, or cytomegalovirus.

No major antibody function has yet been ascribed to IgD. Plasma cells secreting this immunoglobulin have been found in tonsillar and adenoid tissue, but occur rarely in spleen, peripheral lymphoid tissue, and the gut. Using sensitive techniques, IgD-specific binding to penicillin G (Gleich *et al.*, 1969), diphtheria toxoid (Heiner *et al.*, 1969), and insulin (Devey *et al.*, 1970) have been demonstrated at very low levels in selected sera. In both cord blood and blood from patients with chronic lymphocytic leukaemia IgD is the predominant class of surface immunoglobulin found on B lymphocytes and Rowe *et al.* (1973) have suggested that IgD functions as a lymphocytic receptor and is possibly involved in the induction of immunologic tolerance.

3.3 Membrane Transmission

Immunoglobulin transfer from a mother to her young occurs prenatally in man, postnatally in the pig, and during both phases in the rabbit, rat, and mouse. Prenatal transport of IgG occurs across placental membranes in man or yolk-sac membranes in the rat and mouse, whereas postnatal transport involves the passage of intact IgG, which is present in colostrum, across the membranes of the gut. In man, all four IgG subclasses appear to be able to cross the placenta (Wang *et al.*, 1970; Virella *et al.*, 1972), but in ruminants and the pig only the IgG1 sub-class is absorbed through the gut.

Membrane transport has been investigated intensively by Brambell and coworkers who proposed a mechanism to explain their observations (Brambell *et al.*, 1960). According to this hypothesis serum proteins are taken up into pinocytotic vacuoles and IgG molecules become bound selectively through a specific receptor and are protected, whereas other protein molecules remain in the fluid phase and are catabolized. Thus, only IgG molecules, or a fraction of the total IgG in each vacuole, survive the journey across the placental membrane and are released intact on the foetal side. Whatever the mechanism involved, it is generally agreed that in all species it is both selective and saturable. For example, Waldmann *et al.* (1971) investigated the uptake and transport of radiolabelled proteins across segments of the neonatal rat duodenum. Only homologous IgG was transported at a high rate, and both IgG and Fc fragment were bound to surface membranes of purified enterocytes.

For obvious ethical reasons, there are little direct data on the transport of immunoglobulins and their fragments in man. However, Gitlin and coworkers (1964) injected labelled proteins into pregnant women volunteers at various stages of gestation and found that the Fc fragment of IgG was transported more rapidly to the foetus than was the Fab fragment, intact IgG, or any other protein. Work in other animals supports the view that the Fc region is critical, but there are as yet no data on which domain, C_H2 or C_H3, is the most important. For further details of the mechanism of membrane transmission see reviews by Waldmann and Strober (1969), and by Waldmann and Hemmings (1974).

3.4 Regulation of Catabolism

Each immunoglobulin class appears to be distinct metabolically with different synthetic and fractional catabolic rates (Table 8). The serum concentration of a particular protein is a reflection of the balance between synthesis and catabolism. For example, the synthetic rate for IgG (33 mg/Kg day^{-1}) is similar to that for IgA, but the serum concentration of the latter is much lower because of its higher fractional catabolic rate. The subclasses also differ one from another; thus IgG1, IgG2, and IgG4 have similar fractional catabolic rates (7 per cent of the intravenous pool degraded/day) and half lives of about 20 days, whereas IgG3 has a fractional catabolic rate of 17 per cent and a half life of seven days.

For IgG, the fractional catabolic rate is directly proportional to the serum concentration of this protein. Thus, in patients with G myeloma proteins, there is accelerated catabolism and the protein has a short half life, whereas in patients with sex-linked hypogammaglobulinaemia the fractional catabolic rate is reduced. For IgD and IgE, there appears to be an inverse relationship between the serum concentration and catabolic rate, whereas for IgM and IgA the fractional catabolic rate is independent of the serum concentration.

To explain the concentration–catabolism effects observed with IgG, Brambell *et al.* (1964) proposed a saturable protein-protection system specific for IgG molecules. According to this model, which is similar to that proposed to explain membrane transmission (see above), a constant fraction of the IgG molecules is isolated in a catabolic pool separate from the circulating protein pool (possibly within pinocytotic vacuoles). The site of such catabolism is not known; the liver,

Table 8 Metabolic characteristics of human immunoglobulins

Immuno-globulin	Half life (days)	Distribution (per cent intravascular)	Fractional catabolic rate (per cent intravascular pool catabolized/day)	Synthetic rate (mg/kg day^{-1})
IgG1	21 ⎫		7 ⎫	
IgG2	20 ⎬ 45		7 ⎬	
IgG3	7	45	17 ⎬	33
IgG4	21 ⎭		7 ⎭	
IgM	10	80	8·8	3·3
IgA1	6 ⎫	42	25	24
IgA2	6 ⎭			
sIgA	—	—	—	—
IgD	3	75	37	0·4
IgE	2	50	71	0·002

gastrointestinal tract, and kidney have all been implicated, but the process may take place in the reticuloendothelial system all over the body. In any event, it is suggested that IgG molecules become attached to specific receptors from which they are returned to the circulation ultimately. The remaining unbound IgG molecules are degraded by proteolytic enzymes (cathepsins and neutral proteases).

The site of the IgG molecule which controls the rate of catabolism has been shown in several studies to reside in the Fc region (Waldmann *et al.*, 1971). The elimination of Fab and pFc' (equivalent to the C_H3 region) fragments of human IgG occurs rapidly in both man and the mouse. However, Fc fragments have a relatively long half life suggesting that the N-terminal half of the Fc region (equivalent to C_H2) is important in regulating the catabolic rate (Watkins *et al.*, 1971). This also is supported by the work of Dorrington and Painter (1974) who determined the half lives of the C_H2 and C_H3 fragments from human IgG1 injected intravenously into rabbits and compared them with the half lives of Fc, IgG1, and Fab in the same system. The C_H2 fragment, Fc fragment, and IgG have similar half lives of 60–70 hours, while the C_H3 and Fab fragments are eliminated much more rapidly; the half lives are between 16 and 17 hours.

Since Spiegelberg (cited by Waldmann and Hemmings, 1974) has reported that a monoclonal protein characterized as a half molecule of IgG (H + L) is eliminated rapidly from the circulation it appears that both heavy chains are required to provide the necessary conformation for normal catabolism. The present evidence therefore suggests that the dimeric C_H2 region of IgG is critical for the maintenance of a normal circulation time, although whether the mechanism of catabolism involves receptor binding with pinocytotic vacuoles, as envisaged by Brambell *et al.* (1960), is still far from clear.

3.5 Activation of Complement

The first step in the activation of complement by the classical pathway is the

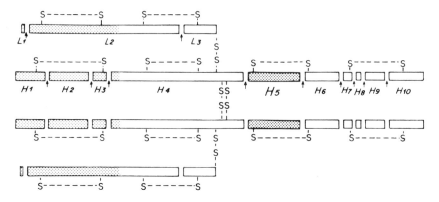

Figure 23 Schematic representation of the structure of a mouse myeloma IgG2a protein (MOPC 173) showing the localization of cyanogen bromide fragments produced by cleavage at the points indicated by the arrows. Peptide fragment (H5) has been shown to fix complement. Reproduced from Kehoe and Fougereau (1969), with permission of publisher

binding of the C1 subcomponent (C1q) to an IgG or IgM antibody. The association of this function with the Fc regions of these immunoglobulins was one of the first examples of the structural basis for the functional duality of antibody molecules (Müller-Eberhard and Kunkel, 1961; Augener *et al.*, 1971).

The further localization of the complement-fixing site has, however, proved difficult. Kehoe and Fougereau (1969) isolated by cleavage with cyanogen bromide a fragment consisting of 60 amino acid residues from the C_H2 region of a monoclonal murine IgG2a protein (Figure 23). This fragment, when absorbed onto polystyrene latex particles, is able to fix guinea-pig complement, although on a molar basis only 3 per cent of the original activity remains.

Attempts to isolate biologically active subfragments from the Fc region of IgG by proteolytic digestion initially gave large fragments from the C_H3 region but much smaller peptides with molecular weights of less than 7000 from the C_H2 region; none of the latter has ever been shown to retain activity. However, Ellerson *et al.* (1972) were able to isolate a dimeric fragment of human IgG1 which corresponds closely to the C_H2 region plus the hinge region (residues 223–234). This was prepared by brief trypsin digestion of acid-treated Fc fragment and was characterized as a covalently bound dimer of the C_H2 region. In the C1q-binding assay of Augener *et al.* (1971), the fragment was found to have the same affinity for C1q as Fc when compared on a molar basis (Dorrington and Painter, 1974). Since reduced and alkylated β-microglobulin (a protein homologous to a single immunoglobulin domain) is able to interact with C1 in the same assay, it appears that little secondary or tertiary folding is required for the existence of an active C1-binding site.

Nevertheless hinge-region inter-heavy chain disulphide bridges are crucial for the binding of C1 by the intact IgG molecule. Isenman *et al.* (1975) have suggested that this effect is not related to the conformation of the active site itself but to the overall rigidity of the whole molecule and particularly the prevention of Fab regions from sterically hindering access of C1 to the site. These workers obtained further evidence in support of this hypothesis in comparative studies of C1 binding by IgG1 and IgG4 proteins and their Fc fragments. It is well established that IgG4 does not bind C1q (see Table 7) and it is surprising therefore that the Fc fragment of this subclass was found to be as active as the Fc fragment of IgG1. It is concluded that the structural features which allow C1 to interact with IgG are present in the IgG4 molecule but are not available in the presence of the Fab regions. It is possible that the heterogeneity of the IgG hinge regions (see Figure 8), with respect to position and number of inter-heavy chain disulphide bridges, is a critical factor in determining whether C1 binding occurs or not.

Further evidence that the C_H2 domain of IgG is involved in C1 fixation comes from work on an unusual fragment of rabbit IgG called Facb (Fragment antigen and complement binding). This is prepared by plasmin digestion of acid-treated IgG (Connell and Porter, 1971) and comprises the two Fab regions linked to the C_H2 region. The fragment lacks the C-terminal 108 amino acids of each heavy chain (that is the C_H3 region). This fragment has been found by Colomb and Porter (1975) to fix C1 by the classical complement pathway as efficiently as whole IgG which had been subjected to the same treatment with acid. Since the $F(ab')_2$ fragment is known not to fix complement, the activity of the Facb fragment again points to a C_H2 location for this function. It is of interest that the hinge region of rabbit IgG is not cleaved by plasmin presumably because the single lysine residue is adjacent to a proline residue. In contrast, human IgG1 has a lysine–threonine bond in the hinge region, and this is hydrolysed by plasmin.

IgM is, perhaps, a more important complement-fixing protein than IgG, but little is known about the structural localization of the complement-fixing site. Wolfenstein-Todel et al. (1973) showed that in the absence of antigen the pentameric $(Fc)_{5\mu}$ fragment is about 20 times more effective (on a molar basis) in complement fixation than the intact immunoglobulin. This suggests that the site is located in either the $C_\mu3$ or $C_\mu4$ domain and that it only becomes accessible after a conformational change brought about by interaction with antigen.

Hurst et al. (1974) studied the fixation of C1 by a monoclonal IgM protein and various fragments obtained by selective proteolysis and chemical degradation. A fragment (molecular weight 6800) from the C-terminal domain $C_\mu4$, and a fragment CNBr5, which contains the $C_\mu3$ and a portion of the $C_\mu4$ domain, were both found to bind C1 effectively. Subsequently, Hurst et al. (1975) characterized the $C_\mu4$ fragment which was obtained by limited tryptic cleavage of $Fc\mu$—itself obtained by reduction of $(Fc)_{5\mu}$. The fragment consists of 24 residues on the N-terminal side of the $C_\mu4$ domain linked by a disulphide bridge to 32 residues on the C-terminal side of the loop, with 23 residues having been cleaved out of the centre of the disulphide loop (Figure 24). The activity of this fragment in a C1-fixation assay is decreased markedly following cleavage of the disulphide bridge, although the isolated A and B peptides do retain a limited ability to fix $C\bar{1}$. Hurst et al. (1975) have suggested that transient binding of C1 by the individual A and B

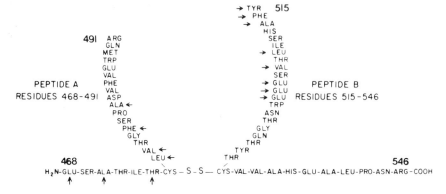

Figure 24 Primary amino acid sequence of the C_H4 fragment from human IgM which has been shown to fix C1. Reproduced from Hurst *et al.* (1975) with permission

peptide chains may be sufficient to activate C1, which in turn consumes C4.

The J chain seems to play no role in classical complement fixation since pentameric IgM reassembled in its absence is only 25 per cent less effective in C1q binding than the pentamer with J chain (Kownatzki and Drescher, 1973). Moreover, the $C_\mu4$ fragment studied by Hurst and coworkers (1975) appears not to contain portions of J chain but to originate solely from the μ chain.

The alternative complement pathway, which does not involve C1, C4, or C2, is known to be activated by various immunoglobulin aggregates such as human IgA, guinea-pig IgG1, and ruminant IgG2. Isolated $F(ab')_2$ fragments from both guinea-pig IgG1 and IgG2 are able to activate the alternative pathway (Sandberg *et al.*, 1971). Similarly, rabbit $F(ab')_2$ fragments have been shown to convert Factor B (Spiegelberg and Götze, 1972). Since Fab fragments are not active, it is possible that a Factor B-binding site exists in the hinge region of these molecules, but no precise localization of such a site has been reported yet.

3.6 Interactions with Cell Membranes

3.6.1 Macrophages and Monocytes

Macrophage cytophilic antibodies were first described by Boyden and Sorkin (1960) who showed that such antibodies are capable of cellular fixation prior to their combination with antigen. Subsequently, Berken and Benacerraf (1966, 1968) have applied the term 'cytophilic' to those antibodies which become bound to macrophages after combination with antigen. These authors considered cytophilia to be a 'property of opsonizing antibody which provides the receptors which permit the binding of the antibody to the macrophage cell membrane in preparation for phagocytosis'. Other authors, notably Tizard (1969), have disputed this view and have claimed the existence of two distinct populations of antibody molecules. This aspect is considered further below.

Cytophilic binding to macrophages has been shown in rabbit (Boyden and Sorkin, 1960), guinea-pig (Berken and Benacerraf, 1966), and man (Lo Buglio *et al.*, 1967). In man, it has been shown that monocytic phagocytosis of erythrocytes coated with anti-Rh antibodies is inhibited by IgG1 and IgG3 myeloma proteins but not by IgG2 or IgG4 proteins (Huber and Fudenberg, 1968; Huber *et al.*, 1971). Similarly, Hay *et al.* (1972) showed that radiolabelled IgG1 and IgG3 myeloma proteins can bind strongly to the surface of the monocyte whereas IgG2 and IgG4 myeloma proteins bind poorly, if at all. Moreover, this binding can be inhibited both by fresh human serum and by soluble immune complexes.

Both Berken and Benacerraf (1966) and Lo Buglio *et al.* (1967) showed that the monocyte-binding activity of IgG is destroyed by digestion of the IgG with pepsin. Since these workers were studying residual $F(ab')_2$ fragments they considered that the results indicated an Fc location for the macrophage-binding site. In another study, Abramson *et al.* (1970) studied the capacity of various IgG fragments to inhibit rosette formation between anti-D-coated erythrocytes and human mononuclear cells. The Fc fragment was strongly inhibitory and the $F(ab')_2$ fragment weakly inhibitory. No inhibition was noted with Fab or with peptic peptides from the Fc region (including the pFc′ fragment). These authors concluded that the peptide portions of IgG which attach to mononuclear cells are located in the N-terminal half of the Fc fragment and require the integrity of inter-heavy chain disulphide bridge. In contrast, however, Yasmeen *et al.* (1973) showed that heterologous binding of human IgG to guinea-pig peritoneal macrophages is a function of the C_H3 domain but not of the N-terminal C_H2 domain. This was demonstrated both by a direct rosetting assay and by an indirect assay which measured the ability of various proteins to inhibit rosette formations between macrophages and erythrocytes coated with IgG. In the indirect assay, IgG, Fc, and C_H3 fragments were strongly inhibitory but C_H2 and Fab fragments are only weakly inhibitory. Using a homologous rosetting system of human monocytes and human erythrocytes coated with incomplete anti-D, Okafor *et al.* (1974) were able to study the inhibitory capacity of pFc′ fragments (equivalent to the C_H3 domain) obtained from all four IgG subclasses. Fragments from IgG1 and IgG3 myeloma proteins were significantly more inhibitory than fragments from IgG2 and IgG4 proteins, in agreement with the earlier work on intact immunoglobulin.

Recently, Ciccimarra *et al.* (1975) have reported that intact C_H3 and a peptide derived from it and provisionally located between residues 407–416 (Eu IgG1 numbering) are able to bind to human monocytes and also to inhibit rosette formation of antibody-coated erythrocytes with human monocytes. The amino acid sequences of IgG1 and IgG4 proteins are identical in this region except for residue 409 where an arginine/lysine substitution occurs. There are, however, no sequence data available for this region of IgG2 or IgG3 molecules to enable further comparisons to be made.

In contrast to the above workers, Holm *et al.* (1974) were unable to inhibit monocyte-mediated haemolysis with C_H3 fragments. These differences cannot at present be reconciled, but it is possible (Turner, 1974) that they relate to the different test system used. Furthermore, the observation of Dorrington and Painter (1974) that β_2-microglobulin is inhibitory in the monocyte-rosetting assay may indicate that cross-reactions occur between the heavy-chain domains.

The data of Hay *et al.* (1972) are consistent with the view first proposed by Berken and Benacerraf that the phagocyte-binding site of opsonizing antibodies is identical to the structure involved in cytophilic binding to macrophages. Thus, the inhibition of IgG1 and IgG3 binding to monocytes by soluble immune complexes is strikingly parallel to the inhibition by IgG1 and IgG3 of phagocytosis of opsonized red cells (Huber and Fudenberg, 1968). Furthermore, it was observed by Hay and coworkers (1972) that immune complexes are more effective than native immunoglobulins as inhibitors of IgG1 and IgG3 adherence. This may arise due to multipoint attachment of the complexes through several Fc regions giving much firmer binding than that established by the single Fc site of an individual IgG molecule. It seems probable, therefore, that uptake of antigen by phagocytic cells is much more likely to occur through an opsonizing antibody pathway than by the less efficient process of cytophilia. However, the site on the immunoglobulin molecule interacting with the macrophage membrane receptor may be identical in both processes.

Recently, Capron *et al.* (1975) have shown that rat IgE antibodies against *Schistosoma mansoni* antigens are able to bind to the schistosomules and also to adhere to peritoneal macrophages. The latter attachment was presumed to be Fc mediated, but further work is required to establish this unequivocally. A role of IgE-mediated macrophage adherence in schistosomiasis and other helminthic diseases is clearly an attractive possibility which would, if established, provide a rational biological function for this class of immunoglobulin.

3.6.2 Neutrophils

A receptor for IgG on the surface of human neutrophils was first reported by Messner and Jelinek (1970). Erythrocytes sensitized indirectly with antibacterial IgG antibodies, after passive sensitization with bacterial antigens, adhered to neutrophil monolayers and this adherence could be inhibited by whole IgG, IgG1, and IgG3 myeloma proteins, and by the Fc fragment but not by the Fab fragment.

Using an assay system based on the release of lysosomal constituents such as β-glucuronidase, Henson *et al.* (1972) concluded that, when aggregated, all four human IgG subclasses react with neutrophils. In addition, aggregated IgA1 and IgA2, but not IgM, IgD, or IgE, were found to be reactive. In a direct binding assay using [^{125}I] immunoglobulins, Lawrence *et al.* (1975) found that neutrophils bind unaggregated myeloma proteins of the subclasses IgG1, IgG3, IgG4, IgA1, and IgA2. Furthermore, a preparation of secretory IgA was shown to bind. After aggregation with a rabbit $F(ab')_2$ anti-human Fab fragment reagent, neutrophils show increased binding of immunoglobulin of all classes.

The binding of IgA to neutrophils is the only known cytophilic property of this immunoglobulin class, although the biological significance of the observation remains to be evaluated. Since no significant cross-inhibition has been observed, it appears that the receptors for IgG and IgA on neutrophils are distinct but further work is clearly required in this field.

It seems likely that the IgG receptor interacting with phagocytic neutrophils is the same as that involved in monocyte/macrophage interactions, but the work of Messner and Jelinek (1970) with different rosetting systems suggests that the density of cell-surface receptors for IgG on neutrophils and monocytes differs.

3.6.3 Lymphocytes

B Lymphocytes usually have detectable surface immunoglobulin thought to be synthesized by the cell itself and T lymphocytes also appear to have small amounts of an IgM-like protein on their surface. In addition, there is evidence that human lymphocyte-like cells have receptors with specificity for both homologous and heterologous IgG (Brain and Marston, 1973; Frøland et al., 1973). Using inhibition of a rosette assay with IgG-sensitized indicator erythrocytes, Frøland et al. (1974) have studied the specificity of these receptors on so-called EA–RFC cells for various Ig subclasses and fragments. Both IgG1 and IgG3 inhibit strongly whereas IgG2 and IgG4 show only weak inhibition. No inhibition occurs using Fab or F(ab')$_2$ fragments, but the Fc fragment and the IgG3 Fch fragment (Fc plus the extended hinge region characteristic of IgG3) are strongly inhibitory. Partial reduction and alkylation reduces the inhibitory capacity of both fragments. The pFc' fragment of IgG (equivalent to the $C_\gamma 3$ region) is not inhibitory in this assay system, and the authors concluded that the $C_\gamma 2$ region is the probable molecular location of the receptor for lymphocyte-like cells. It seems very likely that the effector cells in antibody-dependent cytotoxicity (the K cells) are a subpopulation of these EA–RFC cells.

Lawrence et al. (1975) found that unaggregated IgG1 and IgG3 proteins bind to 'lymphocytes' but not IgG2, IgG4, IgA1, IgA2, IgM, IgE, IgD, or secretory IgA. However, unlike Frøland et al. (1974) who observed no differences following aggregation using a possibly different cell population, Lawrence and coworkers (1975) found that IgG of all subclasses and IgE are able to bind following aggregation with a rabbit F(ab')$_2$–anti-human Fab reagent. Preliminary studies with nylon fibre-purified T lymphocytes and B lymphocytes from a patient with chronic lymphocytic leukaemia suggest that both cell types have a receptor for IgG which is in agrement with other reports of IgG binding to B (Basten et al., 1972) and T lymphocytes of mouse (Anderson and Grey, 1974). Santana and Turk have shown that the binding of aggregated IgG to T cells requires large aggregates of greater than 200 S and that binding is temperature dependent (cited by Turner, 1974).

3.6.4 Basophils and Mast Cells

Immunoglobulin molecules with a capacity to bind to the membranes of basophils and mast cells are known as homocytotropic and have been recognized

Table 9 Properties of three major types of anaphylactic homocytotropic antibody in the guinea-pig

Property	IgE (Reagin)	IgG1	IgG2
Tissue sensitized	isologous	isologous	heterologous
Optimum sensitization time (hr)	50–80	2–4	2–4
Persistance in skin	4 weeks	1–2 days	1–2 days
Heat (56°, 30 min)	labile	stable	stable
C1q fixation	−	−	+

Modified from Stanworth (1970)

for many years. In several species, homocytotropic antibodies have been shown to be associated with two, or even three, distinct immunoglobulin classes (Table 9), but the most important biologically appears to be the reaginic (IgE) type (see reviews by Bennich and Johansson, 1971; Ishizaka and Ishizaka, 1971).

The concentration of IgE in serum is minute, and it is assumed that at any one time the bulk of the body pool is bound to the surface membranes of basophils and mast cells. The recent availability of rat myeloma IgE (Bazin *et al.* 1974) has permitted direct investigation of the interaction of IgE with rat basophilic leukaemic cells (Kulczycki *et al.*, 1974; Kulczycki and Metzger, 1974). From kinetic studies, it is clear that the interaction is described by the equation

$$\text{IgE} + \text{receptor} \underset{k_{-1}}{\overset{k_1}{\rightleftharpoons}} \text{receptor–IgE complex}$$

and that the association is first order both with regard to IgE and receptor concentrations. The reaction is specific, thus human IgE, heated rat IgE, rat IgG, rat IgA, and rat IgM do not bind, sites are saturable, and binding is reversible. The affinity constant ($K_A = k_1/k - 1$) has been calculated to be of the order of 6×10^9 M^{-1} and the number of binding sites per cell was found to be in the range 3×10^5 to more than 1×10^6.

An indirect estimation of k_A for the human IgE–basophil interation (Ishizaka *et al.*, 1973) gives values of 0.1–1.3×10^9 M^{-1} for 12 of 13 preparations and 1.2×10^{10} M^{-1} for the other. In the same study, the number of receptors per cell was found to be in the range 3×10^4–8.5×10^4, although such numbers should be intepreted with caution since they appear to be a variable characteristic of different cell types (Kulczycki and Metzger, 1974) and may also vary with the metabolic state of the cell.

The structural location of the mastcell-binding site of IgE is still under investigation and at the time of writing has not been localized more precisely than the $C_\varepsilon 3$–$C_\varepsilon 4$ regions. Bennich and von Bahr-Lindstrom (1974) have suggested that the binding of an IgE molecule to a mast cell or basophil cell surface membrane may involve two distinct sites in the $C_\varepsilon 3$–$C_\varepsilon 4$ regions. One type of site, which they have termed 'primary', has a recognition function, interacts with a membrane receptor on the basophil or mast cell, and may be located in the $C_\varepsilon 4$

domain. A 'secondary' binding site is proposed also, which may be present in either domain, shows no particular cell specificity, and is capable of interacting with any cell membrane.

It is well established that the ability of IgE to bind to mast cells and basophils is lost following heat treatment at 56° for 30 minutes. The structural changes induced by such treatment were studied by Dorrington and Bennich (1973) using circular dichroism and ultraviolet absorption difference spectra. It was found that intact IgE showed changes in both the aromatic side-chain and peptide-bond spectral regions, which were only partially reversible on cooling. Similar studies were performed with the $F(ab')_2$, Fc'', and Fc fragments of IgE (see Figure 22); the conformational changes induced in $F(ab')_2$ and Fc'' fragments were fully reversible. Furthermore, antigenic determinants known to be located in the Fc'' region were unaffected by prolonged exposure to heat. These studies indicate that the irreversible thermal effects are restricted to the two C-terminal domains, one or both of which are known to carry the cytotropic site.

Recently, Hamburger (1975) has reported that a pentapeptide (Asp-Ser-Asp-Pro-Arg) corresponding in sequence to amino acid residues 320–324 (that is adjacent to the inter-heavy chain disulphide bridge between $C_\varepsilon 2$ and $C_\varepsilon 3$) is able to inhibit *in vivo* passive transfer of IgE-mediated sensitivity in the Prausnitz–Küstner test. Whether or not this represents the mast cell binding site of the IgE molecule is a controversial issue and the focus of much current research.

As stressed earlier there exists, in several species, a second type of homocytotropic antibody which is usually of IgG-type and which characteristically sensitizes homologous tissues for short periods. Established examples of this type of antibody are IgGa of rat, IgG1 of guinea-pig, IgG1 of mouse, and IgS of sheep. Studies of rat homocytotropic antibodies by Bach *et al.* (1971) suggest that IgE and IgGa compete for the same cell receptor although the affinity of IgG is much lower than that of IgE.

Man also appears to have a weak cell-binding, heat-stable, mercaptoethanol-resistant homocytotropic IgG antibody capable of passively sensitizing human or primate skin for two to four hours (Malley and Perlman, 1966; Parish, 1974). An antibody with similar properties to this so-called 'short-term sensitizing antibody' (IgG S–TS) has been described in subjects sensitive to horse serum (Terr and Bentz, 1965) and in asthmatic patients unresponsive to disodium cromoglycate (Bryant *et al.*, 1973). There is no direct evidence that IgG S–TS belongs to any of the known subclasses, although Stanworth and Smith (1973) have reported that an IgG4 myeloma protein is able to block the binding of human IgE to baboon mast cells.

A biologically unimportant homocytotropic antibody activity can be demonstrated in human, rabbit, and mouse IgG. Each of these immunoglobulins can sensitize heterologous (guinea-pig) skin for reverse passive cutaneous anaphylaxis reactions (Ovary, 1960). The subclasses involved—IgG1, IgG3, and IgG4 of man, and IgG2a of mouse and rat (Ovary *et al.*, 1965; Terry, 1966)—do not sensitize isologous skin and are thus generally distinct from the short-term sensitizing IgG homocytotropic antibodies.

3.7 Reactivity with Staphylococcal Protein A

In 1966, Forsgren and Sjöquist reported that a cell-wall protein, called protein A isolated from *Staphylococcus aureus* is able to bind the Fc region of human IgG. This was confirmed by Kronvall (1967) and extended to the IgG of other species, including rabbit (Forsgren and Sjöquist, 1967), guinea-pig IgG1 and IgG2 (Forsgren, 1968), and mouse IgG (Kronvall *et al.*, 1970*a*).

In man, anti-protein A reactivity is confined to the IgG1, IgG2, and IgG4 subclasses (Kronvall and Williams, 1969), while in the mouse IgG2a, IgG2b, and IgG3 are reactive but not IgG1 (Kronvall *et al.*, 1970*a*). Human IgA and IgM were found to be unreactive (Kronvall *et al.*, 1970*c*). In a separate study, a single IgD and a single IgE myeloma protein were also unreactive (Kronvall *et al.*, 1970*a*). (*Note added in proof:* Recent work (Saltvedt and Harboe, 1976) has shown that proteins of the human IgA2 subclass react with staphylococci and that some IgM proteins (provisionally designated IgM2) are also reactive.)

Kronvall and Frommel (1970) used a procedure involving the inhibition of precipitation to show that protein A reactivity is a property of the Fc fragment and heavy chains but not of $F(ab')_2$, Fab, Fc', and pFc' fragments, or of light chains. This suggests that protein A binding is yet another function of the C_H2 domain but this remains to be demonstrated in a direct-binding assay.

Kronvall *et al.* (1970*b*) measured the equilibrium constant of two different IgG myeloma proteins for staphylococcal protein A and found both to be about $4 \times 10^7 \, M^{-1}$. In the same study, the number of protein A residues was estimated to be 80 000/organism, which is four times the density of the blood group A antigen on erythrocytes.

The biological importance of protein A binding is not yet fully understood, but several studies point to a possible involvement in non-immune complement activation. For example, protein A–IgG complexes can fix guinea-pig complement (Sjöquist and Stålenheim, 1969; Kronvall and Gewurz, 1970; Stålenheim and Malmheden-Eriksson, 1971) and also complement from fresh human, pig, and dog sera (Kronvall and Gewurz, 1970). Also, Kronvall and Gewurz (1970) have suggested that protein A is able to bring IgG molecules into the close spatial proximity necessary for activation of C1 esterase. Both dimerization of IgG by protein A and larger structures due to secondary aggregation may produce complement-activating complexes. This suggestion is supported further by the studies of Stålenheim and Castensson (1971) who found that when protein A is added to human serum C3 is converted to C3a and C3b. However, neither protein A nor aggregates of protein A and IgG can convert purified C3. The most probable explanation of these observations is that protein A reacts with the Fc region of IgG and that C1 is then activated by fixation to the protein A–IgG complex. Thus, according to this view the protein A–IgG complex initiates complement fixation by the classical pathway in much the same way as an ordinary antigen–antibody complex.

3.8 Interaction with Rheumatoid Factors

Rheumatoid factors are a group of serum proteins first described by Waaler

(1940) and by Rose *et al.* (1948). Subsequently, they were characterized as IgM antibodies reacting with antigenic determinants of both human and foreign species IgG (Hobson and Gorrill, 1952; Grubb, 1956; Waller and Vaughan, 1956). These antigenic determinants have been shown by several investigators to be located in the Fc region of the molecule—see for example Franklin (1961), Osterland *et al.* (1963), and Henney and Stanworth (1964)—but, although some authors have taken the view that they arise after conformational alteration of IgG, there is no unequivocal evidence to support this.

Several of the Gm allotypic antigens interact with rheumatoid factors and were, in many cases, first described and defined using serum from patients with rheumatoid arthritis (Grubb and Laurell, 1956; Harboe, 1959; Natvig, 1966). More recently, the $nG1m(a)$ and γ_4 non-a antigens, which are antithetic to $G1m(a)$, and the $nG3m(b^1)$ antigen, which is antithetic to $G3m(b^1)$, have been shown to interact with appropriate rheumatoid factors (Gaarder and Natvig, 1972; Natvig *et al.*, 1972). The $nG1m(a)$ and $nG3m(b^1)$ antigens are shared by several subclasses and behave as both allotypic and isotypic antigens. The isotypic Ga antigen (Allen and Kunkel, 1966; Gaarder and Natvig, 1970) is shared by the IgG1, IgG2, and IgG4 subclasses and is probably the most important of all the antigens interacting with rheumatoid factors. It is unrelated apparently to either the $G3m(g)$ or $G3m(b^1)$ antigens which are present on IgG3 molecules. Furthermore, the latter antigens probably occupy different molecular locations in the γ_3 chain since there are antithetic $nG3m(g)$ and $nG3m(b^1)$ markers for each allotype.

A provisional localization of the antigens interacting with serologically defined rheumatoid factors has been achieved using various proteolytic fragments (Natvig and Turner, 1970; Natvig *et al.*, 1972). As shown in Table 10 all the

Table 10 Molecular location of isotypic and allotypic antigens of human IgG known to interact with appropriate rheumatoid factors

Immunoglobulin subclass and allotype			Homology region		
			C_H2	C_H3	
IgG1	G1m(ax)	Ga	$nG3m(b^1)$	G1m(a)	G1m(x)
IgG1	G1m(f)	Ga	$nG3m(b^1)$	nG1m(a)	
IgG2	G2m(n +)	Ga	$nG3m(b^1)$	nG1m(a)	
IgG2	G2m(n −)	Ga	$nG3m(b^1)$	nG1m(a)	
IgG3	G3m(g)	G3m(g)	$nG3m(b^1)$	nG1m(a)	
IgG3	G3m(b)		$G3m(b^1)$	nG1m(a)	
IgG4	a	Ga		γ_4 non-a	
IgG4	b	Ga		γ_4 non-a	

antigens are in the Fc region and the eight known specificities appear to be determined by amino acid substitutions in five antigenic regions. Using pFc′ fragments (equivalent to C_H3 fragments) from each allotypic variant of the four subclasses in a haemagglutination-inhibition assay system, it was possible to demonstrate the presence of the antithetic $G1m(a)$, $nG1m(a)$ and γ_4 non-a antigens in the C_H3 region. From earlier sequence studies, it appears that these

Table 11 Amino acid sequences associated with three antigens interacting with rheumatoid factors

Subclass	Antigen	Sequence number			
		355	356	357	358
IgG1	G1m(a)	Arg	*Asp*	Glu	*Leu*
IgG1 G1m(f)					
IgG2	nG1m(a)	Arg	Glu	Glu	Met
IgG3					
IgG4	γ_4 non-a	*Gln*	Glu	Glu	Met

antigens are specified by amino acid residues located between residues 355 and 358 of the γ chain (following the Eu numbering of Edelman *et al.*, 1969). The sequences and associated antigens are given in Table 11.

There is evidence from studies using antiglobulins obtained from sensitized healthy individuals that the expression of each of these antigens requires the presence of a non-correlative determinant located near the C-terminus of the γ chain (Turner *et al.*, 1969, 1972). Work with a rheumatoid factor interacting with G1m(a) suggests a similar requirement for this antigen-antibody system (Okafor and Turner, 1974). Whether this determinant is actually part of these antigenic sites or merely influences their conformation is not clear.

The G1m(x) antigen also is known to be present in the C_H3 region but there are insufficient sequence data available to permit a more precise localization. By virtue of the failure of pFc' fragments to inhibit the binding of appropriate specific rheumatoid factors the following antigens are presumed to be located in the C_H2 domain: the antithetic G3m(b^1) and nG3m(b^1) antigens; the G3m(g) antigen; and the Ga antigen. With the exception of G3m(g), which may be specified by residue 296 (see Table 6), there are no sequence data for these antigens.

Earlier studies (Normansell, 1970, 1971) have indicated a low binding affinity between a rheumatoid factor of undefined specificity and both native and aggregated IgG. More recently, Steward *et al.* (1973) have measured the binding affinities of rheumatoid factors interacting with the G1m(a), G1m(x), nG1m(a), and γ_4 non-a antigens using single antigen systems of appropriate, isolated C_H3 fragments. All the rheumatoid factors studied show specific binding with the fragments possessing the homologous antigen and the binding affinities of these rheumatoid factors are low—between 10^4 and 10^5 M^{-1}. A similar value has been obtained by Dissanyake *et al.* (unpublished results) using the isolated Fab fragment of an IgM rheumatoid factor and either native or aggregated IgG. The impressive superior reactivity of aggregated IgG with rheumatoid factors is yet another example of the biological amplification effect which is possible when multivalent attachment occurs.

3.9 Future Perspectives

In the preceding sections the evidence for the location of various IgG effector

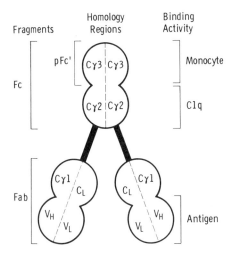

Figure 25 Schematic diagram of human IgG showing homology regions, enzymic fragments, and the location of various biological activities

functions has been reviewed briefly and some data are summarized in Figure 25. It seems likely that in the immediate future the precise localization of the rheumatoid factor antigens will be the most readily achieved since these are antigenic determinants which correlate with specific amino acid sequences found within a single allotype or an isotype with an antithetic marker.

In contrast, a full understanding of the molecular configuration required for binding C_{1q} or for the interaction with cell-membrane receptors will require considerable advances in the X-ray crystallography field. At the present time no effector function site is mapped within the three-dimensional structure in the same detail as the antibody combining site. The recent report (Colman *et al.*, 1976) of the structure of a whole IgG molecule at 0·5 nm resolution is the best source of data available for the Fc region and suggests that there is a degree of flexibility in this region. This is not incompatible with the view that allosteric changes may occur in immunoglobulins following antigen binding to expose a C_{1q} binding site (in the case of IgG and IgM) or perhaps initiate mast cell degranulation (in the case of IgE).

The biological activity of the cell-binding immunoglobulins may prove the most difficult to dissect. The possible involvement of two sites has been proposed in connection with IgE–mast cell interactions (see pp. 46–47) (Stanworth, 1973; Bennich and Bahr-Lindstrom, 1974), and may be applicable to other Ig–cell systems. Cell binding may involve a site in a single domain or it may, conceivably, require co-operation between adjacent domains. This could explain some of the discrepancies observed in the case of monocyte binding.

Although there is at present a dearth of information on the structural basis of immunoglobulin effector functions it is to be expected that current interests in membrane biochemistry and cell-triggering phenomena will act as a stimulus to further investigations in this area of immunochemistry.

REFERENCES

Abramson, N., Gelfand, E. W., Jandl, J. H., and Rosen, F. S. (1970). *J. Exp. Med.*, **132**, 1207.

Allen, J. C., and Kunkel, H. G. (1966). *Arth. Rheumat.* **9**, 758.

Amzel, L. M., Chen, B. L., Phizackerly, R. P., Poljak, R. J., and Saul, F. (1974). In *Progress in Immunology II*, Vol. I, (Brent, L., and Holborow, J., eds.), North Holland Publishing Co., Amsterdam, p. 85.

Anderson, C. L., and Grey, H. M. (1974). *J. Exp. Med.*, **139**, 1175.

Anderson, J. R., and Terry, W. D. (1968). *Nature (Lond.)*, **217**, 174.

Atwell, J. L., and Marchalonis, J. J. (1975). *J. Immunogenetics*, **1**, 391.

Atwell, J. L., and Marchalonis, J. J. (1976). In *Comparative Immunology*, (Marcholonis, J. J., ed.), Blackwell, Oxford. p. 276

Augener, W., Grey, H. M., Cooper, N. R., and Müller-Eberhard, H. J. (1971). *Immunochemistry*, **8**, 1011.

Bach, M. K., Bloch, K. J., and Austen, K. F. (1971). *J. Exp. Med.*, **133**, 752.

Baglioni, C., Alescio-Zonta, L., Cioli, D., and Carbonara, A. (1966). *Science, N.Y.*, **152**, 1517.

Basten, A., Miller, J. F. A. P., Spent, J., and Pye, J. (1972). *J. Exp. Med.*, **135**, 610.

Bazin, H., Querinjean, P., Beckers, A., Heremans, J. F., and Dessy, F. (1974). *Immunology*, **26**, 713.

Bennich, H., and Johansson, S. G. O. (1971). *Adv. Immunol.*, **13**, 1.

Bennich, H., and von Bahr-Lindstrom, H. (1974). In *Progress in Immunology II*, Vol. I, (Brent, L., and Holborow, J., eds.), North Holland Publishing Co., Amsterdam, p. 49.

Berken, A., and Benacerraf, B. (1966). *J. Exp. Med.*, **123**, 119.

Berken, A., and Banacerraf, B. (1968). *J. Immunol.*, **100**, 1219.

Bernier, G. M., Tominaga, K., Easley, C. W., and Putnam, F. W. (1965). *Biochemistry*, **4**, 2072.

Boyden, S. V., and Sorkin, E. (1960). *Immunology*, **3**, 272.

Brain, P., and Marston, R. H. (1973). *Eur. J. Immunol.*, **3**, 6.

Brambell, F. W. R., Hemmings, W. A., and Morris, I. G. (1964). *Nature (Lond.)*, **203**, 1352.

Brambell, F. W. R., Hemmings, W. A., Oakley, C. L., and Porter, R. R. (1960). *Proc. Roy. Soc. Ser. B.*, **151**, 478.

Braun, D. G., Eichmann, K., and Krause, R. M. (1969). *J. Exp. Med.*, **129**, 809.

Bryant, D. H., Burns, M. W., and Lazarus, L. (1973). *Brit. Med. J.*, iv, 589.

Butcher, B. T., Salvaggio, J. E., and Leslie, G. A. (1975). *Clin. Allergy*, **1**, 33.

Capra, J. D., and Kindt, T. J. (1975). *Immunogenetics*, **1**, 417.

Capron, A., Dessaint, J.-P., Capron, M., and Bazin, H. (1975). *Nature (Lond.)*, **253**, 474.

Carrel, S., Morell, A., Skvaril, F., and Barandun, S. (1972). *FEBS Letters*, **19**, 305.

Chapuis, R. M., and Koshland, M. E. (1974). *Proc. Nat. Acad. Sci., U.S.A.*, **71**, 657.

Chodirker, W. B., and Tomasi, T. B. (1963). *Science, N.Y.*, **142**, 1080.

Ciccimarra, F., Rosen, F. S., and Merler, E. (1975). *Proc. Nat. Acad. Sci., U.S.A.*, **72**, 2081.

Cohen, S. (1963). *Biochem. J.*, **89**, 334.

Colman, P. M., Deisenhofer, J., Huber, R., and Palm, W. (1976). *J. Mol. Biol.*, **100**, 257.

Colomb, M., and Porter, R. R. (1975). *Biochem. J.*, **145**, 177.

Connell, G. E., and Porter, R. R. (1971). *Biochem. J.*, **124**, 53P.

De Préval, X., Pink, J. R. L., and Milstein, C. (1970). *Nature (Lond.)*, **228**, 930.
Devey, M., Carter, D., Sanderson, C. J., and Coombs, R.R.A. (1970). *Lancet, ii*, 1280.
Dorrington, K. J., and Bennich, H. (1973). *J. Biol. Chem.*, **248**, 8378.
Dorrington, K. J., and Painter, R. H. (1974). In *Progress in Immunology II*, Vol. I, (Brent, L., and Holborow, J., eds.), North Holland Publishing Co., Amsterdam, p. 75.
Dorrington, K. J., and Rockey, J. H. (1970). *Biochim. Biophys. Acta*, **200**, 584.
Dreyer, W. J., and Bennett, J. C. (1965). *Proc. Nat. Acad. Sci., U.S.A.*, **54**, 864.

Edelman, G. M. (1970). *Biochemistry*, **9**, 3197.
Edelman, G. M., Cunningham, B. A., Gall, W. E., Gottlieb, P. D., Rutishauser, U., and Waxdal, M. J. (1969). *Proc. Nat. Acad. Sci., U.S.A.*, **63**, 78,
Edelman, G. M., and Gall, W. E. (1969). *Ann. Rev. Biochem.*, **38**, 415.
Edelman, G. M., and Gally, J. A. (1962). *J. Exp. Med.*, **116**, 207.
Edelman, G. M., and Poulik, M. D. (1961). *J. Exp. Med.*, **113**, 861.
Ellerson, J. R., Yasmeen, D., Painter, R. H., and Dorrington, K. J. (1972). *FEBS Letters*, **24**, 318.
Edmundson, A. B., Ely, K. R., Girling, R. L., Abola, E. E., Schiffer, M, and Westholm, F. A. (1974). In *Progress in Immunology II*, Vol. I, (Brent, L., and Holborow, J., eds.), North Holland Publishing Co., Amsterdam, p. 103.

Feinstein, A., and Rowe, A. J. (1965). *Nature (Lond.)*, **205**, 147.
Feinstein, D., and Franklin, E. C. (1966). *Nature (Lond.)*, **212**, 1496.
Fleischman, J. B., Pain, R., and Porter, R. R. (1961). *Archs Biochem. Biophys.*, Suppl. 1, 174.
Forsgren, A. (1968). *J. Immunol.*, **100**, 921.
Forsgren, A., and Sjöquist, J. (1966). *J. Immunol.*, **97**, 822.
Forsgren, A., and Sjöquist, J. (1967). *J. Immunol.*, **99**, 19.
Frangione, B., and Milstein, C. (1968). *J. Mol. Biol.*, **33**, 893.
Frangione, B., and Wolfenstein-Todel, C. (1972). *Proc. Nat. Acad. Sci., U.S.A.*, **69**, 3673.
Frank, M. M., and Humphrey, J. H. (1969). *Immunology*, **17**, 237.
Franklin, E. C. (1961). *Proc. 10th Int. Congr. Rheumatol.*, **2**, 804.
Frøland, S. S., Michaelsen, T. E., Wisløff, F., and Natvig, J. B. (1974). *Scand. J. Immunol.*, **3**, 509.
Frøland, S. S., Natvig, J. B., and Wisløff, F. (1973). *Scand. J. Immunol.*, **2**, 83.

Gaarder, P. I., and Natvig, J. B. (1970). *J. Immunol.*, **105**, 928.
Gaarder, P. I., and Natvig, J. B. (1972). *J. Immunol.*, **108**, 617.
Gitlin, D., Kumate, J., Urrusti, J., and Morales, C. (1964). *J. Clin. Invest.*, **43**, 1938.
Gleich, G. J., Bieger, R. C., and Stankievic, R. (1969). *Science, N.Y.*, **165**, 606.
Grabar, P., and Williams, C. A. Jr. (1953). *Biochim. Biophys. Acta*, **10**, 193.
Grey, H. M., Abel, C. A., Yount, W. J., and Kunkel, H. G. (1968). *J. Exp. Med.*, **128**, 1223.
Grey, H. M., Hirst, J. W., and Cohn, M. (1971). *J. Exp. Med.*, **133**, 289.
Grubb, R. (1956). *Acta path. microbiol. scand.*, **39**, 195.
Grubb, R., and Laurell, A. B. (1956). *Acta path. microbiol. scand.*, **39**, 390.

Hamburger, R. (1975). *Science, N.Y.*, **189**, 389.
Harboe, M. (1959). *Acta path microbiol scand.*, **47**, 191.
Hay, F. C., and Torrigiani, G. (1973). *Clin. Exp. Immunol.*, **15**, 517.
Hay, F. C., Torrigiani, G., and Roitt, I. M. (1972). *Eur. J. Immunol.*, **2**, 257.
Heiner, D. C., Saha, A., and Rose, B. (1969). *Fed. Proc.*, **28**, 766.
Henney, C. S., and Stanworth, D. R. (1964). *Nature (Lond.)*, **201**, 511.
Henson, P. M., Johnson, H. B., and Spiegelberg, H. L. (1972). *J. Immunol.*, **109**, 1182.

Heremans, J. F. (1959). *Clin. Chim. Acta*, **4**, 639.

Hill, R. L., Delaney, R., Lebovitz, H. E., and Fellows, R. E. (1966). *Proc. Roy. Soc., Ser. B.*, **166**, 159.

Hilschmann, N., and Craig, L. C. (1965). *Proc. Nat. Acad. Sci., U.S.A.*, **53**, 1403.

Hobson, D., and Gorrill, R. H. (1952). *Lancet*, *i*, 389.

Holm, G., Engvall, E., Hammarström, S., and Natvig, J. B. (1974). *Scand. J. Immunol.*, **3**, 173.

Huber, H., Douglas, S. D., Nusbacher, J., Kochwa, S., and Rosenfield, R. E. (1971). *Nature (Lond.)*, **229**, 419.

Huber, H., and Fudenberg, H. H. (1968). *Int. Archs Allergy*, **34**, 18.

Hurst, M. M., Volanakis, J. E., Hester, R. B., Stroud, R. M., and Bennett, J.C. (1974). *J. Exp. Med.*, **140**, 1117.

Hurst, M. M., Volanakis, J. E., Stroud, R. M., and Bennett, J. C. (1975). *J. Exp. Med.*, **142**, 1322.

Inman, F. P., and Ricardo, M. J. (1974). *J. Immunol.*, **112**, 229.

Isenman, D. E., Dorrington, K. J., and Painter, R. H. (1975). *J. Immunol.*, **114**, 1726.

Ishizaka, K., and Ishizaka, T. (1971), *Clin. Allergy*, **1**, 9.

Ishizaka, K., Ishizaka, T., and Hornbrook, M. M. (1966). *J. Immunol.*, **97**, 75.

Ishizaka, T., Soto, C. S., and Ishizaka, K. (1973). *J. Immunol.*, **111**, 500.

Jefferis, R., Butwell, A. J., and Clamp, J. R. (1975). *Clin. Exp. Immunol.*, **22**, 311.

Kehoe, J. M., and Fougereau, M. (1969). *Nature (Lond.)*, **224**, 1212.

Köhler, H., Shimizu, A., Paul, C., Moore, V., and Putnam, F. W. (1970). *Nature (Lond.)*, **227**, 1318.

Kownatzki, E., and Drescher, M. (1973). *Clin. Exp. Immunol.*, **15**, 557.

Kratzin, H., Altevogt, P., Ruban, E., Kortt, A., Staroscik, K., and Hilschmann, N. (1975). *Hoppe-Seyler's Z. Physiol. Chem.*, **356**, 1337.

Kronvall, G. (1967). *Acta. path. microbiol. scand.*, **69**, 619.

Kronvall, G., and Frommel, D. (1970. *Immunochemistry*, **7**, 124.

Kronvall, G., and Gewurz, H. (1970). *Clin. Exp. Immunol.*, **7**, 211.

Kronvall, G., Grey, H. M., and Williams, R. C., Jr. (1970a). *J. Immunol.*, **105**, 1116.

Kronvall, G., Quie, P. G., and Williams, R. C., Jr. (1970b). *J. Immunol.*, **104**, 273.

Kronvall, G., Seal, U.S., Finstad, J., and Williams, R. C., Jr. (1970c). *J. Immunol.*, **104**, 140.

Kronvall, G., and Williams, R. C., Jr. (1969). *J. Immunol.*, **103**, 828.

Kulczycki, A., Isersky, C., and Metzger, H. (1974). *J. Exp. Med.*, **139**, 600.

Kulczycki, A., and Metzger, H. (1974). *J. Exp. Med.*, **140**, 1676.

Kunkel, H. G., and Prendergast, R. A. (1966). *Proc. Soc. Exp. Biol. Med.*, **122**, 910.

Lawrence, D. A., Weigle, W. O., and Spiegelberg, H. L. (1975). *J. Clin. Invest.*, **55**, 368.

Leslie, G. A., Clem, L. W., and Rowe, D. (1971). *Immunochemistry*, **8**, 565.

Lo Buglio, A. F., Cotran, R. S., and Jandl, J. H. (1967). *Science, N.Y.*, **158**, 1582.

Malley, A., and Perlman, F. (1966). *Proc. Soc. Exp. Biol. Med.*, **122**, 152.

Marchalonis, J. J. (1972). *Nature, New Biol.*, **236**, 84.

Messner, R. P., and Jelinek, J. (1970). *J. Clin. Invest.*, **49**, 2165.

Mestecky, J., Schrohenloher, R. E., and Kulhavy, R. (1974). *Fed. Proc.*, **33**, 747.

Mestecky, J., Schrohenloher, R. E., Kulhavy, R., Wright, G. P., and Tomana, M. (1974). *Proc. Nat. Acad. Sci., U.S.A.*, **71**, 544.

Metzger, H. (1970). *Adv. Immunol.*, **12**, 57.

Michaelsen, T. E. (1973). *Scand. J. Immunol.*, **2**, 523.

Milstein, C. (1966). *Nature (Lond.)*, **209**, 370.

Milstein, C., and Svasti, J. (1971). In *Progress in Immunology*, Vol. I, (Amos, B., ed.), Academic Press, New York and London, p. 35.

Milstein, C. P., Richardson, N. E., Deverson, E. V., and Feinstein, A. (1975). *Biochem. J.*, **151**, 615.

Montgomery, P. C., Dorrington, K. J., and Rockey, J. H. (1969). *Biochemistry*, **8**, 1427.

Morris, J. E., and Inman, F. P. (1968). *Biochemistry*, **7**, 2851.

Müller-Eberhard, H. J., and Kunkel, H. G. (1961). *Proc. Soc. Exp. Biol. Med.*, **106**, 291.

Natvig, J. B. (1966). *Nature (Lond.)*, **211**, 318.

Natvig, J. B., Gaarder, P. I., and Turner, M. W. (1972). *Clin. Exp. Immunol.*, **12**, 177.

Natvig, J. B., and Kunkel, H. G. (1973). *Adv. Immunol.*, **16**, 1.

Natvig, J. B., and Turner, M. W. (1970). *Nature (Lond.)*, **225**, 855.

Nisonoff, A., Hopper, J. E., and Spring, S. B. (1975). *The Antibody Molecule*, Academic Press, New York and London.

Normansell, D. E. (1970). *Immunochemistry*, **7**, 787.

Normansell, D. E. (1971). *Immunochemistry*, **8**, 593.

O'Donnell, I. J., Frangione, B., and Porter, R. R. (1970). *Biochem. J.*, **116**, 261.

Ogra, P. L., and Karzon, D. T. (1969). *J. Immunol.*, **102**, 15.

Okafor, G. O., and Turner, M. W. (1974). *Scand. J. Immunol.*, **3**, 181.

Okafor, G. O., Turner, M. W., and Hay, F. C. (1974). *Nature (Lond.)*, **248**, 228.

Oliveira, B., and Lamm, M. E. (1971). *Biochemistry*, **10**, 26.

Onoue, K., Kishimoto, T., and Yamamura, Y. (1968). *J. Immunol.*, **100**, 238.

Osterland, C. K., Harboe, M., and Kunkel, H. G. (1963). *Vox Sang*, **8**, 135.

Ovary, Z. (1960). *Immunology*, **3**, 19.

Ovary, Z., Barth, W. F., and Fahey, J. L. (1965). *J. Immunol.*, **94**, 410.

Parish, W. E. (1970). *J. Immunol.*, **105**, 1296.

Parish, W. E. (1974). In *Progress in Immunology II*, Vol. IV, (Brent, L., and Holborow, J., eds.), North Holland Publishing Co., Amsterdam, p. 19.

Parkhouse, R. M. E., Askonas, B. A., and Dourmashkin, R. R. (1970). *Immunology*, **18**, 575.

Pink, J. R., Buttery, S. H., De Vries, G. M., and Milstein, C. (1970). *Biochem. J.*, **117**, 33.

Plaut, A. G., and Tomasi, T. B., Jr. (1970). *Proc. Nat. Acad. Sci., U.S.A.*, **63**, 318.

Plaut, A. G., Wistar, R., and Capra, J. D. (1974). *J. Clin. Invest.*, **54**, 1295.

Poger, M. E., and Lamm, M. E. (1974). *J. Exp. Med.*, **139**, 629.

Poljak, R. J. (1975). *Nature (Lond.)*, **256**, 373.

Porter, R. R. (1959). *Biochem. J.*, **73**, 119.

Porter, R. R. (1962). *Symposium on Basic Problems in Neoplastic Disease* (Gelhorn, A., and Hirschberg, E., eds.), Columbia University Press, p. 177.

Putnam, F. W., Florent, G., Paul, C., Shinoda, T., and Shimizu, A. (1973a). *Science, N.Y.*, **182**, 287.

Putnam, F. W., Shinoda, T., Shimizu, A., Paul, C., Florent, G., and Raff, E. (1973b). In *3rd International Convocation on Immunology*, Kargel, Basel, p. 40.

Putnam, F. W., Titani, K., and Whitley, E. (1966). *Proc. Roy. Soc., Ser. B.*, **166**, 124.

Robboy, S. J., Lewis, E. J., Schur, P. H., and Colman, R. W. (1970). *Am. J. Med.*, **49**, 742.

Rose, H. M., Ragan, C., Pearce, E., and Lipman, M. O. (1948). *Proc. Soc. Exp. Biol. Med.*, **68**, 1.

Rowe, D. S., and Fahey, J. L. (1965a). *J. Exp. Med.*, **121**, 171.

Rowe, D. S., and Fahey, J. L. (1965b). *J. Exp. Med.*, **121**, 185.

Rowe, D. S., Hug, K., Forni, L., and Pernis, B. (1973). *J. Exp. Med.*, **138**, 965.

Saltvedt, E., and Harboe, M. (1976). *Scand. J. Immunol.*, **5**, 1103.

Sandberg, A. L., Oliveira, B., and Osler, A. G. (1971). *J. Immunol.*, **106**, 282.

56

Scholz, R., and Hilschmann, N. (1975). *Hoppe-Seyler's Z. Physiol. Chem.*, **356**, 1333.
Schur, P. H. (1972). In *Progress in Clinical Immunology*, Vol. I, (Schwartz, R., ed.), Grune and Stratton, New York, p. 71.
Segal, D. M., Padlan, E. A., Cohen, G. H., Silverton, E. W., Davies, D. R., Rudikoff, S., and Potter, M. (1974). In *Progress in Immunology II*, Vol. I, (Brent, L., and Holborow, J., eds.), North Holland Publishing Co., Amsterdam, p. 93.
Seon, B.-K., and Pressman, D. (1975). *Immunochemistry*, **12**, 333.
Sjöquist, J., and Stålenheim, G. (1969). *J. Immunol.*, **103**, 467.
Solheim, B. G., and Harboe, M. (1972). *Immunochemistry*, **9**, 623.
South, M. A., Cooper, M. D., Wolheim, F. A., Hong, R., and Good, R. A. (1966). *J. Exp. Med.*, **123**, 615.
Spiegelberg, H. L. (1974). *Adv. Immunol.*, **19**, 259.
Spiegelberg, H. L. (1975). *Nature (Lond.)*, **254**, 723.
Spiegelberg, H. L., and Götze, O. (1972). *Fed. Proc.*, **31**, 655.
Spiegelberg, H. L., Prahl, J. W., and Grey, H. M. (1970). *Biochemistry*, **9**, 2115.
Stålenheim, G., and Castensson, S. (1971). *FEBS Letters*, **14**, 79.
Stålenheim, G., and Malmheden-Eriksson, I. (1971). *FEBS Letters*, **14**, 82.
Stanworth, D. R. (1970). *Clin. Exp. Immunol.*, **6**, 1.
Stanworth, D. R. (1973). *Immediate Hypersensitivity*, North Holland Publishing Co., Amsterdam.
Stanworth, D. R., and Smith, A. K. (1973). *Clin. Allergy*, **3**, 37.
Stanworth, D. R., and Turner, M. W. (1973). In *Handbook of Experimental Immunology*, 2nd. Edition (Weir, D. M., ed.), Blackwell Scientific Publications, p. 10.1.
Steward, M. W., Turner, M. W., Natvig, J. B., and Gaarder, P. I. (1973). *Clin. Exp. Immunol.*, **15**, 145.
Strausbauch, P. H., Hurwitz, E., and Givol, D. (1971). *Biochemistry*, **10**, 2231.
Svasti, J., and Milstein, C. (1972). *Eur. J. Biochem.*, **31**, 405.

Terr, A. I., and Bentz, J. D. (1965). *J. Allergy*, **36**, 433.
Terry, W. D. (1966). *J. Immunol.*, **95**, 1041.
Terry, W. D., Fahey, J. L., and Steinberg, A. G. (1965). *J. Exp. Med.*, **122**, 1087.
Thompson, R. A. (1970). *Nature (Lond.)*, **226**, 946.
Tizard, I. R. (1969). *Int. Archs Allergy*, **36**, 332.
Turner, M. W. (1974). In *Progress in Immunology II*, Vol. I, (Brent, L., and Holborow, J., eds.), North Holland Publishing Co., Amsterdam, p. 280.
Turner, M. W., and Bennich, H. (1968). *Biochem. J.*, **107**, 71.
Turner, M. W., Bennich, H., and Natvig, J. B. (1970). *Clin. Exp. Immunol.*, **7**, 603.
Turner, M. W., Komvopoulos, A., Bennich, H., and Natvig, J. B. (1972). *Scand. J. Immunol.*, **1**, 53.
Turner, M. W., Mårtensson, L., Natvig, J. B., and Bennich, H. (1969). *Nature (Lond.)*, **221**, 1166.

Vaerman, J. P., and Heremans, J. F. (1966). *Science, N.Y.*, **153**, 647.
Valentine, R. C., and Green, N. M. (1967). *J. Mol. Biol.*, **27**, 615.
van der Giessen, M. (1975). Doctoral thesis, University of Amsterdam.
Virella, G., Nunes, M. A-S., and Tamagnini, G. (1972). *Clin. Exp. Immunol.*, **10**, 475.

Waaler, E. (1940). *Acta path. microbiol. scand.*, **17**, 172.
Waldmann, T. A., and Hemmings, W. A. (1974). In *Progress in Immunology II*, Vol. I, (Brent, L., and Holborow, J., eds.), North Holland Publishing Co., Amsterdam, p. 230.
Waldmann, T. A., and Strober, W. (1969). *Prog. Allergy*, **13**, 1.
Waldmann, T. A., Strober, W., and Blaese, R. M. (1971). In *Progress in Immunology*, Vol. I, (Amos, B., ed.), Academic Press, New York, p. 891.

Waller, M., and Vaughan, J. H. (1956). *Proc. Soc. Exp. Biol. Med.*, **92**, 198.

Wang, A. C., Faulk, W. P., Stukey, A. M. A., and Fudenberg, H. H. (1970). *Immunochemistry*, **7**, 703.

Wang, A. C., van Loghem, E., and Shuster, J. (1973). *Fed. Proc.*, **32**, 1003.

Watanabe, S., Barnikol, H. U., Horn, J., Bertram, J., and Hilschmann, N. (1973). *Hoppe Seyler's Z. Physiol. Chem.*, **354**, 1505.

Watkins, J., Turner, M. W., and Roberts, A. (1971). In *Protides of the Biological Fluids*, (Peeters, H., ed.), Pergamon Press, Oxford and New York, p. 461.

Wells, J. V., Bleumers, J. F., and Fudenberg, H. H. (1973). *Proc. Nat. Acad. Sci. U.S.A.*, **70**, 827.

Welscher, H. D. (1970). *Nature (Lond.)*, **228**, 1236.

Wolfenstein-Todel, C., Prelli, F., Frangione, B., and Franklin, E. C. (1973). *Biochemistry*, **12**, 5195.

Wu, T. T., and Kabat, E. A. (1970). *J. Exp. Med.*, **132**, 211.

Wolfenstein-Todel, C., Frangione, B., Prelli, F., and Franklin, E. C. (1976). *Biochemical and Biophysical Research Communications*, **71**, 907.

Yasmeen, D., Ellerson, J. R., Dorrington, K. J., and Painter, R. H. (1973). *J. Immunol.*, **110**, 1706.

Yount, W. J., Dorner, M. M., Kunkel, H. G., and Kabat, E. A. (1968). *J. Exp. Med.*, **127**, 633.

CHAPTER 2

Antigen-Combining Region of Immunoglobulins

F. F. Richards, J. M. Varga,
R. W. Rosenstein, and W. H. Konigsberg

1 ANTIBODY COMBINING REGION STRUCTURE

1.1 Combining Region Specificity

Stimulation by antigen evokes the production of immunoglobulins in the serum and secretions of vertebrates. A common property of these induced proteins is the ability to bind antigen. The ligating function of the immunoglobulin molecule is predominantly the property of the combining regions, which are two symmetrical areas at the solvent-exposed ends of the Fab arms of the Y-shaped immunoglobulin molecules. The combining region is situated in the variable (V region) domain, a compact region consisting of the N-terminal half of the light chain and the N-terminal quarter of the heavy chain which are linked by sulphydryl bonds. Between the areas of this domain occupied by the light and heavy chain variable regions is a cleft exposed to the solvent, in or close to which antigens have been shown to bind (Amzel et al., 1974). An induced antibody population is said to be specific because it usually binds most strongly to the immunizing antigen and less strongly to other compounds which structurally resemble the immunogen. Occasionally, antibodies (heteroclitic) are induced which bind more strongly to some determinant other than the immunogen (Mäkelä et al., 1975). In general, antibody populations show a high degree of specificity in that they are able to discriminate between chemical compounds differing by as little as a single functional group, between stereoisomers, or between two proteins differing by as little as a single amino acid residue (Reichlin, 1974, Richards et al., 1975).

The number of individual immunoglobulins in an immune serum may be quite large. It is not unusual to see as many as 50 protein bands on isoelectric focusing, all of which are capable of binding the immunogen, but such a population of immunoglobulins does not behave uniformly with respect to ligand binding. In fact, subpopulations can be identified that bind ligand over a wide range of intrinsic binding constants (K_A) (Eisen, 1964a, Eisen and Siskind, 1964). This, in turn, suggests that the antigen combining sites also show corresponding variations of structure. This structural heterogeneity is further complicated by a degree of temporal heterogeneity, since during the immune response the composition of the antibody population does not remain constant (Steiner and Eisen, 1966; Steiner and Eisen, 1967a, b; Steward and Petty, 1972; Macario and Conway de Macario, 1975). New antibodies appear while others disappear, suggesting that the antibodies expressed at any one time during the immune response are only a small proportion of the total number with complementarity to the immunizing antigen that the animal is capable of producing. Thus, the immune response is very heterogeneous but, when viewed as a population, also highly specific with respect to antigen binding. This chapter will explore the structural basis of antibody specificity.

1.2 General Properties of Combining Regions

The first quantitative assessments of the number of antigen molecules and antibody molecules in antigen–antibody complexes suggested that 7 S antibody molecules are bivalent (Porter and Press, 1962). This conclusion was reinforced by ultracentrifugal studies (Nisonoff and Thorbecke, 1964), and when accurate values for the molecular weights of antibody molecules became available, the dimeric nature of the binding units (Cohen and Porter, 1964) confirmed this hypothesis.

Both heavy and light chains are necessary for optimal binding. Experiments that tested isolated light or heavy chains for their ability to ligate hapten showed that isolated light chains have little ability to bind, although with sensitive methods low-affinity binding of haptens can be detected (Yoo et al., 1967; Painter et al., 1972). Isolated heavy chains are generally insoluble, but when rendered soluble one mole of heavy chain generally binds one mole of antigen. However, the binding affinity of isolated heavy chains is greatly reduced (Utsumi and Karush, 1964), even though the ability to discriminate between related antigens is retained (Haber and Richards, 1967).

Experiments in Porter's laboratory showed that papain digestion of the IgG molecule produces Fab fragments containing the whole light chain and the N-terminal half of the heavy chain. These Fab fragments were shown to bind antigen with a valence of one (Porter, 1958). Pepsin digestion of some myeloma immunoglobulins under controlled conditions gives a fragment which consists of the N-terminal half—or in the nomenclature of Konigsberg and of Edelman, the first domain (Waxdal et al., 1968; Edelman et al., 1969)—of the Fab fragment (Inbar et al., 1972). This fragment (Fv) contains the variable N-terminal half of the light chain and the N-terminal variable quarter of the heavy chain. The Fv fragment retains the binding function of the Fab fragment and carries the idiotypic (or combining region-related) antigenic determinants of the immunoglobulin molecule (Figure 1). Such studies show that the 7 S unit of immunoglobulins has two combining regions located at the N-terminal ends of the Fab fragments and that both the light and heavy chains are necessary for maximal antigen binding.

On the basis of fluorescence polarization studies, Edelman originally proposed that the combining regions were situated at either end of a long, rod-like molecule (Weltman and Edelman, 1967), but the electron micrographs of Feinstein and Rowe (1965), followed by the detailed pictures of bivalent hapten–antigen complexes by Valentine and Green (1967) and by Green, (1969) left little doubt that the molecule is in fact Y-shaped, with the combining regions occupying the ends of the two Fab arms. In addition, the experiments by Valentine and Green

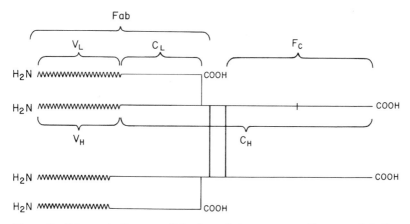

Figure 1 Schematic diagram of the four-chain structure of immunoglobulin. V_L and V_H are the variable regions of the light and heavy chains; C_L and C_H are the constant regions. The antigen-binding sites, one each heavy–light chain pair, are made up of amino acid residues from the variable regions. Fab and Fc are the fragments produced by papain digestion of immunoglobulin

(1967) showed that the site binding the dinitrophenyl hapten (DNP) is some distance below the surface of the molecule, since bivalent DNP antigens, in which the two DNP groups are connected by a short spacer moiety, fail to form head-to-head immunoglobulin polymers. This supports earlier observations indicating a hydrophobic environment for the DNP-binding site, thus suggesting that the site is located below the surface (Little and Eisen, 1967). Other experiments have indicated that the Fab arms are movable with respect to each other and the Fc fragment (Yguerabide *et al.*, 1970; Cathou *et al.*, 1974).

Thus, prior to X-ray crystallographic analysis, a speculative picture had emerged of a combining region located at the ends of the movable Fab arms, containing a cleft or cavity, surrounded by both light and heavy chain variable regions. It is remarkable how accurately the antigen-probe methods were able to predict the probable size and shape of the combining region which have been substantiated by X-ray crystallography.

1.3 Immunological Probes for Combining Regions

The antibody molecule itself is antigenic both when injected into heterologous species (Brient *et al.*, 1971) and when introduced into mice of the same inbred strain from which the immunizing antibody is derived (Sirisinha and Eisen, 1971). In heterologous immunization, the quantitatively dominant immunogenic region is the Fc fragment of the molecule. For instance, an anti-rabbit serum of sheep has most of its binding activity directed against rabbit Fc regions. When homogeneous immunoglobulins are introduced into a homologous inbred mouse line—when a mouse myeloma tumour immunoglobulin derived from a BALB/c mouse is injected repeatedly into other BALB/c mice—levels of antibodies to the Fc region are relatively low in titre and antibodies appear which react with Fab fragments. These antibodies were believed to recognize only the inducing myeloma protein and were therefore called anti-idiotypic (Nisonoff *et al.*, 1975). A characteristic of a proportion of the early anti-idiotype sera is that the idiotype–anti-idiotype interaction is inhibited to some extent by antigen (Brient *et al.*, 1971). The Fv region of a mouse myeloma (derived from tumour MOPC 315) is able to adsorb the anti-idiotypic activity of a mouse serum induced by immunization with protein 315, and that it therefore contains all the idiotypic determinants (Haimovich *et al.*, 1972). The Fv fragments has previously been shown to contain one V region of the light chain and the whole V region. Comparative sequential analysis by Wu and Kabat (1970), and by Capra and Kehoe, (1976) identified three groups of amino acid residues within the V_L and V_H regions which are more variable than other residues in this region. These hypervariable residues were shown by X-ray diffraction analysis to be located on the outside of six polypeptide loops on the free distal region of the N-terminal domain which are accessible to solvent and which surround the antibody combining region (Padlan *et al.*, 1974; Poljak *et al.*, 1974). Isolated light and heavy chains are capable of inhibiting the idiotype–anti-idiotype interaction (Hoessli *et al.*, 1976). From these data, it seems reasonable to deduce that anti-idiotypic sera are directed against the solvent-accessible regions and hypervariable loops of the N-terminal domain. Since whole light chains may be common to two different antibodies and since sequential data suggest that whole hypervariable loops may have structures that resemble each other, anti-idiotypic sera are clearly not anti-idiotypic in the sense that they can characterize only one combining region.

The lack of idiotypy in these determinants also has been recognized experimentally. The literature abounds in terms such as 'shared idiotypic specificities' which have been recognized not only between different mouse strains (Kuettner et al., 1972), but also between different species (Varga et al., 1974). Anti-idiotype antibodies, therefore, are not antibodies which define a unique set on V-region structures. In this chapter the term antibodies to V regions will henceforth be used.

The relationship between the antigen-binding capacity of a single V region and the antibodies raised against the V region has been studied in detail (Potter and Lieberman, 1970; Lieberman et al., 1975). It is concluded that antibodies may be prepared complementary to a region of a myeloma protein binding a determinant such as phosphorylcholine. These antibodies cross-react with some, but generally not with all, myeloma V regions binding the same antigenic determinant. Those myeloma proteins which cross-react with the same anti-V-region serum generally show the same fine specificity, that is, they all bind a series of haptens related to the antigenic determinant. Thus, it appears that there may be several families of antibodies complementary to a single antigen and that such families may be distinguished from each other by anti-V-region sera. Similar considerations apply also to antibodies elicited by antigens (Lieberman et al., 1974).

Antibodies to V regions are inhibited by antigens to different extents, and this can be understood if it is remembered that bound antigens may encroach on different solvent-exposed loops to varying degrees, and that anti-V-region sera are not necessarily directed against all loops to the same degree. An interesting method has been developed by Claflin and his associates (Claflin and Davie, 1975) in which antibodies to V regions are bound to affinity columns containing the requisite V regions attached to the solid support. The bound antibodies are eluted with haptens, thus displacing only those immunoglobulins that are directed against loops in close apposition to the hapten-binding site. By exploiting the multiple binding potential of a single binding region, it should be possible to produce serological probes directed against individual peptides within the combining region, a potentially useful tool for probing the structure of the combining region.

Since antibodies to V regions may bind in the same general area as antigens, they appear to be able to mimic some of the physiological consequences of antigen binding and to induce a limited immune response (Cosenza and Kohler, 1972). Also, they can blanket the combining region, preventing the antigen gaining access, thereby inhibiting the immune response. For this reason, control or suppression of certain antibodies by anti-V-region antibodies has been considered recently. The bimodal nature of the reaction of antibodies to V regions has suggested to some workers that antibodies to the second, third, or perhaps even higher degree may form a network controlling the immune response (Jerne, 1974). Whether or not this theoretical web is anchored firmly remains to be determined. Among the more recent practical uses of anti-V-region antibodies has been an attempt to investigate the nature of antigen-binding receptors on T lymphocytes. The results of these experiments have suggested that V-region antigens are present on, or close to, the antigen-recognition site of T lymphocytes (Binz et al., 1974). This suggests that a recognition mechanism, which has some common features with immunoglobulin V regions, is also present on the T cells. This area is at present under investigation.

1.4 Polymeric Ligand Probes

An important method, which accurately predicted the size of the combining region, was devised originally by Kabat (1960). If there is point-to-point contact with antigen in the antibody combining region, one should be able to raise antibodies to homopolymers of the type $(X-X-X)_n$, where n is a large number. Monomers, dimers, trimers, tetramers, and oligomers of X may be prepared and their ability to inhibit the reaction between the X polymer and the antibody may be determined. It was reasoned that, on a molar basis, the inhibition of the oligomers should increase until the combining region is filled completely, and after this, increasing the size of competing molecule should have no further effect on the inhibition. In his original experiments, Kabat used dextran for immunization and found that polysaccharides containing up to five or six glucose units inhibited maximally and that thereafter, increasing length did not have any further effect on inhibition. From these data he suggested that the combining region could be as large as $3\cdot4 \times 1\cdot2 \times 0\cdot7$ nm, the extended measurement of the isomaltohexaose unit. Kabat also noted that there was evidence of heterogeneity in the type of contact which was made. Using some sera, the isomaltotroise unit is almost as efficient an inhibitor as the isomaltohexaose (Kabat, 1960).

Numerous laboratories have repeated these experiments using other homopolymers, such as polypeptides and polynucleotides, as well as random amino acid copolymers. The conclusions of these studies are that the size of the site is compatible with binding extended polymers of the size range $2\cdot5$–$3\cdot6 \times 1\cdot0$–$1\cdot7 \times 0\cdot6$–$0\cdot7$ nm. More recently, careful quantitative studies using polyalanine (Schechter et al., 1970) and using antibodies to blood group A substance, inhibited by various polysaccharides (Moreno and Kabat, 1969), have substantiated that the binding energy is incremental with each added unit and that antibody–antigen contact in these complexes must extend over a relatively large area.

Similar methods have been used to determine if there is any variation in the average size of the combining region during the changes in antibody population that occur during maturation of the immune response, using polyasparagine was used as antigen. It was concluded that there is some increase in average site dimensions during maturation (Murphy and Sage, 1970).

1.5 Affinity and Photoaffinity Probes

A chemically reactive ligand, which initially is bound by non-covalent interactions at the binding site of a ligating protein, can be induced to react with the protein, resulting in the formation of covalent bonds. If these bonds are sufficiently stable, the protein may be digested chemically or enzymatically into peptides and the location in the primary sequence of the amino acid residues modified by the affinity reagent determined. This method used in enzymology was introduced into immunology by Wofsy et al. (1962) and has been used extensively to study the combining regions of both myeloma proteins and whole antibody populations directed against antigenic determinants (Singer and Doolittle, 1966; Knowles, 1972; Givol, 1974).

Affinity reagents consist of chemically reactive moieties which are attached to, or are an integral part of, a haptenic determinant. Such reagents depend entirely on the higher concentrations of the reagents at, or near, the combining region for differential labelling. No evidence of special reactivity of a single amino acid side chain within the immunoglobulin combining region is available. Since concentration differences are a crucial factor in affinity labelling, high affinity of the immunoglobulin for the hapten and a low molar ratio of ligand to immunoglobulin combining region will favour site-related labelling. At higher ligand levels, local accumulations of ligand in regions of the protein not related to the high-affinity site are likely to increase and may modify the protein in these regions. Protection of the combining region by the hapten itself is used as an index of site-directed labelling. However, when there is a considerable difference in K_A between hapten and the hapten-based affinity reagents, the possibility of nonequivalence of the two binding processes should be considered.

In practice, only two types of reactive groups have been used as affinity reagents with immunoglobulins. Wofsy et al. (1962) used diazonium fluoroborate to label antibody-combining regions. These fluoroborates are relatively stable salts, which react with amino groups of proteins, the ε-amino groups of lysine, and the phenol ring of tyrosine; reaction of this diazonium salt with histidine has also been reported (Wofsy and Parker, 1967). The stability and ease of synthesis recommend this reagent. However, the limited reactivity may mean that the contact site itself may not be labelled, but rather that reaction occurs at the nearest or most reactive tyrosine, lysine, or histidine residue. The haloketone compounds employed as affinity reagents by Givol, Eisen and their associates (Haimovich et al., 1970; Eisen, 1971; Haimovich et al., 1972; Givol, 1974) have similar strengths and weaknesses. Their spectrum of reactivity with amino acids resembles that of the diazonium salts. Since all affinity reagents are introduced into the aqueous solvent and enter the combining site by diffusion, the rate of hydrolysis of such reagents must be slow, thus limiting both the spectrum of reactivity and the concentrations in which the reagent may be used.

If a non-reactive labelling reagent could be placed at the combining site, and if within the combining site the non-reactive labelling reagent could be activated to produce a moiety capable of forming covalent bonds with the antibody protein then some, but by no means all, of the difficulties associated with affinity reagents might be ameliorated. Converse and Richards (1968; 1969) synthesized a DNP-based diazoketone of the type described earlier by Vaughan and Westheimer (1969), which may be photoactivated to a carbene or a ketene, the former authors showed that this reagent with anti-DNP antibodies. Fleet *et al.* (1969) introduced another light-activated compound, an aromatic azide, for the same purpose (Fisher and Press, 1974).

It is possible to isolate antibody–reagent complexes and to activate these specifically, although for this a relatively high binding energy for the hapten–antibody complex is needed. However, the major advantage is that some molecules of these reagents are in contact with the protein very shortly after they are generated and do not first pass through the solvent. Most reagents that are highly reactive with protein will also react with aqueous solvents. By generating highly reactive reagents *in situ*, it is possible to label specifically residue side chains. For instance, the activated carbenes are potentially capable of inserting into any carbon–heteroatomic linkage, and it is probable that the nitrenes generated by light from the aromatic azido compounds have a similar broad range of reactivity. It must be remembered, however, that light will activate not only those molecules of labelling reagent immobilized at the site, but also those in the vicinity of the site. Moreover, if the half life of the activated species is sufficiently long, migration of the activated species may occur (Hew *et al.*, 1973; Yoshioka *et al.*, 1973; Lifter *et al.*, 1974; Richards *et al.*, 1974). It has been suggested that scavenger molecule should be employed to deal with the wandering activated photoaffinity label molecules (Ruoho *et al.*, 1973). However, such molecules may react with the activated reagent bound at the site, and since scavenger molecules may themselves form low-affinity interactions with the protein, there is a possibility at least that an already complex system will become even more complicated due to such corrective measures. A second approach has been to synthesize photoaffinity reagents with shorter chemical half lives, such as the azulene reagents (Smith and Knowles, 1973).

The chemistry of affinity and photoaffinity reagents has been introduced in some detail since it is difficult to interpret results of the exploration of antibody combining regions without adequate knowledge. Although it is probable that no single reagent is ideal, it is hoped that a consensus of the labelling information will provide some understanding of the binding properties of immunoglobulins. However, no easy general conclusions are possible: but in general, modifications occur at, or near, some of the hypervariable regions. There are, however, two reports of labelling outside the accepted hypervariable regions (Franek, 1973; Richards *et al.*, 1974); some residues, such as the tyrosine at position 33 or 34 in the light chain, are modified in a number of different experiments. There is, reasonable doubt that this is a contact amino acid residue, as it is a constant residue within a hypervariable region. Modification of this residue reduces the strength of binding, but does not affect the number of DNP groups which can be bound (Goetzl and Metzger, 1970). The same residue is modified both by nitrophenol affinity reagents in anti-DNP immunoglobulins and by a phosphorylcholine-based reagent in a phosphorylcholine-binding myeloma protein. Also, in labelling experiments on myeloma protein 460, the modified residues may well be so far apart as to make it unlikely that these residues can have been modified by a reagent binding to only a single site within each Fab fragment.

To summarize, it seems likely that affinity reagents do modify amino acid residues in the general combining region. It may be that, in some instances, they modify contact amino acids of a single major binding site. In other cases, a number of different binding sites (perhaps with a wide range of binding affinities) is modified. There is no *a priori* reason why only one high-affinity binding site should be modified (Richards *et al.*, 1974) if others of lower affinity are also present (Haselkorn *et al.*, 1974). While the original expectations of affinity labelling may have been unduly simple, affinity and photoaffinity labelling methods may still be valuable tools for studying the complex geometry of hapten ligation to antibodies.

1.6 Physicochemical Probes of Antibody Combining Regions

The properties of all molecules are affected by their environment. With certain molecules, changes in property between the molecule in solution and the molecule bound to an immunoglobulin combining region may be observed directly. The observed effects of physical and chemical alterations on binding may include differences in ionization (Albertson and Phillipson, 1960), solubility properties (Day *et al.*, 1963), and increases or decreases in fluorescence either of the protein or of the ligand in the rotatory dispersion of light, in the circular dichroism of polarized light, and in the circular dichroism of polarized emitted fluorescent light (Schlessinger *et al.*, 1975). The magnetic properties, as well as the electron spin resonance of ligand and ligating molecule, also may be affected by binding (Dwek *et al.*, 1975a). Sensitive calorimetric methods can measure changes in enthalpy, and indirectly, changes in the entropy during antibody–antigen interaction can be determined (Johnston *et al.*, 1974). Variations in the rotatory behaviour of whole immunoglobulin molecules on binding large antigens can be monitored by the depolarization of emitted fluorescence; even changes in specific molar volume have been observed (Ohta *et al.*, 1970). More recently, the internal patterns of movement of macromolecules (the concerted breaking and reforming of hydrogen bonds which have been described as the 'breathing' of the molecule and which may affect ligand binding) have been observed. This wealth of physicochemical information is discussed by Feinstein and Beale in Chapter 8 of this volume and in other review articles (Day, 1972; Cathou *et al.*, 1974).

It is perhaps disappointing how little direct information this work on combining-region structure and function has yielded in comparison to X-ray diffraction analysis. It seems likely that as with other proteins, the largest and most important contributions these methods may have to make is yet to come. It is in the fine analysis of mechanism of macromolecules whose overall anatomy is understood that these methods are most useful.

The areas in which physicochemical probes have given the most information about the combining region have been the depth and hydrophobicity of the combining sites, the involvement of light and heavy chains in ligand binding, and the unexpected degree to which small ligands stabilize the light–heavy chain interaction. Physicochemical methods also have been a mainstay in the assessment of possible conformational changes secondary to antigen binding.

X-ray crystallographic studies quoted in Section 1.8 show that in the two antibody V regions so far examined both the small ligand (phosphorylcholine) and a larger one (γ-hydroxy vitamin K_1) appear to make contact with both the light and heavy chains. Nevertheless, the area of contact of phosphorycholine with the light chain is small. It is known, however, that light–heavy chain contacts in the V and C_1 domains of the Fab fragment are extensive and involve many amino acid residues. It is, therefore, somewhat surprising that small ligands such as the DNP moiety can stabilize light–heavy chain interaction to a considerable degree. Light and heavy chains may be isolated from reduced and alkylated IgG in dissociating solvents by gel filtration. Metzger and Singer (1963) found that light and heavy chain yields are reduced considerably when the small DNP antigen is present in the mixture. Optical rotatory dispersion studies by Cathou and Haber (1967) and by Cathou and Werner (1970) showed also that the presence of the DNP hapten greatly reduces the unfolding of antibody molecules in the dissociating agent, quanidine hydrochloride. Thus, antibody without the DNP ligand unfolds in the presence of guanidine hydrochloride (2 N), while in the presence of the ligand, binding activity is still intact in the presence of a higher concentration of guanidine hydrochloride (4 N). Yet isolated heavy chains derived from DNP antibodies still show binding activity, albeit with a greatly reduced K_A, which may be due to the presence of new structures resembling the combining regions formed from heavy-chain dimers (Stevenson, 1973).

When tryptophan is excited by ultraviolet light at 280 nm, it fluoresces at 345 nm. Tryptophan residues are found in close association with the combining region. Introduction of a DNP or a folic acid group into the combining region will absorb emitted tryptophan fluorescence usually. The quenching of fluorescence has been used both as a structural tool and as an indication of hapten binding. The wavelength of maximal absorption of incident light exhibited by ligands such as DNP also may be red-shifted by binding to the protein (Eisen, 1964b). The observed spectral changes have suggested to some workers that charge–transfer complexes may be formed between aromatic ligands and residues such as tryptophan. However, convincing evidence for the presence of charge–transfer complexes remains elusive (Rubinstein and Little, 1970). It is now well recognized that a large number of different V regions may bind small ligands such as DNP with K_0 ranging from 10^{-11} to 10^{-4} M. It is unlikely that such a wide range of binding energies can be consistent with one type of DNP-binding site.

Optical spectrophotometric evidence for conformational changes secondary to antigen binding has been dealt with elsewhere (see Schlessinger *et al.*, 1975. The introduction of electron spin resonance probes (Stryer and Griffith, 1965; Hsia and Piette, 1969; Piette *et al.*, 1972) has added an additional tool for the study of combining regions. These workers used haptens which had been linked previously to moieties containing the nitroxide spin label. When the hapten is firmly fixed to the nitroxide spin label, it can be shown that the complex is firmly bound. By producing molecules in which the hapten and the spin label are separated by chemical spacer groups of various lengths, the degree of rotational freedom of the spin label can be estimated as a function of spacer length. Some information on the size or depth of the combining region can be extrapolated from this information.

The lanthanide element series bind both to the Fc and Fv region of antibody molecules. In rabbit IgG, the Fc binding constant is around 5×10^{-6} M, while those in the combining region have a K_0 of around 10^{-4} M for gadolinum. It has been shown that, in a DNP-binding IgA myeloma protein, the gadolinum (Gd III)-binding site is close to that of DNP and that the binding of DNP weakens the attachment of lanthanide (Dower *et al.*, 1975; Dwek *et al.*, 1975b). The same workers have shown also by using Piette's technique that the portion of the combining region binding DNP probably measures $1 \cdot 1 \times 0 \cdot 9 \times 0 \cdot 6$ nm, based on nitroxide spin labels. Proton nuclear magnetic resonance spectroscopy at 270 MH gives a paramagnetic difference spectrum, which suggests that about 30 aliphatic and 30 aromatic residues are involved around the DNP-combining site.

1.7 Electron Microscopic Probes

Although early biophysical studies had suggested that the viscosity of the IgG molecule was consistent with the interpretation that was composed of three independently moving units with molecular weights of approximately 50 000 (Noellsen *et al.*, 1965), the first convincing demonstration that it is, in fact, Y-shaped and that the two combining regions are located at the ends of the two movable arms of the Y, came from electron microscopy. The studies of Lafferty and Oertelis (1963) and of Almeida and Waterson (1969) showed viruses with thread-like structures which formed U-shaped bands on the viral surface, while Feinstein and Rowe (1965) demonstrated ferritin molecules held together by thin, angled molecules. Valentine and Green (1967) used bifunctional DNP haptens which were separated from each by carbon skeletons of various lengths. With the bifunctional antigen containing an eight-carbon skeleton, $DNP–NH–(CH_2)_8–NH–DNP$, excellent cross-linked complexes were obtained in which the combining region of one molecule was joined head-to-head with the combining region of the next molecule (Figure 2). The electron microscopic field at a magnification of $\times 400\ 000$ shows predominantly ring-shaped structures of various sizes with knobs protruding outwards. These rings are composed of two, three, four, or more molecules of IgG joined by their combining regions and held together by the bifunctional antigen. The knob can be removed with pepsin, an enzyme known to cleave the Fc fragment from the dimeric $F(ab)_2$ fragment. When bifunctional DNP antigens with a carbon skeleton of five or less were tested with protein 315, an anti-DNP mouse IgA myeloma protein, no ring structures were produced.

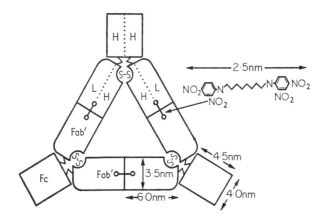

Figure 2 Diagrammatic representation of complexes of anti-DNP–IgG with bivalent DNP ligands. The electron micrographs on which this diagram is based gave the major dimensions of the IgG molecule, and the locations of the combining regions and the Fc fragment. The electron micrographs also demonstrated the flexibility of the Fab region at the hinge region of the molecule. By courtesy of Dr. N. M. Green and the Journal of Molecular Biology

These dramatic electron micrographs show (*i*) that the IgG and IgA molecules are Y-shaped, and (*ii*) that the arms are movable about a hinge-like region. Unlike previous studies, deformation of the molecule due to fixation on the carbon grid cannot be invoked to explain the different angles which Fab segments exhibited with respect to each other. The circular structures had clearly closed prior to fixation on the grid, demonstrating that flexibility of the Fab fragments with respect to each other is a functional feature of the molecule. The failure to form circular structures with short bifunctional haptens suggests that the DNP-binding site is at least 1·5 nm below the surface of the protein and that a cleft or cavity is probably present at the free end of the Fab fragment (Green, 1969). The major dimensions of the molecule can be measured from the electron micrographs. The Fab fragment containing the combining region has been estimated as 6·0 nm long and 3·5 nm broad. Careful examination of the IgA protein 315 molecules and of the IgG molecules showed that each Fab region is composed of two compact, round structures, giving visual evidence of the immunoglobulin sulphydryl-linked molecule domains which had been proposed on structural grounds by Edelman, Konigsberg, and their collaborators (Waxdal *et al.*, 1968). More recently, electron micrographs of a human IgG1 myeloma protein crystal using an optical averaging method have confirmed the Y-shaped structure of the whole molecule and the dimensions of the Fab fragment (Labow and Davies, 1971).

1.8 X-Ray Crystallography of Combining Regions

Northrop (1942) described the first crystalline preparation derived from trypsin-treated antibody and a number of investigators subsequently reported crystalline antibodies or antibody fragments (see, for example, Nisonoff *et al.*, 1967; Hochman *et al.*, 1973). The first Fab fragment crystals, however, which had potential for high resolution X-ray analysis only became available in the late 1960s. A human IgG1 myeloma, protein NEW, was analysed at 0·2 nm resolution by Poljak *et al.* (1974) and a mouse IgA myeloma protein derived from the McPc 603 tumour was studied by Segal *et al.* (1974) at a resolution of 0·2 nm. A third myeloma protein has been studied extensively by Edmundson, Schiffer, and their collaborators (Schiffer *et al.*, 1973; Edmundson *et al.*, 1974); this is a λ light-chain dimer associated with the McG human myeloma protein. In addition, Fehlhammer *et al.* (1975) and Epp *et al.* (1975) have compared the structure at 0·2 nm resolution of two κ light-chain dimers, Au and Rei, which differ in structure by only 16 amino acid residues.

At the time of writing, detailed information is available about the antigen-combining region complex of one human IgG myeloma (NEW), one mouse γA combining region–antigen complex (McPc 603), and three light-chain dimer models of the combining region (from Mcg, Au, and Rei).

Knowledge of the three-dimensional structure of the combining region has answered or potentially can answer a number of questions about antibody specificity. (*i*) What is the extent of the region complementary to antigen? (*ii*) Can several diverse antigen-binding sites be demonstrated in the combining region? (*iii*) The V region has a common folding pattern associated with areas of conserved amino acid sequence, in spite of which, it shows very large variation of antigen-binding specificity. By what mechanism is structural variation in binding sites created? (*iv*) Why is antigen binding predominantly to the combining region? What physical characteristics found in this region only, facilitate binding? (*v*) What are the structural consequences of antigen ligation? Are physiologically important conformational changes found secondary to antigen binding? If so, are these conformational signals transmitted to the Fc region or does some other mechanism occur?

A comparison of the structure of the variable domain shows some striking similarities between proteins NEW and McPc 603 (Poljak, 1975). Firstly, the basic immunoglubulin fold of the V-region polypeptides is essentially the same in both proteins, the same fold being found in the V_L and the V_H regions. The only difference is that the second light-chain hypervariable region is absent from NEW and the polypeptide backbone bridges across the base of the loop. A single disulphide bond links cysteine residues at loci equivalent to positions 26 and 85 on the light chain. The polypeptide backbone is principally in parallel folds in the form of β-pleated sheets, and there are no substantial α-helical segments. There are two sets of loops at either end of the V region of each chain (see Figures 3 and 4). One set of loops makes contact with the first constant domain; the other set are free in the sense that they are exposed to solvent. These three solvent-exposed

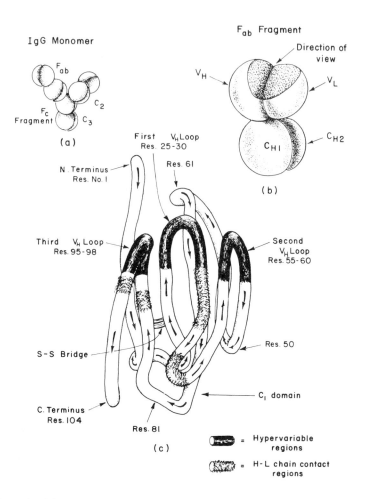

Figure 3 (a) The arrangement of the six domains of the antibody molecule with respect to each other. (b) An exploded diagram of the variable domain showing the V_L-V_H contact surface. (c) The polypeptide backbone fold of the heavy chain indicating the areas in contact with the light chain and the approximate location of the hypervariable regions. Redrawn from data on the NEW immunoglobulin molecule from Poljak *et al.* (1973) and Poljak (1975)

loops correspond approximately to the hypervariable regions. Hypervariable regions centre on residues 25–30, 50, and 95–100 of the light chain and residues 30, 55–60, and 105–110 of the heavy chain. It must be remembered that these are not rigidly bounded areas, the extent of hypervariability will depend on whether all light chains, κ or λ, or chains within each κ or λ subgroups are compared. The greater the difference between the groups and subgroups, the more extensive the region of hypervariability. While hypervariable residues in mouse and man occur in the area of the combining region there is no evidence to suggest that these are

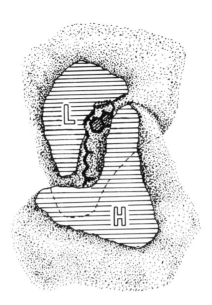

Figure 4 Scheme of the combining region of protein NEW looking into the long axis of the Fab fragment. The areas labelled L and H are occupied by the light and heavy chain, respectively. Between lies a depression approximately 0·5–0·6 nm deep in which the γ-hydroxy of vitamin K_1 molecule is located

obligatory contact residues for antigens. The X-ray evidence indicates that some hypervariable residues are in contact with antigen, while others are close and still more do not make contact. Contact is also made by antigen with regions other than the hypervariable ones (Poljak, 1975). In the rabbit, the relationship between hypervariability and antigen contact is even less certain (Haber *et al.*, 1975). It is probable that hypervariability does not reflect only the variation in amino acid sequence needed to bind directly to antigen. Compensatory sequence changes in regions away from the contact residues may also give rise to hypervariability. The predictions made from analysis of variability have proved very valuable in showing the general area in which antigen binding takes place.

In other regions of the back-bone polypeptide fold, the side chains of residues are involved in heavy–light chain interactions. These include residues 35, 37, 42, 43, 86, and 99 in the V_L and C_L, and residues 37, 39, 43, 45, 47, 95, and 108 in the V_H region of protein NEW (Poljak, 1975). These interacting residues are mainly, although not exclusively, hydrophobic and their presence does not appear to correlate with the heavy or light chain subgroup or light chain class, suggesting that there is no rigid restriction on the recombination of heavy and light chains. The V_L and V_H regions are essentially similar in shape. On association, they interact to form a roughly spherical domain, with the solvent-exposed distal end forming an approximately flat plate fringed by the hypervariable loops. Between the areas occupied by the light and heavy chains on this plate runs a cleft which is approximately 1·5–1·7 nm long. In the protein NEW, this cleft is shallow (Figure 5), perhaps 0·5–0·6 nm deep, while in protein 603 it is 1·2 nm deep, 1·5 nm wide, and 2·0 nm long (Poljak *et al.*, 1974). The light chain of protein 603 is of the κ type and has an insertion of six residues at, or close to, the first hypervariable region. This has the effect of forcing apart the V_L and V_H regions and increasing the depth and width of the cleft. In the case of λ light-chain dimer studied, one light chain takes on a rotational position corresponding to the 'heavy' chain; the other adopts the light-chain position (Schiffer *et al.*, 1973; Edmundson *et al.*, 1974). The cleft in these dimers is much deeper, forming a funnel with a cavity at the

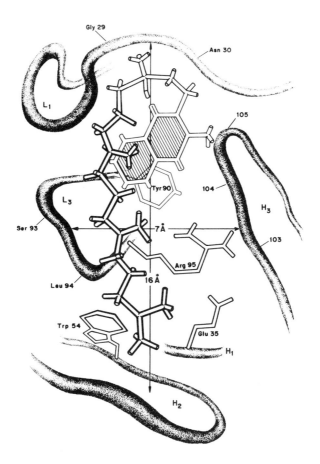

Figure 5 γ-Hydroxy Vitamin K_1 bound to the combining region of the human myeloma IgG molecule NEW. L_1 and L_3 are the first and third light-chain hypervariable regions. (L_2 is deleted in this molecule.) H_1, H_2, and H_3 are the three hypervariable regions of the heavy chain

bottom whose floor is approximately 1·6–1·7 nm below the entrance to the cleft. The κ-chain dimers, Au and Rei, also have a large cavity between the light and 'heavy' chain regions. An important difference in this region is the presence, in Au, of trytophan at position 96 instead of the tyrosine residue found in Rei. The indole ring of this residue protrudes into the cavity, suggesting that it might impede access to a considerable part of the cavity by a moderately large presumptive hapten (Epp *et al.*, 1975; Fehlhammer *et al.*, 1975).

The mouse IgA myeloma, protein 603, binds the small molecule phosphorylcholine approximately in the middle of the cleft. The phosphate moiety touches only the heavy chain at tyrosine 33 and arginine 52. The choline moiety lies at the bottom of the cleft, making contact with residues 102–103 of the heavy chain and residues 91–94 of the light chain; the contact region seems to be composed predominantly of heavy chain and it is of interest that phosphorylcholine-binding myeloma proteins, which do not share the TEPC 15 idiotype, may have light chains that have little resemblance to those found on protein 603 (Poljak, 1975). This suggests that conditions for binding of this small determinant may be relatively non-stringent and are not dependent on a particular light chain, whereas some larger antigens making substantial contact with both light and heavy chains may show a considerable degree of stringency. It is noteworthy that the hypervariable loops form a very extensive region which frames the site of hapten attachment. The third hypervariable region of the heavy chain and the second hypervariable region of the light chain do not make contact with the hapten.

The human IgG myeloma protein NEW binds a γ-hydroxyl derivative of vitamin K_1 (Figure 5) with K_A of $1·7 \times 10^5 \, M^{-1}$. Fab fragment-ligand complexes have been crystallized and analysed by Fourier difference maps (Amzel *et al.*, 1974; Poljak *et al.*, 1974). The vitamin derivative K_1 is a large molecule consisting of a naphthoquinone moiety and a long hydrophobic phytyl side chain. The whole molecule nestles in the cleft, almost completely filling it. The naphthoquinone residue lies obliquely on the floor of the cleft making contact with tyrosine residue 90 of the light chain, with the backbone and side chain of heavy chain residue 104, and with L chain residues 29 and 30. When 2-methyl-1:4-naphthoquinone—the vitamin K molecule without the phytyl tail is bound to protein NEW, it occupies an identical site to that of vitamin derivative K_1 derivative. Of the total binding energy (approximately 7·2 kcal/mole at 20°), the naphthoquinone rings provide approximately 4·2 kcal/mole, thus by difference the phytyl tail provides 3·0 kcal/mole. The phytyl tail loops upward and around, making close contact with the light chain at glycine 29 and asparagine 30. It then proceeds downward and superficially makes contact with the light chain at residues 93 and 94, and with the heavy chain at residue 104. At the free end of the chain, contact is made with a constant heavy-chain tryptophan residue at position 54. Approximately 10–12 amino acid residues make contact with the antigen, and contact is made extensively with both heavy and light chains over a maximal dimension of perhaps 1·5 nm (Amzel *et al.*, 1974; Poljak *et al.*, 1974).

The Mcg λ light-chain dimer appears to have at least three distinct binding sites. One is located on the rim of the funnel-shaped cleft, a second is at the constriction between funnel and cavity, and a third at the bottom of the cavity. These sites bind a whole range of compounds including ε-dansyllysine, colchicine, 1,10-phenanthroline, methadone, morphine, meperidine, 5-acetyluracil, caffeine, theophylline, menadione, and triacetin (Schiffer *et al.*, 1973).

1.9 Conclusions from X-Ray Crystallography and Remaining Problems

Certain general principles are beginning to emerge from the studies so far carried out. These answer, in part, the questions set (see p. 71). It is, however, distinctly possible that further structural elucidation could modify these conclusions.

(*i*) Antigen binding so far observed occurs in the solvent channel between the light- and heavy-chain areas of the V domain. Since only two antigens in actual combining regions have been mapped so far, it is not yet known whether antigen binding is confined to the channel or can extend outside it. Certainly the light-chain dimer model of the combining region suggests that very deep hapten-binding clefts and cavities may exist in some antibodies. More mapping with antibody–antigen complexes will be required before all the region involved in ligation of antigen can be defined.

(*ii*) Analysis of the protein Fab NEW–Vitamin K_1OH complex suggests strongly that antigen binding is not confined to a small, localized contact point, but consists of multipoint contact over an extensive area of the immunoglobulin molecule. This is an observation consistent with the existence of multiple binding sites. If the Mcg model of the immunoglobulin combining region resembles light–heavy chain combining regions, the clustering of binding sites also may be found in antibodies.

(*iii*) It is now clear that both the light and heavy regions as well as the C regions have a common polypeptide fold. Each light and each heavy folded unit has a relatively flat surface which makes contact with the other unit. On assembly each unit makes an angle with the other, that is the two units are not completely symmetrical, but show one dyad axis. At the free end of the Fv domain, the heavy and light chains are not in contact, thus creating a solvent-filled channel. Antigens have been shown to bind to the walls of this channel. The walls of the cleft are composed of six loops, or five in the case of the protein NEW, the tips of which bear hypervariable residues. The nature of the insertions or deletions of amino acid sequence apparently alters the depth of the cleft. For instance, the insertion of six amino acid residues in the first hypervariable loop in κ light chain of the McPc 603 protein forces apart the heavy- and light-chain regions and gives rise to a deeper cleft. From the three-dimensional models, it has been predicted that variations in the length of the third hypervariable loop (around residue 105) would have the same effect. The pattern of amino acid residue variability found at the tips of the loops resembles the pattern of variable or 'permissive' residues found when cytochromes from different species are compared. Here also the loci of greatest variation are found at the tips of outside polypeptide loops. This variability may be permissive in the sense that compensatory change for differences in cleft structure are visible here. It is, however, equally likely that residues at the tips of the loops have some direct functional significance. Haptens appear to bind along the walls of the cleft and not only at the hypervariable residues. The present scanty evidence does not rule out the possibility that the binding region could be much more extensive. It appears that the depth of the cleft can be modulated, exposing new binding sites, and that this may be one method of introducing variability in antigen binding. The light-chain dimers show an extremely wide and deep cleft in which a very large number of determinants binds. Light-chain dimers found in human myelomas show strong affinity for tissue components, infiltrating tissues in the form of amyloid deposits. This effect may be related directly to the large number of combining sites exposed.

(iv) It is not clear why antigen binding occurs primarily at the Fab combining region, or why most of the ligand binding observed, for example, in an enzyme molecule such as lysozyme, should occur in the cleft in which the substrate binds. Since it is known that deep cavities are not required for ligand binding in immunoglobulins, a number of crevices, folds, and channels elsewhere in the molecule might be thought to serve equally well. Richards (1974) has considered a similar problem in the case of ribonuclease and has calculated that the atomic packing densities within the substrate-combining cleft are considerably less than at other solvent-exposed regions of the molecule. This suggests that the vibratory modes of various functional groups in the combining region could occur with greater degrees of freedom, and that this may be associated with greater ligating potential. Similar studies carried out with the immunoglobulin molecule would be of great potential interest.

2 RELATIONSHIP BETWEEN ANTIBODY STRUCTURE AND FUNCTION

2.1 Binding Specificity and Amino Acid Sequence

Antibodies of different ligand-binding specificities may have large regions of the primary sequence in common. It is, therefore, reasonable to suggest that in these antibodies those regions which show amino acid sequence variability are those concerned with binding antigens. However, it does not follow from this proposition, that those amino acid residues which show the greatest sequence variability are necessarily the contact residues at which antigens bind. Wu and Kabat (1970) analysed light-chain sequences for variability and plotted variability at each amino acid position *versus* position and obtained a graph showing three regions of greatest sequence variability which they termed 'hypervariable' regions. Capra and Kehoe (1975) performed a similar analysis on heavy-chain variable region sequences and were also able to demonstrate hypervariable regions.

2.2 Groups and Subgroups of the Variable Region

Early studies comparing partial amino acid sequences of different myeloma immunoglobulins showed that if one made an attempt to maximize amino acid residue homology, the variable regions of both the κ and λ light-chain groups could be divided into a number of subgroups. Five human λ (V_λ I–V) and three human κ (V_κ I–III) subgroups have been described (Smith *et al.*, 1971). In the V regions of human heavy chains, three analogous subgroups V_H I–III have been delineated. Similar analyses on mouse κ chains show that the number of subgroups and sub-subgroups is rather large (Hood *et al.*, 1973).

With each group or subgroup, there are amino acid residues which are subgroup specific, (for example, found only in the V_κ I subgroup), group specific (found only in k chains), chain specific (found only in light chains), and species specific (found only in dog light chains).

2.3 Ligand Contact Residues and Hypervariability

Several groups of research workers have compared both monoclonal immunoglobulins and antibody populations of known specificity to see if the amino acid sequence in the hypervariable regions can be correlated with antigen-binding specificity. Cebra *et al.* (1974) have compared the amino acid sequence in the hypervariable regions of guinea-pig anti-DNP and anti-arsonate antibodies, using purified antibodies from strain 13 guinea-pigs. The hypervariable regions were additionally identified by attachment of radioactive affinity reagents. It was found that distinct sequences occur in the hypervariable regions which correlate with DNP binding and other sequences which correlate with the ability to bind arsonate.

Capra *et al.* (1971) examined the light chains from some homogeneous antibodies derived from patients with hypergammaglobulinaemic purpura, all of which had IgG-ligating activity. The amino acid residue sequence are identical in some antibodies up to residue #40; in others there are only infrequent amino acid differences. The hypervariable regions of most of these proteins closely resemble each other.

In contrast to this work is that in which rabbits were hyperimmunized with type VIII staphylococcal polysaccharide. A percentage of such rabbits shows the clonal dominance phenomenon in which the normally heterogeneous antibody becomes highly restricted or monoclonal. Using this phenomenon, a large number of homogeneous rabbit antibodies having specificity for the type VIII staphylococcal polysaccharide has been isolated. These show the normal variations in binding constants for the antigen. The primary structure of a number of V_L and some V_H regions from these monoclonal immunoglobulins has been determined (Margolies *et al.*, 1975). Cluster analysis was carried out using both the specific anti-staphylococcal antibodies and control monoclonal antibodies. A computer was used to search the sequences for groups or clusters of amino acid residues which are consistent within the experimental (anti-type VIII polysaccharide) group and which are different from these sequences in the control group. No such clusters could be demonstrated, suggesting that in the rabbit system many different combining regions contribute to the binding of polysaccharide staphylcoccal.

These results are by no means mutually incompatible. If one considers a set of immunoglobulins on neighbouring branches of an evolutionary tree, these will have diverged from each other only by a few residues. Among the multiple specificities represented in the combining region, it is quite likely that one function will not have been altered by the few amino acid replacements in the V region. Neighbouring branches on such a generic tree will have a set of proteins with V-region structures which closely resemble each other and which have a common antigen-binding specificity.

Since, however, other sets of contact amino acids also may bind the same antigen, several dissimilar sets of immunoglobulins will be distributed widely over non-adjacent branches of the tree since they have no necessary close evolutionary kinship. Depending on the method used for selecting the immunoglobulins, either sets of immunoglobulins with similar or dissimilar V regions can be obtained. It is also conceivable that some antigens may be so stringent in their binding requirements that only one set of evolutionarily related clones on adjacent branches may be able to bind the antigen. In brief, it is a fallacy to believe that, because antibodies with similar V regions bind a common antigen, this antigen can be bound *only* by that type of V region.

2.4 Conservation of Variable Regions

When initial comparisons were made between partial light-chain amino acid sequences in mouse and man, it was noted that more sequence homology exists between certain mouse and human light-chains than between certain V_L-region sequences of two light chains within the species (Smith, 1973). Later work showed great similarity in structure between V regions of inbred and outbred animals of the same species and between the V regions of similar specificity raised in guinea-pigs and mice (Capra and Kehoe, 1974). This similarity is not surprising and may represent, for instance, the retention of certain sequences which ligate some persisting pathogens and thus may be subject to selective pressure. Alternatively, it may represent an example of parallel evolution, or the development of the same lighting sequence from two originally different sequences under the selective pressure exerted by, perhaps, a common pathogen.

2.5 Correlation between Structure and Function

The relationship between primary amino acid sequence in the V region and antibody specificity is, on the one hand, very simple; related structures share specificities. On the other hand, it is very complex, since many different unrelated V regions may bind a single antigenic determinant with different degrees of affinity. It is probably naive to expect to find a common structural feature in the V regions of all antibodies to a small determinant X. There may be several anti-X families which need bear little resemblance to each other, although within each family the members will have close similarities, sharing idiotypes, and perhaps the ability to bind other antigens. The ability to bind X by itself is a poor indication of 'consanguinity' since it is the property of many families of antibodies. A large, site-filling antigen, which requires interaction at several points and demands stringent binding conditions, is more likely to select a smaller set of antibody-producing cell clones, perhaps only one family or even only one clone, which is able to meet these conditions. Similarly non-stringent selection conditions which select for binding of a small determinant over a wide range of binding energies will demand a relatively large heterogeneous collection of antibody-producing cell clones which can meet these non-stringent conditions.

2.6 Polyfunctional Antibody-Combining Regions

In recent years, two lines of evidence have suggested that a single immunoglobulin may have antibody-combining regions which are complementary to several structurally dissimilar antigens. Haimovich and Du Pasquier (1973) have shown that the tadpole has approximately 1×10^6 lymphocytes, yet it is able to mount a specific humoral response against the DNP determinant (anti-DNP). The response to single haptens is usually heterogeneous, involving many different clones of cells which produce anti-DNP antibody. In order that the antibody reaches detectable levels, the number of cells involved in this specific anti-DNP response must be a very considerable proportion of the total. There is no doubt that the tadpole can respond to many antigens, thus there seems to be too few cells at any one time to account for the range of immune responses observed. In addition, clonal-dilution studies, which indicate the presence of many antibodies complementary to one antigenic determinant, have been carried out (Williamson, 1972).

All this work may be summarized by stating that if there is only one anti-hapten specificity per antibody molecule (or per cell), there do not appear to be enough lymphoid cells to account for the number of antigenic specificities. Reciprocally, there appears to be a very large number of clones involved in the production of antibodies against a single haptenic determinant. Over the last decade, homogeneous myeloma proteins which bind antigens have become available and an early finding was that a number of these myeloma proteins can bind more than one haptenic determinant. This binding is competitive, and since only one determinant can be bound at a time to a single combining region, it has been assumed that there are common structural features in the competing determinants that are bound to a single locus on the protein.

Rosenstein and his coworkers (Rosenstein *et al.*, 1972; Jackson and Richards, 1974) examined the combining region of protein 460, a mouse γ A myeloma protein which binds competitively the haptens DNP and menadione. These workers found a sulphydryl group in relation to the combining region. When this group is substituted with a bulky reagent, the ability of protein 460 to bind

DNP   menadione

menadione is impaired, while the ability to bind DNP remains intact. When the protein is partially denatured using 4·3 M guanidine hydrochloride and then allowed to refold partially, the ability to bind DNP is ablated, while menadione binding remains intact. Other methods for differentially affecting one binding activity have been described by these authors.

This work suggests, but does not prove, that there are spatially separated sites within the combining region. Later work on the same protein using the technique of fluorescent energy transfer between donor fluorescent probes placed on the sulphydryl groups and the DNP and menadione molecules bound to their sites shows that there is a minimul separation of 1·2–1·4 nm between the DNP and the menadione binding site (Manjula et al., 1976). To support these findings, dextran bead–spacer–DNP and dextran bead–spacer–menadione columns were constructed with spacer molecules of varying length. The shortest spacer–determinant combination needed to hold protein 460 to the column was determined both for DNP and menadione. The difference in length between the two shortest molecules is 1·25 nm, a finding consistent with the separation distance calculated from the energy transfer experiments (Rosenstein and Richards, 1976). There appears to be reasonable evidence that there is substantial spatial separation between two combining sites within the antibody combining region, making it probable that the combining region is in fact a mosaic of determinant-binding sites.

Even though an individual antibody combining region may bind diverse determinant at different sites, this is not, by itself, proof that multiple binding is physiologically significant. It is, for instance, possible that binding at only one subsite of the V-region cell-surface receptor induces cell proliferation and antibody production. Experiments, however, have shown that this objection does not appear to be true. In rabbits (Varga et al., 1973) and in mice (Varga et al., 1974), isoelectric focusing can pick out individual immunoglobulin bands which bind two dissimilar haptens. In the same animals, the similar double-binding bands can be induced by either of the two antigens (Figure 6), indicating that the binding of both antigens induces cell proliferation and antibody production within the cell clone which binds both antigens (Varga et al., 1973).

Double-binding myeloma proteins appear to have V regions which resemble those of some of the induced antibodies binding the same antigens. Anti-idiotypic sera raised against determinants in the V region of myeloma proteins cross-react with their naturally induced counterparts. They will even do this occasionally

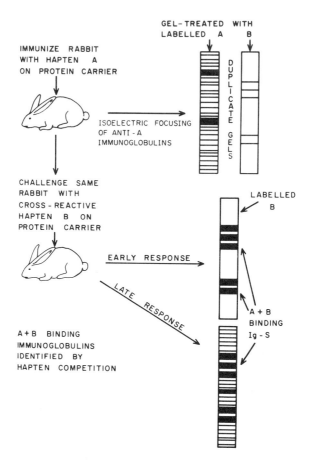

Figure 6 Experimental protocol for determining the presence of immunoglobulins with polyfunctional combining regions in anti-hapten antisera

when the double-binding myeloma proteins arise in one species and the 'natural' double-binding antibodies are induced in another species (Varga *et al.*, 1974), stressing that considerable conservation of the V region between species, or perhaps that parallel evolution, has occurred in the combining region.

It is not yet clear how many different antigens are complementary to a single combining region. It has been estimated that when random antigens are screened, interactions with a K_0 of approximately $1 \times 10^5 \text{ M}^{-1}$ occur once in about 140 compounds screened, while weaker interactions in the $1 \times 10^3 \text{ M}^{-1}$ range occur much more frequently (once in 20 compounds screened) (Varga, Lande and Richards, 1974). Clearly these figures are only approximate since the choice of antigens can never be really random. Nevertheless, the general principle is that the higher the interaction energy, the less frequently cross-reactions are found. It is intuitively clear that if high energy cross-reactions were very common, antibody populations would be like glue, sticking together all biological structures are showing no population specificity.

The high degree of specificity of an immune serum has been discussed earlier. It has assumed frequently that if a population of antibodies has apparently exclusive specificity for one antigen, the individual antibodies constituting that population must show the same exclusive specificity. In a perceptive article, Talmage (1959) showed that this need not be true and that an apparently highly specific population could be derived from members having different specificities. It is known now that in myeloma proteins individual hapten-combining sites have, in fact, a high degree of specificity and will, for instance, distinguish DNP from mononitrophenols and trinitrophenols (Haimovich and Du Pasquier, 1973). At the same time, protein 460 will bind a number of unrelated haptens at other sites within the combining region. The consequence of this, however, are exactly as Talmage first suggested.

Assuming that a single V region may bind 100 different determinants, if the animal is immunized with determinant A, all those cells producing A-binding immunoglobulins of sufficient affinity will respond to the antigenic stimulus by cell proliferation and antibody production. Thus, all antibody species produced

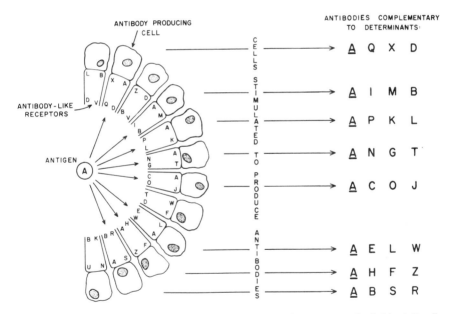

Figure 7 Immune serum specificity as a population phenomenon. Individual B cell receptors are shown as having properties similar to immunoglobulin-combining regions. It is assumed that each is complementary to four different antigens; it is supposed that this figure is in fact much larger. Stimulation by antigen A causes the cells with A specificity to divide and produce antibodies directed against A. The immune serum produced will therefore react in high titre with antigen A. Each immunoglobulin also has other specificities, but because these need not be the same in every molecule, the other specificities, B–Z, will be diluted out and will react only in low titre

bind A. Each antibody will also bind 99 other determinants, but these need not be the same for each antibody and such ligating activity will be present only at a lower level (for example, 1 per cent) in the antibody population and will be diluted out. Thus, antibody specificity is, in essence, a population phenomenon, an average characteristic, rather than the property of each member of the population (see Figure 7).

3 CONCLUSION

In the great complexity of the humoral immune system, a pattern is discernible. Antibody combining regions, although tremendously diverse, are made out of two chains, light and heavy, whose diversity is less than that of the assembled product. Both light and heavy chains give evidence of having evolved over millennia and many of the evolved forms are retained by vertebrates. This retention of many diverse patterns in certain animals serves to create hetero-geneous populations of antibodies which as a whole are effective in ligating complex and simple antigens. Combining regions appear to have many common characteristics, judging by the limited number of examples which has so far been analysed. Differences in antibody specificity may depend on quite limited variations in amino acid primary sequence, such as short deletions and insertions which make different parts of the combining region accessible to antigens. The evolutionary process, by numerous step-wise changes of a basic pattern, has created an efficient and adaptable system for combating infection.

ACKNOWLEDGEMENTS

The authors would like to thank the U.S. Public Health Service, the National Science Foundation, and the American Heart Association for their support of this work. This chapter was completed while F.F.R. was a Senior Faculty Fellow of the Josiah Macy Foundation at Glasgow University, Scotland. Most of all, thanks are due to Mrs. Valerie Vishno whose skill and patience in putting together this manuscript is acknowledged with much gratitude.

REFERENCES

Albertson, P., and Phillipson, L. (1960). *Nature (Lond.)*, **185**, 38.
Almeida, J. D., and Waterson, A. P. (1969). *Adv. Virus Res.*, **15**, 307.
Amzel, L. M., Poljak, R. J., Saul, F., Varga, J. M., and Richards, F. F. (1974). *Proc. Nat. Acad. Sci., U.S.A.*, **71**, 1427.

Binz, H., Lindemann, J., and Wigzell, H. (1973). *Nature (Lond.)*, **246**, 146.
Binz, H., Lindemann, J., and Wigzell, H. (1974). In *The Immune System, Genes, Receptors, Signals*, (Sercarz, E. E., Williamson, A. R., and Fox, C. F., eds.), Academic Press, New York and London, 533.
Brient, B. W., Haimovich, J., and Nisonoff, A. (1971). *Proc. Nat. Acad. Sci., U.S.A.*, **68**, 3136.

Capra, J. D., and Kehoe, J. M. (1974). *Proc. Nat. Acad. Sci., U.S.A.*, **71**, 4032.
Capra, J. D., and Kehoe, J. M. (1975). *Adv. Immunol.*, **20**, 1.
Capra, J. D., Winchester, R. J., and Kunkel, H. G. (1971). *Medicine*, **50**, 125.
Cathou, R. E., and Haber, E. (1967). *Biochemistry*, **6**, 513.
Cathou, R. E., Holowka, D. A., and Chan, L. M. (1974). In *Progress in Immunology II*, Vol. I, (Brent, L., and Holborow, J., eds.), North Holland Publishing Co., Amsterdam, p. 63.
Cathou, R. E., and Werner, T. C. (1970). *Biochemistry*, **9**, 3149.
Cebra, J. J., Koo, P. H., and Ray, A. (1974). *Science*, **186**, 263.
Claflin, J. L., and Davie, J. M. (1975). *J. Immunol.*, **114**, 70.
Cohen, S., and Porter, R. R. (1964). *Adv. Immunol.*, **4**, 287.
Converse, C. A., and Richards, F. F. (1968). *Fed. Proc.*, **27**, 683.
Converse, C. A., and Richards, F. F. (1969). *Biochemistry*, **8**, 4431.
Cosenza, H., and Kohler, H. (1972). *Proc. Nat. Acad. Sci., U.S.A.*, **69**, 2701.

Day, E. D. (1972). *Advanced Immuhochemistry*, Williams and Wilkins, Baltimore.
Day, L. A., Sturtevant, J. M., and Singer, S. J. (1963). *Ann. N.Y. Acad. Sci.*, **103**, 611.
Dower, S. K., Dwek, R. A., McLaughlin, A. C., Mole, L. M., Press, E. M., and Sunderland, C. A. (1975). *Biochem. J.*, **149**, 73.
Dwek, R. A., Jones, R., Marsh, D., McLaughlin, A. C., Press, E. M., Price, N. C., and White, A. I. (1975*a*). *Roy. Soc. Lond., Ser. B*, **272**, 53.
Dwek, R. A., Knott, J. C. A., Marsh, D., McLaughlin, A. C., Press, E. M., Price, N. C., and White, A. I. (1975*b*). *Eur. J. Biochem.*, **53**, 25.

Edelman, G. M., Cunningham, B. A., Gottlieb, P. D., Rutishauser, U., and Waxdal, M. J. (1969). *Proc. Nat. Acad. Sci., U.S.A.*, **63**, 78.
Edmundson, A. B., Ely, K. R., Girling, R. L., Abola, E. E., Schiffer, M., Westholm, F. A., Fausch, M. D., and Deutsch, H. F. (1974). *Biochemistry*, **13**, 3816.
Eisen, H. N. (1964*a*). In *Immunology*, Harper and Row, Hagerstown.
Eisen, H. N. (1964*b*). In *Methods in Medical Research*, (Eisen, H. N., ed.), Vol. 10, Year Book Medical Publishers, Chicago, p. 115.
Eisen, H. N. (1971). In *Progress in Immunology*, Vol. 1, (Amos, B., ed.), Academic Press, New York and London, p. 243.
Eisen, H. N., and Siskind, G. W. (1964). *Biochemistry*, **3**, 996.
Epp, O., Lattman, E. E., Schiffer, M., Huber, R., and Palm, W. (1975). *Biochemistry*, **14**, 4943.

Fehlhammer, H., Schiffer, M., Epp, O., Colman, P. M., Lattman, E. E., Schwager, P., Steigemann, W., and Schramm, H. J. (1975). *Biophys. Struct. Mechan.*, **1**, 139.
Feinstein, A., and Rowe, A. J. (1965). *Nature (Lond.)*, **205**, 147.
Fisher, C. E., and Press, E. M. (1974). *Biochem. J.*, **139**, 135.
Fleet, G. W., Knowles, J. R., and Porter, R. R. (1969). *Nature (Lond.)*, **224**, 511.
Franek, F. (1973). *Eur. J. Biochem.*, **33**, 59.
Freedman, M., Merret, T. R., and Pruzanski, W. (1976). *Immunochemistry*, **13**, 193.

Givol. D. (1974). In *Essays in Biochemistry*, Vol. **10**, Biochemical Society, London, p. 73.
Goetzl, E. J., and Metzger, H. (1970). *Biochemistry*, **9**, 3826.
Green, N. M. (1969). *Adv. Immunol.*, **11**, 1.

Haber, E., Margolies, M. N., Cannon, L. E., and Rosenblatt, M. S. (1975). In *Molecular Approaches to Immunology*, Academic Press, New York and London, p. 303.
Haber, E., and Richards, F. F. (1967). *Proc. Roy. Soc. Lond.*, **166**, 176.
Haber, E., Richards, F. F., Spragg, J., Austen, K. F., Valloton, M., and Page, L. B. (1967). *Cold Spring Harbor Symp. Quant. Biol.*, **32**, 299.

Haber, E., and Stone, M. (1969). *Israel J. Med. Sci.*, **5**, 332.

Haimovich, J., and Du Pasquier, L. (1973). *Proc. Nat. Acad. Sci.*, *U.S.A.*, **70**, 1898.

Haimovich, J., Eisen, H. N., Hurwitz, E., and Givol, D. (1972). *Biochemistry*, **11**, 2389.

Haimovich, J., Givol, D., and Eisen, H. N. (1970). *Proc. Nat. Acad. Sci.*, *U.S.A.*, **67**, 1656.

Haselkorn, D., Friedman, S., Givol, D., and Pecht, I. (1974). *Biochemistry*, **13**, 2210.

Hew, C.-L., Lifter, J., Yoshioka, M., Richards, F. F., and Konigsberg, W. H. (1973). *Biochemistry*, **12**, 4685.

Hochman, J., Inbar, D., and Givol, D. (1973). *Biochemistry*, **12**, 1131.

Hoessli, D., Olander, J., and Little, J. R. (1976). *J. Immunol.*, **113**, 1024.

Hood, L., McKean, D., Farnsworth, V., and Potter, M. (1973). *Biochemistry*, **12**, 741.

Hsia, J. C., and Piette, L. H. (1969). *Archs Biochem. Biophys.*, **129**, 296.

Inbar, D., Hochman, J., and Givol, D. (1972). *Proc. Nat. Acad. Sci.*, *U.S.A.*, **69**, 2659.

Jackson, P., and Richards, F. F. (1974). *J. Immunol.*, **112**, 96.

Jerne, N. K. (1974). *Ann. Immunol. Inst. Pasteur*, **125c**, 373.

Johnston, M. F. M., Barisas, B. G., and Sturtevant, J. M. (1974). *Biochemistry*, **13**, 390.

Kabat, E. A. (1960). *J. Immunol.*, **84**, 82.

Knowles, J. R. (1972). *Ac. Chem. Res.*, **5**, 155.

Kuettner, M. C., Wang, A. L., and Nisonoff, A. (1972). *J. Exp. Med.*, **135**, 579.

Labow, L. W., and Davies, D. R. (1971). *J. Biol. Chem.*, **246**, 3760.

Lafferty, K. J., and Oertelis, S. (1963). *Virology*, **21**, 91.

Lieberman, R., Potter, M., Humphrey, W., Jr., Mushinski, E. B., and Vrana, M. (1975). *J. Exp. Med.*, **142**, 106.

Lieberman, R., Potter, M., Mushinski, E. B., Humphrey, W., Jr., and Rudikoff, S. (1974). *J. Exp. Med.*, **139**, 983.

Lifter, J., Hew, C.-L., Yoshioka, M., Richards, F. F., and Konigsberg, W. H. (1974). *Biochemistry*, **13**, 3567.

Little, J. R., and Eisen, H. N. (1967). *Biochemistry*, **6**, 3119.

Macario, A. J. L., and Conway de Macario, E. (1975). *Curr. Top. Microbiol. Immunol.*, **71**, 125.

Mäkelä, O., and Imanishi, T. (1975). *Eur. J. Immunol.*, **5**, 202.

Manjula, B. N., Richards, F. F., and Rosenstein, R. W. (1976). *Immunochemistry*, **13**, 929.

Margolies, M. N., Cannon, L. E., III, Strosberg, A. D., and Haber, E. (1975). *Proc. Nat. Acad. Sci.*, *U.S.A.*, **372**, 2180.

Metzger, H., and Singer, S. (1963). *Science*, **142**, 674.

Moreno, C., and Kabat, E. A. (1969). *J. Exp. Med.*, **129**, 871.

Murphy, P. D., and Sage, H. J. (1970). *J. Immunol.*, **105**, 460.

Nisonoff, A., Hopper, J. E., and Spring, S. B. (1975). *The Antibody Molecule*, Academic Press, New York and London, p. 448.

Nisonoff, A., and Thorbecke, G. J. (1964). *Ann. Rev. Biochem.*, **33**, 355.

Nisonoff, A., Zappacosta, S., and Jureziz, R. (1967). *Cold Spring Harbor Symp. Quant. Biol.*, **32**, 89.

Noellsen, M. E., Nelson, C. A., Buckley, C. E., III, and Tanford, C. (1965). *J. Biol. Chem.*, **240**, 218.

Northrop, J. A. (1942). *J. Gen. Physiol.*, **25**, 465.

Ohta, Y., Gill, T. J., III, and Leung, C. S. (1970). *Biochemistry*, **9**, 2708.

Padlan, E. A., Segal, D. M., Cohen, G. A., and Davis, D. R. (1974). In *The Immune System, Genes, Receptors, Signals*, (Sercarz, E. E., Williamson, A. R., and Fox, C. F., eds.), Academic Press, New York and London, p. 7.

Painter, R. G., Sage, H. J., and Tanford, C. (1972). *Biochemistry*, **11**, 1327.

Piette, L. H., Kiefer, E. F., Grossberg, A. L., and Pressman, D. (1972). *Immunochemistry*, **9**, 17.

Poljak, R. J. (1975). *Nature (Lond.)*, **256**, 373.

Poljak, R. J., Amzel, L. M., Avey, H. P., Chen, B. L., Phizackerly, R. P., and Saul, F. (1973). *Proc. Nat. Acad. Sci., U.S.A.*, **70**, 3305.

Poljak, R. J., Amzel, L. M., Chen, B. L., Phizackerley, R. P., and Saul, F. (1974). *Proc. Nat. Acad. Sci., U.S.A.*, **71**, 3440.

Porter, R. R. 1958). *Nature (Lond.)*, **182**, 670.

Porter, R. R., and Press, E. M. (1962). *Ann. Rev. Biochem.*, **31**, 621.

Potter, M., and Lieberman, R. (1970). *J. Exp. Med.*, **132**, 737.

Reichlin, M. (1974). *Immunochemistry*, **11**, 21.

Richards, F. F. (1974). *J. Mol. Biol.*, **82**, 1.

Richards, F. F., Konigsberg, W. H., Rosenstein, R. W., and Varga, J. M. (1975). *Science, N.Y.*, **187**, 130.

Richards, F. F., Lifter, J., Hew, C.-L., Yoshioka, M., and Konigsberg, W. H. (1974). *Biochemistry*, **13**, 3572.

Richards, F. F., Sloane, R. W., Jr., and Haber, E. (1967). *Biochemistry*, **6**, 476.

Rosenstein, R. W., Musson, R. A., Armstrong, M. Y. K., Konigsberg, W. H., and Richards, F. F. (1972). *Proc. Nat. Acad. Sci., U.S.A.*, **69**, 877.

Rosenstein, R. W., and Richards, F. F. (1976). *Immunochemistry*, **13**, 939.

Rubinstein, W. A., and Little, J. R. (1970). *Biochemistry*, **9**, 2106.

Ruoho, A. E., Kiefer, H., Roeder, P. E., and Singer, S. J. (1973). *Proc. Nat. Acad. Sci., U.S.A.*, **70**, 2567.

Schechter, B., Schechter, I., and Sela, M. (1970). *J. Biol. Chem.*, **245**, 1438.

Schiffer, M., Girling, R. L., Ely, K. R., and Edmundson, A. B. (1973). *Biochemistry*, **12**, 4620.

Schlessinger, J., Steinberg, I. Z., Givol, D., Hochman, J., and Pecht, I. (1975). *Proc. Nat. Acad. Sci., U.S.A.*, **72**, 2775.

Segal, D., Padlan, E. A., Cohen, G. H., Rudikoff, S., Potter, M., and Davies, D. R. (1974). *Proc. Nat. Acad. Sci., U.S.A.*, **71**, 4298.

Singer, S. J., and Doolittle, R. F. (1966). *Science, N.Y.*, **153**, 13.

Sirisinha, S., and Eisen, H. N. (1971). *Proc. Nat. Acad. Sci., U.S.A.*, **68**, 3130.

Smith, G. P. (1973). *The Variation and Adaptive Expression of Antibodies*. Harvard University Press, Cambridge, Mass.

Smith, G. P., Hood, L., and Fitch, W. M. (1971). *Ann. Rev. Biochem.*, **40**, 969.

Smith, R. A. G., and Knowles, J. R. (1973). *J. Am. Chem. Soc.*, **95**, 5072.

Steiner, L. A., and Eisen, H. N. (1966). *Bacteriol. Rev.*, **30**, 383.

Steiner, L. A., and Eisen, H. N. (1967a). *J. Exp. Med.*, **126**, 1161.

Steiner, L. A., and Eisen, H. N. (1967). *J. Exp. Med.*, **126**, 1185.

Stevenson, G. T. (1973). *Biochem. J.*, **133**, 827.

Steward, M. W., and Petty, R. E. (1972). *Immunology*, **23**, 881.

Stryer, L., and Griffith, O. H. (1965). *Proc. Nat. Acad. Sci., U.S.A.*, **54**, 1785.

Talmage, D. W. (1959). *Science*, **129**, *Immunochemistry*, **12**, 173.

Utsumi, S., and Karush, F. (1964). *Biochemistry*, **3**, 1329.

Valentine, R. C., and Green, N. M. (1967). *J. Mol. Biol.*, **27**, 615.
Varga, J. M., Konigsberg, W. H., and Richards, F. F. (1973). *Proc. Nat. Acad. Sci.*, *U.S.A.*, **70**, 3269.
Varga, J. M., Lande, S., and Richards, F. F. (1974). *J. Immunol.*, **112**, 1565.
Varga, J. M., Rosenstein, R. W., and Richards, F. F. (1974). *Fed. Proc.*, **33**, 810.
Vaughan, R. J., and Westheimer, F. H. (1969). *J. Am. Chem. Soc.*, **91**, 217.

Waxdal, M. J., Konigsberg, W. H., and Edelman, G. M. (1968). *Biochemistry*, **7**, 1967.
Weil, E., and Felix, A. (1916). *Wien. Klin. Wochenschr.*, **29**, 974.
Weltman, J. K., and Edelman, G. M. (1967). *Biochemistry*, **6**, 1437.
Williamson, A. R. (1972). *Biochem. J.*, **130**, 325.
Wiswesser, W. J. (1973). *Aldrichim. Acta*, **6**, 41.
Wofsy, L., Metzger, H., and Singer, S. J. (1962). *Biochemistry*, **1**, 1031.
Wofsy, L., and Parker, D. A. (1967). *Cold Spring Harbor Symp. Quant. Biol.*, **32**, 111.
Wu, T. T., and Kabat, E. A. (1970). *J. Exp. Med.*, **132**, 211.

Ygerabide, J., Epstein, H. F., and Stryer, L. (1970). *J. Mol. Biol.*, **51**, 573.
Yoo, T. J., Roholt, O. A., and Pressman, D. (1967). *Science, N.Y.*, **157**, 707.
Yoshioka, M., Lifter, J., Hew, C.-L., Converse, C. A., Armstrong, M. Y. K., Konigsberg, W. H., and Richards, F. F. (1973). *Biochemistry* **12**, 4679.

CHAPTER 3

Biosynthesis of Immuno-globulins

R. M. E. Parkhouse

1 INTRODUCTION

The production of circulating antibodies by warm-blooded vertebrate animals is the consequence of cell interactions under the stimulating influences of an immunogenic challenge. Although these cell interactions are poorly understood, the major types of cells involved are the B and T lymphocytes (Cooper *et al.*, 1966; Miller and Mitchell, 1969), the latter being capable of aiding or suppressing an immune response (Mitchison, 1971; Gershon, 1975; Tada *et al.*, 1975). Macrophages also may play an accessory role in the response, thereby increasing the complexity of the system. What is clear is that the precursors of high-rate antibody-secreting cells are B lymphocytes, while T lymphocytes never develop into cells which secrete immunoglobulin. This article therefore is confined to the expression and production of immunoglobulins by B lymphocytes and their progeny.

2 STRUCTURE AND GENETICS OF IMMUNOGLOBULINS

The structure and genetics of immunoglobulins are both discussed elsewhere in this volume: structure by Turner (Chapter 1) and genetics by both Sogn and Kindt (Chapter 4) and by Williamson (Chapter 5). However, for clarity and completeness, a brief discussion of these aspects of immunoglobulins will be considered here.

Immunoglobulins are multichain proteins built up from two basic types of polypeptide chain—heavy and light chains. In its simplest arrangement, an immunoglobulin molecule consists of two heavy chains and two light chains assembled through disulphide bridges. Such a structure is commonly called a monomer and is typical of the IgG, IgD, and IgE classes. Higher molecular weight forms may be constructed by forming disulphide-linked polymers from the monomer subunits. When this occurs, as in the case of the IgM and IgA classes, a further polypeptide, the J chain (Inman and Mestecky, 1974; Koshland, 1975) is required. Typically, IgM is secreted as a polymer consisting of five monomer (IgMs) units, whereas IgA may be secreted in a variety of forms—monomeric, dimeric, trimeric, or tetrameric. However, the important point is that whatever the size of the polymer, only one J chain is incorporated (Chapuis and Koshland, 1974). Furthermore, the immunoglobulin found in mucous secretions (sIgA) is a dimeric form which includes one J chain and a further polypeptide chain termed the secretory component (Tomasi and Grey, 1972).

The distinction between different immunoglobulin classes and subclasses resides in their heavy chains. Nomenclature reflects this fact; thus, the heavy chains of IgG are referred to as γ chains, of IgA as α, of IgM as μ, and so on. Subclasses are defined as, for example in the human, γ_1, γ_2, γ_3, and γ_4. Light chains may be classified into two classes, κ and λ, either of which may be found in random association with any class of heavy chain. A given immunoglobulin molecule is always symmetrical consisting entirely of light chains of the same class and heavy chains of the same class (or subclass).

A fundamental feature of immunoglobulin polypeptide chains became apparent as a result of amino acid sequential studies. In both heavy and light chains, the N-terminal region, comprising about 100 residues, is almost always unique and comprises the variable (V) region (V_H for the heavy chain, V_L for the light chain). The antibody combining site results from interaction between V_H and V_L. Thus, antibody diversity reflects the diversity of variable regions. The remaining C-terminal sequence of the heavy and light chains is invariant and distinct for a given classification, and is therefore called the constant (C) region. The constant regions of light chains, for example, will therefore show one or other invariant sequence characteristic of either κ or λ. Similarly, constant regions of human IgG subclasses may be $C_\gamma 1$, $C_\gamma 2$, $C_\gamma 3$, or $C_\gamma 4$.

The fact that immunoglobulin polypeptide chains are composed of C and V regions complicates genetic studies. The major problem is that of how can many V regions be associated with the same C-region sequence, and it is basically this which is responsible for the 'two gene—one polypeptide chain' proposal for immunoglobulins. This concept is well established now and there is considerable experimental evidence to support it. Nonetheless, the majority of genetic studies centre on those genes coding for C regions.

Each defined C region of a heavy or light chain is under the control of a classical Mendelian locus. Genes specifying the various C_H genes (C_μ, $C_\gamma 1$, $C_\gamma 2$, and so on) are linked closely, but C_κ and C_λ genes are unlinked to C_H genes or to each other. In the rabbit, the V_H and C_H genes are linked closely, and there are recent indications that a similar situation exists in mice. Strong evidence now points to integration of the information for V and C regions at the DNA level and this will be discussed below. All C_H-region genes are drawn from the same pool of V-region genes. There are, however, two further pools of V-region genes, one for C_κ and the other for C_λ.

Answers to the questions of the size of the V-region pool and the mechanism of its generation are not known. At best, informed—and sometimes prejudiced—guesses can be made, and arguments still rage as to whether all V regions are carried in the germ line or whether they arise from a few germ-line genes by somatic diversification. It is suggested that the reader refers to reviews by Kindt and Sogn (Chapter 4) and by Williamson (Chapter 5) in this volume, with the warning that the issue is not settled definitively.

For many C-region gene loci there are allelic alternatives and these are referred to as allotypes. An animal may be homozygous or heterozygous with respect to a given allotype system. In heterozygous animals, although the serum contains both allotypic variants, analysis at the level of the individual cell reveals a remarkable specialization, namely that a single cell synthesizes only one of the two allelic alternatives. In an individual cell there is, therefore, exclusive expression of one allele at each immunoglobulin locus. The genetic basis of this phenomena of allelic exclusion is not understood. Nonetheless, the consequence is an expression of one unique heavy–light chain pair, and thus one antibody combining site.

The structure and genetics of immunoglobulin molecules has been the subject of a number of recent reviews to which the reader is referred (Lennox and Cohn, 1967; Herzenberg et al., 1968; Fudenberg and Warner, 1970; Milstein and Munro, 1970; Milstein and Pink, 1970; Pink et al., 1971; Gally and Edelman, 1972; Capra and Kehoe, 1975; Hood et al., 1975; Williamson, 1975).

3 THE LYMPHOCYTE

A characteristic feature of B lymphocytes is the presence of easily detectable immunoglobulin on their surfaces (Raff et al., 1970), and it is this material that acts as the receptor for antigen (Walters and Wigzell, 1970; Strayer et al., 1975). Following this interaction, and perhaps with help from T lymphocytes and macrophages, proliferation and differentiation results in the production of memory cells and high-rate immunoglobulin-secreting cells. The mechanism by which such cells are stimulated to divide and differentiate is still unknown. Equally mysterious is the non-specific, or polyclonal, stimulation of B lymphocytes by mitogens.

It is clear from some recent experiments using the fluorescence-activated cell sorter (FACS) that allotype exclusion occurs in normal lymphocytes (Jones et al., 1974a). Lymphocytes from rabbits heterozygous at the b allotype locus were reacted with fluorescent-labelled, monospecific anti-allotype antibodies, and then were separated into fluorescent and nonfluorescent populations. When tested either in an in vivo transfer system, or by stimulation with pokeweed antigen *in vitro*, lymphocytes with a particular b locus allotype on their surfaces give rise to cells secreting the same (and no other) b locus allotype. Earlier suggestions that allotypic exclusion may not operate in lymphocytes are due, presumably, to problems associated with passive absorption by lymphocytes of immunoglobulin from serum.

Contentious issues are the number and physiological role of lymphocytes bearing IgG or IgA on their surfaces. Biochemical analysis (Abney and Parkhouse, 1974; Parkhouse *et al.*, 1976; Abney *et al.*, 1976; Melcher *et al.*, 1974; Vitetta *et al.*, 1975) indicates that there is little IgG or IgA expressed on the surface of murine lymphocytes. Instead, the major classes represented are IgD and IgM. The available evidence suggests that a similar situation exists in man and that many cells apparently bearing surface IgG do so as a result of absorption from the serum (Kurnick and Grey, 1975; Winchester *et al.*, 1975). It therefore appears that the number of lymphocytes actually synthesizing membrane IgG and IgA is small, and their exact role in immune responses is not clear.

A crucial question which remains to be resolved is if IgG and IgA-secreting cells are derived from lymphocytes with those immunoglobulins present on their surfaces. At present there is no firm evidence to exclude the derivation of at least some cells secreting IgA and IgG from lymphocytes bearing IgM and/or IgD. In fact, there is evidence that, in the rabbit, there are precursors of IgA-secreting cells which have neither IgA nor IgM on their surfaces (Jones *et al.*, 1974*b*). It seems likely that, in this case, the cell-surface immunoglobulin will prove to be the rabbit equivalent of IgD. Furthermore, the failure to suppress expression of IgG by treatment of lymphocytes with antisera to γ-chain determinants (Mage, 1975) may simply reflect the fact that precursors of IgG-secreting cells do not have IgG on their surface.

An intriguing observation is the simultaneous presence of IgM and IgD on the surface of the same lymphocyte in humans (Knapp *et al.*, 1973; Rowe *et al.*, 1973) and mice (Parkhouse *et al.*, 1976; Abney *et al.*, 1976). It is of particular interest that in such cells the V region is identical in both immunoglobulin classes (Pernis *et al.*, 1974; Salsano *et al.*, 1974; Fu *et al.*, 1975). This observation raises an important question, the solution of which will have implications for the mechanism of V–C-gene integration. The question is: Does the simultaneous expression of two C-region genes—C_μ and C_δ—sharing one V-region sequence result from the presence of two integrated heavy-chain genes (V–C_μ and V–C_δ) in the chromosome? An alternative explanation could be based on the persistence of mRNA for μ chain, for example, in a cell containing only the integrated V–C gene. The former possibility demands the simultaneous integration of C_μ and C_δ genes with the same V-region gene, while in the latter case, there would be successive gene integration events. Should simultaneous integration be demonstrated for C_μ and C_δ, then the possibility of simultaneous integration of all C_H regions is raised. Resolution of this problem requires the demonstration of mRNA synthesis for immunoglobulin heavy chains in those cells with cell-surface IgM and IgD. However, the fact that many long-lived chronic lymphatic leukaemic cells do have IgM and IgD present simultaneously on their surfaces

(Salsano *et al.*, 1974; Fu *et al.*, 1975) does suggest that two integrated heavy-chain genes exist in these cells.

By incubating lymphocytes with radiolabelled amino acids or sugars, it has been possible to demonstrate unequivocally the synthesis of surface immunoglobulin (Melchers and Andersson, 1973; Vitetta and Uhr, 1973, 1974; Parkhouse, 1975). These observations and other studies using cells externally labelled with ^{125}I (Cone *et al.*, 1971; Vitetta and Uhr, 1972; Melchers *et al.*, 1975), also indicate that there is turnover of membrane immunoglobulin. Loss of immunoglobulin *in vitro* occurs by a process termed 'shedding' (Vitetta and Uhr, 1972), since the immunoglobulin released from lymphocytes has been found complexed to fragments of plasma membrane. Whether or not this process occurs *in vivo* is uncertain. The analysis of surface immunoglobulin turnover is complicated by the heterogeneity of lymphocyte populations usually used in these studies. In a recent review (Melchers *et al.*, 1975), have divided lymphocytes into two subpopulations. One cell-type is large and releases cell-surface immunoglobulin with a half life of one to three hours. On the other hand the second subpopulation is small and releases surface immunoglobulin at an appreciably slower rate; the half life is 20–28 hours. It has been suggested that the smaller cell is derived from the larger (Melchers *et al.*, 1975). Clearly, the distribution of IgM and IgD on these different cell populations should be determined.

Unlike the plasma cell, the lymphocyte is not characterized by the secretory apparatus of intracellular membranes so typical of other secretory cells. The question of how surface-membrane constituents, including immunoglobulins, reach their final site in the plasma membrane is not well understood. It is possible (Vitetta and Uhr, 1974), but certainly not proven, that surface immunoglobulin is translated and transported within the cell on membrane elements, as is the case in plasma cells. What is interesting is that immunoglobulin may be secreted, as it is by plasma cells, or may be associated with the surface membrane as in the case of lymphocytes. It is reasonable to ask, therefore, if there is anything to distinguish between membrane-associated and secreted immunoglobulin. There are two obvious differences. One is that a large proportion of surface immunoglobulin is IgD, an immunoglobulin which at best is only a minor component of serum. Secondly, IgM found on the surface of B lymphocytes is in the monomeric form (IgMs), whereas secreted IgM is generally in the pentameric form (Vitetta *et al.*, 1971; Marchalonis *et al.*, 1972).

Unfortunately, these differences do not help to explain the mode of insertion of immunoglobulin into cell membranes. In the absence of sequential data for IgD, it is impossible to say whether its association with cell membranes is correlated with particular structural characteristics, for example a hydrophobic C-terminal sequence. However, the sequence of IgM known (Putnam *et al.*, 1973) and does not indicate C-terminal hydrophobicity. Furthermore, under certain conditions—admittedly pathological in the human (Solomon and Kunkel, 1967) but not so in elasmobranchs—(Marchalonis and Edelman, 1965) monomeric IgMs is secreted into the serum. A suggestion that surface IgM is deficient in galactose and fucose (Melchers and Andersson, 1973) has been contradicted subsequently (Vitetta and Uhr, 1974). At present, small structural differences between surface and secreted immunoglobulin cannot be ruled out, but their demonstration constitutes a formidable task. The actual interaction of surface immunoglobulin with the membrane is another intriguing feature about which little is known. The solution of this problem could well have implications for the mechanism of antigenic stimulation.

4 THE PLASMA CELL

Mature plasma cells are specialized in their cellular organization and the uniqueness of their secretory product. Like most secretory cells, the plasma cell has a highly organized endoplasmic reticulum consisting of both rough and smooth membranes. The rough membrane, so-called because it is studded with ribosomes on the cytoplasmic surface, comprises an extensive network of tubules (cysternae) within the cytoplasm. The smooth, often called the golgi zone, is a mass of vacuoles usually situated towards one pole of the cell. Under normal circumstances, the plasma cell represents a terminal differentiation stage. The immunoglobulin which it secretes is homogeneous and contains the identical V_H–V_L pair expressed on the original precursor lymphocyte. Thus, the antibody specificity of the lymphocyte is preserved in its progeny, exactly as would be predicted from Burnet's theory of clonal selection. A given plasma cell expresses only one C_H and C_L, but examples of plasma cell which secrete one or other of all C-region sequences can be found in the general population (Mäkelä and Cross, 1970). If plasma cells secreting IgG and IgA are derived from lymphocytes with IgM and/or IgD, then there must be a switch in immunoglobulin gene expression during the development of such clones. Experiments in which administration of anti-IgM antibodies *in vivo* abolishes the appearance of IgG and IgA strongly suggest the existence of this sort of phenotypic switch (Kincade *et al.*, 1970).

For many biochemical approaches, the cellular heterogeneity of lymphoid organs poses a major problem. Fortunately, it is possible experimentally to produce myeloma tumours in mouse which can be propagated by serial transplantation (Potter, 1967). These tumours are composed of plasma cells which, unlike their naturally occurring counterparts, divide vigorously. Each myeloma represents the product of a single neoplastic cell, and is therefore a clone of plasma cells secreting a unique homogeneous immunoglobulin. Most studies on the biosynthesis of immunoglobulins have been carried out using these tumour cell lines.

4.1 Synthesis and Assembly of Four-Chain (H_2L_2) Molecules

It is now well established that immunoglobulin heavy and light chains are synthesized independently on polyribosomes in immune tissue and myeloma cells (Scharff and Uhr, 1965; Askonas and Williamson, 1966; Bevan *et al.*, 1972). This is consistent with genetic evidence, which indicates non-linkage between genes for heavy and light chains. The polyribosomes responsible for heavy and light-chain synthesis sediment at about 300 S and 200 S, respectively. Direct visualization of the polyribosomes by electron microscopy (De Petris, 1970) indicates that heavy and light-chain polyribosomes are composed of 11–18 and four to five ribosomes, respectively. As would be expected, experiments in which myeloma cells are exposed to radiolabelled amino acids for short periods demonstrate sequential growth of the polypeptide chain from the N-terminus (Lennox *et al.*, 1967). The actual time of synthesis is short, being about one minute for a light chain and two minutes for a heavy chain.

Given two genes for one polypeptide chain, integration could be at the DNA, RNA, or protein level. The demonstration of sequential growth of heavy and light chains from the N to the G terminus, however, rules out the last possibility (Lennox *et al.*, 1967). A similar conclusion was drawn from experiments with cell-free systems and a 9–13 S fraction of RNA isolated from a light chain-producing myeloma tumour (Stavnezer and Huang, 1971). An RNA of this size would be sufficient to code for an entire light chain. When added to a cell-free system derived from rabbit reticulocytes, the product synthesized gives pepetides almost identical to the light chains synthesized by the myeloma tumour *in vivo*. The most compelling evidence, however, comes from the work of Milstein and his colleagues (1974*a*) who were able to isolate the mRNA for a light chain in a sufficiently pure form to establish conclusively that it exists as a single molecule. In addition to the poly A sequence of 200 residues and the bases required for specifying the amino acid sequence of the light chain, there are two untranslated base sequences. One of 150 residues is at the 5′-end preceding the V-region sequence, and the other of 200 residues is at the 3′-end interposed between the C-region sequence and the poly A. The function of these untranslated sequences is not known. One obvious possibility is that part of the untranslated sequence ensures that translation occurs on membrane-bound polyribosomes. It is equally possible, however, that the 'extra' RNA sequences control more generalized functions, such as transport from the nucleus. Finally, somatic cell hybrids formed between xenogeneic (Cotton and Milstein, 1973) or syngeneic (Köhler and Milstein, 1975) immunoglobulin-synthesizing cells only produce the parental heavy or light chains. In other words, there is no evidence for scrambling of the C and V regions of heavy and light chains contributed by each of the parental cell lines. Thus, V–C integration cannot possibly result from cytoplasmic events.

The sum total of evidence therefore, strongly points to integration of V and C genes at the level of DNA. What cannot be ruled out formally at present is integration during the transcription of separate V and C genes. This possibility is rather unlikely, however, since there are plasma cells which secrete abnormal heavy chains with part of both the C and V regions deleted (heavy-chain disease) (see Stanworth, Chapter 6). It is difficult to see how such proteins could arise given an integration event at the RNA level. The most probable explanation for heavy-chain disease proteins is that a deletion occurs during or after fusion of V and C genes. On the other hand, it has to be admitted that a suitably large deletion could produce the same result even if the V and C genes were not integrated.

The major impetus for the isolation of mRNA molecules for immunoglobulin is their use as probes for nucleic acid hybridization studies in order to measure directly the size of the V-gene pool. This aspect is discussed by Williamson in this volume (Chapter 5). In the course of establishing the purity of the mRNA (a prerequisite for all hybridization studies), it is usual to examine the product formed when the mRNA is used to programme translation in a cell-free system. A number of workers have made the same interesting observation (Milstein *et al.*, 1972; Swan *et al.*, 1972; Mach *et al.*, 1973; Tonegawa and Baldi, 1973; Schmeckpeper *et al.*, 1974; Green *et al.*, 1975). They have found that the translation product of light-chain mRNA in a cell-free system is larger than the secreted light chain. This enlarged light chain (pro-light chain) is thought to be a precursor to the secreted form. It contains an extra 15–20 amino acids at the N-terminus which are cleaved presumably *in vivo*. The biological significance of the precursor form is not understood, but one suggestion by Milstein *et al.* (1972) is that the extra N-terminal sequence could determine that translation takes place on membrane-bound ribosomes.

In the case of the heavy chain the product of the cell-free system is, if anything, slightly smaller than the secreted form, but it has been argued that a similar situation exists. It has been suggested that, although there is a precursor segment, heavy chain translated in the cell-free system is devoid of carbohydrate (Cowan and Milstein, 1973; Cowan *et al.*, 1973; Green *et al.*, 1975). These two factors would essentially cancel each other out with the consequent similarity in mobility between precursor and secreted heavy chains.

In many, but not all, cases, the synthesis of heavy and light chains is balanced, so that the only secretory product of plasma cells is fully assembled immunoglobulin (Askonas and Williamson, 1969; Baumal and Scharft, 1973a). It would seem likely that this balance is achieved at the transcriptional rather than at the translational level.

The immediate event following the completion of the synthesis of heavy and light chains is their assembly into four-chain structures. In the case of IgA and IgM synthesis, this is followed by the addition of the J chain and the formation of polymeric structures, while for the class of IgA found in the mucosal secretions (sIgA) another polypeptide, the secretory component is added (Tomasi and Grey, 1972). The addition of secretory component takes place after secretion of dimeric IgA molecule from plasma cells, secretory component being synthesized by epithelial cells rather than by plasma cells. Assembly is accompanied or followed by almost invariably the addition of carbohydrate at various points on the polypeptide chain.

In the majority of species in which biosynthetic assembly has been studied, the four-chain structures are held together by both covalent disulphide bridges and non-covalent linkages. It is experimentally feasible to study the former (but not the latter) and to define the order of disulphide bridge formation. This proves to be variable for immunoglobulins as a whole, but is characteristic and constant for a given immunoglobulin class or subclass (Bevan *et al.*, 1972; Baumal and Scharff, 1973a). The first disulphide-linked intermediate formed in the assembly of an H_2L_2 structure can be either H_2 or H–L. Conversion to the four-chain molecule then takes place either by addition of light chains to H_2 or by dimerization of H–L.

In practice, cell suspensions are incubated for relatively short times and then intracellular immunoglobulin and immunoglobulin subunits are isolated and characterized by gel electrophoresis. Absolutely essential, however, is the demonstration that a given Ig subunit is an intermediate in the biosynthesis of the secreted immunoglobulin. To achieve this, pulse–chase experiments are carried out, and then the flow of label from one intermediate to another can be shown. From this type of analysis, it is clear that covalent assembly to the H_2L_2 structure is, like synthesis of the polypeptide chain, relatively rapid, taking between five and 15 minutes.

In the mouse, most IgG is formed *via* the H_2 intermediate, whereas IgM is assembled from HL subunits. The absence of disulphide bonds between the heavy and light chains of mouse IgA means that H_2 is the only possible disulphide bonded intermediate. Interestingly, the pattern of disulphide bridge formation within the cell correlates with the lability of the disulphide bonds to reducing conditions (Bevan *et al.*, 1972). Thus, in molecules which assemble via H–L intermediates the H–H disulphide bond is more susceptible to cleavage by reduction than is the H–L disulphide bridge and *vice versa*. Thus, by simply studying the reduction intermediates of an immunoglobulin, it is possible to predict the biosynthetic pathway.

One should not be misled into thinking that the order of disulphide bond formation between the chains is necessarily the same as the order of interactions of the polypeptide chains. The order of non-covalent chain interaction is more difficult to define. However, a feature of immunoglobulin heavy and light chains is their strong non-covalent interactions, which are strong enough to give a functional, antigen-binding H_2L_2 structure in the absence of covalent linkages. On this basis, then, given a mixture of heavy and light chains within the cell, a reasonable prediction would be the immediate formation of non-covalently linked H_2L_2 entitites. The heavy and light chains being appositely placed would, of course, be favourably positioned for formation of inter-chain disulphide bonds.

4.2 Immunoglobulin Secretion and the Addition of Carbohydrate

The plasma cell is a typical secretory cell with a well-developed endoplasmic reticulum. Typically, such cells secrete only immunoglobulin and yet immunoglobulin accounts for only 20–40 per cent of the total protein manufactured by these cells. The problem that arises, therefore, is how to segregate the immunoglobulin for export from those proteins synthesized for intracellular use. A solution to this question came originally from work with other secretory cells such as pancreatic (Jamieson and Palade, 1967a, b) and hepatic tissue (Campbell, 1970). From this work a general mechanism for secretory cells and a functional role for the endoplasmic reticulum has been established.

In general, molecules destined for secretion are translated on polyribosomes associated with the endoplasmic reticulum. The polypeptide chain is then extruded as it is synthesized into the cysternae of the endoplasmic reticulum (vectorial release), from where it passes to the exterior milieu *via* the golgi apparatus. With this knowledge gained from studies made on other cells, it was then a relatively simple matter to confirm that similar events occurred in the secretion of immunoglobulin.

From a series of meticulously conducted experiments, conclusive evidence has been presented to show that immunoglobulin synthesis occurs on polysomes associated with the endoplasmic reticulum (Ciopi and Lennox, 1973). The vectorial release of immunoglobulin peptides into the cysternae of the rough endoplasmic reticulum has also been demonstrated (Vassalli *et al.*, 1967; Bevan, 1971*a*). Data from cell fractionation, coupled with carbohydrate analysis (Melchers, 1969; Uhr and Schenkein, 1970; Melchers, 1971*a*, Choi *et al.*, 1971*a*, *b*), and electron microscopic autoradiography of galactose-labelled immunoglobulin has shown the passage of immunoglobulin from the rough endoplasmic reticulum to the golgi zone (Zagury *et al.*, 1970). Immunoglobulin probably is associated with membranes during the whole of its intracellular life.

Studies of the transit time for an immunoglobulin to pass from the site of synthesis to the exterior yield estimates which vary according to the myeloma tumour used. An average half-life value is 90–150 minutes. However, some molecules spend only 30 minutes within the cell, while others remain inside for two hours or more (Scharff *et al.*, 1967; Melchers, 1970; Parkhouse, 1971*a*; Choi *et al.*, 1971*a*, *b*). This appears to be the consequence of a large mixing pool of immunoglobulin within the rough endoplasmic reticulum. As a result, attempts to follow the passage of immunoglobulin from the rough endoplasmic reticulum to the golgi apparatus are inherently difficult, although this type of experiment has been performed. The data of Choi *et al.* (1971*a*, *b*) suggest that an immunoglobulin molecule spends about two-thirds of its intracellular life within the rough endoplasmic reticulum and the remaining third in the golgi apparatus.

A major problem, still unsolved, is how to explain the remarkable selectivity of the secretion mechanism. Some authors have speculated that secreted proteins have 'transport-recognition sequences' (Schubert and Cohn, 1968*b*), or that carbohydrate may label the protein for secretion (Eylar, 1966; Melchers and Knopf, 1967). However, amino acid sequential studies have not identified a transport sequence and many proteins, including immunoglobulin light chains, are devoid of carbohydrate and yet are still secreted (Winterburn and Phelps, 1972). The simplest and most likely explanation is that mRNAs for secretory proteins contain a non-translatable nucleotide sequence with an affinity for membrane-bound ribosomes or ribosomal subunits. In murine myeloma cells, newly synthesized 60 S ribosomal subunits bind directly to membranes and the 40 S ribosome–mRNA complex then binds to the membrane-bound 60 S particle (Baglioni *et al.*, 1971). There are, therefore, certain constraints on any proposed model.

During passage of immunoglobulin molecules through the membranous elements of the cell, carbohydrate residues are added at discrete intracellular sites. Whether the carbohydrate is a prerequisite for secretion is not proven conclusively but, as mentioned above, the existence of secreted light chains lacking in carbohydrate is certainly an argument against an obligatory role for carbohydrate in secretion.

Studies on the incorporation of radiolabelled monosaccharides into immunoglobulin have been carried out using normal rabbit lymphoid cells (Swenson and Kern, 1968; Cohen and Kern, 1969), mouse myeloma cells (Melchers, 1970, 1971b; Schenkein and Uhr, 1970; Uhr and Schenkein, 1970; Choi et al., 1971a; Parkhouse and Melchers, 1971; Cowan and Robinson, 1973; Della Corte and Parkhouse, 1973a), and mitogen-stimulated B lymphocytes (Melchers and Andersson, 1973). The rates of appearance of radioactive immunoglobulin inside and outside the cell, in the presence or absence of an inhibitor of protein synthesis, indicate that glucosamine and mannose are added close to the time of synthesis of the polypeptide chains as well as later. However, galactose is added later during passage through the golgi apparatus, while sialic acid and fucose are added close to the time of secretion. The one exception is IgM, in which case galactose is added very close to the time of secretion.

It has been suggested that the 'bridge sugar' N-acetylglucosamine is attached to growing immunoglobulin chains on the polyribosomes (Moroz and Uhr, 1967; Sherr and Uhr, 1969), as has been claimed for the glycoproteins synthesized by rat liver (Molnar et al., 1965; Robinson, 1969). The evidence for this is not conclusive as no special precuations were taken to overcome the problem of the ribosomes absorbing completed immunoglobulin chains. The discovery of a case of human myeloma with both Bence–Jones protein and IgG (Edmundson et al., 1968) bears on this point. Although the Bence–Jones protein and light chain isolated from the intact IgG had the same primary amino acid sequence, carbohydrate was only present on the Bence–Jones protein. This observation is difficult to reconcile with the addition of the bridge sugar to the nascent chain, as also is the presence of carbohydrate on the C_H2 region of only one of the two heavy chains comprising rabbit IgG (Fanger and Smyth, 1972).

4.3 Polymeric Immunoglobulin

A major immunoglobulin observed on the B lymphocyte membrane is IgMs, perhaps reflecting its origins in ontogeny and phylogeny. It is interesting to consider how such a large molecule is assembled and secreted by plasma cells while also functioning as a receptor for antigen on lymphocytes. Based on the possibility that the normal process of assembly and secretion might be arrested at some stage in lymphocytes with surface IgMs, this section will concentrate on terminal events in the biosynthesis of polymeric immunoglobulins. An interesting problem which arises is why secreted IgM is a uniform pentameric product whereas IgA is secreted as a heterogeneous mixture of monomer and polymers.

The most characteristic feature in the assembly of murine polymeric immunoglobulins is the conversion of 7 S (H_2L_2) subunits to polymers just before, or simultaneously with, secretion (Parkhouse and Askonas, 1969; Bevan, 1971b;

Parkhouse, 1971*a*, *b*, 1975; Bargellesi *et al.*, 1972; Buxbaum and Scharft, 1973; Della Corte and Parkhouse, 1973*a*; Parkhouse and Della Corte, 1974). This conclusion is based on the observation that the major species of immunoglobulin found in polymer-secreting plasmacytoma and normal lymphoid cells is the 7 S subunit; the amounts of intracellular polymer are low, if detectable at all. Thus, polymerization of the subunits and exit to the exterior must be closely linked if not simultaneous events. In man, studies with myeloma cells have shown a similar picture for the secretion of IgA (Buxbaum *et al.*, 1974*a*), but a considerable number of human myeloma tumour cells secreting IgM contain easily detectable quantities of the 19 S polymeric form (Buxbaum *et al.*, 1974).

Isolated intracellular 7 S IgMs does not polymerize spontaneously unless first treated with a reducing agent, suggesting that the cysteine residues responsible for inter-subunit linkage are blocked within the cell (Askonas and Parkhouse, 1971). Removal of the block, perhaps with the participation of an enzyme-mediating disulphide interchange, may form the basis of a control mechanism for the final polymerization step. Other events that take place at the time of polymerization, just before secretion of polymeric immunoglobulins, are the incorporation of the J chain into the molecule (Halpern and Coffman, 1972; Parkhouse, 1972) and the addition of terminal carbohydrate residues (Parkhouse and Melchers, 1971; Cowan and Robinson, 1972; Melchers, 1972; Della Corte and Parkhouse, 1973*a*; Melchers and Andersson, 1973; Parkhouse, 1975). The polymerization therefore requires the integration of several defined biochemical events. An interruption at this stage of biosynthesis may establish whether IgM molecules become surface associated rather than being secreted.

Given that the majority of lymphocytes bear surface IgM, key questions to ask concern molecular events following antigenic stimulation. In the study of these processes, the small number of responding cells to a given antigen presents a major problem. However, it is now possible to overcome this difficulty using stimulants that can activate a large number of bone marrow-derived lymphocytes into proliferation and differentiation resulting in IgM-secreting cells (Parkhouse *et al.*, 1972; Melchers and Andersson, 1973). It is to be hoped that biochemical investigations of such inductive systems will lead to an understanding of the molecular mechanism of antigenic stimulation.

In order to explain the control of polymerization, one must consider possible roles for addition of carbohydrate and J chain, an enzyme mediating disulphide interchange, and non-covalent association between subunits.

Carbohydrate does not play a critical role in polymerization because intracellular monomeric forms of IgA and IgM, precursors of the secreted polymers, can be polymerized *in vitro* (Della Corte and Parkhouse, 1973*b*). Since intracellular monomeric subunits have been shown to lack fucose and to be deficient in galactose (Parkhouse and Melchers, 1971; Cowan and Robinson, 1972; Melchers, 1972; Della Corte and Parkhouse, 1973*a*; Melchers and Andersson, 1973; Parkhouse, 1975), addition of these terminal carbohydrate residues is unlikely to be necessary for polymerization. Furthermore, in a murine myeloma secreting monomeric and polymeric forms of IgA, all secreted molecular species have an identical carbohydrate composition (Della Corte and Parkhouse, 1973a).

A mandatory role for J chain (reviewed by Koshland, 1975 and by Inman and Mestecky, 1974) in the assembly of murine polymeric immunoglobulins was shown in a series of experiments in which radiolabelled intracellular or secreted immunoglobulin subunits were polymerized *in vitro* (Della Corte and Parkhouse, 1973b). Both IgA and IgM can be polymerized from subunits previously prepared by reduction of polymeric forms, and from intracellular or secreted monomeric subunits. Monomeric IgM is converted to the pentamer, and monomeric IgA to the dimer. In all cases, polymerization is total, there being no residue of the monomeric form. Polymerization only occurs when both murine J chain and a purified disulphide-interchange enzyme are available. In the absence of the enzyme, and provided that the concentration of immunoglobulin is relatively high, IgM, but not IgA, can be polymerized from subunits prepared by mild reduction (Parkhouse *et al.*, 1970, 1971; Askonas and Parkhouse, 1971). The importance of the disulphide-interchange enzyme is emphasized therefore by the fact that low concentrations of both IgA and IgM subunits can be polymerized in the presence of the enzyme provided that J chain is supplied.

These experiments infer, but do not demonstrate conclusively, a role for the disulphide-interchange enzyme within the intact secreting cell. While it is true that IgM subunits prepared by reduction will polymerize *in vitro* in the absence of J chain (Kownatski, 1973; Eskeland, 1974), it is important to note that the product is not pentameric IgM, but, a mixture of molecular sizes. It must be concluded, therefore, that the J chain is essential for the accurate assembly of IgM molecules.

The J chain is not simply a catalyst since all J chain released from IgM by reductive cleavage is incorporated back into reassembled polymer (Della Corte and Parkhouse, 1973b). On the basis of these experiments, the J chain therefore appears to be an essential structural requirement for polymeric immunoglobulins. However, the possibility of rare exceptions to this rule cannot be excluded. Indeed, a human 19 S myeloma IgM (Eskeland and Brandtzaeg, 1974) and certain fish IgM molecules (Weinheimer *et al.*, 1971) appear to be devoid of J chain. However, such rare exceptions do not prove that J chain is not a structural requirement for polymerization of normal IgM. Similarly, the presence of heavy-chain disease myeloma proteins which do not have light chains does not provide proof that light chains are an optional requirement for fully functional immunoglobulin structures.

A remarkable degree of specificity in polymerization has been demonstrated (Della Corte and Parkhouse, 1973b). Not only do reduced albumin and IgG fail to interfere with polymerization, but IgA and IgM subunits can be reassembled simultaneously into specific polymeric forms without the formation of hybrid molecules. Thus, subunits of IgM cannot interact with subunits of IgA, in spite of the fact that the same J chain can mediate polymerization of both immunoglobulin classes.

Assuming that the J chain travels from its site of synthesis by the same route as heavy and light chains, that is through the membranous elements of the cell, then an important factor in the control of polymerization may be the demonstrated lack of measurable non-covalent interactions between J chain and intracellular 7 S subunits. Further control may be due to the fact that the cysteine residues responsible for inter-subunit disulphide bridging are blocked within the cell, suggesting an obvious role for the disulphide-interchange enzyme. High levels of this enzyme are found in the golgi apparatus and plasma membrane, whereas the enzyme is present in the rough endoplasmic reticulum but is inactive (Williams *et al.*, 1968; Della Corte and Parkhouse, 1973*b*). Therefore, during the passage of immunoglobulin subunits through the rough endoplasmic reticulum formation of polymers would not be expected to occur. Within the golgi vesicles, however, the enzyme is present, and so the failure to find appreciable quantities of intracellular polymer is explained perhaps by a short transit time of 7 S subunits through the golgi apparatus. This suggestion gains credence from the low levels of galactose found attached to intracellular monomers (Parkhouse and Melchers, 1971; Melchers and Andersson, 1973; Parkhouse, 1975) and from the fact that galactosyl transferase is located primarily within the golgi apparatus. On the other hand, there is no experimental evidence to rule out a segregation of J chain from 7 S subunits until the assembly site is reached. It is interesting to speculate that the presence of 19 S IgM within some, but not all, human IgM-secreting myeloma cells (Buxbaum *et al.*, 1971) might be due to a prolonged sojourn of such molecules within the golgi apparatus. If this were true, appreciable amounts of galactose-labelled IgM would be expected within the cells. Alternatively, the occurrence of 19 S IgM intracellularly could result from a derangement of a normal control mechanism which segregates the J chain from 7 S subunits.

An intriguing question is why secreted IgM is essentially all uniform pentamer, whereas IgA is secreted as a heterogeneous mixture of the monomer and polymers. Since it is clear that the IgA-producing cells contain the biochemical machinery necessary for polymerization and since secreted (or intracellular) IgA monomer can be polymerized *in vitro*, it is possible that the amount of intracellular J chain could be a critical factor. That this is indeed the case has been demonstrated by the fact that in cells secreting IgM, the synthesis of J chain and 7 S IgM is balanced normally so that neither is produced in excess. In cells secreting IgA, however, there is a deficiency in J chain, resulting in secretion of the monomeric form (Parkhouse and Della Corte, 1973).

Given the fact that J chain is limiting in IgA-secreting cells, formation of larger polymers similar to IgM might appear to offer an economical use of J chain. However, in murine plasma cell tumour MOPC 315, for example, only about 15 per cent of the secreted IgA is accounted for by molecules larger than the dimer (Della Corte and Parkhouse, 1973*a*). Two clues help to rationalize this problem. The first is the finding that J chain is located as a disulphide 'clasp' between only two monomeric subunits in pentameric IgM (Chapuis and Koshland, 1974) and polymeric IgA (Hauptman and Tomasi, 1975). The second is the demonstration of non-covalent interactions between subunits of IgM produced by reduction and alkylation (Tomasi, 1973; Parkhouse, 1974). Partially reduced and alkylated IgM contains material which sediments at 19 S under non-dissociating conditions, but which is dissociated by sodium dodecyl sulphate into oligomeric material (probably the dimer) and 7 S subunits. Thus, alkylated 7 S IgM can associate with oligomeric IgM through non-covalent forces to form a molecule which sediments at 19 S. In contrast, monomeric and dimeric forms of IgA produced by MOPC 315 cells sediment independently. The obvious conclusion is, therefore, that in the polymerization of both IgA and IgM the initial step is the formation of a dimer with the inclusion of J chain. For IgM, further polymerization is promoted by non-covalent interactions between the dimer and monomeric subunits. In the IgA system, such interactions are presumably infrequent, thus further polymerization is not favoured. An explanation for the degree of polymerization, which is characteristic and stable for a given IgA myeloma protein, should then be sought in the intracellular levels of J chain and in the presence or absence of non-covalent interaction between reduced subunits of large polymers.

The exact mechanism of polymerization has been discussed in detail by Koshland (1975) and by Inman and Mestecky (1974). Basically, the proposals involve interaction between J chain and monomeric subunits, and a succession of disulphide-exchange reactions.

An interesting finding has been the detection of J chain in murine (Kaji and Parkhouse, 1974, 1975; Mossman and Baumal, 1975) and human (Brandtzaeg, 1974) plasma cells not secreting polymeric immunoglobulin. Comparable amounts of J chain were found in murine myeloma cells secreting IgG and polymeric IgA or IgM, although it is absent in marine L cells. It is possible that J chains are degraded within IgG-producing cells, since they cannot be detected in culture supernatants of cells incubated for five hours *in vitro*. Furthermore, J chains are also found in murine myeloma cells which synthesize but do not secrete monomeric IgA. Thus the expression of J chain is not related to secretion of polymeric immunoglobulin or even to secretion itself.

What is the significance of J chain present in myeloma cells secreting IgG? While other interpretations must be considered (for example, that the cells studied are neoplastic), it is possible to speculate that intracellular J chain in IgG-secreting cells represents a relic from a previous commitment to IgM synthesis, which would allow the same progenitor cell line to switch from IgG to IgA synthesis. Such a developmental succession of immunoglobulin-class expression has been postulated by Cooper *et al.* (1972). Accordingly, the genes for heavy and J chain would not be expected to be controlled co-ordinately. This appears to be the case, since J chain has been found in myeloma variants with grossly suppressed synthesis of heavy chains (Kaji and Parkhouse, 1974, 1975; Mosman and Baumal, 1975); in these myelomas the major secretory product is light chains. In a murine myeloma tumour with suppression of both heavy and light-chain synthesis, however, J chain is absent. Whether this means that J and light chain synthesis are under co-ordinate control is difficult to say, due to the aneuploid nature of mouse myeloma cells. More work will have to be done before such a conclusion can be drawn. It is certainly intriguing that J chain is synthesized by cells not producing polymer immunoglobulin, but a full explanation of this observation is not immediately apparent. Interestingly, J chain was not detected in two murine leukaemia cell lines, one T cell-like and the other B cell-like. This stresses the different nature of the stimuli responsible for conversion of lymphocytes to immunological function or neoplastic state.

4.4 Defective Synthesis of Immunoglobulin

The argument of whether the V-gene pool is carried in the germ line or is amplified by somatic variation has prompted a search for variant immunoglobulin arising as a result of mutation in cultures of murine myeloma cells. Thus, a study of somatic mutation in this type of system could help possibly in understanding the generation of antibody diversity. It is equally possible, however, that myeloma cells, being fully differentiated, are not the cells of choice and that precursors of antibody-secreting cells should form the basis of the investigations. This is easy to say but difficult to do, and until there are culture lines of precursor cells there is little hope of tackling this problem.

Given tissue-cultured adapted myeloma cells, the first task is to select variants. Two procedures have been described. In one, myeloma cells are seeded at low cell density in a semi-solid, agar medium (Coffino and Scharff, 1971). Each cell grows into a clonal colony and then the secreted product of each clone is revealed by the application of appropriate antibodies. Most clones continue to secrete immunoglobulin and, as a result, an immune precipitate forms between the clonal product and their anti-immunoglobulin. Some, however, do not secrete immunoglobulin and are recognized by the absence of an immune precipitate using either anti-heavy or anti-light-chain reagents. Others are distinguished by secreting only light chains and this is the most common event observed when IgG-secreting myelomas are screened in this way. The spontaneous loss of heavy-chain expression occurs at the rate of 1×10^{-3} per cell per generation, and this is followed by the loss of light-chain expression at the rate of $4 \cdot 5 \times 10^{-4}$ per cell per generation (Baumal et al., 1973). When mutagens are added to the cell cultures, the rate of change increases and occasionally altered heavy chains (for example with a C-terminal deletion) are found (Preud'homme et al., 1973; Birshtein et al., 1974). In such cases, it is probable that a mutation event is responsible for the phenotypic change. Alternative explanations, such as post-transcriptional defects or activation of a previously unexpressed gene cannot be ruled out formally. Not all non-secreting clones have ceased to synthesize immunoglobulin (Cowan et al., 1974). Both heavy and light chains can be found intracellularly although no secretion takes place. In addition, several examples are available of spontaneously occurring or mutagen-induced myeloma cell variants which synthesize heavy chains in the absence of light chains, but which do not secrete them. The heavy chains may be as large as those of the parental cell, but sometimes they are smaller. In one study by Cowan et al. (1974), the absence of light-chain synthesis was attributed to a defective mRNA for the light chain.

An alternative approach for recognizing variants arising in cultures of myeloma cells has been used by Milstein and his colleagues (Cotton *et al.*, 1973). In this method, the clones are selected randomly and the presence or absence of secreted and intracellular immunoglobulin is screened by isoelectric focusing of cells or culture supernatants of $[^{14}C]$ lysine cultures. The major advantage of this procedure is that small variants in both the V and C regions might be recognized by the screening procedure. Again, non-secreting variants and cells secreting short heavy chains have been identified (Secher *et al.*, 1973; Cowan *et al.*, 1974; Milstein *et al.*, 1974b). One major difference in this system is the failure to detect variants secreting only light chains, which is particularly difficult to understand since myeloma tumours secreting either excess light chains or light chains only are observed frequently in mice (Potter, 1972; Baumel and Scharff, 1973b) and in man (Osserman and Takatsoki, 1963). The non-secreting variants are interesting as they all contain a heavy chain shorter than the parental type. To discover the exact structural lesion would be a formidable task, since only very small quantities are available for characterization. The altered heavy chains which are secreted result from deletions, either internally or at the C terminus.

Perhaps the most disappointing feature of this work is the failure to find any alterations in the V regions. With more variants available for analysis it is possible that some will arise. In addition, and although the numbers are small, the frequency of mutations that are best accounted for by chain-termination events are much higher than those explained by substitutions; this would not be expected from simple random point mutations. Of course, the detection of one or a few amino acid substitutions in an immunoglobulin molecule is much more difficult than the detection of gross size differences due to deletions; thus, the distinction may be more apparent than real.

Defective immunoglobulin synthesis is not infrequent in cases of multiple myeloma in man (see Stanworth, Chapter 6). As mentioned previously, one of the most common defects is production of excess light chains. It is arguable whether this represents the normal situation in murine lymphoid tissue; opinions and results vary on this issue. For example, Askonas and Williamson (1967a, b), and Askonas (1974) stress that in normal lymphoid tissue the synthesis of heavy and light chains is balanced so that the only secretory product is fully assembled immunoglobulin. In contrast Baumal and Scharff (1973b) argue that, while synthesis of heavy and light chains can be balanced in normal lymphoid tissue, there is almost invariably some excess light chain produced. Analysis of a large number of murine myeloma tumours has shown that most secrete excess light chains. Some, however, are balanced with respect to heavy and light-chain synthesis, whereas others synthesize excess light chain but do not secrete it (Baumal and Scharff, 1973b). When production of excess light chain does occur in a myeloma tumour it may result from unbalanced synthesis of heavy and light chains within all the cells of the tumour (Parkhouse, 1971a, b; Baumal and Scharff, 1973), or from the presence of variants secreting only light chains (Schubert and Cohn, 1968a). In normal lymphoid tissue, the absence of cells containing only light chains (Cebra, 1969) would argue that excess light-chain production, when it occurs, results from unbalanced synthesis of heavy and light chains rather than the presence of variants secreting solely light chains.

In many examples of human myelomatosis, expression of genes for heavy chains is suppressed completely and only light chains are produced. These chains are found characteristically in the urine as Bence–Jones protein. Similarly, myelomas secreting abnormal heavy chains have been described (Seligmann *et al.*, 1969; Frangione and Franklin, 1973).

5 HYBRID CELLS

Hybridization of immunoglobulin-producing cells offers the possibility of analysing some of the problems of gene expression. For example, it may be possible to show unequivocally that V and C genes cannot be transcribed on separate mRNAs (Cotton and Milstein, 1973; Köhler and Milstein, 1975). In general, somatic cell hybrids formed between immunoglobulin-producing cell lines and fibroblasts produce little, if any, immunoglobulin (Periman, 1970; Coffino *et al.*, 1971). At present one cannot conclude that immunoglobulin synthesis has been switched off under the influence of the fibroblast partner in the hybrid. Careful karyotype analysis is required to ensure that the myeloma chromosome(s) carrying the information for immunoglobulin is present in the hybrid cell. When murine myeloma cells have been fused with peripheral human lymphocytes not forming detectable immunoglobulins, the resultant hybrid secrete both murine and human immunoglobulins (Schwaber and Cohen, 1974). Assuming that the human contribution to the hybrids is definitely non-secreting lymphocytes (which has not been established critically), then lymphocytes can be turned on to immunoglobulin synthesis by fusion with high-rate immunoglobulin-secreting cells.

Fusion of immunoglobulin producing cells in xenogeneic (Cotton and Milstein, 1973), allogeneic (Bloom and Nakamura, 1974) or syngeneic (Köhler and Milstein, 1975) combinations give hybrid cells which secrete immunoglobulin of both parental types. Analysis of the products shows that, while random assortment of the heavy and light chains can occur, there is no evidence for scrambling V and C regions.

The most spectacular hybridization system is one in which spleen cells from mice primed to sheep erythrocytes are hybridized with murine myeloma cells from the same strain (BALB/c) (Köhler and Milstein, 1975). Hybrids are formed at quite high frequency and secrete, in addition to the myeloma protein, specific antibody to the sheep red blood cells. Although most, if not all, heavy-chain classes are represented in the antibody secreted by a mixture of hybrids, upon cloning only one isotope is expressed by a given isolate. There is, therefore, the possibility of preparing hybrid clones secreting specific antibody of all the known heavy-chain classes. Furthermore, since the fusion has been conducted between syngeneic cells, one of which is a myeloma cell, the hybrid can be transplanted serially in mice. Köhler and Milstein (1975) noted that it should be a relatively simple matter to prepare similar hybrids which do not secrete the myeloma protein, either by using a non-immunoglobulin-producing myeloma variant for hybridization or by selecting hybrids which do not express the myeloma protein. In addition, the antibody specificity can, of course, be selected simply by what is injected into the mouse prior to preparation of the spleen cells for the hybridization.

REFERENCES

Abney, E. R., Hunter, I. R., and Parkhouse, R. M. E. (1976). *Nature (Lond.)*, in press.

Abney, E. R., and Parkhouse, R. M. E. (1974). *Nature (Lond.)*, **252**, 600.

Askonas, B. A. (1974). *Ann. Immunol. (Inst. Pasteur)*, **125**, 253.

Askonas, B. A., and Parkhouse, R. M. E. (1971). *Biochem. J.*, **123**, 629.

Askonas, B. A., and Williamson, A. R. (1966). *Proc. Roy. Soc., Ser. B*, **166**, 232.

Askonas, B. A., and Williamson, A. R. (1967a). *Nobel Symposium*, Vol. **3**, (Killander, J., ed.), John Wiley and Sons, London, p. 369.

Askonas, B. A., and Williamson, A. R. (1967b). *Cold Spring Harbor Symp. Quant. Biol.*, **32**, 223.

Askonas, B. A., and Williamson, A. R. (1969). *Antibiot. Chemother.*, **15**, 64.

Baglioni, C., Bleiberg, I., and Zauderer, M. (1971). *Nature, New Biol.*, **232**, 8.

Bailey, L. K., Hannestad, K., and Eisen, H. N. (1973). *Fed. Proc.*, **32**, 1013.

Bargellesi, A., Periman, P., and Scharff, M. D. (1972). *J. Immunol.*, **108**, 126.

Baumal, R., Birshtein, B. K., Coffino, P., and Scharff, M. D. (1973). *Science, N.Y.*, **182**, 164.

Baumal, R., and Scharff, M. D. (1973a). *Transplant. Rev.*, **14**, 163.

Baumal, R., and Scharff, M. D. (1973b). *J. Immunol.*, **111**, 448.

Bevan, M. J. (1971a). *Biochem. J.*, **122**, 5.

Bevan, M. J. (1971b). *Eur. J. Immunol.*, **1**, 133.

Bevan, M. J., Parkhouse, R. M. E., Williamson, A. R., and Askonas, B. A. (1972). *Prog. Biophys. Mol. Biol.*, **25**, 131.

Birshtein, B. K., Preud'homme, J.-L., and Scharff, M. D. (1974). *Proc. Nat. Acad. Sci., U.S.A.*, **71**, 3478.

Bloom, A. D., and Nakamura, F. T. (1974). *Proc. Nat. Acad. Sci., U.S.A.*, **71**, 2689.

Brandtzaeg, P. (1974). *Nature, (Lond.)*, **252**, 418.

Buxbaum, J. N., and Scharff, M. D. (1973). *J. Exp. Med.*, **138**, 278.

Buxbaum, J. N., Zolla, S., Scharff, M. D., and Franklin, E. C. (1971). *J. Exp. Med.*, **133**, 1118.

Buxbaum, J. N., Zolla, S., Scharff, M. D., and Franklin, E. C. (1974). *Eur. J. Immunol.*, **5**, 367.

Campbell, P. N. (1970). *FEBS Letters*, **7**, 1.

Capra, J. D., and Kethoe, J. M. (1975). *Adv. Immunol.*, **20**, 1.

Cebra, J. J. (1969). *Bacteriol. Rev.*, **33**, 159.

Chapuis, R. M., and Koshland, M. E. (1974). *Proc. Nat. Acad. Sci., U.S.A.*, **71**, 657.

Choi, Y. S., Knopf, P. M., and Lennox, E. S. (1971a). *Biochemistry*, **10**, 659.

Choi, Y. S., Knopf, P. M., and Lennox, E. S. (1971b). *Biochemistry*, **10**, 668.

Ciopi, D., and Lennox, E. S. (1973). *Biochemistry*, **12**, 3211.

Coffino, P., and Scharff, M. D. (1971). *Proc. Nat. Acad. Sci., U.S.A.*, **68**, 219.

Coffino, P., Knowles, B., Nathenson, S. G., and Scharff, M. D. (1971). *Nature, New Biol.*, **231**, 87.

Cohen, H. J., and Kern, M. (1969). *Biochim. Biophys. Acta*, **188**, 255.

Cone, R. E., Marchalonis, J. J., and Rolley, R. T. (1971). *J. Exp. Med.*, **134**, 1373.

Cooper, M. D., Lawton, A. R., and Kincade, P. W. (1972). *Clin. Exp. Immunol.*, **11**, 143.
Cooper, M. D., Peterson, R. D., South, M. A., and Good, R. A. (1966). *J. Exp. Med.*, **123**, 75.
Cotton, R. G. H., and Milstein, C. (1973). *Nature, (Lond.)*, **244**, 42.
Cotton, R. G. H., Secher, D. S., and Milstein, C. (1973). *Eur. J. Immunol.*, **3**, 135.
Cowan, N. J., Harrison, T. M., Browlee, G. G., and Milstein, C. (1973). *Biochem. Soc. Trans.*, **1**, 1247.
Cowan, N. J., and Milstein, C. (1973). *Eur. J. Biochem.*, **36**, 1.
Cowan, N. J., and Robinson, G. B. (1972). *Biochem. J.*, **126**, 751.
Cowan, N. J., Secher, D. S., and Milstein, C. (1974). *J. Mol. Biol.*, **90**, 691.

Della Corte, E., and Parkhouse, R. M. E. (1973*a*). *Biochem. J.*, **136**, 589.
Della Corte, E., and Parkhouse, R. M. E., (1973*b*). *Biochem. J.*, **136**, 597.
De Petris, S. (1970). *Biochem. J.*, **118**, 385.

Edmundson, A. B., Sheber, F. A., Ely, K. R., Simonds, N. B., Hutson, N. K., and Rossiter, J. L. (1968). *Archs. Biochem. Biophys.*, **127**, 725.
Eskeland, T. (1974). *Scand. J. Immunol.*, **3**, 757.
Eskeland, T., and Brandtzaeg, P. (1974). *Immunochemistry*, **11**, 161.
Eylar, E. H. (1966). *J. Theoret. Biol.*, **10**, 89.

Fanger, M. W., and Smyth, D. G. (1972). *Biochem. J.*, **127**, 767.
Frangione, B., and Franklin, E. C. (1973). *Semin. Haematol.*, **10**, 53.
Fu, S. M., Winchester, R. J., and Kunkel, H. G. (1975). *J. Immunol.*, **114**, 250.
Fudenberg, H. H., and Warner, N. L. (1970). *Adv. Human Genet.*, **1**, 131.

Gally, J. A., and Edelman, G. M. (1972). *Ann. Rev. Genet.*, **6**, 1.
Gershon, R. K. (1975). *Transplant. Rev.*, **26**, 170.
Green, M., Graves, P. N., Zehavi-Willner, T., McInnes, J., and Pestka, S. (1975). *Proc. Nat. Acad. Sci., U.S.A.*, **72**, 224.

Halpern, M. S., and Coffman, R. L. (1972). *J. Immunol.*, **109**, 674.
Hauptman, S. P., and Tomasi, T. B. (1975). *J. Biol. Chem.*, **250**, 3891.
Herzenberg, L. A., McDevitt, H. O., and Herzenberg, L. A. (1968). *Ann. Rev. Genet.*, **2**, 209.
Hood, L., Campbell, J. M., and Elgin, S. C. R. (1975). *Ann. Rev. Genet.*, **9**, 305.

Inman, F. P., and Mestecky, J. (1974). In *Contemporary Topics in Immunochemistry*, Vol. 3, (Ada, G. L., ed.), Plenum Press, New York, p. 111.

Jamieson, J. D., and Palade, G. E. (1967*a*). *J. Cell. Biol.*, **34**, 577.
Jamieson, J. D., and Palade, G. E. (1967*b*). *J. Cell. Biol.*, **34**, 597.
Jones, P. P., Cebra, J. J., and Herzenberg, L. A. (1974*a*). *J. Exp. Med.*, **139**, 581.
Jones, P. P., Craig, S. W., Cebra, J. J., and Herzenberg, L. A. (1974*b*). *J. Exp. Med.*, **140**, 452.

Kaji, H., and Parkhouse, R. M. E. (1974). *Nature, (Lond.)*, **249**, 45.
Kaji, H., and Parkhouse, R. M. E. (1975). *J. Immunol.*, **114**, 1218.
Kinkade, P. W., Lawton, A. R., Buckman, D. E., and Cooper, M. D. (1970). *Proc. Nat. Acad. Sci., U.S.A.*, **67**, 1918.
Knapp, W., Bolhuis, R. L. H., Radl, J., and Hijmans, W. (1973). *J. Immunol.*, **111**, 1295.
Köhler, G., and Milstein, C. (1975). *Nature, (Lond.)*, **256**, 495.
Koshland, M. E. (1975). *Adv. Immunol.*, **20**, 41.
Kownatski, E. (1973). *Immunol. Commun.*, **2**, 105.

Kurnick, J. T., and Grey, H. M. (1975). *J. Immunol.*, **115**, 305.

Lennox, E. S., and Cohn, M. (1967). *Ann. Rev. Biochem.*, **36**, 365.
Lennox, E. S., Knopf, P. M., Munro, A. J., and Parkhouse, R. M. E. (1967). *Cold Spring Harbor Symp. Quant. Biol.*, **32**, 249.

Mach, B., Faust, C., and Vassalli, P. (1973). *Proc. Nat. Acad. Sci., U.S.A.*, **70**, 451.
Mage, R. G. (1975). *Fed. Proc.*, **34**, 40.
Mäkelä, O., and Cross, A. M. (1970). *Prog. Allergy*, **14**, 145.
Marchalonis, J. J., Cone, R. E., and Atwell, J. L. (1972). *J. Exp. Med.*, **135**, 956.
Marchalonis, J., and Edelman, G. M. (1965). *J. Exp. Med.*, **122**, 601.
Melcher, U., Vitetta, E. S., McWilliams, M., Lamm, M. E., Philips-Quagliata, J. M., and Uhr, J. W. (1974). *J. Exp. Med.*, **146**, 1427.
Melchers, F. (1969). *Biochemistry*, **8**, 938.
Melchers, F. (1970). *Biochem. J.*, **119**, 765.
Melchers, F. (1971*a*). *Biochemistry*, **10**, 653.
Melchers, F. (1971*b*). *Biochem. J.*, **125**, 241.
Melchers, F. (1972). *Biochemistry*, **11**, 2204.
Melchers, F., and Andersson, J. (1973). *Transplant. Rev.*, **14**, 76.
Melchers, F., and Knopf, P. M. (1967). *Cold Spring Harbor Symp. Quant. Biol.*, **32**, 255.
Melchers, F., von Boehmer, H., and Philips, R. A. (1975). *Transplant. Rev.*, **25**, 26.
Miller, J. F. A., and Mitchell, G. F. (1969). *Transplant. Rev.*, **1**, 3.
Milstein, C., and Munro, A. J. (1970). *Ann. Rev. Microbiol.*, **24**, 335.
Milstein, C., and Pink, J. R. L. (1970). *Prog. Biophys. Mol. Biol.*, **21**, 209.
Milstein, C., Adetugbo, K., Cowan, N. J., and Secher, D. S. (1974*a*). In *Progress in Immunology II*, Vol. I, (Brent, L., and Holborrow, J., eds.), North Holland Publishing Co., Amsterdam, p. 157.
Milstein, C., Brownlee, C. G., Cartwright, E. M., Jarvis, J. M., and Proudfoot, N. J. (1974*b*). *Nature*, (*Lond.*), **252**, 354.
Milstein, C., Brownlee, G. G., Harrison, T. M., and Mathews, M. B. (1972). *Nature, New Biol.*, **239**, 117.
Mitchison, N. A. (1971). *Eur. J. Immunol.*, **1**, 10.
Molnar, J., Robinson, G. B., and Winzler, R. J. (1965). *J. Biol. Chem.*, **240**, 1882.
Moroz, C., and Uhr, J. W. (1967). *Cold Spring Harbor Symp. Quant. Biol.*, **32**, 263.
Morrison, S. L., and Scharff, M. D. (1975). *J. Immunol.*, **114**, 655.
Mosmann, T., and Baumal, R. (1975). *J. Immunol.*, **115**, 955.

Osserman, E. F., and Takatsoki, K. (1963). *Medicine*, **42**, 357.

Parkhouse, R. M. E. (1971*a*). *Biochem. J.*, **123**, 635.
Parkhouse, R. M. E. (1971*b*). *FEBS Letters*, **16**, 71.
Parkhouse, R. M. E. (1972). *Nature, New Biol.*, **236**, 9.
Parkhouse, R. M. E. (1974). *Immunology*, **27**, 1063.
Parkhouse, R. M. E. (1975). *Transplant. Rev.*, **14**, 131.
Parkhouse, R. M. E., and Askonas, B. A. (1969). *Biochem. J.*, **115**, 163.
Parkhouse, R. M. E.. Askonas, B. A., and Dourmashkin, R. R. (1970). *Immunology*, **18**, 575.
Parkhouse, R. M. E., and Della Corte, E. (1973). *Biochem. J.*, **136**, 607.
Parkhouse, R. M. E., and Della Corte, E. (1974). In *The Immunoglobulin A System*, (Mestecky, J., and Lawton, A. R., eds.), Plenum Press, New York, p. 139.
Parkhouse, R. M. E., Hunter, I. R., and Abney, E. R. (1976). *Immunology*, **30**, 409.
Parkhouse, R. M. E., Janossy, G., and Greaves, M. F. (1972). *Nature, New Biol.*, **235**, 21.
Parkhouse, R. M. E., and Melchers, F. (1971). *Biochem. J.*, **125**, 235.

Parkhouse, R. M. E., Virella, G., and Dourmashkin, R. R. (1971). *Clin. Exp. Immunol.*, **8**, 581.

Periman, P. (1970). *Nature, (Lond.)*, **228**, 1086.

Pernis, B., Brouet, J. C., and Seligman, M. (1974). *Eur. J. Immunol.*, **4**, 776.

Pink, J. R. L., Wang, A.-C., and Fudenberg, H. H. (1971). *Ann. Rev. Med.*, **22**, 145.

Potter, M. (1967). *Meth. Cancer Res.*, **2**, 105.

Potter, M. (1972). *Physiol. Rev.*, **52**, 631.

Preud'homme, J.-L., Buxbaum, J. N., and Scharff, M. D. (1973). *Nature, (Lond.)*, **245**, 320.

Putnam, F. W., Florent, G., Paul, C., Shinoda, U., and Shimizu, A. (1973). *Science, N.Y.*, **182**, 287.

Raff, M. C., Sternberg, M., and Taylor, R. B. (1970). *Nature, (Lond.)*, **225**, 553.

Robinson, G. B. (1969). *Biochem. J.*, **115**, 1077.

Rowe, D. S., Hug, K., Forni, L., and Pernis, B. (1973). *J. Exp. Med.*, **138**, 965.

Salsano, P., Froland, S. S., Natvig, J. B., and Michaelsen, T. E. (1974). *Scand. J. Immunol.*, **3**, 841.

Secher, D. S., Cotton, R. G. H., and Milstein, C. (1973). *FEBS Letters*, **37**, 311.

Seligman, M., Mihaesco, E., Hurez, D., Mihaesco, C., Preud'homme, J.-L., and Rambaud, J.-C. (1969). *J. Clin. Invest.*, **48**, 2374.

Scharff, M. D., Shapiro, A. L., and Ginsberg, B. (1967). *Cold Spring Harbor Symp. Quant. Biol.*, **32**, 235.

Scharff, M. D., and Uhr, J. W. (1965). *Science, N.Y.*, **148**, 646.

Schenkein, J., and Uhr, J. W. (1970). *J. Cell. Biol.*, **46**, 42.

Schmeckpeper, B. J., Cory, J., and Adams, J. M. (1974). *Mol. Biol. Reps.*, **1**, 355.

Schubert, D., and Cohn, M. (1968a). *J. Mol. Biol.*, **38**, 263.

Schubert, D., and Cohn, M. (1968b). *J. Mol. Biol.*, **38**, 273.

Schwaber, J., and Cohen, E. P. (1974). *Proc. Nat. Acad. Sci., U.S.A.*, **71**, 2203.

Sherr, C. J., and Uhr, J. W. (1969). *Proc. Nat. Acad. Sci., U.S.A.*, **64**, 381.

Solomon, A., and Kunkel, H. G. (1967). *A. J. Med.*, **42**, 958.

Stavnezer, J., and Huang, R. C. C. (1971). *Nature, New Biol.*, **230**, 172.

Strayer, D. S., Vitetta, E. S., and Köhler, H. (1975). *J. Immunol.*, **114**, 722.

Swan, D., Aviv, H., and Leder, P. (1972). *Proc. Nat. Acad. Sci., U.S.A.*, **69**, 1967.

Swenson, R. M., and Kern, M. (1968). *Proc. Nat. Acad. Sci., U.S.A.*, **59**, 546.

Tada, T., Taniguchi, M., and Takemori, T. (1975). *Transplant. Rev.*, **26**, 106.

Tomasi, T. B. (1973). *Proc. Nat. Acad. Sci., U.S.A.*, **70**, 3410.

Tomasi, T. B., and Grey, H. M. (1972). *Prog. Allergy*, **16**, 81.

Tonegawa, S., and Baldi, I. (1973). *Biochem. Biophys. Res. Commun.*, **51**, 81.

Uhr, J. W., and Schenkein, I. (1970). *Proc. Nat. Acad. Sci., U.S.A.*, **66**, 952.

Vassalli, P., Lisowska-Bernstein, B., Lamm, M. E., and Benacerraf, B. (1967). *Proc. Nat. Acad. Sci., U.S.A.*, **58**, 2422.

Vitetta, E. S., Baur, S., and Uhr, J. W. (1971). *J. Exp. Med.*, **134**, 242.

Vitetta, E. S., Melcher, U., McWilliams, M., Lamm, M. E., Philips-Quagliata, J. M., and Uhr, J. W. (1975). *J. Exp. Med.*, **147**, 206.

Vitetta, E. S., and Uhr, J. W. (1972). *J. Exp. Med.*, **136**, 676.

Vitetta, E. S., and Uhr, J. W. (1973). *Transplant. Rev.*, **14**, 50.

Vitetta, E. S., and Uhr, J. W. (1974). *J. Exp. Med.*, **139**, 1599.

Walters, C. S., and Wigzell, H. (1970). *J. Exp. Med.*, **132**, 1233.

Weinheimer, P. F., Mestecky, J., and Acton, R. T. (1971). *J. Immunol.*, **107**, 1211.

Williams, D. J., Gurari, D., and Rabin, B. R. (1968). *FEBS Letters*, **2**, 133.

Williamson, A. R. (1976). *Ann. Rev. Biochem.*, **45**, 467.

Winchester, R. J., Fu, S. M., Hoffman, T., and Kunkel, H. G. (1975). *J. Immunol.*, **114**, 1210.

Winterburn, P. J., and Phelps, C. F. (1972). *Nature*, (*Lond.*), **236**, 147.

Zagury, D., Uhr, J. W., Jamieson, J. D., and Palade, G. E. (1970). *J. Cell. Biol.*, **46**, 52.

CHAPTER 4

Genetics of Immunoglobulins

J. A. Sogn and T. J. Kindt

1 INTRODUCTION

An individual is capable of synthesizing a large number of antibody molecules, each with a different specificity for one of the many antigens encountered in its lifetime. A major problem in immunogenetics concerns the nature of the genes which direct the synthesis of this large array of molecules. Basic questions concerning the genetic origin of antibody diversity are discussed in this volume by Williamson (see Chapter 5). Although many questions remain unanswered, there exists a body of experimental data which gives an indication of the nature of the antibody genes. In this chapter, studies on the immunogenetic markers of immunoglobulins, allotypes and more recently idiotypes, which have contributed to the majority of these data will be discussed.

Allotypes have been defined as intraspecies antigenic determinants present on immunoglobulins. Many of these serologically detected markers for immunoglobulins have been shown to correlate with variations in amino acid sequence and, therefore, may be considered as markers for primary gene products. Idiotypes, which may be considered antigenic markers for antibody binding sites, have been found in recent studies similarly to correlate with primary structure. With an increase in the amount of sequence data available, non-antigenic, structurally defined markers are being recognized, thus adding significantly to the allotypes and idiotype data.

Studies on allotype inheritance have supplied specific information such as the autosomal codominant nature of immunoglobulin genes (Oudin, 1960a, b) and the absence of linkage relationships between antibody heavy and light-chain allotypes (Dubiski et al., 1962). In addition to this specific information, these studies have yielded results that have implications beyond the field of immunoglobulin inheritance. The presence of common V-region genetic markers on immunoglobulin heavy chains of different classes has opened the possibility that two or more genes interact prior to the synthesis of a complete heavy chain (Feinstein, 1963; Todd, 1963; Kindt and Todd, 1969). These associations of rabbit V_H allotypes with different immunoglobulin classes suggest an exception to the 'one gene—one polypeptide chain' axiom. Similarly, the observation that antibody-producing cells synthesize only one of the two possible immunoglobulin alleles (Pernis et al., 1965; Weiler, 1965) provided the first example of allelic exclusion for an autosomal trait. While allelic exclusion has been observed for X-linked characteristics (Lyon, 1961), these observations suggested a more general occurrence of this phenomenon.

The majority of the immunogenetic studies to be discussed here has been carried out using rabbit and mouse allotypes and idiotypes; these systems will be briefly described. Structural data available concerning allotypic correlates will be emphasized. Detailed reviews covering allotypy in these species have appeared recently (Mage et al., 1973; Kindt, 1975). Much important immunogenetic information has come from studies of human allotypes, but these will not be discussed directly. For a thorough review of human allotypy, the reader is referred to an article by Natvig and Kunkel (1973). Rat allotypes will not be considered, although recent descriptions of the classes, structures, and allotypes of rat immunoglobulins indicate that this system might provide valuable material for future immunogenetic studies (Bazin et al., 1973, 1974a, b; Nezlin et al., 1974).

Linkage relationships between the allotypes and idiotypes within the rabbit or the mouse system will be delineated, and an attempt will be made to integrate these data into a current picture of the nature and interrelationship of the genes controlling antibody synthesis. The phenomenon of allelic exclusion as it exists in immunoglobulin-producing cells will be described and compared to the more fully characterized phenomenon of X-chromosome inactivation in females. A model, proposed by Riggs (1975) for X-chromosome inactivation, will be considered in this context.

The discussion of allotypes as genetic markers normally proceeds under the assumption that the immunoglobulin allotype genes are allelic structural genes. Recently, however, several reports have described deviations from simple allelic behaviour for allotypes (Bosma and Bosma, 1974; Strosberg et al., 1974; Mudgett et al., 1975). Possible explanations for this behaviour will be considered, along with their implications for current concepts of immunoglobulin genetics.

2 EXPERIMENTAL ALLOTYPIC SYSTEMS

Well-established and long-studied allotypic systems exist in man, rabbit, and mouse. Each system has unique features of interest and has provided key information in the development of current concepts of immunogenetics. The ready availability of human Bence–Jones and myeloma proteins at an early stage in the study of immunoglobulin structure and genetics made them the source of many key initial observations. Particularly significant in this respect were the discoveries that heavy and light chains are under independent genetic control (Harboe et al., 1962a; Franklin et al., 1962) and that light chains themselves are under the control of at least two genes (Hilschmann and Craig, 1965). Although the human system remains a productive one, technical advances in the ability to manipulate responses in the rabbit and the mouse, combined with the obvious advantages of working with experimental animals, have made the latter systems currently very attractive.

2.1 Allotypes of the Rabbit

At present, the major importance of the rabbit in immunogenetic studies rests on the variety and multiplicity of allotypes which have been described for rabbit immunoglobulins (Mage et al., 1973; Kindt, 1975). Allotypes are available for each region of the molecule with the exception of the V_L region, and preliminary studies indicate that there may be suitable markers for this region (Thunberg et al., 1973). An area of active interest which will be emphasized here is the correlation of allotype with primary structure.

Although rabbit myeloma proteins have not been available for use in structural studies, an adequate substitute became available when injection with bacterial vaccines was shown to induce homogeneous antibody in large quantities (Krause, 1970). Bacterial injections are now being used to obtain homogeneous rabbit antibodies and amino acid sequential data are rapidly becoming available (Chen et al., 1974; Fleischman, 1971; Jaton, 1974a, b; Margolies et al., 1974). Inbred strains of rabbits have been developed and work has begun on histocompatibility antigens (Chai, 1974; Cohen and Tissot, 1974; Tissot and Cohen, 1974). These developments will enhance the value of the rabbit in future immunogenetic studies.

2.1.1 Immunoglobulins of the Rabbit

Five heavy-chain classes have been described for the rabbit. These are IgG, IgA1, IgA2, IgM, and IgE. There is some evidence for the existence of subclasses of IgG, but these have not been described in detail (Florent *et al.*, 1973).

The rabbit IgG molecule is different from that of human and mouse in several respects. Figure 1 depicts a molecule of rabbit IgG with κ light chains, indicating the disulphide bridges and the various regions of the heavy and light chains. Rabbit light chains may be either κ or λ type; the former comprises more than 90 per cent of the chains in normal circulation. The majority of rabbit κ light chains has seven half-cystine residues (K_B subtype) (Reisfeld *et al.*, 1968). There is a second smaller population of κ chains which has five half-cystine residues (K_A subtype) (deVries *et al.*, 1969; Rejnek *et al.*, 1969; Zikan *et al.*, 1967).

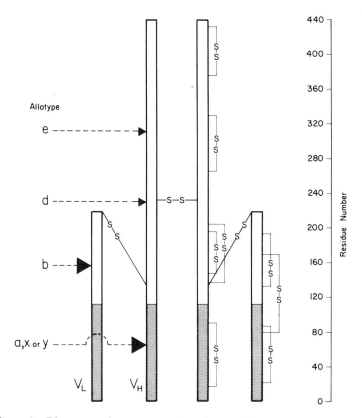

Figure 1 Diagrammatic representation of a rabbit IgG with a K_B light chain. The rabbit light chain differs from the human in having a third disulphide bridge, linking the C_L and V_L domains (Poulsen *et al.*, 1972). The $C_H I$ domain also has an additional intra-chain disulphide bridge and there is only one inter-heavy chain disulphide bond (O'Donnell *et al.*, 1970). The general locations of the known correlates of the various IgG allotypes are shown to the left

Variable region subgroups of κ chains have been described by N-terminal sequential analysis of the chains from homogeneous antibodies to streptococcal carbohydrate (Hood *et al.*, 1970). There is evidence for the existence of at least six κ subgroups (Kindt *et al.*, 1974; Thunberg and Kindt, unpublished results).

2.1.2 Rabbit Allotypes

Rabbit allotypes were first described by Oudin (1956), who coined the name for these intraspecies antigenic determinants. Table 1 summarizes the major allotypic specificities of the rabbit. These specificities will be discussed in more detail below.

Table 1   Major allotypes of rabbit immunoglobulins*

Molecular location	Allotypic group	Allotypes	Correlates
H Chain			
V Region	a	1, 2, 3	complex, see text
	x	32	not known
	y	33	not known
C Region-IgG	d	11, 12	d11-methionine (225)
			d12-threonine (225)
	e	14, 15	e14-threonine (309)
			e15-alanine (309)
C Region-IgA	f	68, 70, 71, 72, 73	not known
C Region-IgA	g	74, 75, 76, 77	not known
C Region-IgM	n	81, 82	not known
κL Chain			
C Region	b	4, 5, 6, 9	complex, see text
λL Chain			
C Region	c	7, 21	not known
Secretory component	t	61, 62	not known

* For complete references, see Kindt (1975)

Rabbit allotypic determinants are expressed by a small letter designating the group (or locus) followed by a number for the allele. The original proposal for the allotype nomenclature (Dray *et al.*, 1962) included an A before every notation (for example, Aa1, Ab4), but it is usual to omit this. A unique number is assigned to each allotype. Phenotypes are written with an oblique stroke separating the groups, such as a1a2/b4/d11d12. Genotypes are written with the alleles as superscripts, for example, $a^1a^2/b^4b^4/d^{11}d^{12}$. Allotypes not assigned to a group are written with an A preceding the number. For instance, the early reports of allotypes d11 and d12 would have referred to them as A11 and A12.

2.1.3 Structural Correlates of Allotypes

The validity of allotypes as genetic markers rests on the supposition that they are primary gene products. That is to say, the differences that the allotypic antisera recognize must reside in the primary structure of the immunoglobulin. Correlation of primary structure with allotypy is rather more complicated than a superficial examination of the problem would indicate (Todd, 1972). Detection of structural differences in allotypically different proteins is not proof that these are the differences which give rise to allotypic determinant. Furthermore, several kinds of variations other than allotypic variations have been described for antibody chains, including class, subclass, subgroup, and the binding site-associated hypervariable regions. Each type of variation must, of course, be recognized and taken into consideration. Therefore, to assign accurately allotypic correlates, a considerable background information on the general structural features of immunoglobulin chains in question is needed.

Amino acid substitutions that are present on chains of one allotype and that are different on chains of a second allotype are called correlates. Todd (1972) has pointed out that a correlate need not be involved in the antigenic determinant of the allotype. Proof that a given substitution in the amino acid sequence is indeed an allotypic determinant requires the isolation of homologous peptides and the subsequent demonstration that one peptide has one allotype and the second another. Such proof has been obtained in very few instances for rabbit allotypes (McBurnett and Mandy, 1974).

2.1.4 V_H Allotypes

The rabbit is unique in having allotypic markers present in the variable region of the heavy chain. Of these, the group a markers are by far the most thoroughly studied. While sequential studies of rabbit heavy chains are complicated by the fact that most of the chains are blocked at the N-terminus, sequence differences between group a allotypically defined pooled heavy chains have been demonstrated, as shown in Figure 2. The substitutions are extensive and in some instances, most notable in the peptide from residues 69–73, two of the allotypes are identical and the third different. This situation would be expected if allotypes represent mutants of a common ancestral gene (Kindt, 1975). Cross-reactions have been observed (Brezin and Cazenave, 1975) between a1 and a3 heavy chains which were recognized only by antisera prepared in a^2a^2 rabbits. These cross-reactions could be explained possibly by the type of substitutions observed at positions 69–73 in the heavy chains.

In certain cases, as shown in Figure 2, heavy chains from homogeneous antibodies have been observed to carry substitutions other than those observed for the pooled heavy chains (Jaton et al., 1973). Similarly, it has been shown that group a allotypic specificities expressed by homogeneous antibodies are immunologically deficient with respect to those of IgG pools (Kindt et al., 1973c). These findings suggest that group a allotypy may comprise a group of subspecificities in the V_H region.

That certain heavy chains lack group a allotypes has been recognized for some time (Dray and Nisonoff, 1963). In homozygous allotype suppression experiments, David and Todd (1969) were able to raise the level of group a-negative IgG

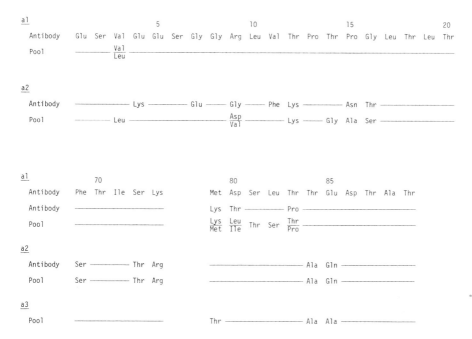

Figure 2 Sequences from V_H regions showing variation correlated with group a allotype. The regions are 1–20, 69–73, and 79–89. The sources of the sequences shown are pools (Mole *et al.*, 1971; Porter, 1974; Mole, personal communication); a1 antibodies (Jaton and Braun, 1972; Jaton *et al.*, 1973; Jaton, 1974*a*); and a2 antibody (Fleischman, 1971, 1973; Jaton, 1975)

molecules to nearly 100 per cent. Also, in several instances, homogeneous antibodies produced by streptococcal injection have been shown to lack group a allotypes (Kindt *et al.*, 1970*b*, 1973*a*). The a-negative heavy chains have been shown to have distinct structural features, including amino acid composition (Tack *et al.*, 1973) and N-terminal sequence. Amino acid composition differences were shown to be limited to the N-terminal half of the heavy chain. The distribution of N-terminal peptides recovered from a1, a2, a3, and three a-negative ($\bar{a}$) preparations derived by allotype suppression in a homozygote of each allotype is shown in Table 2.

Table 2 Distribution of N-terminal peptides in different allotypes

Peptide	Yield (moles of peptide/mole of heavy chain)					
	a1	a2	a3	$\bar{a}$(a1)	$\bar{a}$(a2)	$\bar{a}$(a3)
pGlu-Ser-Val-Glu	0·67	0·38	0·16	0·05	0·15	0·03
pGlu-Ser-Leu-Glu	0·06	0·34	0·63	0·03	0·09	0·06
pGlu-Glu-Glu	0·10	0·17	0·09	0·77	0·77	0·67

Distinct groups of allotypic markers also have been found on a-negative heavy chains (Kim and Dray, 1972, 1973). At least two allotypes in distinct groups (x32 and y33) are present on different populations of a-negative molecules. It should be emphasized that x32 and y33 are not allelic either to each other or to the allotypes a1, a2, or a3.

2.1.5 C_H Allotypes

The IgG C-region allotypes d11, d12, e14, and e15 are the only rabbit allotypes for which simple structural correlates are known. The group d allotypes were shown to correlate with methionine (d11)—threonine (d12) interchange at position 225 of the γ chain (Prahl *et al.*, 1969). McBurnett and Mandy (1974) have demonstrated that a hinge region peptide having the methionine substitution has d11 antigenic activity.

Group e allotypy was shown also to correlate with a single amino acid interchange in the C_γ region (Appella *et al.*, 1971). These allotypes were correlated with threonine (e14) and alanine (e15) at position 309. No other differences among tryptic peptides from the Fc fragments have been noted.

No structural correlates have been reported as yet for the allotypes of rabbit IgA or IgM.

2.1.6 C_L Allotypes

The group b allotypes, found in the C region of chains of both kappa subtypes, appear from preliminary sequential studies to correlate with multiple amino acid substitutions, like the group a allotypes. Unlike the group a allotypes, however, the serological specificities of the group b allotypes appear to be identical on homogeneous antibodies and among IgG pools (Kindt *et al.*, 1972). The first allotypically different peptides reported for group b allotypes were at the C terminals of the light chains (Appella *et al.*, 1969; Frangione, 1969; Goodfleisch, 1975) (Figure 3).

Figure 3 Light chain C-terminal peptide sequences of group b allotypes

b4	Asn- Arg- Gly- Asp- Cys
b5	Ser ——Lys- Asx ——
b6	Ser ——Lys- Ser ——
b9	——————

Other significant differences have been reported among the b4, b5, and b9 peptides containing cysteine 171 (Lamm and Frangione, 1972; Chen *et al.*, 1974; Goodfleisch, 1975). More recently, studies on b9 light chains in several laboratories have demonstrated extensive differences between b4 and b9 in positions 110–130 (Hood *et al.*, 1975; Zeeuws and Strosberg, 1975; Thunberg, unpublished results). As shown in Figure 4, the b9 sequences differ from the b4 in at least seven positions, and they differ from one another in at least one position. In the authors' laboratory, a b4 light chain from a homogeneous anti-streptococcal antibody (4539) has been found which differs from the prototype b4 sequence at two positions, including 121 where it has the serine residue

L CHAIN SEQUENCES – POSITIONS 110–130

	110				115					120					125					130
b4 4135[a]	Asp Pro Val	[ ]	Ala Pro Thr	Val	Leu Ile Phe	Pro	Pro Ala Ala	Asp Gln	Val Ala Thr	Gly Thr Val
b4[b]	——————						Ser ————	Leu	——————	
b9[c]	———— Gln	Ile	————————		Leu ————		Ser ————		Glx Leu Thr	Gly Glx
b9[d]	———— Xxx	Ile	————————		Leu ————		Ser ————		—— Leu Thr	—— Glu

Figure 4 C_L sequences of two b4 and two b9 chains in the region 110–130. [a]Chen et al. (1974); [b]Sogn, unpublished results; [c]Zeeuws and Strosberg (1975); [d]Hood et al. (1975) for b9 pool and Thunberg (unpublished results) obtained for a homogeneous antibody light chain

associated only with b9 (Sogn, unpublished results). Antibodies of the b4 allotype show considerable variation in sequence at position 174 (Strosberg *et al.*, 1972; Appella *et al.*, 1973). The complication of intra-allotype C-region sequential variation, combined with the extensive interallotype differences, makes identification of residues involved in the allotypic determinant as yet impossible.

Allotype suppression has been used to increase the relative concentration of λ chains in rabbits to levels which allow more detailed studies (Appella *et al.*, 1968; Rejnek *et al.*, 1969; Chersi and Mage, 1973). The two markers described for these chains, c7 and c21, (Mage *et al.*, 1968) have been shown to be pseudoalleles (Gilman-Sachs *et al.*, 1969). No structural correlates are available.

2.1.7 Genetic Markers for the V_L Region

Structural and serological evidence suggests that the V_L region is not involved in group b allotypic variation (Appella *et al.*, 1969; Frangione, 1969; Kindt *et al.*, 1972). While no V_L allotypes have been described, genetic variants detected by sequential analysis, which do not give rise to antigenic differences, are known. Studies of these sequence variations have shown them to be associated preferentially with different group b allotypes.

Studies by Waterfield *et al.* (1973) on the N-terminal sequences of allotypically defined light-chain pools indicate allotype-related variation of a quantitative nature, which is sufficiently reproducible to allow 'typing' of the b allotypes by this method. Furthermore, Thunberg *et al.* (1973) have detected a glutamate residue at position N16 of certain homogeneous b9 light chains, a substitution never previously reported for light chains of any species. This substitution was found in b9 light chain pools only obtained from rabbits descended from one of two b9 progenitor rabbits in the colony. Thus, the glutamate 16 substitution may represent an inherited difference in the rabbit V_L region.

Other substitutions, which occur in light chains of allotype b4, but not b9, have been reported at position 2 (tyrosine) and at positions 12 and 13 (glutamate). These substitutions occur in b4 light chains over three generations in one family, and in b4 IgG pools. In addition, they have been found in roughly the same frequency on a list of 41 homogeneous b4 light-chain N-terminal sequences as found in pooled IgG.

Since none of the substitutions described above is found in all chains of the allotype with which they are associated, they are unlikely to be allotype related. If they represent subgroup differences, then their allotype-related absences are difficult to explain. It seems more likely that these substitutions indicate the presence of a finite number of V_L genes linked to the C_L genes.

2.2 Allotypes of the Mouse

The mouse has several advantages over the rabbit for genetic studies. These include the obvious ones of smaller size and a shorter gestation period, as well as the availability of inbred and congenic strains. In addition, transplantable plasmacytomas, which can produce immunoglobulins in sufficient amounts for structural studies, are induced readily in the mouse (Potter, 1967). Immunogenetic studies in mice have been limited by the fact that allotypic markers have been identified only for the C_H regions. This shortcoming has been circumvented partially by the use of idiotypes as V_H markers in conjunction with the C_H allotypes to obtain information on organization of immunoglobulin genes in this species. Furthermore, a genetic marker for the V_H region of mouse chains, detectable by structural means, has been described (Edelman and Gottlieb, 1970).

Structural correlates for mouse allotypes have not been described, but the recent completion of the amino acid sequence of a murine IgG heavy chain (Bourgois *et al.*, 1974) indicates that such data should be available in the near future.

2.2.1 Immunoglobulins of the Mouse

There are six heavy-chain immunoglobulin classes in the mouse. These are referred to by different designations. Most reports use one of the following notations

γM	IgM	
γA	IgA	
γ1	IgF	IgG1
γ2a	IgG	IgG2a
γ2b	IgH	IgG2b
γ3	IgI	IgG3

The general structural features of mouse immunoglobulins are similar to those in man. The light chains have two intra-chain disulphide bridges and the heavy chains have four. The light chains of the mouse may either be κ or λ. As with the rabbit, the former comprises the large majority (97 per cent) of the light chains in normal circulation. The number of V_L subgroups for mouse κ chains may be greater than 20 based on sequential studies utilizing κ chains from BALB/c plasmacytomas (Hood *et al.*, 1973). Two λ V-region subgroups have been described (Mage *et al.*, 1973).

2.2.2 Mouse C_H Allotypes

Allotypes have been described for the C region of mouse immunoglobulin classes F, G, H, and A. No allotypes have been described for classes IgI or IgM. In addition, there is a group of allotypes which have not yet been assigned to any heavy chain class. The early work on mouse allotypes has been reviewed by Potter and Lieberman (1967), and by Herzenberg *et al.* (1968). Mage *et al.* (1973) have presented more recently a thorough review.

The mouse allotypes have been named by two different systems. Each uses a designation for the heavy-chain class on which the allotype is expressed, followed

Table 3 Alignment of mouse allotypes reported by different investigators*

IgG		IgH		IgF		IgA	
1	2	1	2	1	2	1	2
G^1	1·10	H^9	3·4	F^{19}	4·1	A^{12}	2·2
G^3	1·3	H^{11}	3·2	F	4·2	A^{13}	2·3
G^5	1·11	H^{16}	3·9	F^8		A^{14}	2·4
G^4		H^4				A^{15}	
G^6	1·12	H^{22}				A^{17}	
G^8							
G^{3+8}							

1. The nomenclature of Potter and Lieberman (1967). 2. The nomenclature of Herzenberg *et al.* (1968). Only the allotypes 2 which have counterparts in the system 1 are listed here
* In addition to the determinants listed here, there are determinants 2, 10, 18, 21, and 24 which have not been assigned to a heavy-chain class

by a number to describe the determinant. In the system used by Potter and Lieberman (1967), the class designations are G, A, H, and F: that is, the same as the immunoglobulin classes. The determinants are then numbered in order of their discovery, using a unique number for each determinant. Therefore, the allotype G^1 is an IgG allotypic determinant, presumably the first observed by these workers. If the same number is used twice with different letters (for example, G^8 and F^8) this means that the same determinant has been detected on two different classes of immunoglobulin.

A second system (Herzenberg *et al.*, 1968) uses a number for the class (IgG = 1, IgA = 2, IgH = 3, and IgF = 4) and a second number, separated from the first by a full stop, for the determinant. The numbers are repeated for each set of determinants. Therefore, in this system, 1.1 and 2.1 are not the same, but rather would indicate different determinants on IgG and IgA, respectively.

Mage *et al.* (1973) published a table showing alignment of the allotype determinants as named by the different systems. This useful alignment is reproduced in a simpler form (Table 3) omitting allotypes for which the class has not been ascertained yet and omitting the determinants of Herzenberg *et al.* (1968), which do not have a corresponding determinant in the system of Potter and Lieberman.

The mouse allotypes are often referred to by the inbred strain in which they occur. For example, the complete BALB/c allotype ($G^{1, 6, 7, 8}$, $A^{12, 13, 14}$, $H^{9, 11, 22}$, $F^{8, 19}$) is too cumbersome therefore often it is called the BALB/c allotype. This refers to the entire C_H-gene complex present in the BALB/c strain. This notation is convenient when congenic strains are being discussed.

The determinants for a single class within a single strain may be designated also by a condensed notation using the Herzenberg number for class designation with a small letter as a superscript for the allele. The BALB/c IgG allotype ($G^{1, 6, 7, 8}$) is written as 1^a and the C57BL/6(G^-) as 1^b. In some reports these may be written as

IgG^a and IgG^b, or even as G^a and G^b. A listing of alleles present in various inbred strains is given by Mage *et al.* (1973).

2.2.3 *Genetic Marker for the Variable Region of Mouse κ Chains*

Edelman and Gottlieb (1970) observed that a peptide detected by autoradiography from the V$_L$ region of certain mouse κ chains would serve as a genetic marker. This marker was found in three of 17 strains surveyed. More recently, Gottlieb (1974) has shown correlation between this marker, called I$_B$-peptide marker, and the thymocyte cell-surface antigen Ly-3.1. This finding, which represents the first report of linkage between an immunoglobulin gene and another characteristic, would place the putative V$_L$ gene in linkage group XI on chromosome 6 of the mouse (Itakura *et al.*, 1972).

3 IDIOTYPES AS VARIABLE-REGION MARKERS

The presence of serological markers in both C and V regions of an immunoglobulin chain enables studies to be made concerning the number and nature of the genes for antibody V regions and the relationships between these genes and those encoding C regions. C-region allotypes are quite readily available in both rabbits and mice, but the only V-region allotype described is the rabbit group a in the V$_H$ region. Structurally defined genetic markers, such as those described earlier for rabbit and mouse V$_L$ regions, offer an alternative to V-region allotypes. A second alternative is the use of idiotypes. Idiotypic phenomena have been reviewed recently by Capra and Kehoe (1975).

The individual antigenic specificity of human myeloma proteins was recognized initially by Slater *et al.* (1955), who used absorbed rabbit antibodies to detect the differences between myeloma proteins. Oudin and Michel (1963) observed that rabbit antibodies to bacterial vaccines also possessed very restricted antigenic determinants. The antisera of Oudin were prepared in allotypically matched rabbits (Oudin and Michel, 1969*a, b*). Oudin named this phenomenon *idiotypy*.

Idiotypic determinants are binding-site related and some idiotypic reactions may be inhibited by haptens against which the antibodies are raised (Brient and Nisonoff, 1970; Weigert *et al.*, 1974). Many idiotypes have been shown to require specific heavy–light chain combinations for expression (Grey *et al.*, 1965). The idiotypes of two human myeloma proteins with anti-IgG activity have been related recently to near identity of amino acid sequences in heavy-chain hypervariable regions (Capra and Kehoe, 1974). While it may be premature, it is tempting to define idiotypes as antigenic determinants related to hypervariable regions of immunoglobulins.

Use of idiotypes as markers became possible when studies on idiotypes of homogeneous antibodies in rabbit families (Eichmann and Kindt, 1971) established that idiotypes are genetically transmitted. Further work on the idiotypes of rabbit antibodies showed linkage of group a allotypes to idiotypes

(Kindt *et al.*, 1973*b*, *c*; Kindt and Krause, 1974). In addition, the association of an idiotype with an infrequently occurring V_κ subgroup has been demonstrated in these same rabbit families (Klapper and Kindt, 1974). Genetic experiments on the idiotypes of the mouse which have extended the original observations will be discussed in the following section.

4 RELATIONSHIPS BETWEEN IMMUNOGLOBULIN GENES

4.1 General Considerations

Investigations of immunoglobulin allotypes have placed the genes coding for immunoglobulin synthesis at three distinct loci. These loci code for the heavy chains, the κ light chains, and the λ chains. The original observation was made by Dubiski *et al.* (1962), who noted that the two groups of allotypic markers for heavy chains and κ light chains (Oudin, 1956, 1960*a*, *b*) showed independent assortment. Genetic studies on the group c allotypes of the λ chains have added the third unlinked group (Gilman-Sachs *et al.*, 1969). The recent observation of secretory-piece allotypes, which are not linked to any of the other allotypes, may add a fourth locus (Knight *et al.*, 1974*b*).

All the C_H and V_H allotypes so far observed for the rabbit heavy chain are linked to one another. Likewise, mouse C_H allotypes are linked to each other and to the idiotypes which have been used as V_H gene markers. Because serological markers for genetic variants in V_L regions are not available, there is no similar linkage information for the κ and λ light-chain loci. Data on structurally detected markers of the V region of the rabbit κ light chains (Thunberg *et al.*, 1973; Waterfield *et al.*, 1973; Thunberg, 1974) suggest that the light-chain gene complex consists of few C-region genes closely linked to larger numbers of V-region genes.

4.2 Heavy-Chain Gene Complexes

The availability of allotypic markers for several mouse heavy-chain classes has made it possible to test the linkage between the genes encoding the different C regions. In back-crosses involving 2371 progeny, no recombinant types were observed, indicating a very low recombination frequency among the genes which encode the C_H allotypes. The existence of allotypic combinations in wild mice which do not occur in inbred strains suggests that crossovers can and have occurred among these closely linked genes (Lieberman and Potter, 1969).

Data obtained on the linkage of rabbit allotypes in the C_H region concur with these conclusions. That is, in the rabbit as well as in the mouse, the C_H genes are very closely linked. Again, the existence of various combinations of the rabbit C_H genes indicates that at some time crossovers have occurred among them. The presence of a limited number of possible linkage groups, called 'allogroups', has been observed in both species. For example, the rabbit IgA allotypic groups f and g have five and four alleles, respectively, but of the twenty possible combinations,

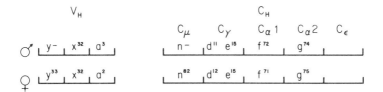

Figure 5 The complete heavy-chain typing of a single rabbit. The allogroup inherited from the paternal side is at the top and that from the maternal side is at the bottom

only five have so far been observed (Hanly and Knight, personal communication).

A striking example of restriction is obtained by considering the entire heavy-chain allogroup of the rabbit (Figure 5), with its three V_H-region (a, x, and y) and five C_H-region (d, e, f, g, and n) allotypic groups. The total number of possible combinations may be estimated by multiplying the number of alleles in each group (see Table 1). In this manner, an estimate of 2880* different allogroups is obtained. Of these 2880 possibilities, only 12 have been observed (Mage *et al.*, 1973)—less than 0·5 per cent of the maximum number of combinations.

Such restriction of possible gene combinations which seems to be the rule for the rabbit and the mouse systems has also been observed with human immunoglobulin allotypes (Natvig and Kunkel, 1973). The reason for the existence of so few allogroups is obscure. It may be that certain combinations are deleterious and are, therefore, selected against. Alternatively, the linkage of the C_H genes may be so close that very few of the theoretically possible crossovers can occur in practice.

4.3 V_H and C_H Allotypes and Idiotypes

The genetic relationships between the allotypes of the C_H and V_H regions have implications beyond the field of immunology. The original observation of Todd (1963) that IgM and IgG have in common a V-region allotype suggests that two or more genes interacted prior to the synthesis of a single polypeptide chain. The presence of these V-region allotypes was demonstrated subsequently for rabbit IgA (Feinstein, 1963) and IgE (Kindt and Todd, 1969). The observation of identical idiotypes on human myeloma proteins with different heavy-chain classes (Penn *et al.*, 1970; Wang *et al.*, 1970) has provided strong independent confirmation of the 'two gene—one polypeptide' hypothesis. Also pertinent to the relationships of V_H and C_H genes is the observation of Fu *et al.* (1975), who have recently shown that the IgM and IgD molecules on the surface of human lymphocytes have the same idiotypic determinants. This simultaneous presence on one cell of two different chains with identical V regions must be taken into

* This is a conservative estimate because the number of alleles in several groups is not known and only one additional allotype has been allowed for these. Furthermore, the existence of subclasses and allotypes of other classes not yet well described in the rabbit (IgE, IgD) would raise this number.

128

account in molecular mechanisms which seek to explain the production of antibody heavy chains by translocation events.

The genetic relationships between V and C-region genes were tested experimentally with the discovery of rabbit heavy-chain C-region allotypes (Mandy and Todd, 1968; Dubiski, 1969a). It was soon shown (Zullo et $al.$, 1968; Dubiski, 1969b) that the C-region allotypes of group e and group d are linked to the V-region allotypes of group a. Subsequently, linkage of idiotypes to C_H allotypes has been demonstrated in the mouse for a large number of idiotypes. Crossovers between the C and V-region allotypes have been documented for rabbit families (Mage et $al.$, 1971; Kindt and Mandy, 1972; Hamers-Casterman and Hamers, 1975), thus providing further evidence for the involvement of two separate genes in antibody heavy-chain synthesis. The crossover frequency for the C_H and V_H genes of the rabbit based on these observed recombinations has been estimated to be 0·3 per cent (Mage et $al.$, 1973). Low recombination frequencies also have been reported for mouse idiotypes and C_H allotypes (Blomberg et $al.$, 1972; Eichmann and Berek, 1973; Pawlak et $al.$, 1973; Lieberman et $al.$, 1974).

By studying combinations of V and C allotypes present on the molecules from rabbits doubly heterozygous for these markers, it was observed that a high percentage of the heavy chains retains the combinations of markers inherited from the parents (Kindt et $al.$, 1970a). That is, the majority of syntheses are directed by genes in the coupling phase. In the example given in Figure 6 the majority of molecules in the offspring's circulation with allotype a1 would express d11; those with a2 would express d12. Similarly, in the mouse, Eichmann (1973) showed that idiotypically related antibodies produced in allotypically heterozygous mice always have the same allotype–idiotype combination. This indicates that usually mouse idiotypes, like rabbit allotype, are synthesized from

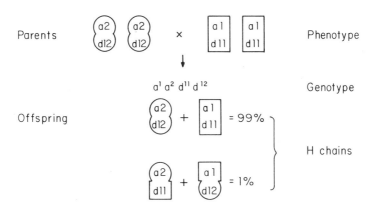

Figure 6 An illustration of the preference in a rabbit for heavy-chain synthesis using V and C genes inherited on the same chromosomes. Parental chromosomes (or heavy chains) are shown at the top. In the offspring, 99 per cent of circulating heavy chains have the same allotypic combination as one or the other of the parents

information present on the same chromosome as the C_H gene with which they are transmitted genetically.

In rabbits, the estimates of molecules with recombinant types obtained by the selective absorption experiments of Landucci-Tosi and Tosi (1973) agree well with the estimate of 1 per cent which Pernis *et al.* (1973) obtained using double fluorescent staining techniques. More recent experiments have measured the percentage of recombinant molecules utilizing IgA C-region allotypes in combination with the allotypes of group a. The numbers obtained are slightly higher than those for IgG (Knight *et al.*, 1974a). It is not known whether the recombinant molecules result from synthesis directed by genes in repulsion or by genes on chromosomes which result from mitotic crossovers between C_H and V_H genes.

The recognition of a number of idiotypes in inbred mouse strains makes it possible, by examining recombinants among the idiotypes and the allotypes to which they are linked, to begin to map the area of the chromosome where these genes are found and thereby to estimate the number of V_H genes present. For example, one study involved the linkage between two different mouse idiotypes (A5A and ARS), both linked to the A/J C_H allotype (Eichmann *et al.*, 1974). The observation of a crossover between the A5A idiotype and the BALB/c allotype in one male mouse provided the opportunity to test the linkage between the two idiotypes. The crossover mouse was bred and the new haplotype (allogroup) was shown to be inherited without the ARS idiotype. On the basis of this data, the chromosomes of the BALB/c, A/J and recombinant might be as represented as shown in Table 4.

Table 4   Crossing over in V-region genes between BALB/c and A/J mice

	V_H Idiotypes		C_H Allotypes
A/J	A5A$^+$	ARS$^+$	l.e
BALB/c	A5A$^-$	ARS$^-$	l.a
Recombinant	A5A$^+$	ARS$^-$	l.a

Such an observation would suggest that V-region genes are present in sufficient numbers to observe crossovers among them. Whether the ARS and A5A idiotypes occur in heavy chains with the same or different V_H subgroups is not known. A more complete survey of mapping data in the mouse has been presented by Eichmann (1975).

4.4 Interaction of Multiple Genes in the Synthesis of Single Immunoglobulin Variable Regions

As discussed in Section 4.3, the synthesis of a single immunoglobulin chain is probably directed by more than one gene. The existence of separate V and C

130

genes has been most firmly established by allotypic and structural studies of heavy chains (Todd, 1963; Dreyer and Bennett, 1965). More recently, structural and serological data on V regions have led to the further suggestion that V-region synthesis may be directed by multiple genes. The experiments supporting this hypothesis have been discussed by Capra and Kindt (1975), who suggested that three types of genes interact in the synthesis of a single antibody chain: (*i*) C-region genes which specify isotypes; (*ii*) the V genes which specify the relatively invariant, or framework residues of the V region, including subgroup-specific residues and any allotypic determinants; and (*iii*) the V genes which specify the hypervariable regions and the idiotype.

Structural studies on the V regions of antibodies in myeloma proteins indicate that hypervariable regions are interspersed between V-region sequences which show very little or even no variation among immunoglobulins from different individuals or distinct species (Wu and Kabat, 1970; Capra and Kehoe, 1975). Because of the problem of genetic load (Ohno, 1970), the existence of these invariant portions may be explained best by theories based on few genes, while structural studies showing conservation of hypervariable regions in genetically dissimilar individuals may best be explained by multigene theories. Gene-interaction theories explain this constancy and variability within the same polypeptide chain by the existence of multiple gene segments which interact to synthesize a single V region.

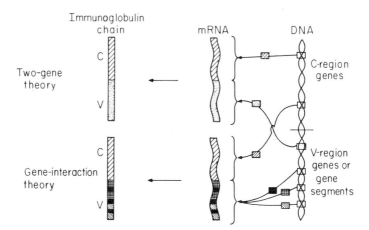

Figure 7   An example of a gene interaction theory, as compared to a two-gene theory. In the two-gene theory, one C-region gene and one V-region gene together code for a mRNA specifying a complete immunoglobulin chain. In the gene-interaction theory, multiple V-region gene segments interact with one C-region gene to yield the mRNA. In the example, three types of V-region gene segments are suggested to be involved, one for the N-terminal half of the V-region, one for the C-terminal half and one for the hypervariable sections. Other formulations are possible within the framework of the gene-interaction hypothesis

Results supporting gene-interaction theories have been obtained in serological studies on combinations of V_H allotypes and idiotypes (Kindt *et al.*, 1973*a*). It has been shown that two antibodies with identical idiotypes differ in their V-region allotypes and N-terminal sequences (Waterfield *et al.*, 1972). Structural studies on myeloma proteins with shared idiotypic specificities similarly have supported the interaction theory (Kunkel *et al.*, 1973). Sequential analysis of the V_H regions of two idiotypically similar myeloma proteins from non-related individuals indicates differences in eight positions. Only three of these differences occur in the hypervariable regions (Capra and Kehoe, 1974). Randomly selected myeloma proteins from the same V-region subgroup will differ by an average of 33 of the 42 hypervariable positions. More recently, studies on localization of variable residues within the framework residues of the V region have shown that variability associated with subgroup or species is confined to the N-terminal portions of this region. Positions toward the C-terminal end of the V region show no such pattern. Such an observation argues that these regions may be encoded by separate genes.

There is no direct evidence for gene interaction or for any other theory of V-region diversity. There is a precedent, however, for gene interaction from studies on V and C-region genes. The upper portion of Figure 7 depicts the synthesis of a single immunoglobulin chain from separate V and C-region genes. In the lower portion of Figure 7 this well-accepted event is extended to include interaction between V-region gene segments. While mechanisms for the proposed inter-actions are conjectural, there is evidence to suggest that translocation events occur prior to translation (Capra and Kindt, 1975).

5 SELECTIVE EXPRESSION OF ALLOTYPE GENES

Although individual plasma cells may produce and simultaneously express immunoglobulins of several classes on their membranes (Warner, 1974), in allotypic heterozygotes a single plasma cell uses only one of the two allotypes available in each allotypic group in its genome. Thus, immunoglobulin-producing cells may be said to exhibit a mosaic of phenotypes. Because the genes coding for heavy and light chains are unlinked at least two different loci, perhaps on different chromosomes, must be involved. This phenomenon, generally referred to as allelic exclusion, was first proposed on the basis of allelic restriction observed for myeloma proteins (Harboe *et al.*, 1962*b*). This was demonstrated subsequently at the cellular level for rabbit allotypes by Pernis *et al.* (1965) and for mouse allotypes by Weiler (1965). The term allotype selection will be used here in preference to allelic exclusion as recent data, to be discussed in Section 6, indicate a strong possibility that at least some allotypic groups are not composed of true alleles. Regardless of the nomenclature, the phenomenon, as a unique example of co-ordinated selective gene activation or inactivation at multiple loci, is an important component of the mechanism regulating the immune response.

While an individual antibody-producing cell in the rabbit exhibits only one allele of each group, any combination of paternal or maternal allotypes may be observed. Because the allotypes of group a and b are unlinked and presumed to be on different chromosomes, this situation necessitates the activation, or inactivation, of genes at two distinct loci. If the allotypes of the λ light chains and the secretory component are taken into consideration, then the activation or inactivation process must take place in an antibody-producing cell at four distinct loci, perhaps on four different autosomes. The fact that the synthesis of 99 per cent of heavy chains utilizes information from genes in coupling also must be taken into account (see Figure 6). The gene-activation process may then have specificity for genes on the same chromosome (Tosi *et al.*, 1974). If this were the case, the low percentage of molecules expressing non-linked markers would be synthesized by cells in which somatic crossovers have occurred.

Another example of selective gene expression, and one which has points in common with allotype selection, is the utilization of only one X-chromosome in somatic cells of female mammals. A female with two X chromosomes, at a certain developmental state, randomly activates (or inactivates) one of the two chromosomes in each cell. When this was first postulated by Lyon (1961), the major evidence cited was the occurrence of the 'mottled' or 'dappled' coat colour phenotypes in heterozygous female mice and the existence of normal XO females. This has been confirmed in many subsequent studies using a number of X-linked traits, some of which can be assayed at the level of single cells. For example, Beutler *et al.* (1962) demonstrated that single erythrocytes from human females heterozygous for glucose 6-phosphate dehydrogenase deficiency exhibit either the normal or the deficient phenotype.

In both cases of selective gene expression, certain conclusions may be drawn. Firstly, it is likely that the process involves activation rather than inactivation. Individuals with more than the normal complement of X chromosomes have only one which is activated. It is much simpler to postulate a mechanism for the selective activation of one set of immunoglobulin genes than for inactivation of the many not used. Secondly, it is a random event in that either X chromosome may be activated and any of the many possible immunoglobulins may be synthesized. Immunoglobulin-gene activation may not be completely random, since studies have shown an imbalance of one allotype in pre-immune serum for allotypically heterozygous animals (Kindt, 1975). One of the possible explanations for these findings is the preferential activation of one locus. Thirdly, it is a permanent event. The progeny cells are committed to maintain their specific state of activation throughout all successive cell divisions and differentiative processes. It is reasonable to postulate because of these similarities that the same mechanism underlies both the autosomal and X-linked phenomena.

No mechanism yet proposed for either case of selective gene expression has received any significant experimental support. However, the model recently proposed by Riggs (1975) for selective activation of X chromosomes is particularly promising, but requires experimental verification.

In this model, Riggs has proposed that DNA methylation is the mechanism for X-chromosome activation. Enzymes, which are present in *Escherichia coli*, have been shown to methylate DNA forming N-6-methyladenine or 5-methylcytosine.

The methylation rate for DNA that has the opposing strand methylated is 10^3 times faster than the rate for strands which are not methylated. The methylated bases do not interfere, however, with pairing of DNA strands. Riggs has postulated that the methylation of an inactivation centre (a specifically recognized base sequence) on one X chromosome renders this chromosome active. In all subsequent cell divisions, the same centre would be rapidly methylated because one strand is already methylated. Thus, randomness and permanence are explained easily by this model. Prevention of methylation during oogenesis or spermatogenesis would allow formation of the derivatives to be reversed.

Riggs' model also may be applied to autosomal activation phenomena with minor changes. The major difference lies in the necessity for inactivation centres at several loci that may serve to inactivate only portions of the chromosomes on which they reside. A positive aspect of the Riggs model for selective gene activation is that it can be tested by the measurement of methylated bases in DNAs from various cells and by determining the presence of specific methylating enzymes.

6 NATURE OF ALLOTYPE GENES

It is assumed tacitly in many immunogenetic arguments that allotype and idiotype synthesis is controlled by structural genes. There is, however, some recent evidence suggesting that this may not be the case. One alternative might be that regulator genes exist and that these are inherited as autosomal codominant alleles. In this case, the information for all allotypic variants would reside in each individual and the expression of a set of allotypes would depend on the inheritance of the appropriate regulator genes. The mode of action of the regulator gene could involve specific activation or repression of the structural genes encoding the immunoglobulins.

Data consistent with such a model have come from the studies of Bell and Dray (1971), who showed that RNA extracts from rabbit spleen can induce synthesis of the donor's allotype in spleen cells from genetically different rabbits. Similarly, Rivat *et al.* (1973) showed that non-specific stimulation of cultured human lymphocytes gives rise to allotypes which have not been observed in the individual cell donors.

Members of a congenic mouse strain having the C57BL/ka allotype on a BALB/c background have been shown recently by Bosma and Bosma (1974) to express the BALB/c (IgG^a) allotype in a transient and unpredictable manner. These animals had been selected for homozygosity for the C57BL/ka allotype. Only the BALB/c allotype for immunoglobulins of the IgG classes were expressed. No other BALB/c allotypes were observed in these animals. Because the appearance of the so-called 'hidden allotype' in the homozygous animals appeared to coincide with general debilitation, it is considered possible that a virus causes the deviation from allelic behaviour. An alternative suggestion

134

invokes the presence of regulator genes which somehow became derepressed in the homozygotes and allow synthesis of the unexpected BALB/c allotype.

Data obtained from studies on rabbit allotypes also may be interpreted in terms of gene regulation. Strosberg *et al.* (1974) observed recently that a rabbit with allotype a^1a^3/b^4b^5 produced antibodies with allotypes a2 and b6 after immunization with *Micrococcus lysodeikticus*. The a2 and b6 allotypes were not necessarily on the same antibodies since the time of their appearances did not coincide. In addition to the rabbit producing these antibodies, two other rabbits in the Strosberg colony were found simultaneously to express three group a allotypes. The a2 allotype from the a^1a^3 was shown to be immunologically identical to normal a2 IgG using Ouchterlony analysis and by inhibition of radiobinding assays.

In the authors' colony, an a^1a^2 rabbit produced antibody of allotype a3 upon immunization with streptococcal C vaccine. Quantitative allotypic determination carried out on non-immune sera from a large number of rabbits representing different populations detected low levels of group a allotypes not identified by qualitative typing or anticipated from breeding data (latent allotypes) in 50 per cent of sera tested (Mudgett *et al.*, 1975). Allotype inhibition curves given by dilutions of a non-immune serum from an adult rabbit with nominal allotype a^2a^2 are depicted in Figure 8. This serum shows an appreciable concentration of IgG with allotype a3 and to a lesser extent a1. The latent allotypes, which are serologically identical to allotypes of pooled IgG, have been detected in sera from rabbits with all possible combinations of group a allotypes. Expression of latent allotypes in individual rabbits is transitory and sporadic.

Although the data of Strosberg *et al.* (1974) and the related findings in the authors' rabbits can be explained readily by failures in the postulated regulatory mechanisms, other explanations must be considered also. Among these is the

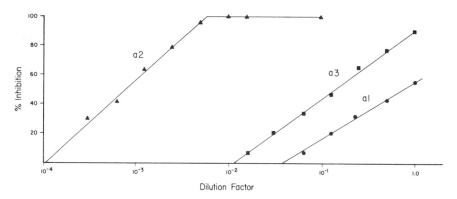

Figure 8   Inhibition of binding of 0·25 µg of radioiodinated a1b4, a2b4, or a3b4 IgG to *N*-hydroxysuccinimide-activated Sepharose immobilized anti-a1, anti-a2, or anti-a3, respectively, by dilutions of non-immune serum from rabbit 4120 (nominal allotype a2). Carrier proteins used in these assays include an excess of immunoglobulins with all a and b allotypes except that being measured. From Mudgett *et al.* (1975)

possibility that crossovers between V_H genes give rise to chromosomes simultaneously carrying genes for two different allotypes. Such an event would be more likely if there were many V_H genes in the germ line carrying the group a allotypes. Failure to observe rabbits with three group a allotypes has been used as an argument against the existence of multiple V_H genes in the germ line (Todd, 1972).

Whatever the exact nature of the allotype genes, the relationships between them as described in the previous sections must be taken into consideration. That is to say, a complete theory of immunoglobulin synthesis must take into account (i) the possible existence of separate V_H and C_H genes, (ii) the associations of V_H and C_H markers in the molecules of heterozygotes, and (iii) allelic exclusion of allotypes. Explanation of these phenomena must involve novel mechanisms, whether the postulated genes are structural or regulatory in nature.

7 CONCLUSION

The goal of the genetics of immunoglobulin is to determine the number and nature of the genes that interact and code for immunoglobulins, the arrangement of these genes in the genome, and the mechanisms behind the regulatory processes which determine what immunoglobulin will be produced by a single plasma cell. All of these remain current problems, but studies to date put significant constraints on any proposed model.

It is known that the genes which code for the allotypes of heavy chains, and κ and λ light chains are not linked, placing immunoglobulin genes at a minimum of three distinct loci. Genes encoding different C_H-region allotypes are linked closely and inherited as gene complexes called allogroups. Only a limited number of the many possible combinations of C_H genes has been observed in allogroups. There is good evidence that separate but tightly linked genes code for the V and C regions of a single immunoglobulin chain.

The number and nature of the V and C-region genes are unclear. All estimates indicate one, or very few C-genes, exist for each C-region allotype, but recent descriptions of polymorphisms within allotypically identical C regions must be taken into account. Competing theories suggest the presence of either few or many V-region genes for each group. Alternatively, there is appreciable evidence which suggests that V regions themselves may be the product of interaction between two or more distinct gene segments.

Evidence shows that about 99 per cent of γ and α heavy chains are synthesized from C_H and V_H genes interacting in coupling phase. This overwhelming preference for intra-chromosomal interaction puts constraints on any mechanism proposed for gene interaction. Additional constraints are imposed by the finding that individual cells can display simultaneously membrane IgM and IgD with the same idiotype. This implies that the same V_H gene may be utilized with two different C_H genes to synthesize these heavy chains.

Allotypically heterozygous single plasma cells express only one of the alternative allotypes available within each allotype group. This 'allotype exclusion' is required if clonal expansion is to lead to a specific response to antigenic expansion. The mechanism underlying this example of selective gene activation is unknown but intriguing hypotheses have been proposed. Description of regulatory mechanisms in immunoglobulin synthesis is further complicated by data which suggest that allotypes and hence immunoglobulin structural genes are not allelic. Since allotypes are inherited generally as simple Mendelian codominant alleles, it has been suggested that allelism is at the level of regulator genes and not structural genes. The unexplained complexities of immunoglobulin synthesis are such that it would certainly not be surprising to discover several levels of as yet undescribed regulator control over this vital physiological function.

ACKNOWLEDGEMENTS

This work was supported by PHS grants from the NIAID, AI 11995 and AI 11439. J.A.S. is a fellow of the Arthritis Foundation.

REFERENCES

Appella, E., Chersi, A., Mage, R. G., and Dubiski, S. (1971). *Proc. Nat. Acad. Sci., U.S.A.,* **68**, 1341.

Appella, E., Mage, R. G., Dubiski, S., and Reisfeld, R. A. (1968). *Proc. Nat. Acad. Sci. U.S.A.,* **60**, 975.

Appella, E., Rejnek, J., and Reisfeld, R. A. (1969). *J. Mol. Biol.,* **41**, 473.

Appella, E., Roholt, O. A., Chersi, A., Radzimski, G., and Pressman, D. (1973). *Biochem. Biophys. Res. Commun.,* **53**, 1122.

Bazin, H., Beckers, A., Deckers, C., and Moriame, M. (1973). *J. Nat. Cancer Inst.,* **51**, 1359.

Bazin, H., Beckers, A., and Querinjean, P. (1974a). *Eur. J. Immunol.,* **4**, 44.

Bazin, H., Beckers, A., Vaerman, J. P., and Heremans, J. F. (1974b). *J. Immunol.,* **112**, 1035.

Bell, C., and Dray, S. (1971). *Science, N.Y.,* **171**, 199.

Beutler, E., Yeh, M., and Fairbanks, V. F. (1962). *Proc. Nat. Acad. Sci., U.S.A.,* **48**, 9.

Blomberg, B., Geckeler, W. R., and Wiegert, M. (1972). *Science, N.Y.,* **177**, 178.

Bosma, M. J., and Bosma, G. C. (1974). *J. Exp. Med.,* **139**, 512.

Bourgois, A., Fougereau, M., and Rocca-Serra, J. (1974). *Eur. J. Biochem.,* **43**, 423.

Brezin, C., and Cazenave, P. A. (1975). *Immunochemistry,* **12**, 241.

Brient, B. W., and Nisonoff, A. (1970). *J. Exp. Med.,* **132**, 951.

Capra, J. D., and Kehoe, J. M. (1974). *Proc. Nat. Acad. Sci., U.S.A.,* **71**, 4032.

Capra, J. D., and Kehoe, J. M. (1975). *Adv. Immunol.,* **20**, 1.

Capra, J. D., and Kindt, T. J. (1975). *Immunogenetics,* **1**, 417.

Chai, C. K. (1974). *Immunogenetics,* **1**, 126.

Chen, K. C. S., Kindt, T. J., and Krause, R. M. (1974). *Proc. Nat. Acad. Sci., U.S.A.,* **71**, 1995.

Chersi, A., and Mage, R. G. (1973). *Immunochemistry,* **10**, 277.

Cohen, C., and Tissot, R. G. (1974). *Transplantation,* **18**, 150.

David, G. S., and Todd, C. W. (1969). *Proc. Nat. Acad. Sci., U.S.A.,* **62**, 860.

deVries, G. M., Lanckman, M., and Hamers, R. (1969). *Eur. J. Biochem.*, **11**, 370.
Dray, S., Dubiski, S., Kelus, A., Lennox, E. S., and Oudin, J. (1962). *Nature, (Lond.)*, **195**, 785.
Dray, S., and Nisonoff, A. (1963). *Proc. Soc. Exp. Biol. Med.*, **113**, 20.
Dreyer, W. J., and Bennett, J. C. (1965). *Proc. Nat. Acad. Sci., U.S.A.*, **54**, 864.
Dubiski, S. (1969a). *J. Immunol.*, **103**, 120.
Dubiski, S. (1969b). *Protides Biol. Fluids Proc. Colloq.*, **17**, 117.
Dubiski, S., Rapacz, J., and Dubiska, A. (1962). *Acta Genet.*, **12**, 136.

Edelman, G. M., and Gottlieb, P. D. (1970). *Proc. Nat. Acad. Sci., U.S.A.*, **67**, 1192.
Eichmann, K. (1973). *J. Exp. Med.*, **137**, 603.
Eichmann, K. (1975). *Immunogenetics*, **2**, 491.
Eichmann, K., and Berek, C. (1973). *Eur. J. Immunol.*, **3**, 599.
Eichmann, K., and Kindt, T. J. (1971). *J. Exp. Med.*, **134**, 532.
Eichmann, K., Tung, A., and Nisonoff, A. (1974). *Nature, (Lond.)*, **250**, 509.

Feinstein, A. (1963). *Nature, (Lond.)*, **199**, 1197.
Fleischman, J. B. (1971). *Biochemistry*, **10**, 2753.
Fleischman, J. B. (1973). *Immunochemistry*, **10**, 401.
Florent, G., deVries, G. M., and Hamers, R. (1973). *Immunochemistry*, **10**, 425.
Frangione, B. (1969). *FEBS Letters*, **3**, 341.
Franklin, E. C., Fudenberg, H., Meltzer, M., and Stanworth, D. R. (1962). *Proc. Nat. Acad. Sci., U.S.A.*, **48**, 914.
Fu, S. M., Winchester, R. J., and Kunkel, H. G. (1975). *J. Immunol.*, **114**, 250.

Gilman-Sachs, A., Mage, R. G., Young, G. O., Alexander, C., and Dray, S. (1969). *J. Immunol.*, **103**, 1159.
Goodfleisch, R. M. (1975). *J. Immunol.*, **114**, 910.
Gottlieb, P. D. (1974). *J. Exp. Med.*, **140**, 1432.
Grey, H. M., Mannik, M., and Kunkel, H. G. (1965). *J. Exp. Med.*, **121**, 561.

Hamers-Casterman, C., and Hamers, R. (1975). *Archs Int. Phys. Biochim.*, **83**, 188.
Hanly, W. C., Lichter, E. A., Dray, S., and Knight, K. L. (1973). *Biochemistry*, **12**, 733.
Harboe, M., Osterland, C., and Kunkel, H. G. (1962a). *Science, N.Y.*, **136**, 979.
Harboe, M., Osterland, C., Mannik, M., and Kunkel, H. G. (1962b). *J. Exp. Med.*, **116**, 719.
Herzenberg, L. A., McDevitt, H., and Herzenberg, L. A. (1968). *Ann. Rev. Genet.*, **2**, 209.
Hilschmann, N., and Craig, L. C. (1965). *Proc. Nat. Acad. Sci., U.S.A.*, **53**, 1403.
Hood, L., Campbell, J. H., and Elgin, S. C. R. (1975). *Ann. Rev. Genet.*, **9**, 305.
Hood, L., Eichmann, K., Lackland, H., Krause, R. M., and Ohms, J. J. (1970). *Nature, (Lond.)*, **228**, 1040.
Hood, L., McKean, D., Farnsworth, V. and Potter, M. (1973). *Biochemistry*, **12**, 741.

Itakura, K., Hutton, J. J., Boyse, E. A., and Old, L. J. (1972). *Transplantation*, **13**, 239.

Jaton, J. C. (1974a). *Biochem. J.*, **141**, 1.
Jaton, J. C. (1974b). *Biochem. J.*, **141**, 15.
Jaton, J. C. (1975). *Biochem. J.*, **147**, 235.
Jaton, J. C., and Braun, D. E. (1972). *Biochem. J.*, **130**, 539.
Jaton, J. C., Braun, D. G., Strosberg, A. D., Haber, E., and Morris, J. E. (1973). *J. Immunol.*, **111**, 1838.

Kim, B. S., and Dray, S. (1972). *Eur. J. Immunol.*, **2**, 509.
Kim, B. S., and Dray, S. (1973). *J. Immunol.*, **111**, 750.
Kindt, T. J. (1975). *Adv. Immunol.*, **21**, 35.

138

Kindt, T. J., Klapper, D. G., and Waterfield, M. D. (1973a). *J. Exp. Med.*, **137**, 636.
Kindt, T. J., and Krause, R. M. (1974). *Ann. Immunol. (Inst. Pasteur)*, **125C**, 369.
Kindt, T. J., and Mandy, W. J. (1972). *J. Immunol.*, **108**, 1110.
Kindt, T. J., Mandy, W. J., and Todd, C. W. (1970a). *Immunochemistry*, **7**, 457.
Kindt, T. J., Seide, R. K., Boksich, V. A., and Krause, R. M. (1973b). *J. Exp. Med.*, **138**, 522.
Kindt, T. J., Seide, R. K., Lackland, H., and Thunberg, A. L. (1972). *J. Immunol.*, **109**, 735.
Kindt, T. J., Seide, R. K., Tack, B. F., and Todd, C. W. (1973c). *J. Exp. Med.*, **138**, 33.
Kindt, T. J., Thunberg, A. L., Mudgett, M., and Klapper, D. E. (1974). In *The Immune System: Genes, Receptors, Signals*, (Sercarz, E. E., Williamson, A. R., and Cox, C. F., eds.), Academic Press, New York and London, p. 69.
Kindt, T. J., and Todd, C. W. (1969). *J. Exp. Med.*, **130**, 859.
Kindt, T. J., Todd, C. W., Eichmann, K., and Krause, R. M. (1970b). *J. Exp. Med.*, **131**, 343.
Klapper, D. G., and Kindt, T. J. (1974). *Scand. J. Immunol.*, **3**, 483.
Knight, K. L., Malek, T. R., and Hanly, W. C. (1974a). *Proc. Nat. Acad. Sci., U.S.A.*, **71**, 1169.
Knight, K. L., Rosenzweig, M., Lichter, E. A., and Hanly, W. C. (1974b). *J. Immunol.*, **112**, 877.
Krause, R. M. (1970). *Adv. Immunol.*, **12**, 1.
Kunkel, H. G., Agnello, V., Joslin, F. G., Winchester, R. J., and Capra, J. D. (1973). *J. Exp. Med.*, **137**, 331.

Lamm, M. E., and Frangione, B. (1972). *Biochem. J.*, **128**, 1357.
Landucci-Tosi, S. L., and Tosi, R. M. (1973). *Immunochemistry*, **10**, 65.
Lieberman, R., and Potter, M. (1969). *J. Exp. Med.*, **130**, 519.
Lieberman, R., Potter, M., Mushinski, E. B., Humphrey, W., and Rudikoff, S. (1974). *J. Exp. Med.*, **139**, 983.
Lyon, M. F. (1961). *Nature, (Lond.)*, **190**, 372.

Mage, R., Lieberman, R., Potter, M., and Terry, W. D. (1973). In *The Antigens*, (Sela, M., ed.), Academic Press, New York, p. 300.
Mage, R. G., Young, G. O., and Reisfeld, R. A. (1968). *J. Immunol.*, **101**, 617.
Mage, R. G., Young-Cooper, G. O., and Alexander, C. (1971). *Nature, New Biol.*, **230**, 63.
Mandy, W. J., and Todd, C. W. (1968). *Vox Sang.*, **14**, 264.
Margolies, M. N., Strosberg, A. D., Fraser, K. J., Perry, D. J., Brauer, A., and Haber, E. (1974). *Fed. Proc.*, **33**, 809.
McBurnette, S. K., and Mandy, W. J. (1974). *Immunochemistry*, **11**, 255.
Mole, L. E., Jackson, S. A., Porter, R. R., and Wilkinson, J. M. (1971). *Biochem. J.*, **124**, 301.
Mudgett, M., Fraser, B. A., and Kindt, T. J. (1975). *J. Exp. Med.*, **141**, 1448.

Natvig, J. B., and Kunkel, H. G. (1973). *Adv. Immunol.*, **16**, 1.
Nezlin, R. S., Vengerova, T. I., Rokhlin, O. V., and Machulla, H. K. G. (1974). *Immunochemistry*, **11**, 517.

O'Donnell, I. J., Frangione, B., and Porter, R. R. (1970). *Biochem. J.*, **116**, 261.
Ohno, S. (1970). *Evolution by Gene Duplication*, Springer Verlag, New York.
Oudin, J. (1956). *C. R. Acad. Sci., Paris*, **242**, 2606.
Oudin, J. (1960a). *J. Exp. Med.*, **112**, 107.
Oudin, J. (1960b). *J. Exp. Med.*, **112**, 125.

Oudin, J., and Michel, M. (1963). *C.R. Acad. Sci., Paris*, **257**, 805.
Oudin, J., and Michel, M. (1969*a*). *J. Exp. Med.*, **130**, 595.
Oudin, J., and Michel, M. (1969*b*). *J. Exp. Med.*, **130**, 619.

Pawlak, L. L., Mushinski, E. B., Nisonoff, A., and Potter, M. (1973). *J. Exp. Med.*, **137**, 22.
Penn, G. M., Kunkel, H. G., and Grey, H. M. (1970). *Proc. Soc. Exp. Biol. Med.*, **135**, 660.
Pernis, B., Chiappino, G., Kelus, A., and Gell, P. G. H. (1965). *J. Exp. Med.*, **122**, 853.
Pernis, B., Forni, L., Dubiski, S., Kelus, A. S., Mandy, W. J., and Todd, C. W. (1973). *Immunochemistry*, **10**, 281.
Porter, R. R. (1974). *Ann. Immunol. (Inst. Pasteur)*, **125C**, 85.
Potter, M. (1967). *Meth. Cancer Res.*, **2**, 105.
Potter, M., and Lieberman, R. (1967). *Cold Spring Harbor Symp. Quant. Biol.*, **32**, 187.
Poulsen, K., Fraser, K. J., and Haber, E. (1972). *Proc. Nat. Acad. Sci., U.S.A.*, **69**, 2495.
Prahl, J. W., Mandy, W. J., and Todd, C. W. (1969). *Biochemistry*, **8**, 4935.

Reisfeld, R. A., Inman, J. K., Mage, R. G., and Appella, E. (1968). *Biochemistry*, **7**, 14.
Rejnek, J., Appella, E., Mage, R. G., and Reisfeld, R. A. (1969). *Biochemistry*, **8**, 2712.
Riggs, A. D. (1975). *Cytogenet. Cell Genet.*, **14**, 9.
Rivat, L., Gilbert, D., and Ropartz, C. (1973). *Immunology*, **24**, 1041.

Slater, R. J., Ward, S. M., and Kunkel, H. G. (1955). *J. Exp. Med.*, **101**, 85.
Strosberg, A. D., Fraser, K. J., Margolies, M. N., and Haber, E. (1972). *Biochemistry*, **11**, 4978.
Strosberg, A. D., Hamers-Casterman, C., van der Loo, W., and Hamers, R. (1974). *J. Immunol.*, **113**, 1313.

Tack, B. F., Feintuch, K., Todd, C. W., and Prahl, J. W. (1973). *Biochemistry*, **12**, 5172.
Thunberg, A. L. (1974). Doctoral Dissertation, The Rockefeller University, New York, N.Y.
Thunberg, A. L., Lackland, H., and Kindt, T. J. (1973). *J. Immunol.*, **111**, 1755.
Tissot, R. G., and Cohen, C. (1974). *Transplantation*, **18**, 142.
Todd, C. W. (1963). *Biochem. Biophys. Res. Commun.*, **11**, 170.
Todd, C. W. (1972). *Fed. Proc.*, **31**, 188.
Tosi, R. M., Landucci-Tosi, S., and Chersi, A. (1974). *J. Immunol.*, **113**, 876.

Wang, A. C. Wilson, S. K., Hopper, J. E., Fudenberg, H. H., and Nisonoff, A. (1970). *Proc. Nat. Acad. Sci., U.S.A.*, **66**, 337.
Warner, N. L. (1974). *Adv. Immunol.*, **19**, 67.
Waterfield, M. D., Morris, J. E., Hood, L. E., and Todd, C. W. (1973). *J. Immunol.*, **110**, 227.
Waterfield, M. D., Prahl, J. W., Hood, L. E., Kindt, T. J., and Krause, R. M. (1972). *Nature, New Biol.*, **240**, 215.
Weigert, M., Raschke, W. C., Carson, D., and Cohn, M. (1974). *J. Exp. Med.*, **139**, 137.
Weiler, E. (1965). *Proc. Nat. Acad. Sci., U.S.A.*, **54**, 1765.
Wu, T. T., and Kabat, E. A. (1970). *J. Exp. Med.*, **132**, 211.

Zeeuws, R., and Strosberg, A. D. (1975). *Archs Int. Physiol. Biochim.*, **83**, 41.
Zikan, J., Skarova, B., and Rejnek, J. (1967). *Folia Microbiol.*, **12**, 162.
Zullo, D. M., Todd, C. W., and Mandy, W. J. (1968). *Proc. Can. Fed. Biol. Soc.*, **11**, 111.

CHAPTER 5

Origin of Antibody Diversity

A. R. Williamson

1 INTRODUCTION

The origin of antibody diversity can be sought at three major levels: protein structure, cellular synthesis, and structural genes. This chapter sets forth the evidence for antibody diversity at each of these levels. Also, the various hypotheses that have been proposed to account for the antibody diversity are discussed.

The most basic question, which has been asked repeatedly, is whether the information for antibody synthesis precedes the challenge by antigen. This is the situation at the level of protein structure and at the level of cellular synthesis. At the genetic level, however, the question of whether information precedes antigenic challenge has not been answered completely. The uncertainty which remains concerns the proportion of the total pool of antibody structural genes expressed in a mature animal which is inherited in the germ line. Another way of posing this question is to ask to what extent the forces of mutation, recombination, and selection, which determine the diversity of the antibody gene pool, act either during evolution of the germ line or as somatic processes to amplify inherited diversity during the life of the individual.

2 STRUCTURAL BASIS OF ANTIBODY SPECIFICITY

2.1 Introduction

The best understood aspect of antibody diversity and specificity is the underlying structural basis. The fact that very similar immunoglobulin molecules can exhibit such a wide range of antibody specificities presented a paradox which has now been explained in terms of the amino acid sequences in each chain of each immunoglobulin molecule. It is accepted generally that the amino acid sequence of a protein determines its three-dimensional structure, and the specific demonstration of this fact for antibody molecules implies that a functional diversity of amino acid sequence is required to provide a set of different antibody combining sites. Antibodies of a different class have many physical and biological properties in common. This fact implies that considerable portions of the antibody molecule must have a common amino acid sequence. For each isotypic polypeptide chain the regions of constant amino acid sequence have been defined now. The region of amino acid sequence that varies from one immunoglobulin chain to the next has been the major focus of attention for those seeking to explain antibody diversity. Comparison of V-region amino acid sequences reveals a pattern of variability. Individual positions show a wide range of statistical variation. For each species, V-region sequences can be grouped into three distinct groups, corresponding to the κ, λ, and heavy chain C regions (Mage *et al.*, 1973). Within each set of V regions particular individual amino acids are invariant. The three-dimensional structure of two different immunoglobulin molecules indicates that a number of the constant amino acids are involved in making contact between the light and heavy chains (Davies and Padlan, 1975; Poljak, 1975). Other invariant or conservatively varied amino acids determine the characteristic folding for the peptide chain of each V region. This folding shows a great degree of similarity to that of each C-region domain.

2.2 Hypervariable Regions

The positions showing the highest degree of variability within each V region are found to be clustered together in three or four short portions which have been termed 'hypervariable regions' (Wu and Kabat, 1970; Capra and Kehoe, 1974*b*; Figure 1). The affinity-labelling data are provided in Table 1. The sequence in these hypervariable regions can be linked to the specificity of the antibody combining site.

(*i*) From these observations it is logical to deduce that a large proportion of the variation in sequence and V regions should contribute to functional diversity. Therefore, a role for the hypervariable regions in controlling antibody specificity might be expected.

(*ii*) Affinity-labelling studies using a variety of antibodies and myeloma proteins have identified many different positions in both V_L and V_H sequences as being close to or in the antibody combining site (Table 1). When these data are assembled together with a plot of variability, it can be seen that affinity-labelled amino acids or peptides lie in or adjacent to hypervariable regions (see Figure 1).

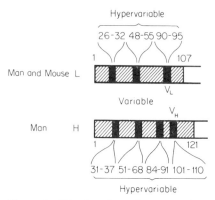

Figure 1 The location of some amino acids or peptides identified by affinity labelling relative to the hypervariable regions of V_H and V_L. (a)

In the case of protein MOPC 315 which binds DNP, a special affinity label having two active groupings was designed in order to show that the tyrosine 34 of the light chain and the lysine 54 of the heavy chain could be labelled simultaneously (Givol *et al.*, 1971). In this covalent joining of the two V regions, the distance between the tyrosine and lysine must be of the order of 0·5 nm.

(*iii*) In addition, correlation of the hypervariable-region sequence with antibody specificity has been shown in certain cases. Three examples are given here.

(*a*) *Human immunoglobulin M anti-γ globulins.* Some mixed cryoglobulins have been shown to consist of IgM antibodies specific for and complexed with IgG. From a group of 40 such IgM antibodies described by Williams *et al.* (1968), the

Table 1 Affinity-labelling data for location of some amino acids or peptides to the hypervariable regions of V_H and V_L

Species	Antibody specificity	Affinity-labelled positions	Reference
Light Chain			
Rabbit	DNP	Tyr 86	*a*
Pig	DNP	Tyr 33, Tyr 93	*b*
Mouse (TEPC15)	PC	Tyr 32	*c*
Mouse (MOPC315)	DNP	Tyr 34	*d*
Heavy Chain			
Rabbit	NAP	29–34, 95–114	*e*
Mouse (MOPC315)	DNP	Lys 54	*f*
Guinea-pig	DNP	Tyr 32, Tyr 60, Tyr (99–119)	*g*

a, Singer and Thorpe (1968); *b*, Franek (1971); *c*, Chesebro and Metzger (1972); *d*, Goetzl and Metzger (1972); *e*, Fisher and Press (1974); *f*, Givol *et al.* (1973); *g*, Ray and Cebra (1972). DNP, 2,4-dinitro phenyl; PC, phosphorylcholine; NAP, 2-nitro-4-azo-phenyl

Table 2 Structural differences between human non-selected V_HIII regions and V regions selected by cross-idiotypy

	Total sequence (124)	Hypervariable regions (41)	Non hypervariable regions (83)
V_HIII myelomas			
(Tie, Was, Jon, Zap	33	27	6
Tur, Gal, Nie) average range	28–45	25–32	3–13
Pom/Lay IgM anti-γ-globulins	8	3	9

Data from Capra and Kehoe 1974*c*

proteins Lay and Pom were selected for sequential analysis of the V regions (Capra and Kehoe, 1974*c*). These two proteins show extensive cross-idiotypic specificity, but each contains unique determinants (Kunkel *et al.*, 1973). The proteins Lay and Pom differ at only eight positions in their V_H regions. The distribution of these differences is striking for only three occur within the statistically defined hypervariable regions. Comparing the differences between Lay and Pom with differences between any two of the seven other human V_HIII sequences (each of a human myeloma protein of unknown specificity), it can be seen that outside of hypervariable regions Lay and Pom are as different as any two other V_HIII sequences (Table 2). The correlation between antibody specificity and the hypervariable-region sequence is clear. Indeed, two complete hypervariable regions are common to both proteins. This study also underlines the value of idiotypy as a marker for hypervariable region sequence and, in some instances, for the combining site of an antibody.

(*b*) *Pooled guinea-pig antibody sequences.* Amino acid sequential analysis of the heterogeneous collection of V regions found in pooled normal immunoglobulin can yield a single amino acid sequence corresponding to the most prevalent amino acid at each position. The number of alternative amino acids detected at each position depends upon the sensitivity of the analysis. In such an analysis, the hypervariable regions can be detected because of the lack of any single prevalent amino acid at those steps in the sequence. On this basis, the hypervariable regions of guinea-pig heavy chains has been defined as 31–35, 48–59, and 99–118 (Birshtein and Cebra, 1971). Cebra *et al.* (1974) used groups of inbred guinea-pigs to raise and purify antibodies specific for three different haptens—dinitrophenyl (DNP), *p*-azobenzenearsonate (ARS), and *p*-azobenzenetrimethylammonium (TMA). A single major sequence was determined for the first 83 positions of the V regions of each of these three antibody pools. The three sequences correspond to each other and to the non-hypervariable sequence of normal pooled IgG, except that each of the antibodies shows a characteristic major sequence through the first two hypervariable regions as well as showing differences at positions 2, 16, and 79 (Figure 2). Those positions showing a different amino acid characteristic of the given antibody specificity are 16, 35, 50, 52, 54, and 59. The last five

Guinea-pig (a)

Normal

```
            1                                          10                                          20
Glu– υ –Gln–Leu–Val–Glu–Ser–Gly–Gly–Leu–Val–Gln–Pro–Gly– υ –Ser–Leu–Arg–Leu–Ser–Cys–Val–Ala–Ser–Gly–
```

Anti ARS ——————— Glu
Anti DNP ——————— Glu
Anti TMA ——————— Val ——————————————— Ser
——————————————————————————— Ala
——————————————————————————— Lys

Mouse (b)

Anti ARS

```
            1                                          10                                          20
Glu–Val–Gln–Leu–Gln–Ser–Gly–Ala–Glu–Leu–Val–Lys–Pro–Gly–Ser–Ser–Val–Lys–Met–Ser–Cys–Ser–Ala–Thr–Gly–
```

```
    30                                          40                                          50
–Phe–Thr–Phe–Ser– υ – υ – υ – υ –Trp–Ile–Arg–Gln–Ala–Pro–Gly–Lys–Gly–Leu–Glu–Trp– υ –Thr– υ –Ile– υ – υ – υ –Gly– υ –Asx–Ile– υ
```

Ser–Tyr–Thr–Met–Tyr ——————— Ile–Ser–Tyr ——— Ser–Ser–Ser–Ser–Tyr ——— Lys
Ser–Tyr–Tyr–Met–Ala ——————— Val–Thr–Trp ——— Gly–Asn–Thr–Gly–Gly–Ser ——— Gly
Asn–Tyr–Trp–Met–Asn ——————— Ile–Ser–Ala ——— Asn–Ser–Asp–Gly–Ser–Ser ——— Tyr

Tyr–Thr–Phe–Ser–Tyr–Gly–Leu–Tyr–Trp–Val–Arg

```
    60                                          70
Tyr–Ala–Asx–Ser–Val–Lys–Gly–Arg–Phe–Thr–Ile–Ser–Arg–Asp–Asp–Gly–Lys–Asn–Thr–Leu–Gln–Met
```

——————————————————————— Val ———————

Figure 2 Sequences of anti-hapten antibodies from guinea-pig and mouse. Sequences identical to the normal protein are indicated by straight line; υ indicates that no major amino acid could be detected at that position. (a) N-terminal amino acid sequences of V_H regions of guinea-pig normal IgGa and three antibodies to haptens. From Cebra *et al.* (1974). (b) N-terminal amino acid sequence of V_H region of mouse antibody to the hapten ARS; the antibody was raised in strain A/J mice and shows an idiotype characteristic of the strain. From Capra *et al.* (1975)

positions lie within the hypervariable regions statistically defined from mouse and human sequences. A correlation of hypervariable region sequence with antibody specificity can even be drawn between species. The first hypervariable region of a homogeneous mouse anti-ARS heavy chain (Capra *et al.*, 1975) also is shown in Figure 2. Of particular importance is the presence of tyrosine at position 35.

(*c*) *Mouse myeloma proteins binding phosphorylcholine.* Seven mouse myeloma proteins, each capable of binding phosphorylcholine, have been isolated independently and the V_H-region amino acid sequences determined (Figure 3). These data illustrate the subtlety of antibody diversity at the level of amino acid sequence. The overall similarity of the sequences is striking. The hypervariable regions defined for human V_H regions are marked and it can be seen that each of the proteins has the same sequence in the first hypervariable region. Most of the sequence differences between these seven proteins occur in the second and fourth hypervariable regions. Indeed, comparison of these sequences shows two short hypervariable regions from 53 to 58a and from 99 to 108. These regions show insertions and deletions as well as amino acid substitutions. The major sequence identity correlates with the similar gross specificity of these seven proteins, while the two hypervariable regions identified in proteins 603, 511, and 167 correlate with fine specificity differences between these proteins and the other four (Leon and Young, 1971). The sequences can also be correlated with the pattern of shared and unique idiotypes (see Section 4.4.7).

(*iv*) The detailed role of the hypervariable region amino acids in defining the antibody-combining site has been revealed by the determination of the three-dimensional structures of the Fab fragments of two myeloma proteins—the human protein NEW, and the mouse protein McPc 603 (Davies and Padlan, 1975; Poljak, 1975). There is a striking similarity between these two structures, the basis of which is the β-pleated structures of each domain. This structure has been termed the basic immunoglobulin fold; it also has been found to occur in two light chain dimers (Schiffer *et al.*, 1973; Epp *et al.*, 1974). In all cases, the hypervariable regions exist outside the basic immunoglobulin fold. In each of the two Fab structures, five of the seven hypervariable regions of the light and heavy chains are close to one end of the Fab, are exposed fully to solvent, and surrounding the cavity. This cavity has been defined as the antibody combining site on the basis of ligand binding. Several different ligands can be bound into the cavity of protein NEW, and subsites within the cavity have been defined (Amzel *et al.*, 1974). The contact points for each ligand are the side chains of individual amino acids within the hypervariable regions of both light and heavy chains.

This is the best evidence that the complementarity of the combining site can be determined by the pattern of amino acids in hypervariable regions. The mystery of the origins of antibody diversity will be clarified greatly if it is possible to determine the origin of hypervariable regions. A valid explanation must account

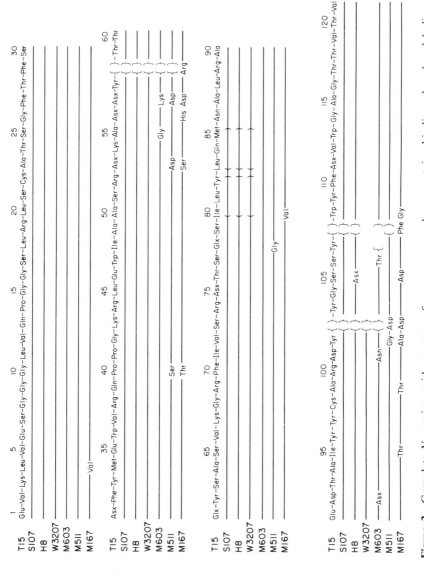

Figure 3 Complete V_H amino acid sequences from mouse myeloma proteins binding phosphorylcholine. Sequences identical to T15 are indicated by straight lines; deletions are indicated by brackets; and parentheses indicate where only compositional data is available. From Hood *et al.* (1976)

not only for the hypervariable sequences around the antibody combining site, but also for those regions remote from the combining site and playing no obvious role in defining antibody specificity.

2.3 Implications of Structure for the Origin of Antibody Diversity

At the molecular level, the origin of antibody diversity is clearly defined. The information needed to make a given antibody molecule is contained entirely within the sequences of the necessary heavy and light chains independent of any encounter with an antigen. The properties of the antibody-combining site can now be summarized, and some of the implication for antibody diversity delineated.

(*i*) The V regions of both light and heavy chains contribute to the combining site in a pseudo-symmetrical way. The arrangement of two V_L regions in a light-chain dimer also forms a pseudo-combining site (Schiffer *et al.*, 1973). The constancy (or conservative replacement) of the amino acid involved in contact between V_L and V_H regions should ensure that the maximum number of combining sites can be formed from a given number of V_L and V_H sequences (Poljak, 1975).

(*ii*) The overall size of the antibody-combining site can be varied by inserting or deleting one, or more, amino acid in those hypervariable regions proximal to the cavity. It is relevant to the origin of diversity that insertions or deletions are confined largely to those hypervariable regions surrounding the cavity.

(*iii*) In each combining site, the exact shape and specificity is determined primarily by a few (and not the same few each time) amino acid side chains rather than by all of the amino acids in the hypervariable regions. Thus, certain positions within or adjacent to each hypervariable region can be defined as complementarity-determining amino acids but these positions will differ according to the antibody. Indeed for the same V region contributing to different antibodies it is likely that different positions will contribute complementarity-determining amino acids.

(*iv*) Each antibody combining site can accommodate many structurally dissimilar compounds and can be said to exhibit multiple shared specificities. It is probable—but not proven—that for all interactions of easily measurable affinity the specific antibody combining site would contribute to a humoral immune response induced by the given haptenic group; the antibody can then be described as polyfunctional (Richards *et al.*, 1975). The prediction that identical antibody molecules will be found contributing to immune responses elicited by dissimilar haptens is consistent with available evidence. Polyfunctionality reduces the total repertoire of antibody molecules necessary to account for observed antibody diversity. This subject is discussed in greater detail by Richards *et al.* in Chapter 2 of this volume.

(*v*) A corollary to the notion of multiple shared specificities is that many different antibody combining sites can accommodate a given hapten. The nature of the interaction and the degree of fit of the hapten will vary for different combining sites, giving rise to a series of antibodies with varying affinity for a given hapten. The size of the repertoire of antibodies binding a given hapten is of particular interest for theories of the origin of antibody diversity. The prediction can be made that increasing the complexity of the hapten will place more stringent demands on the nature of the antibody combining site so that the repertoire of antibodies binding that hapten will be proportionally smaller.

3 CELLULAR BASIS OF ANTIBODY DIVERSITY

3.1 Introduction

The facts and hypotheses concerning the control of antibody synthesis at a cellular level are drawn together in this section. The details of antibody biosynthesis have been covered in an earlier chapter (see Parkhouse, Chapter 3). The historical development of the present understanding of the cellular basis of antibody diversity can be traced in the writings of Ehlich (1900), Landsteiner (1945), and Burnet (1959).

The basic question of whether information precedes antigenic encounter is answered satisfactorily at the cellular level by the clonal selection hypothesis. A selectional hypothesis operating at the molecular level was proposed by Jerne (1955), but his model still contains elements of an instructional hypothesis. The complete transition to a selectional hypothesis was made independently by Talmage (1957) and by Burnet (1957). Subsequently, the theory of clonal selection was worked out at some length by the latter (Burnet, 1959).

The clonal selection hypothesis envisages a population of cells each restricted to making a single type of antibody. Each antigen interacts with the cell or cells making a complementary antibody and the interaction of the antigen with the appropriate cell leads to cell proliferation. The resultant clonal expansion then increases production of the selected antibody. The precedent for clonal selection was the observation of selection of mutant clones in micro-organisms by appropriate environmental conditions. Thus clonal selection was linked to the idea that genes coding for antibodies are mutating and that each different clone represents a new somatic mutant. The basic hypothesis of clonal selection has survived the necessary modifications occasioned by more recent data. A current, though not necessarily final, version of the selection model is outlined here and has been reviewed in more detail elsewhere (Williamson et al., 1976).

3.2 Cells Involved in the Antibody Response

3.2.1 Stem Cells

Multipotential lymphopoietic stem cells are envisaged as a common precursor to all lymphocytes. These stem cells do not synthesize antibody and are not precommitted for the production of any particular antibody.

3.2.2 Committed Precursor Lymphocytes

These cells arise when stem cells become committed to the production of a specific antibody. The antibody is produced in small amounts (10^4–10^5 molecules/cell) and is used entirely as a receptor on the cell surface. Synthesis of receptor antibody occurs prior to, and independently of, exposure to antigen. The class of this receptor antibody is thought to be usually IgM or IgD.

3.2.3 Memory Cells

These lymphocytes are replicas of the precursor cells generated by antigen-driven clonal expansion. They differ from their progenetors mainly in being less short lived. Each is capable of giving rise to more memory cells by antigen-driven clonal expansion. Memory cells apparently can carry receptor antibody of any class or subclass.

3.2.4 Antibody-Secreting Cells

Each secretory cell produces and secretes approximately 2000 molecules of a single specificity antibody of any class or subclass per second. These cells arise by antigen-driven clonal expansion from either committed precursor lymphocytes or memory cells.

3.2.5 Conclusion

It is inherent in the above description that all cells at each stage in the expansion of a single clone produce antibody of identical specificity, although the class of antibody may vary between cells arising from the same precursor lymphocyte.

3.3 Control of Gene Expression

The essence of clonal selection is the idea of one clone—one antibody, which therefore leads to the observation of one cell—one antibody. The idea that this uniqueness of the product is due solely to mutation of antibody genes is no longer tenable (see Section 6). There are many V genes each of which can be coexpressed with any of the appropriate unique C genes (see Turner, Chapter 1 and Sogn and Kindt, Chapter 4). The restriction of antibody production in a single cell or a single clone probably involves the functional pairing of one V gene for each of the two chains of the antibody molecule. The evidence presented in the chapter on biosynthesis of antibodies (Parkhouse, Chapter 3) points to the joining of V and C genes directly at the DNA level.

The process of commitment whereby a stem cell gives rise to a precursor lymphocyte can be viewed most simply at the genetic level in terms of the joining of one V_H gene with one C_H gene, and one V_L gene with one C_L gene. The synthesis of antibody of identical specificity, but different class, by different cells arising within the same clone requires a mechanism for the movement of the selected V_H gene from its conjunction with one C_H gene to another conjunction with a new C_H gene. The simultaneous expression in one cell of the same V-gene product linked to two different C_H phenotypes requires a mechanism for duplicating the V_H gene. The mechanisms that have been suggested for the rearrangement of V and C genes have been reviewed elsewhere (Williamson and Fitzmaurice, 1976).

3.4 Diversity of Receptor Antibodies

Primotype has been defined as the total repertoire of receptor antibodies expressed on lymphocytes throughout the lifetime of an individual (Gally and Edelman, 1970). The diversity within the primotype will be much larger than the diversity of the germ-line genotype if somatic mutations contribute to the extent of antibody diversity. Whether or not the diversity of the genome in somatic cells exceeds the diversity of the genome in the germ line, it is probable that only a fraction of the primotype is expressed at any one time during the life of an individual. Most studies on the extent of the antibody phenotype utilize secreted antibodies or immunoglobulins which are the products of the ultimate cells in clonal expansion. This subfraction of antibodies available for examination thus depends upon the working of clonal selection (and in the case of myeloma proteins upon the vagaries of the neoplastic process).

The immune response to most antigens consists of a heterogeneous population of antibodies, each antibody representing the product of a single clone. Moreover, the pattern of antibodies produced in the response changes during the course of the response (Macario and Conway de Macario, 1975). In response to simple haptens, this change can be measured in terms of an increase in affinity in the later antibody. Measurements of the affinity of receptor antibodies on cells prior to exposure to the hapten suggest that receptor antibodies of both high and low affinities are present (Lefkovitz, 1974). The difference in the response between early and late periods therefore lies in the fraction of the clones which contribute antibody-secreting cells to the response. A variety of selective influences appears to direct clonal expansion either towards memory cells or towards antibody-secreting cells so that at different times during a response different clones will contribute the major portion of the secreted antibody. In certain instances, conditions may favour a single clone over all other clones. This phenomenon has been termed 'clonal dominance' (Haber, 1968; Askonas and Williamson, 1972). A special case of this is seen in the phenomenon of preferential primary selection. In this instance, the initial response to a given antigen is dominated by a particular clone (Williamson *et al.*, 1976). Preferential primary selection is inherited as a dominant genetic trait.

4 EXTENT OF ANTIBODY DIVERSITY

4.1 Introduction

The extent of diversity must be determined at the level of the antibody phenotype and of the antibody genotype. At the level of the genome, differences between the germ-line genotype and the somatic genotype are important.

All vertebrates are capable of synthesizing antibodies. In all cases tested, antibodies could be produced against any chemical grouping. The ability of the immune response to produce antibodies against novel chemical groupings was seen initially in the work of Lansteiner (1945). These conclusions came as a surprise to those who thought of antibodies solely as a defence mechanism. Any attempt to define the extent of diversity by cataloguing the number of possible antigens is confused by the fact that each antibody also can function as a specific antigen. Therefore, a limit to the extent of antibody diversity can be set only in a closed system in which the number and diversity of antibody sites are sufficient to include an antibody specific for each of the other antibodies.

A variation in this approach of determining the extent of antibody diversity is to look for gaps in the range of immune responsiveness. Specific non-responsiveness to particular antigens can be observed but in most instances it is found not to be due to the absence of antibody of a given specificity, but rather due to the failure of clonal expansion.

In view of the many ways in which an antibody site can be constructed to fit any given epitope, and the multiple specificity of an antibody combining site, the absence of gaps in the repertoire is hardly surprising.

4.2 The Antibody Phenotype

Studies on the antibody phenotype have progressed from demonstrations of diversity, through measurements of the extent of diversity, to attempts to deduce the extent of diversity of the germ-line genotype from the measurements of the phenotype.

The diversity of the antibody phenotype has been demonstrated in terms of the enormous variety of specificities and in terms of the heterogeneity of antibodies elicited by a single antigen. The term antibody, as it is generally used, refers to a population of molecules each having in common specificity for the eliciting antigen. Individual antibody molecules having widely different affinities for the same antigen can be elicited and most antisera contain molecules having different affinities (see Steward, Chapter 7). Antibody diversity may be demonstrated by measurement of affinity constants but the number of antibody molecules of different affinity present in a population can not be deduced directly from these measurements. The extent of diversity of antibody having a defined specificity has been measured using isoelectric focusing, often coupled with biological cloning techniques, to separate and to identify each antibody species. Examples of these measurements will be given below. Idiotypy and the fine specificity of an antibody combining site are powerful markers for the identification of particular antibodies. The examples quoted below conform to the rule that as the fine specificity of the selected subset of antibodies is defined more stringently then the size of the antibody repertoire decreases. This is understandable in terms of the smaller number of ways of making an antibody combining site of a more exactly defined specificity. It is particularly important to define such small subsets of antibodies since it is then possible to determine whether the necessary V regions are encoded by germ-line genes.

The size of an antibody repertoire is estimated by measuring the frequency with which identical antibody molecules are elicited in independent events. The identity of two antibodies can only be stated with complete certainty if the complete amino acid sequences are known. Estimates of the repertoire of myeloma proteins, chosen at random independently of antibody specificity, have relied almost entirely upon amino acid sequence. For most of the studies on specific antibody repertoires, antibody identity has been assessed using as phenotypic markers isoelectric spectrotype, idiotype, or fine specificity. It is important to note that antibodies can be indistinguishable by one or more of these criteria and yet can differ in amino acid sequence.

4.3 Myeloma Protein Repertoires

4.3.1 BALB/c Mouse Myeloma Proteins

Myeloma tumours are inducible and transplantable in BALB/c mice. Considerable effort has been, and is still being, expended on sequencing the V regions of light and heavy chains of BALB/c myeloma proteins. It is assumed that using myeloma proteins obtained from a single inbred strain of mice eliminates polymorphisms which may exist within a species.

4.3.1.1 V_κ Sequences. In the mouse, κ chains constitute 95 per cent of all light chains. Partial or complete data on amino acid sequence are available for almost 50 myeloma κ chains. One way of handling these data is to organize them into subgroups each defined by sequence homology, using gaps where necessary to maximize homology. With increasing numbers of sequences being determined, the definition of subgroup has come to depend upon the genetic interpretation placed upon them (see Section 6). Hood *et al.* (1974) has pointed out that as the number of known N-terminal sequences (first 23 positions) of V_κ regions has accumulated it has not become possible to see a limit for sequence diversity being reached. However, two identical V_κ sequences have been established. The frequency of two identical sequences occurring in the 50 proteins examined allows a statistical estimate of the extent of V_κ sequence diversity; with 90 per cent confidence the number of such sequences lies between 700 and 10 000.

4.3.1.2 V_λ Sequences. Only 5 per cent of mouse light chains are of the λ-type. The V regions of 18 λ myeloma chains have been sequenced completely. This has been both possible and important because of the limited amount of diversity found in these λ sequences. Twelve of the V_λ sequences are identical, four sequences differ from this by unique single base changes, one sequence differs by two base changes, and the last differs by four base changes. The pattern of diversity is particularly interesting since all nine amino acid replacements are found in positions analogous to the hypervariable regions of the V_κ chains (Cohn *et al.*, 1974).

4.3.1.3 V_H Sequences. Only a small amount of V_H-sequence data has so far been obtained and most of it comes from myeloma proteins chosen because of their antigen-binding specificity. The tentative indication from these data is that V_H-region sequential diversity may be less than the diversity of V_κ regions (Barstad *et al.*, 1974).

4.3.2 Human Myeloma Proteins

Details of these proteins may be obtained from reviews by Hood and Talmage (1970), Pink *et al.* (1971) and Dayhoff (1972).

4.3.2.1 V_κ Sequences. In excess of 50 partial or complete V_κ sequences have been obtained. On the basis of the first 20 positions, these sequences can be divided into three subgroups (I, II, and III). A further subdivision of the $V_\kappa I$ subgroup also has been suggested. The sequences show considerable diversity, although this may be less than observed for the V_κ sequences in mouse. Human light chains are approximately 67 per cent κ and 33 per cent λ type.

4.3.2.2 V_λ Sequences. The 25 partial or complete V_λ sequences can be divided into four clear subgroups (I–IV). Sequence diversity is extensive and strikingly greater than in the mouse V_λ family.

4.3.2.3 V_H Sequences. More than 20 partial or complete sequences are available (Capra and Kehoe, 1974*a*). These can be classified into four subgroups on the basis of partial N-terminal sequences. Complete V-region sequences of nine $V_H III$-subgroup proteins have been obtained. The concentration of attention on this subgroup is because of the unblocked N-terminal amino acid which makes the sequences immediately accessible by automated procedures. The conservation of sequential homology between proteins of the $V_H III$ subgroup is quite striking with two exceptions. The first exception is that variation of sequence within the hypervariable regions of this subgroup appears to be greater than that seen within the hypervariable regions of light chains. The second is that diversity increases considerably in the last 25 per cent of V_H sequences, and in fact, no subgroup specific amino acids have been found after position 82.

4.4 Specific Antibody Repertoires

4.4.1 Anti-NIP in CBA/H Mice

This repertoire was measured by using a spleen-cell transfer system at limiting cell dilution to separate the various antibody-forming clones which have been activated in mice immunized with hapten NIP (3-iodo-4-hydroxy-5-nitrophenyl) conjugated to a protein (Kreth and Williamson, 1973). A poisson distribution of memory cells was confirmed by counting the numbers of monoclonal spectrotypes of the NIP-binding antibodies present in the sera of recipient mice. Comparison of clonal spectrotypes was used to screen for similar antibodies in different donor mice. Using four donor mice, 337 spectrotypes were counted (omitting repeated occurrences of a given spectrotype from a single donor) and between donors only five pairs of spectrotype were indistinguishable. From these data the number of different NIP-binding V_H–V_L can be estimated statistically at 5000 with 90 per cent confidence limits of 2700–16 000.

This very large repertoire of antibodies showing specificity for a single hapten was rationalized by the idea of multiple-shared specificities (Williamson, 1973). This idea has gained credence with the demonstration that a single antibody combining site will bind many different antigenic determinants (Richards *et al.*, 1975). It is estimated conservatively that each antibody combining site may bind of the order of 100 different haptens. Thus, each antibody counted as having anti-NIP specificity would also be specific for 99 other epitopes. In any one mouse, something of the order of 200 different clones may be expanded by immunization with NIP–protein and 50–100 of these may contribute antibody to the response at any one time. The specificity of this population of antibody molecules depends upon the fact that they have in common a specificity for the eliciting hapten NIP. The probability that any substantial fraction of the population will share a second specificity will depend upon the degree to which the second epitope is related structurally to NIP. Thus only conventional cross-reactions predictable on a structural basis may be expected. The cross-reactivity of individual antibody combining sites for structurally dissimilar epitopes would not be observed using populations of antibody molecules.

Natural antibodies which display NIP specificity may on the basis of the foregoing reasoning, be present in normal sera in the same proportion as NIP-binding antibodies are represented in the total antibody repertoire. In a large pool of sera from non-immunized CBA/H mice, 0·09 per cent of the total immunoglobulin appears to be NIP-binding antibodies (Inman, 1974). This measurement leads to an estimate of almost 6×10^6 for the total antibody repertoire.

4.4.2 Anti-DNP/TNP in CBA/H and C3H/HE Mice

Each antibody combining site can be characterized by cataloguing the set of shared specificities for that site. If sites are selected on the basis of two shared specificities, the size of the repertoire determined should be considerably smaller than that for site selected for a single specificity. An example of this is seen in a modification of the NIP-repertoire experiment. The donor mice—either CBA/H, or the closely related strain C3H/HE—were immunized with a DNP–protein conjugate but in the recipient mice the transferred clones were challenged with TNP conjugated to the same carrier protein. The repertoire of antibody combining sites exhibiting this dual DNP/TNP fine specificity was estimated at approximately 500 (Pink and Askonas, 1974).

4.4.3 Anti-NP/NIP in C57BL/6 Mice

The fine specificity of antibody combining sites can be characterized in a more discriminating fashion by determining the binding constants of a series of structurally related compounds. This approach can be used to define a small subset of antibodies whose number then can be counted by conventional techniques. A good example of this approach is the demonstration in C57BL/6 mice of a subset of anti-nitrophenyl antibodies which show a higher affinity for NIP or NNP than for the homologous hapten (Imanishi and Mäkelä, 1974; McMichael *et al.*, 1975). Subsets with such properties have been called heteroclitic antibodies. Subsequent analysis of the spectrotypes of such antibodies shows that the repertoire of V_H–V_L combinations with this particular fine specificity is very small (certainly less than 10) with a single clone contributing predominantly to the response.

The way in which the definition of specificity of a combining site affects the observed size of the repertoire of antibodies is well illustrated by comparison of the three specific examples given above (Figure 4). On the reasonable assumption that the total repertoires for DNP in CBA/H mice and for nitrophenol in C57BL/6 mice are similar in extent to that of NIP in CBA/H mice, only 10 per cent of their repertoire can bind a second, structurally similar hapten. Only about 0·1 per cent of the repertoire of antibodies elicited by a hapten exhibits the peculiar property of a higher affinity for structurally related haptens than for the eliciting hapten. The fraction of any specific repertoire that will show binding of any other structurally dissimilar epitope is presumably similar to or less than the fraction exhibiting heteroclitic properties.

4.4.4 Anti-α-DNP–Deca-L-Lysine in Guinea-Pigs

The effectiveness of haptens, such as DNP and NIP, stems from the fact that they constitute the immunodominant portion of a complete antigenic determinant, the remainder of which is contributed by topographically adjacent parts of the carrier protein molecule. Immunodominant haptens contribute disproportionately to the binding energy when compared with the proportion of the space which they fill within the antibody combining site. This is illustrated in a

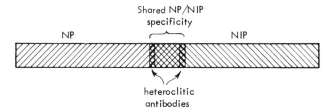

Figure 4   Probable relationships of repertoire size and overlap for antibodies to two related haptens. Heteroclitic antibodies are those elicited by one hapten but which bind the other hapten more strongly

158

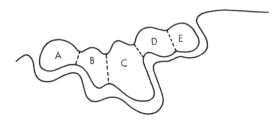

Figure 5 Model of a hypothetical antibody combining site holding a complete epitope. The parts of the epitope are labelled A, B, C, D, and E. Group C is the immunodominant part of the epitope

simplified way in Figure 5. The immunodominant hapten is designated C. Selection for the binding of C defines only one of the several subsites within the antibody combining site. If each part of the complete antigenic determinant (A, B, C, D, E) is defined exactly then the repertoire of complementary antibody combining sites should be very limited. The examples given in this and Sections 4.4.5 and 4.4.6 are consistent with this notion.

A single DNP group presented on polylysine constitutes a simple immunogen with DNP as the dominant group (Schlossman and Williamson, 1972). In guinea-pigs, α-DNP–oligolysines with a chain length of greater than seven lysines are immunogenic. The response to these oligomers, which are of the order of size expected for a complete antigenic determinant, is invariably simple consisting of one, two, or three antibodies each exhibiting a distinct spectrotype. Comparison of the spectrotypes elicited in 33 guinea-pigs of strains 2 and 13 revealed a pattern of repeats, which are catalogued in Table 3. In a total of 51 spectrotypes, only 19 different patterns could be distinguished with seven occurring several times (making up 76 per cent of the observed spectrotypes), while each of the remaining 12 spectrotypes was observed in only one response. A small repertoire of seven antibodies particularly specific for α-DNP-deca-L-lysine appears to be available

Table 3 Spectrotypes in guinea-pigs

Frequency (n)	Number* of clones (C)	$C \times n$
20	1	20
4	1	4
3	5	15
1	12	12
Total	19	51

* Number of anti-α-DNP-deca-L-lysine clones (C) found in all guinea-pigs (that is poly-L-lysine responder and poly-L-lysine non-responder animals) with a frequency n. Sera from 33 guinea-pigs immunized with α-DNP-deca-L-lysine are included in this analysis. Among the 51 monoclonal spectra compared, 19 different spectra are represented. Data from Williamson (1975)

in all guinea-pigs. The total repertoire of antibodies, which include the DNP group in their specificity, has not been determined in the guinea-pig.

Isoelectric focusing studies of antibodies elicited in response to DNP conjugated to proteins show complex spectra. In apparent contrast to this, amino acid sequential analysis of the heavy chains of such anti-DNP antibodies has failed to reveal substantial heterogeneity even in the first two hypervariable regions (Figure 2). If the total repertoire of DNP-binding antibodies is as large in the guinea-pig, as it appears to be in the mouse, then the third hypervariable region (99–118) of the heavy chain and the light chains must contribute considerably to the diversity.

4.4.5 Anti-(DNP)$_2$-Gramicidin S in Rabbits

Gramicidin S is a highly ordered, cyclic decapeptide made up of two identical amino acid sequences arranged in two-fold symmetry. Each half of the molecule is an ideal candidate to act as a complete antigenic determinant. For convenience, the two free amino groups have been coupled to DNP which then serves as the immunodominant part of the antigen.

This presentation of DNP is immunogenic in about 65 per cent of randomly bred rabbits (Montgomery et al., 1975a, b). In each responder rabbit, the antibody obtained has a simple isoelectric spectrum. Comparison of the spectrotypes of the antibody obtained in different rabbits shows many similarities but each spectrotype is unique. Despite this, chain recombination studies using the antibodies produced in two different rabbits supports the hypothesis that the two antibodies have identical combining sites. The genetic basis of non-responsiveness remains to be proved. The intriguing possibility exists that non-responder rabbits may lack structural genes coding for antibodies capable of being elicited in response to (DNP)$_2$–gramicidin S. Since the evidence points to there being an extremely small repertoire of such antibodies in most rabbits, the loss of the necessary V genes in some members of the population would be probable.

4.4.6 Anti-Group A Streptococcal Polysaccharides in BALB/c Mice

Many polysaccharides contain a simple repeating pattern of monomers which, from an immunological point of view, is a multiple presentation of identical complete antigenic determinants. Antibody responses to such polysaccharides are frequently of restricted heterogeneity. Bacterial vaccines are excellent immunogenic presentations of bacterial polysaccharides.

Inbred strains of mice have been characterized as high or low-responders to each polysaccharide. Sufficiently simple responses (two to four clones) to permit analysis of the isoelectric spectrotypes have been obtained in high-responder mice by giving multiple injections of bacterial vaccine. This regime results in clonal dominance being established. Since it is not understood how the properties of a given antibody affect whether or not the clone producing that antibody can

Table 4 V-region antigenic markers (idiotypes) on phosphorylcholine-binding myeloma proteins and anti-phosphorylcholine antibodies of murine origin

Idiotype	Source of anti-idiotype serum	Ig-bearing idiotype		Location of idiotypic determinant
		Anti-PC	Myeloma	
T15	A/J or CE mice anti-T15	Only raised in Ig–1a mice (also on natural antibody Ig–1a mice)	TEPC 15 HOPC 8 M299 S63 S107 Y5170 Y5236	Not site-related (V_H site because linked to C_H-allotype)
$H8_S$	Rabbit anti-H8. Serum absorbed onto H8 and eluted with PC	Raised in any mouse	TEPC 15 HOPC 8[a] CBPC 2[b]	Binding-site specific, requires both V_H and V_L
H_V–PC	Rabbit anti-H8, detected by inhibition of reaction with M167	Raised in any mouse	TEPC 15 HOPC 8[a] CBPC 2 M511[c] M603[c] M167[c]	Entirely on V_H, binding-site related

PC = phosphoryl choline
[a] Other myelomas in T15 group not tested
[b] CBPC2 is a PC-binding myeloma originating in a CB-20 mouse, congenic to BALB/c but with Ig–1b C_H-allotype
[c] Each of these proteins also has unique V-region determinants
Composed from Lieberman *et al.* (1974), Claflin and Davie (1974, 1975a, b)

achieve dominance, it must be assumed that the repertoire of dominant antibodies may be less than the total repertoire of antibodies of similar specificity. On the basis of repeated spectrotypes elicited by group A streptococcal vaccine in BALB/c mice, the repertoire of dominant antibodies was estimated to be between 30 and 40 (Cramer and Braun, 1974). In another high-responder strain, A/J mice, the dominant response showed an indistinguishable monoclonal spectrotype (A5A) in nine out of 10 mice (Eichmann, 1972, 1973). Other spectrotypes are seen in the sera of A/J mice prior to the establishment of clonal dominance.

4.4.7 Anti-Phosphorylcholine in Mice

Phosphorylcholine is a constituent of the capsular polysaccharide of certain pneumococcal strains and which acts as an immunodominant hapten. The availability of seven murine myeloma proteins showing specificity for phosphorylcholine has facilitated greatly the study of the immune response to this hapten (Claflin *et al.*, 1975). Three idiotypes detected on phosphorylcholine-binding myeloma proteins also are present on natural anti-phosphorylcholine antibody (Table 4).

The complete amino acid sequences of the V_H regions of seven of the phosphorylcholine-binding myeloma proteins (see Figure 3) suggest a basis for the idiotypy. The first hypervariable region is identical in all seven proteins and thus correlates with the common heavy-chain idiotype H_V–PC (it should be noted that the third hypervariable region, as defined for human myeloma proteins, is common to all seven sequences). The identity of hypervariable region 2 for proteins T15, S107, and H8 correlates with the $H8_S$ idiotype, but it is known that light-chain sequences also must contribute to this idiotype. The T15 idiotype behaves as a private allotypic specificity present on anti-phosphorylcholine antibodies in Ig-1a mice but not in Ig-1b mice (Lieberman *et al.*, 1974). The myeloma protein CBPC2 (having the C_H allotype Ig-1b) has been sequenced through position 36 of both the heavy and the light chain (Claflin *et al.*, 1975). Comparison with the corresponding sequences of T15 shows only two differences, at positions 14 (Ser → Pro) and 16 (Arg → Gly) of the heavy chain. These differences outside of a hypervariable region could well account for the non-site-related idiotype T15.

The binding site-related idiotype $H8_S$ correlateds with the fine specificity of the antibody combining site as determined by affinity and pattern of cross-reactivity for hapten analogues (Leon and Young, 1971). By the criteria of idiotypy and fine specificity, phosphorylcholine-specific antibodies of many different inbred mouse strains and of wild *Mus musculus* share an identical combining site. On this evidence, the repertoire of anti-phosphorylcholine antibodies in any mouse would appear to be one. The existence of myeloma proteins M511, M603, and M167 points to a larger repertoire. Phosphorylcholine fills only a small portion of the combining site of M603 and is therefore not a complete antigenic determinant. This may be one explanation why M603 and the related proteins are not detected in the immune response elicited by phosphorylcholine-containing bacterial vaccines. Immunization with phosphorylcholine coupled by a tripeptide spacer to a protein does elicit a larger repertoire of antibodies (Gearhart *et al.*, 1975). The response has been cloned and expressed in splenic fragment culture *in vitro*. Between 2 and 50 per cent of clones from different individual BALB/c mice produce phosphorylcholine-binding antibodies which lacked the T15 idiotype.

5 ANTIBODY GENOTYPE

5.1 Deductions from Phenotype

Structural genes coding for antibodies may be mapped by conventional genetics if those genes are carried in the germ line. Studies of the inheritance of allotypic markers, amino acid sequential analysis, and molecular hybridization are each consistent with the hypothesis that a single C gene codes for each C-region sequence (see Sogn and Kindt, Chapter 4). The diversity of antibody V-region sequences led to somatic hypotheses based on the proposition that only certain basic V genes are inherited and that the phenotype represents the sum of the selected mutants of these V genes (see Section 6). It is therefore necessary to ask whether each V-region sequence is encoded by a germ-line V gene or whether it is encoded by a somatic variant V gene arising in a single cell and selected by antigen to give rise to a clone of antibody-secreting cells. Inheritance studies have used a variety of V-region markers, but usually not the most definitive one of complete amino acid sequences.

5.2. Genotype Deduced from Amino Acid Sequences

It is not feasible to investigate the germ-line basis of myeloma V-region sequences by inheritance studies. Therefore, amino acid sequences have been compared with respect to the degree and type of sequence variation in order to deduce the minimum number of germ-line V genes necessary to give rise to the observed diversity.

5.2.1 V-Region Subgroups

Once it was recognized that V-region sequences within a family are too diverse to have arisen by somatic mutations of a single V gene, the sequences were divided into subgroups. The minimum number of V genes in each family was then one for each subgroup. Subgroup assignments based on partial N-terminal sequential analysis have proved to be an oversimplification. Complete V-region sequences have been analysed by more systematic application of the subgroup principle.

5.2.2 Genealogical Analysis

V-Region sequences both within and between families have been shown to be related to each other in a genealogical pattern (Smith *et al.*, 1971; Hood, 1973). This pattern or tree is a putative map of the minimum number of genetic events necessary to have evolved the observed sequences from a single ancestral sequence. The genealogical trees drawn for antibody V regions resemble those drawn for a homologous set of proteins from many different species. The pattern obtained for homologous proteins in turn resembles the classically determined phylogenetic tree relating the species from which each of the proteins was derived. A set of V-region sequences from the same inbred strain could, it is assumed, have been expressed totally within one member of that inbred strain. In this case, each V-region sequence can be considered as arising from a single V gene whose expression is limited to a particular clone of antibody-forming cells. Thus, the genetic events relating different V-region sequences could have occurred within an evolutionary time period (V-gene duplication followed by mutational events) or during the extensive cell division necessary to produce the population of clones found within a single animal (somatic mutational events).

As with subgroup analysis, the most meaningful genealogical trees are produced using complete V-region amino acid sequences. Such an analysis for the V-regions of human myeloma proteins is shown in Figure 6. The κ, λ, and

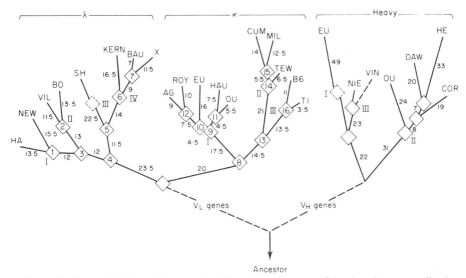

Figure 6 Genealogical tree for complete V-region sequences of the three human antibody families. The numbers of amino acid substitutions occurring between branch points are shown. Nodal sequences that have been deduced are indicated by numbers in diamonds. From Hood *et al.* (1976)

heavy-chain families can be seen to be related distantly. The division of sequences into subgroups can also be seen clearly in this analysis. In deciding upon the level at which sequence variation has arisen, genealogical analysis of myeloma sequences arising in an outbred human population are less useful than the sequences of BALB/c mouse myeloma tumours.

Genealogical analysis of the partial N-terminal sequence (23 positions) of the BALB/c κ-chain yields a tree with more than 25 branches. Only a portion of this genealogical tree can be drawn using complete V-region sequences (Figure 7). Three of these V_κ chains (M70, M321, and T124) have identical N-terminal sequences through to position 23, while M63 differs from this sequence only at position 1. Complete sequence analysis reveals that M70 differs from M321 at 22 positions, while M63 is different from M321 at only eight positions (Figure 7).

The simplest explanation of this genealogical tree is that the sequences are encoded by a minimum of three germ-line genes which arise by duplication and diversion by mutation during evolution (Hood *et al.*, 1976). This analysis is arrived at by discounting the possibility of parallel mutations, which would be required for instance if M63, M21, and T124 each represented variants of a single germ-line V gene. The argument against parallel mutations is that 'no selective forces are known which might employ random somatic mutation and select from the many variants generated two V genes with multiple identical substitutions' (Hood *et al.*, 1976). In contrast, it has been argued that structural constraints, including the antibody fold, can provide a sufficiently strong selective force for parallel mutations to be preserved (Novotny, 1973). It should however be borne

164

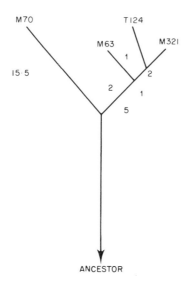

Figure 7 Genealogical tree for four mouse V regions with similar amino acid sequences. The minimum number of base changes separating each protein from the nearest common nodal ancestor is shown. From McKean *et al.* (1973)

in mind that as the requirements for a functional V-region become more stringent the wastefulness of a somatic mutation process will increase. If parallel somatic mutations are disallowed completely, most V_κ diversity must exist in the germ-line genome of BALB/c mice. Likewise, genealogical analysis leads to the conclusion that most of the sequence differences seen for BALB/c V_H regions require that they be coded by separate germ-line genes. For sequences as similar as the V_κ regions of M321 and T124, or the family of 18 V_λ myeloma sequences, genealogical analysis can not distinguish whether the mutational events occurred during evolution or somatically.

5.2.3 Framework and Complementarity-Determining Amino Acids

The pattern of variation seen in the V_λ sequences of 18 BALB/c mice has led to the hypothesis that the positions at which variation are seen represent complementarity-determining amino acids. This conclusion was arrived at because each of the variations occurs within one of the three hypervariable regions defined for V_κ sequences. The invariant stretches of V_κ sequence have been called the framework. The hypothesis has been advanced (Cohn, 1974; Cohn *et al.*, 1974) that 'amino acid replacements in the framework are due principally to mutation and selection of germ-line V genes, whereas replacements

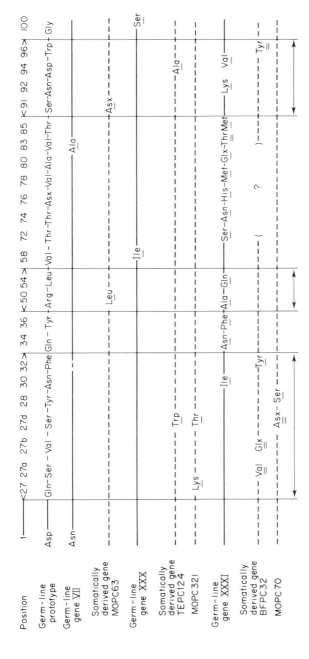

Figure 8 Predicted sequences encoded by three germ-line V_κ genes VII, XXX, and XXXI, and the V_κ products assumed to have been derived by mutation and selection of complementarity-determining positions (Cohn, 1974). Positions indicated ↔ are designated as complementarity-determining amino acids

of complementarity-determinants arise principally because of mutation and selection of somatically derived V genes'. In applying this hypothesis to the interpretation of other families of V-region sequences, the original argument was used to assign V_λ amino acid replacements to complementarity-determining positions has been reversed and all hypervariable region amino acids are assumed to supply complementarity determinants. The framework is taken to be those sequences separating the hypervariable regions, and a different germ-line V gene is assigned for each variation in framework sequence. From the sequences of the hypervariable regions associated with a given framework the sequence of the inherited germ-line gene is predicted. This process is illustrated in Figure 8 for the germ-line genes needed to code for the same set of proteins shown in Figure 7. The prediction of three germ-line genes is the same as the minimum estimate made on the basis of genealogical analysis.

Applying the analysis of framework variation to the known partial sequences of V_κ chains (excluding those from proteins selected previously for binding activity) a statistical estimate of the total number of germ-line V_κ genes can be made (see Table 5). Since the sequences analysed in Table 5 constitute only about a quarter of the total framework, it can be estimated that the total number of genes will be two to four times greater (150–300). Since this hypothesis was inspired by the V_λ-sequence data, it is axiomatic to the hypothesis that all 18 known V_λ sequences are the products of a single germ-line gene.

Estimates of the extent of genotype diversity based on myeloma protein sequences will be too low if myeloma proteins do not represent a random

Table 5 Distribution of unselected V_κ sequences

V_κ gene	Class	Total	Myeloma
I–XXIII	Single	23	LPC 1, MPOC 35, TEPC 157, MOPC 379, HOPC 5, MOPC 21, MPOC 63, MOPC 173, MOPC 41, MOPC 149, McPc 600, MOPC 47A, MOPC 316, BFP 61, McPc 674, McPc 843, TEPC 29, MOPC 29, TEPC 153, MPC 37, MOPC 31C, TEPC 173, 611
XXIV–XXIX	Double	12	MOPC 313, MOPC 178; MPC 11, 641 M, RPC 23; MOPC 46, MOPC 172; MOPC 467, MOPC 37; MOPC 265, MOPC 773
XXX and XXXI	Quintuplet	5	TEPC 124, MOPC 321, 613, BFPC 32, MOPC 70

$$\text{Calculated total genes} = \frac{\text{total sequences}}{2} \quad \frac{\text{singles}}{\text{doubles}} = \frac{40}{2} \quad \frac{23}{6} = 77$$

The sequences of only the first 23 amino acids have been compared for the mouse myeloma κ chains. A gene is assigned to each different sequence. An estimate of the total number of genes is calculated from the frequency with which sequences are found twice. This estimate of gene number must be corrected upwards to account for sequences of complete κ chains (see text). Adapted from Cohn (1974)

selection of the antibody repertoire. Comparison of available myeloma protein sequences with the pattern of amino acids found at each position in the sequence or with a normal pool of serum immunoglobulin reveals both qualitative and quantitative differences. These differences suggest that either the myeloma proteins represent a selected subset of the antibody repertoire or that a sample of 44 myeloma proteins is too few to be representative of a very extensive repertoire.

5.3 Characterization of Specific V_H Genes by Inheritance Studies

The phenotypic markers, idiotype, fine specificity, and spectrotype have been followed in breeding studies to show the inheritance of specific V_H genes. The linkage of these individual V_H genes to the C_H gene, followed by allotypic markers, is consistent with the linkage previously shown by following V_H allotypic markers in the rabbit (see Sogn and Kindt, Chapter 4). The V_H genes so far defined in the mouse are DEX(J558), T15, A5A, ARS, S117, NP(N1), and NBrP. The mapping of these genes has been described in Chapter 4 reviewed elsewhere (Eichmann, 1975).

The identification and mapping of a small number of V_H genes may account for only a tiny fraction of the germ-line V-gene pool. The distances measured by the combination between V_H and C_H genes, ranging from 0·4 to about 3 per cent, would allow space for a very large number of germ-line V genes either between the distal and proximal V genes (relative to C_H), or even between the proximal V_H gene and the C_H gene cluster.

5.4 Molecular Hybridization

Direct assessment of the nature of the germ-line V and C genes can be assessed by RNA–DNA or DNA–DNA hybridization. Several approaches are possible,

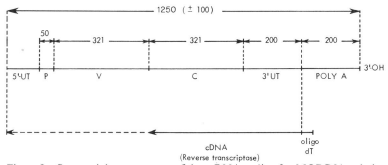

Figure 9 Sequential arrangement of the mRNA coding for MOPC 21 κ chain. The lengths of the total mRNA and its regions are given as the numbers of bases. Lengths of poly A and 3′-untranslated region (3′-UT) have been estimated from partial sequence data. The 5′UT region was estimated only by difference (Milstein et al., 1974). The direction of synthesis of complementary DNA (cDNA) starting from an oligo-DT primer and catalysed by viral reverse transcriptase (RNA-directed DNA polymerase) is shown below the mRNA model

but all ideally require an isogenic mRNA preparation. Hybridization experiments using mRNA of moderate purity can lead to misleading interpretation when the nature of the impurities is unknown. The hybridization probe used may be either mRNA labelled biosynthetically or by radioiodination. Alternatively, a radioactive complementary DNA (cDNA) may be employed, which is prepared by copying mRNA using a viral reverse transcriptase (see Figure 9). There are technical difficulties in obtaining DNA transcripts complementary to the complete mRNA molecule. Partial cDNA molecules are complementary to the sequence of the 3'-untranslated region of the mRNA and the constant region of the polypeptide chain (Figure 9). Such cDNA probes have proved useful in counting the number of C genes.

Most attempts to measure the frequency of immunoglobulin genes have used the technique of hybridization driven by a vast excess of genome DNA (Melli *et al.*, 1971; Bishop, 1972). Reannealing of genome DNA follows second-order kinetics·with individual gene sequences hybridizing at a rate determined by the number of copies of that gene present, thus allowing the frequency of repeated DNA sequences to be estimated. A trace quantity of a probe (mRNA or cDNA) specific for a given gene when added to reannealing DNA forms a hybrid with the complementary genomic DNA strand following pseudo-second-order kinetics and at a rate dependent on the gene frequency.

There are numerous technical problems associated with this technique. The main one is that of obtaining a probe with sufficiently high specific activity so that it can be used in the trace quantities necessary to ensure that single copy genes (representing about one part in 10^7 of genome DNA) are present in excess over the probe. When this condition is fulfilled, an approximate estimate of gene frequency can be made. For the antibody genes another problem arises, namely that the V genes in each family are homologous, but non-identical. Such mismatched sequences will cross-hybridize, although at a slower rate than the rate of annealing of identical sequences. A given V-region sequential probe can count only identical or very similar V genes, even if all V sequences are present as germ-line genes. On the other hand, if the chosen V-region probe represents a somatic variant of a germ-line gene, there will be no germ-line DNA sequence identical to the probe (Williamson and Fitzmaurice, 1976).

Hybridization experiments with probes specific for the C regions of murine κ, λ, or heavy chains reveal complementary gene sequences in non-repetitive genome DNA (reviewed by Williamson and Fitzmaurice, 1976). These results are consistent with genetic data which state that there are single copies of these genes. The data from probes including V-region sequences are less easy to interpret. The purest mRNA κ preparations used as ^{131}I-labelled probes hybridize entirely to non-repetitive DNA sequences; the extent of hybrid formation may be assessed by the resistance of the probe to ribonuclease digestion (Tonegawa, 1976). A cDNA prepared from highly purified mRNA κ (MOPC 21) and of sufficient length to include the entire V-region sequence, forms a duplex stable to deoxyribonuclease S1 with only non-repetitive DNA sequences (Rabbitts and Milstein, 1975). However, when the extent of hybridization of the same cDNA preparation was assayed by binding to hydroxyapatite, partial hybridization to repetitive DNA sequences occurred. These hybrids may represent mismatched sequences, but it is not yet clear whether the sequence involved is the V region, the 5'-untranslated mRNA sequence, or a non-κ-chain impurity in the probe preparation.

A series of experiments using $[^{131}\mathrm{I}]$mRNA probes for the κ chains of MOPC 321 and MOPC 70 showed no hybridization to repetitive DNA—except that due to impurities in certain preparations of mRNA (Tonegawa, 1976). On the assumption that either of these probes should detect both genes (and related genes—see Figures 7 and 8), it was concluded that MOPC 321 and MOPC 70 are somatic variants of the same germ-line V gene. This conclusion is at variance with the deduction based on the analysis of amino acid sequences (see Figures 7 and 8). Calculation of the effect of sequence mismatching on the rate of hybridization of the MOPC 70 V-region sequence to the MOPC 321 V gene, or *vice versa*, suggests that separate germ-line genes coding for 70 and 321 could exist and yet not be counted by hybridization kinetics (Williamson and Fitzmaurice, 1976).

The mouse λ system also has been investigated by molecular hybridization. Leder *et al.* (1975) used a cDNA molecule of sufficient length to include most of the V_λ sequences, while Tonegawa (1976) employed $[^{131}\mathrm{I}]$mRNA λ as the probe. In both cases, the probes hybridized to non-repetitive DNA sequences. The simplest interpretation of these results is that there is only a single V_λ gene in the mouse. The similarity of known V_λ amino acid sequences would allow a nucleic acid probe for one sequence to be used to count all gene sequences unless the gene and mRNA sequences differ by a number of silent mutations.

6 MODELS PROPOSED TO EXPLAIN ANTIBODY DIVERSITY

6.1 Introduction

In order to assess the various models proposed to explain the origin of antibody diversity, the current evidence will be summarized as a list of statements which must form the constraints of any model.

(*i*) The information required for the synthesis of an antibody molecule is present, and is expressed in the form of a receptor antibody, prior to the exposure to antigen. (*ii*) Each antibody polypeptide chain is the product of two structural genes, one coding for the V and the other for the C region. (*iii*) Each cell is programmed to make a single antibody specificity, defined by the combination of one V_L sequence with one V_H sequence. (*iv*) The joining of V and C-gene information occurs at the DNA level, *not* at the RNA or protein level. (*v*) A V gene can only be joined with a C gene on the same chromosome, that is the process is *cis*. (*vi*) There is a single C gene coding for each C_L and C_H region. (*vii*) There are three families of V genes: one linked to the cluster of C_H genes; one linked to the C_κ gene(s); and the third is linked to the C_λ gene(s). (*viii*) Each V_H gene can be expressed sequentially (and possibly simultaneously) in conjunction with each of the C_H genes.

Several of the models considered below are of historical interest only since they are clearly incompatible with the available evidence. Instructional hypotheses and hypotheses invoking errors in translation or transcription are not discussed, since they are no longer tenable and are irrelevant to current thinking. Each model will be discussed and its present standing evaluated.

6.2 Germ-Line Hypotheses

A germ-line hypothesis maintains that somatic processes do not play an essential part in increasing the extent of antibody diversity available from germ-line V genes. In its simplest form this hypothesis states that for each antibody polypeptide chain which an individual can synthesize a structural gene must be transmitted in the germ-line DNA (Hood and Talmage, 1970). This is held usually to be the most conventional of the hypotheses in that it assumes that each antibody gene has evolved by the same processes as the structural genes for other proteins. Successive gene duplications and subsequent diversification of the duplicates by mutation during evolutionary time are general processes in protein evolution.

The discovery of V and C-region sequences in each antibody polypeptide chain has resulted in two variations of this basic hypothesis. The first proposal was that each antibody polypeptide chain is encoded by two germ-line genes, one V and one C gene (Dreyer and Bennett, 1965). In this model, the germ-line DNA would contain a structural gene coding for each V region and one for each C region. Thus, for mouse κ chains something of the order of 1000 V-region genes and only a single C-region gene would be co-inherited. For the production of a κ chain the information from one of the V genes would need to be joined to the C-gene information. It was proposed initially that this might take place at the DNA level. In a reaction against the unconventional idea of two genes coding for a single polypeptide chain, the stringent germ-line hypothesis was restated by Brown (1972) in terms of equal numbers of V and C genes being inherited as single units. The biological precedent for the inheritance of multiple genes with alternate V and C-region nucleotide sequences came from the tandem array of 5 S RNA genes in *Xenopus laevis*. The molecular studies which have shown that there is a single haploid copy of each C gene have eliminated the stringent germ-line hypothesis (see Section 5.4).

The concept of two genes contributing to each antibody polypeptide chain now is accepted as the basis for any viable model of antibody diversity. It is not in itself sufficient for the germ-line hypothesis. On the basis of the current evidence any viable hypothesis must start from the proposition that there are multiple V genes inherited in the germ line. In the germ-line hypothesis, the term 'multiple V genes' is equated with the total repertoire. An acceptable germ-line hypothesis must, therefore, account for the pattern of diversity in V genes, the extent of the repertoire of V genes in which gaps are infrequent, and the stable inheritance of a large multiple gene family. Discussion of these points (see Section 6.4.3) will be delayed until the various somatic hypotheses have been considered.

6.3 Somatic Hypotheses Using a Small Number of Genes

The basic assumption in this class of hypotheses is that the majority of antibody diversity arises by somatic variation of a limited number of germ-line V genes. The germ-line contribution to diversity is very limited.

6.3.1 Hypermutation

A small number of V genes inherited in the germ line is subjected to special mutational events during the proliferation of stem cells. Each mutation is tested as a receptor antibody; successful mutants are those that can be selected by antigen and driven to proliferate into a clone of antibody-forming cells. The original idea was that clones of antibody-forming cells arose in a similar way to mutant clones of micro-organisms (Lederberg, 1959). As understanding of the structural basis of antibody diversity has increased so hypermutation theories have evolved to account for these data. One solution is to postulate directed mutation. Hypervariable regions might be created by an accumulation of errors in a DNA-repair process or by the random generation of short structures of DNA sequence (see, for example, Brenner and Milstein, 1966).

6.3.2 Special Selection

The alternative to directed mutation was to invoke special selection. Hypotheses of this type depend upon a special selective pressure inherent in the developing antibody system. The operation of this selection during ontogeny ensures that the necessary antibody diversity is generated by a normal mutation rate.

The most cogently argued hypothesis of this type is that of Jerne (1971), who suggested that the germ-line V genes code only for antibodies specific for the histocompatibility antigens of the species. The products of these genes would be of two types: those specific for histocompatibility antigens possessed by the individual animal; and those specific for histocompatibility antigens of the species not found in the individual animal. The special selective pressure is exhibited by self-histocompatibility antigens acting during ontogeny to suppress the expression of antibodies against such self-antigens. It was postulated that this pressure only allows the expression of mutants of the germ-line V genes originally coding for self-histocompatibility antigens. The functional immune system would comprise this selected set of spontaneous random somatic mutants together with the germ-line encoded antibodies against alloantigens.

Bodmer (1972) has pointed out a major difficulty associated with Jerne's hypothesis. The model requires a strict parallel evolution, at the population level, of genes coding for the histocompatibility antigens and for immunoglobulin V genes, but these two sets of genes are unlinked. Bodmer, therefore, modified the hypothesis of Jerne by suggesting that the V genes coding for antibodies against self-antigens are directed against differentiation antigens. These antigens characterize different differentiated cell types that are common to all individuals of a species.

6.3.3 Somatic Recombination

The simplest form of this hypothesis was the one-and-a-half gene model proposed by Smithies (1967). A single V–C pair (one gene) and a single V gene (half gene) have been proposed as the germ-line genes. Diversity of the V–C product was postulated to arise by recombination events between the two V-gene sequences. This hypothesis may be easily disproven since it predicts that only two alternative amino acids would be found at each position (except when recombination occurs within a codon).

The hyper-recombinational hypothesis of Gally and Edelman (1970) proposed that the germ-line DNA contains a tandem array of V genes which can undergo haploid, generalized recombination. This recombination would be effected simply by the formation of a V-region episome in any register, without the need for a specific excision sequence. The V-gene episome was postulated to be integrated subsequently with the nearby C gene on the same chromosome; integration was seen as being a highly specific event analogous to the integration of λ phage. Generalized recombination between a small number of V genes cannot explain the known amino acid sequences. It cannot be ruled out that recombination processes play some role in the generation of antibody diversity, but a large number of V genes must be involved. Moreover, it is necessary to divide these V genes into subgroup clusters with intra-subgroup recombination being permitted, while inter-subgroup recombination is forbidden. Even with these conditions there is no direct evidence for somatic recombination mechanisms contributing to antibody diversity.

Specific arguments against the special selection and the recombination somatic hypotheses have been discussed by Cohn (1971).

6.3.4 Clonal Variation

The accepted idea that diversity at the cellular level precedes exposure to antigen (see Section 3.4) appears to have been challenged by Cunningham (1974). His hypothesis of clonal variation consists of mutation and antigenic selection postulated to occur during antigen-driven clonal expansion. This short time scale demands a very high rate of mutation and it has been claimed that, in single clones of antibody-forming cells, variants have been observed to arise at the rate of one in 30 cell divisions. Cunningham (1974) has proposed that the variants are due to point mutations, however there is no physicochemical evidence in support of this. Two types of evidence have been offered. (i) Changes in antibody production by single cells have been deduced from changes in the morphology of plaques (due to lysis of erythrocytes) formed around antibody-secreting cells. The factors governing plaque morphology are complex and differences can be seen in the absence of any variation in the antibody secreted. (ii) Diversity of antibody-forming cells has been observed within selected clones. Such experiments do not eliminate completely the presence in the selected population of silent precursor cells that can give rise subsequently to antibody-forming cells independently of the selected clones.

None of the hypotheses seeking to explain diversity by somatic variation of less than 10 V genes is now tenable, since available sequential data require more than 100 germ-line V genes.

6.4 Current Hypotheses Using Multiple V Genes

6.4.1 Subgroups

The minimum number of V genes needed to account reasonably for known V-region amino acid sequences has increased steadily as sequential data have accumulated, and it does not appear that a limit has been reached yet. By ordering mouse V_κ sequences into a genealogical tree as many new branches for the most recently determined set of 20 sequences have been revealed as for the first 20 sequences obtained (Hood et al., 1974).

A major stage in the ordering of V-region amino acid sequential data was the recognition of subgroups of sequences sharing a similar pattern of amino acids, or gaps introduced to maximize homology. This convenient classification has been interpreted in terms of one V gene for each subgroup with intra-subgroup variation being attributed to somatic diversification processes. The definition of the degree of sequence variation necessary to define a subgroup has varied. Whatever the criterion, a V region usually has been assigned to a subgroup on the basis of only the N-terminal amino acid sequence. On this basis, the human heavy chains each fall into one of four distinct subgroups each characterized by a highly conserved N-terminal sequence. Complete V_H-region sequences show that (i) subgroup-specific amino acids are confined to the 82 N-terminal positions, and (ii) sequential diversity increases in the last 25 per cent of V_H regions (Capra and Kehoe, 1974a). The most precise definition of subgroups—and therefore the one with most predictive value—states that identical amino acid sequences outside the hypervariable regions identify sequences of the same subgroup (see Section 5.2.3). The origin of antibody diversity may then be resolved into the mechanism for generating hypervariable regions. Any valid hypothesis must account for the origin of hypervariable regions of germ-line V genes and also for subsequent localization of somatic variation, if such is postulated. Three hypotheses will be considered.

6.4.2 Somatic Mutation with Antigenic Selection

The following postulates have been advanced by Cohn et al. (1974).

(i) The germ-line complement of V genes, consisting of the order of 100 V_L and 100 V_H genes, has been selected during evolution to code for antibodies specific for pathogens. Such antibodies may afford the immediate survival of the neonate.

(ii) Selection would only act upon about 200 of the maximum number of combining sites (10^4) which the germ-line V genes could generate. In effect, all 10^4 antibodies would show germ-line inheritance although only a small fraction would be selected positively.

174

(*iii*) In the mature animal, mutations of V genes would be expressed if a viable V_L-V_H combination could be made.

(*iv*) Mutants of complementarity-determining amino acids will affect the specificity of the combining site and can be positively or negatively selected by antigenic encounter.

(*v*) Selection must be stepwise with sequential selection acting upon each mutation.

(*vi*) Ten new V genes must be generated somatically and selected to give a minimal mature repertoire of 10^6 antibodies. A rate of 10^{-3}–10^{-5} functional variants/cell division would be necessary (Cohn, 1974). At this rate of generation of new V genes, it follows that in the repertoire of antibodies studied in the mature individual the variation seen in complementarity-determining amino acids will be largely due to somatic mutations of germ-line sequences. Hypervariable regions

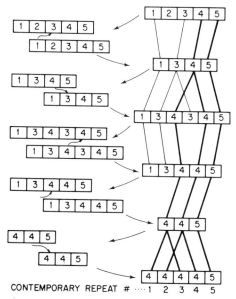

CONTEMPORARY REPEAT # ···· 1 2 3 4 5

Figure 10 Mechanism by which unequal crossing-over can lead to the horizontal spread of mutation (crossover fixation) and the maintenance of multiple gene sets. Each repeated gene is represented by a box. The numbers inside each box allow each gene to be followed and its descendants traced. The descent of contemporary repeats is followed by bold lines. The original genes may be identical. A point mutation in gene number 4 will be spread to four out of five of the contemporary repeat genes by unequal crossing over, thus maintaining a nearly identical set of genes (from Smith, 1973)

are assumed, therefore, to be stretches of amino acids residues whose side chains determine, or potentially determine, complementarity; in any antibody molecule, only a few side chains are involved in contact with the epitope (Davies and Padlan, 1975).

In considering this hypothesis it is important to note that direct evidence for selected somatic point mutations is lacking. Mouse λ-chain sequences are consistent with somatic mutations of a single germ-line V_λ gene, and the RNA–DNA hybridization evidence tends to support this (see Section 5.4). There is no evidence, however, that the mutant phenotypes seen have been expanded due to antigenic selection. The known variants of murine V_λ show amino acid differences at positions analogous to the hypervariable regions of mouse κ chains. However, 40 per cent of the base changes fixed in V_λ correspond to the second hypervariable region of V_κ—the region which is not involved in complementarity in either MCPc 603 or NEW combining sites.

Somatic mutations will occur at a normal rate and the accumulation of mutations in V genes will be more rapid because of the multiplicity of V genes.

6.4.3 Hypothesis for the Inheritance of a Complete Antibody Repertoire

A germ-line hypothesis for antibody diversity currently accounts for the data available (Hood et al., 1974; Williamson, 1976).

(i) Almost all V regions are encoded by germ-line genes. Some somatic variants might be expected, but these are irrelevant to the extent of antibody diversity.

(ii) The differences between V genes are the result of point mutations, deletions, and insertions accumulated during evolution.

(iii) One selective pressure for divergence of V-gene sequence is to stabilize the multiple gene family. This is achieved by decreasing the frequency with which haploid recombination eliminates V genes.

(iv) Framework (non-hypervariable) sequences are conserved by the selective pressure for V_L and V_H association.

(v) Hypervariable sequences result from the lack of selective pressure on these parts of the V-region structure. Mutations in hypervariable regions are thus neutral and are fixed at the rate at which they occur (Kimura, 1968).

(vi) One of the major forces maintaining the multiple V-gene families is unequal crossing-over between sister chromatids (Smith, 1973). The horizontal spread of mutation among a V-gene family can be accomplished by unequal crossing-over and subgroups of related V genes can be produced (Figure 10). Mutations fixed at a rate greater than the rate of unequal crossing-over will accumulate, that is neutral or positively selected mutations.

The maintenance of a multiple V gene system is currently best explained by unequal crossing-over. The idea that hypervariable regions arise due to lack of selection can apply equally to germ-line or somatic mutations. The family of murine V_λ regions could all be neutral variants of a basic sequence, irrespective of when the mutations occur, rather than being antigenically selected variants.

Maximal extimates for the number of germ-line V genes are sufficient to account for antibody diversity. The evidence for the presence of latent V genes (Sogn and Kindt, Chapter 4) suggests that the number of V genes in the germ line may exceed estimates based on phenotype.

6.4.4 Hypotheses Invoking Multiple Gene Interactions

In its clearest form, this type of model invokes insertion of episomes, coding for binding-site sequences, into the hypervariable regions of V genes coding for framework sequences (Wu and Kabat, 1970). The episomes might be scrambled somatically to give extensive antibody diversity.

Capra and Kindt (1974) have proposed that a set of hypervariable episomes is inherited together with individual framework V genes. This hypothesis is invoked to explain the finding of identical or cross-reactive idiotypes associated with V_H regions of different allotype in rabbits (Kindt et al., 1974). The alternate explanation of these data is parallel evolution. Whatever the V-region allotype of a rabbit, a full range of antibody diversity is available. In such an extensive generation of diversity, parallel evolution of similar (see Section 2.2), or even identical hypervariable regions, is understandable and is a simpler explanation than the interaction of five or six genes to give a single polypeptide chain. Cohn (1974) has pointed out that mouse V_κ sequential data support the idea of co-evolution of hypervariable region and framework sequences, and he strongly argues against multiple gene-interaction models. Co-evolution of framework and combining site has been shown by following the inheritance of idiotype and spectrotype for the N1 V_H gene (Williamson and McMichael, 1975).

7 EVOLUTIONARY ORIGIN OF ANTIBODY DIVERSITY

7.1 Evidence from Phylogeny

The importance of antibodies can be argued from their ubiquitous presence in modern vertebrates, the most primitive representative being the cyclostomes—hagfish and lamprey—(see review by Marchalonis, 1975). Diversity of specificity is an essential feature of antibodies and is observed in all vertebrates. It is valid to examine the primitive vertebrates for gaps in the antibody repertoire, but so far there is no evidence that the range of antibody diversity is any less in the latter.

Variation in the number of V genes expressed in the λ or κ families is seen between species (Hood et al., 1967). Furthermore, the proportion of V_H regions of a given subgroup is also characteristic of a species (Capra et al., 1973).

Immunologically related mechanisms in invertebrates are currently under study. It is proposed to attempt to deduce the origin of the antibody system. At present, this is still a highly speculative field.

7.2 Structural Evidence

Sequence homology units (domains) appear to be the basis of evolution of all

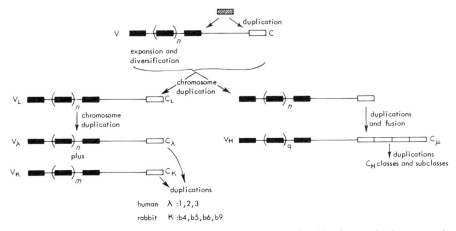

Figure 11 Putative steps in the evolution of antibody gene families from a single ancestral gene of domain size

immunoglobulin genes (see review by Hood, 1973). Possible common evolutionary pathways for modern V and C-gene families are shown in Figure 11. Gene duplication, chromosome duplication (or chromosomal translocation), and fusion of contiguous gene duplicates must be invoked. Expansion and contraction of V-gene families can be effected by unequal crossing-over (see Section 6.4.3(vi)), and the species differences in size of V_κ or V_λ pools can be accounted for by expansion and contraction. The same processes can spread

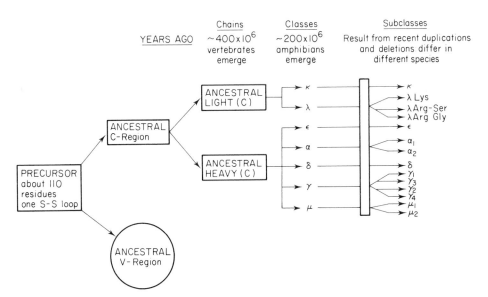

Figure 12 Scheme for the evolution of immunoglobulin C-region genes with an approximate time scale. From Milstein and Munro (1973)

mutations horizontally, thus accounting for framework sequence identities such as the rabbit V-region allotypes (Figure 10).

Diversification of V genes was probably an early event in the evolution of the immune system. Amino acid sequences of V genes from various species suggest that divergence of V subgroups preceded speciation (Wasserman *et al.*, 1974). Moreover, this comparison reveals that V-region sequences show greater conservation between species than do C-region sequences. Since the V regions contain the active site of antibodies the greater conservation of V-region sequence parallels the conservation of active-site sequences in enzymes.

The evolution of classes and subclasses of C regions has occurred subsequent to the divergence of V and C genes. An approximate time scale is given in Figure 12. Only IgM-type antibody is found in the most primitive vertebrates (Marchalonis, 1975). In the chicken, ontogeny recapitulates phylogeny and IgM production commences before IgG production, with IgA production being even later (Cooper *et al.*, 1972).

7.3 Is There a Second Diversity System for Antigen Receptors on T Lymphocytes

The origin of antibody diversity is an important event in evolution. Nevertheless, it seems unlikely that two diversity systems could have arisen independently. The question of a second system only arises because of the controversy over the presence or absence of antibody-like molecules on the surface of T lymphocytes (see Parkhouse, Chapter 3). Moreover the detection of antigen-binding molecules completely distinct from antibodies has been reported in studies on T-helper cells (Munro and Tausig, 1975).

It is reassuring that in two systems idiotypic antigens of T-cell receptors are indistinguishable from the idiotypes of conventional antibody of the same specificity. Binz *et al.* (1974) have shown that an antibody raised against alloantigen-specific T-cell receptors reacts with humoral alloantibody and blocks T-cell reactivity in a graft-*versus*-host assay. Eichmann and Rajewsky (1975) showed an anti-idiotypic antibody raised against A5A anti-streptococcal polysaccharide as a carrier of hapten.

The nature of the receptor molecule carrying the idiotype remains unknown. The presence in that receptor molecule of V gene products is strongly implied, and it would follow that both B and T cells use the same diversity system.

REFERENCES

Amzel, L. M., Poljak, R. J., Saul, F., Varga, J. M., and Richards, F. F. (1974). *Proc. Nat. Acad. Sci., U.S.A.*, **71**, 1427.

Askonas, B. A., and Williamson, A. R. (1972). *Nature, (Lond.)*, **238**, 339.

Barstad, P., Weigert, M., Cohn, M., and Hood, L. (1974). *Proc. Nat. Acad. Sci., U.S.A.*, **71**, 4096.

Binz, H., Lindenmann, J., and Wigzell, H. (1974). *J. Exp. Med.*, **140**, 731.

Birshtein, B. K., and Cebra, J. J. (1971). *Biochemistry*, **10**, 4930.

Bishop, J. O. (1972). In *Gene Transcription in Reproductive Tissue*, p. 247.

Bodmer, W. F. (1972). *Nature, (Lond.)*, **237**, 139.

Brenner, S., and Milstein, C. (1966). *Nature, (Lond.)*, **211**, 242.

Brown, D. D. (1972). In *Molecular Genetics and Developmental Biology*, (Sussman, M., ed.), Prentice Hall, New Jersey, 101.

Burnet, F. M. (1957). *Aust. J. Sci.*, **20**, 67.

Burnet, F. M. (1959). *The Clonal Selection Theory of Acquired Immunity*, Cambridge University Press, Cambridge.

Capra, J. D., and Kehoe, J. M. (1974*a*). *Adv. Immunol.*, **20**, 1.

Capra, J. D., and Kehoe, J. M. (1974*b*). *Proc. Nat. Acad. Sci., U.S.A.*, **71**, 845.

Capra, J. D., and Kehoe, J. M. (1974*c*). *Proc. Nat. Acad. Sci., U.S.A.*, **71**, 4032.

Capra, J. D., and Kindt, T. J. (1974). *Immunogenetics*, **1**, 417.

Capra, J. D., Tung, A. S., and Nisonoff, A. (1975). *J. Immunol.*, **114**, 1548.

Capra, J. D., Wasserman, R. L., and Kehoe, J. M. (1973). *J. Exp. Med.*, **138**, 410.

Cebra, J. J., Koo, P. H., and Ray, A. (1974). *Science, N.Y.*, **186**, 263.

Chesebro, B., and Metzger, H. (1972). *Biochemistry*, **11**, 766.

Claflin, J. L., and Davie, J. M. (1974). *J. Exp. Med.*, **140**, 673.

Claflin, J. L., and Davie, J. M. (1975*a*). *J. Exp. Med.*, **141**, 1073.

Claflin, J. L., and Davie, J. M. (1975*b*). *J. Immunol.*, **114**, 70.

Claflin, J. L., Schroer, J. A., and Cavie, J. M. (1975). In *Proceedings of the 9th Leukocyte Culture Conference*, (Rosenthal, A. S., ed.), Academic Press, New York and London, p. 153.

Cohn, M. (1971). *Ann. N.Y. Acad. Sci.*, **190**, 529.

Cohn, M. (1974). In *Progress in Immunology II*, Vol. I, (Brent, L., and Holborow, J., eds.), North Holland Publishing Co., Amsterdam, p. 261.

Cohn, M., Blomberg, B., Geckeler, W., Raschke, W., Riblet, R., and Weigert, M. (1974). In *The Immune System: Genes, Receptors, Signals*, (Sercarz, E. E., Williamson, A. R., and Fox, C. F., eds.), Academic Press, New York and London, p. 89.

Cooper, M. D., Lawton, A. R., and Kincade, P. W. (1972). In *Contemporary Topics in Immunobiology*, Vol. I, (Hanna, M. G., ed.), Plenum Press, New York, p. 33.

Cramer, M., and Braun, D. G. (1974). *J. Exp. Med.*, **139**, 1513.

Cunningham, A. J. (1974). *Contemp. Top. Mol. Immunol.*, **3**, 1.

Davies, D. R., and Padlan, E. A. (1975). *Ann. Rev. Biochem.*, **44**, 639.

Dayhoff, M. O. (1972). *Atlas of Protein Sequence and Structure*, National Biomedical Research Foundation, Silver Spring, Maryland.

Dreyer, W. J., and Bennett, J. C. (1965). *Proc. Nat. Acad. Sci., U.S.A.*, **54**, 864.

Ehlich, P. (1900). *Proc. Roy. Soc. Secr. B.*, **66**, 424.

Eichmann, K. (1975). *Immunogenetics*, **2**, 491.

Eichmann, K., and Rajewsky, K. (1975). *Eur. J. Immunol.*, **5**, 661.

Epp, O., Colman, P., Fehlhammer, H., Bode, W., Schiffer, M., and Huber, R. (1974). *Eur. J. Biochem.*, **45**, 513.

Fisher, C. E., and Press, E. M. (1974). *Biochem. J.*, **139**, 135.

Franek, F. (1971). *Eur. J. Biochem.*, **19**, 176.

Gally, J. A., and Edelman, G. M. (1970). *Nature, (Lond.)*, **227**, 341.

Gearhart, P. J., Sigal, N. H., and Klinman, N. R. (1975). *J. Exp. Med.*, **141**, 56.

Givol, D., Strausbauch, P. H., Hurwitz, E., Wilchek, M., Haimovich, J., and Eisen, H. N., (1971). *Biochemistry*, **10**, 3461.

Goetzl, E. J., and Metzger, H. (1970). *Biochemistry*, **9**, 3862.

Haber, E. (1968). *Ann. Rev. Biochem.*, **37**, 497.

Hood, L. (1973). *Stadler Symp.*, **5**, 73.

Hood, L., Barstad, P., Loh, E., and Nottenburg, C. (1974). In *The Immune System: Genes, Receptors, Signals*, (Sercarz, E. E., Williamson, A. R., and Fox, C. F., eds.). Academic Press, New York and London, p. 119.

Hood, L., Campbell, J. H., and Elgin, S. C. R. (1976). *Ann. Rev. Genet.*, **9**, 305.

Hood, L., Gray, W., Sanders, B., and Dreyer, W. (1967). *Cold Spring Harbor Symp. Quant. Biol.*, **32**, 133.

Hood, L., and Talmage, D. (1970). *Science, N.Y.*, **168**, 325.

Imanishi, T., and Mäkelä, O. (1974). *J. Exp. Med.*, **140**, 1498.

Inman, J. K. (1974). In *The Immune System: Genes, Receptors, Signals*, (Sercarz, E. E., Williamson, A. R., and Fox, C. F., eds.), Academic Press, New York, p. 37.

Jerne, N. K. (1955). *Proc. Nat. Acad. Sci., U.S.A.*, **41**, 849.

Jerne, N. K. (1971). *Eur. J. Immunol.*, **1**, 1.

Kimura, M. (1968). *Nature, (Lond.)*, **217**, 624.

Kindt, T. J., Thunberg, A. L., Mudgett, M., and Klapper, D. G. (1974). In *The Immune System: Genes, Receptors, Signals*, (Sercarz, E. E., Williamson, A. R., and Fox, C. F., eds.), Academic Press, New York and London, p. 69.

Kreth, H. W., and Williamson, A. R. (1973). *Eur. J. Immunol.*, **3**, 141.

Kunkel, H. G., Agnello, V., Joslin, F. G., Winchester, R. J., and Capra, J. D. (1973). *J. Exp. Med.*, **137**, 331.

Landsteiner, K. (1945). *The Specificity of Serological Reactions*, Harvard University Press, Cambridge, Mass.

Leder, P., Honjo, T., Swan, D., Packman, S., Nau, M., and Norman, B. (1975). In *Molecular Approaches to Immunology*, (Smith, E. E. and Ribbons, D. S., eds.), Academic Press, New York and London.

Lederberg, J. (1959). *Science, N.Y.*, **129**, 1649.

Lefkovits, I. (1974). *Curr. Top. Microbiol. Immunol.*, **65**, 21.

Leon, M. A., and Young, N. M. (1971). *Biochemistry*, **10**, 1424.

Lieberman, R., Potter, M., Mushinski, E. B., Humphrey, W., Jr., and Rudikoff, S. (1974). *J. Exp. Med.*, **139**, 983.

Macario, A. J. L., and Conway de Macario, E. (1975). *Immunochemistry*, **12**, 249.

Mage, R., Lieberman, R., Potter, M., and Terry, W. D. (1973). In *The Antigens*, (Sela, M., ed.), Vol. 1, Academic Press, New York and London, p. 299.

Marchalonis, J. J. (1975). In *Progress in Immunology II*, Vol. II, (Brent, L., and Holborow, J., eds.), North Holland Publishing Co., Amsterdam, p. 249.

McKean, D., Potter, M., and Hood, L. (1973). *Biochemistry*, **12**, 760.

McMichael, A. J., Phillips, J. M., Williamson, A. R., Imanishi, T., and Mäkelä, O. (1975). *Immunogenetics*, **2**, 161.

Melli, M., Whitfield, C., Rao, K. V., Richardson, M., and Bishop, J. O. (1971). *Nature, New Biol.*, **231**, 8.

Milstein, C., Brownlee, G. G., Cartwright, E. M., Jarvis, J. M., and Proudfoot, N. J. (1974). *Nature, (Lond.)*, **252**, 354.

Milstein, C. and Munro, A. J. (1973). In *Defence and Recognition*, (Porter, R. R., ed.), Butterworths, London, p. 199.

Montgomery, P. C., Kahn, R. L., and Skandera, C. A. (1975a). *J. Immunol.*, **115**, 904.

Montgomery, P. C., Skandera, C. A., and Kahn, R. L. (1975b). *Nature, (Lond.)*, **256**, 138.

Munro, A. J., and Taussig, M. J. (1975). *Nature, (Lond.)*, **256**, 103.

Novotny, J. (1973). *J. Theoret. Biol.*, **41**, 171.

Pink, J. R. L., and Askonas, B. A. (1974). *Eur. J. Immunol.*, **4**, 426.
Pink, J. R. L., Wang, A.-C., and Fudenberg, H. H. (1971). *Ann. Rev. Med.*, **22**, 145.
Poljak, R. J. (1975). *Nature*, (*Lond.*), **256**, 373.

Rabbitts, T. H., and Milstein, C. (1975). *Eur. J. Biochem.*, **52**, 125.
Ray, A., and Cebra, J. J. (1972). *Biochemistry*, **11**, 3647.
Richards, F. F., Konigsberg, W. H., and Rosenstein, R. W. (1975). *Science, N.Y.*, **187**, 130.

Schiffer, M., Girling, R. L., Ely, K. R., and Edmundson, A. B. (1973). *Biochemistry*, **12**, 4620.
Schlossman, S. F., and Williamson, A. R. (1972). In *Genetic Control of Immune Responsiveness*, (McDevitt, H. O., and Landy, M., eds.), Academic Press, New York and London, p. 54.
Singer, S. J., and Thorpe, N. O. (1968). *Proc. Nat. Acad. Sci., U.S.A.*, **60**, 1371.
Smith, G., Hood, L., and Fitch, W. (1971). *Ann. Rev. Biochem.*, **40**, 969.
Smith, G. P. (1973). *Cold Spring Harbor Symp. Quant. Biol.*, **38**, 507.
Smithies, O. (1967). *Cold Spring Harbor Symp. Quant. Biol.*, **32**, 161.

Talmage, D. W. (1957). *Ann. Rev. Med.*, **8**, 239.
Tonegawa, S. (1976). *Proc. Nat. Acad. Sci., U.S.A.*, **73**, 203.

Wasserman, R. L., Kehoe, J. M., and Capra, J. D. (1974). *J. Immunol.*, **113**, 954.
Williams, R. C., Kunkel, H. G., and Capra, J. D. (1968). *Science, N.Y.*, **161**, 379.
Williamson, A. R. (1973). *Biochem. J.*, **130**, 325.
Williamson, A. R. (1975). In *Isoelectric Focusing*, (Arbuthnott, J. P., and Beeley, J. A., eds.), Butterworths, London, p. 291.
Williamson, A. R. (1976). *Ann. Rev. Biochem.*, **45**, 467.
Williamson, A. R., and Fitzmaurice, L. C. (1976). In *The Generation of Antibody Diversity*, (Cunningham, A. J., ed.), Academic Press, New York and London, 183.
Williamson, A. R., and McMichael, A. J. (1975). In *Molecular Approaches to Immunology*, (Smith, E. E., and Ribbons, D. W., eds.), Academic Press, New York and London, p. 153.
Williamson, A. R., Zitron, I. M., and McMichael, A. J. (1976). *Fed. Proc.*, **35**, 2195.
Wu, T., and Kabat, E. (1970). *J. Exp. Med.*, **132**, 211.

CHAPTER 6

Immunoglobulinopathies

D. R. Stanworth

1 INTRODUCTION

Disorders grouped under the term immunoglobulinopathies have proved to be considerably more complex than was originally suspected. Initially, it was demonstrated using strip electrophoresis or ultracentrifugation that there was an overabundance or a lack of γ-globulin in the serum. With the advent of

183

immunological techniques, it has become customary to classify these diseases, which involve qualitative and/or quantitative abnormalities in the immunoglobulins, into two main categories. This classification depends upon the elevation or reduction of levels of one or more immunoglobulin constituent. When the increase is restricted to a single subclass or subunit, it is conveniently considered separately as a monoclonal gammopathy. Emphasis in this chapter will be placed on those immunochemical characteristics that permit such classifications and that have been of assistance in elucidating the structure and function of normal immunoglobulins (Turner, Chapter 1).

Another area of interest which will be considered in some depth, is the development of laboratory models for various immunoglobulinopathies. Such models eventually lead to a better understanding of the aetiology of the human diseases, besides providing further valuable aids for those studying the synthesis and role of normal immunoglobulins. These include experimental animal systems, in which plasma-cell neoplasms and/or paraproteinaemias occur spontaneously or are induced experimentally, and the *in vitro* culture of myeloma cell lines that continue to secrete monoclonal immunoglobulin over long periods.

2 HYPERIMMUNOGLOBULINOPATHIES

2.1 Classical Paraproteinopathies

Although the term paraprotein was used initially (Apitz, 1940) when referring to abnormal protein products of myeloma cells detectable in blood, urine, and tissues, it has been applied since to any immunoglobulin-type product of an immunocyte dyscrasia or of a malignant lymphoma. Monoclonal gammopathies, such as myeloma and Waldenström's macroglobulinaemia, are the most prominent; and paraproteins found at high levels in the sera of such patients have often been referred to as M proteins. This term has been extended to include immunoglobulin subunits, such as Bence–Jones protein—light-chain structures—produced in a relatively high proportion of patients with lymphoplasmacytic dyscrasias, half light-chain fragments (C_1), and the products of heavy-chain disease, comprising incomplete immunoglobulin structures detectable in the patients' serum and urine. Thus, the paraproteinopathies offer a

Table 1   Abnormal proteins in hyperimmunoglobulinopathies

Parapraproteinopathy	Abnormal protein
Multiple myeloma	IgA, IgG, IgD, IgE, Bence–Jones protein, V_L, C_L, or deleted forms
Primary Waldenström macroglobulinaemia	IgM, Bence–Jones protein
Heavy-chain (Franklin's) disease	γ, α, μ chain or deleted forms
Light-chain disease	Bence-Jones protein

rich and varied source of material for the immunochemist. These major abnormalities are summarized in Table 1.

2.1.1 Incidence

2.1.1.1 Distribution among Immunoglobulin Classes and Subclasses. The frequency of documentation of paraproteinopathies depends, not unexpectedly, on the nature of the population screened and on the technique employed. The screening of blood donors, the most common group of subjects to be investigated, has revealed an overall incidence of 0·2 per cent; while a somewhat higher incidence of paraproteinopathies has been reported in other supposedly normal populations. For instance, 64 out of 6995 people (0·9 per cent) living in a Swedish county have been shown to possess an M component in their serum when it was examined by electrophoresis (Axelsson *et al.*, 1966). The distribution of this component within the three main immunoglobulin classes was: 61 per cent IgG, 27 per cent IgA, 8 per cent IgM. In serum samples from three subjects, M components of two different immunoglobulin classes were detected.

A similar ratio of IgG to IgA M component (53:25) has been observed in a relatively large group of 212 patients with myeloma (Hobbs, 1969). Only one of which was an IgD myeloma and 19 per cent were cases of light-chain disease. Of a group of 400 patients with paraproteinaemia investigated at two New York hospitals over several years, 10 per cent were proved to be suffering from Waldenström macroglobulinaemia (Osserman and Takatsuki, 1964). In a more recent study by Jancelwicz *et al.* (1975), 0·8 per cent of M components in general, were observed to be IgD; and 2 per cent of cases of myeloma in particular. The

Table 2 Comparison of features of cases of IgE myelomatosis so far documented

Patient	Sex	Age	Serum M component (g/100 ml)	Light-chain type	Bence–Jones protein	Plasma-cell leu-kaemia	Osteo-lytic lesions	Reference
N.D.	M	50	4·5	λ	+	+		Bennich and Johansson (1967)
P.S.	M	60	7·5	λ	+	+		Ogawa *et al.* (1969)
D.M.				κ				Stoice, personal communication
Hea	F	65	2·7	κ	−		+	Fishkin *et al.* (1972)
Yu	M	51		κ	−		+	Stefani and Mokeeva (1972)
Be.				κ				Penn, personal communication
K.G.				κ				Senda and Snai, personal communication
F.K.	M	59	2·1	κ	−		−	Mills *et al.* (1976)
Ka.M.	F	48	6·3	κ	−			Knedel *et al.* (1976)

Table 3 Comparison of the proportion of monoclonal myeloma proteins observed in each IgG subclass with normal serum concentrations

Source of sera	Number studied	IgG1 (per cent)	IgG2 (per cent)	IgG3 (per cent)	IgG4 (per cent)	Reference
Myeloma patients	64	60–70		15	6	Grey and Kunkel (1964)
	191	77	11	9	3	Terry et al. (1965)
	108	82	10	7	1	Bernier et al. (1967)
	n.s.	70	18	8	3	Natvig et al. (1967)
	471	78	13	6	3	Terry (1968)
	147	68	14	10	8	Virella and Hobbs (1971)
	121	74	10	12	4	Virella and Hobbs (1971)
	848	77	14	6	3	Schur et al., unpublished results
	Mean	75*	13*	8*	4*	
Normal adults	10	64	28	5	3	Leddy et al. (1970)
	n.s.	66	23	7	4	Yount et al. (1970)
		64–70	23–28	4–7	3–4	Schur (1972)
	111	72	19	8	1	Shakib et al. (1975)

* Excluding incomplete data of Grey and Kunkel
n.s. = not stated

incidence of IgE myeloma is much lower than this; only a handful of cases having been reported (Table 2). This incidence has been calculated to be of the order of 0·002 per cent of all myeloma cases on the basis of the relative levels of IgE compared with those of IgG, IgA, and IgD in sera of normal subjects.

Some assessment of the reliability of using the relative proportions of immunoglobulins in the sera of normal individuals as a guide to the incidence of different types of monoclonal gammopathy can be obtained by examining the frequency of myeloma paraproteins of different IgG subclass. Data recently obtained in the author's laboratory (Shakib et al., 1975) on the relative proportions of IgG subclasses in the sera of 111 healthy adults correspond reasonably well with the relative incidence of monoclonal IgG paraproteins of the four subclasses observed by other workers (Table 3), particularly with that reported by Natvig and associates (1967). There appear, as yet, little comparable data available on the relative incidence of myelomas belonging to different IgA subclasses.

Biclonal paraproteinaemia has been observed occasionally in cases of myelomatosis, and polyclonal paraproteinaemia has been reported even less frequently. The classification and typing of the M component in 10 multiple

Table 4 Classification and typing of M components in biclonal gammopathies

M component I		M component II		Frequency
Class	Type	Class	Type	
IgG	κ	Bence–Jones	λ	$1 \times$
IgG	κ	IgA	κ	$2 \times$
IgA	κ	IgM	κ	$2 \times$
IgG	κ	IgM	κ	$1 \times$
IgG	κ	IgG	λ	$1 \times$
IgG	λ	IgA	λ	$1 \times$
IgM	κ	IgM	λ	$1 \times$
IgG	λ	IgA	λ	$1 \times$

From Ballieux *et al.* (1968)

myeloma cases with biclonal gammopathy was studied by Ballieux and associates (1968) (see Table 4). Moreover, quantitative immunodiffusion determinations recently performed in the author's laboratory on the sera of 62 patients with IgG myelomatosis (Shakib, 1976) have revealed that 11 possessed abnormally high levels of two subclasses. The most common biclonal combination was IgG1–IgG2 (8 cases), with 2 cases of IgG1–IgG4 and 1 case of IgG2–IgG4.

2.1.1.2 Influence of Age and Sex. The incidence of paraproteinaemia increases with advancing years, reaching as high as 14 per cent in patients over 95 years old (Radl, 1974). By comparison, healthy subjects in the old-age group (60–90 years) show a frequency of around 3 per cent, but very few cases of overt myeloma. M proteins were detected in nine out of 294 Swedish subjects who were older than 70 and apparently in good health (Hällén, 1963). It has been suggested by Osserman and Kohn (1974) that, with advancing years, the number of available antibody clones may decline and therefore on stimulation only a limited number may be available, thus resulting in a restricted heterogeneity of secreted immunoglobulin.

Whereas the mean age at diagnosis of cases of IgG and IgA myeloma is in the 60s (Table 5), that of IgD (and probably IgE) myeloma seems to be somewhat younger. In a relatively large group (133) of IgD myeloma cases studied (see Table 5), 65 per cent were less than 60 years old at diagnosis; whilst the average age at diagnosis was 57 for the small group of IgE myeloma cases so far studied in depth (Table 2). IgD myeloma, unlike that involving IgG or IgA-producing plasma cells, is seen about three times more frequently in males than females. In addition, macroglobulinaemia is twice as frequent in males than in females but, in contrast to the myelomatoses, the onset of this condition occurs at an older age—between 60–80 years (Martin, 1970).

2.1.1.3 Co-existence with Other Conditions. Although the co-existence of paraproteinaemia with other pathological conditions often has been observed, the

Table 5 Comparison of clinical manifestations of IgD with other myelomas

Manifestation	IgD	IgG	IgA	IgE§	Light chains only
Mean age at diagnosis (years)	56·2	62·62*	64·65	57	56·69
Male:female ratio	3:1	1:1	1:1	2:1	1:1
Blood urea nitrogen (BUN) value of 30 mg/100 ml	67	14	33		78
Serum Ca^{2+} level of 11 mg/100 ml	30	8·33†	47–59		33–62
Mean serum M component, g/100 ml	1·7	4·3	2·8		±
Light chains of M components $\kappa:\lambda$ ratio	1:9	2:1	2:1	7:2	1·3:1
Bence–Jones proteinuria (per cent)	92	60	70	33	100
Osteolytic lesions (per cent)	79	57	65		78
Medium survival time,‡ (months)	9	κ 35	κ 22		κ 28
		λ 25	19		λ 11

* Two values for two different series.
† Range of means from five different series
‡ Survival time for 54 patients with fatal myeloma IgD was from the time of diagnosis; for IgG, IgA, and light chains only, the survival time was from the first nelphalan treatment
§ Summary of six well-documented cases referred to in Table 5 (modified from Jancelwicz et al., 1975)

significance of such associations is still far from clear. It is interesting that they are seen in malabsorption states sometimes; for instance, in his original description of primary macroglobulinaemia Waldenström (1944) described one patient with diarrhoea. Other macroglobulinaemic patients with this symptom have been recorded since. One such case investigated in the author's laboratory (Bradley et al., 1968) presented with steatorrhoea. Analytical ultracentrifugation of the serum (Figure 1) revealed a moderately raised serum 19 S peak. In addition, M protein, which proved to be monoclonal by light-chain analysis was detected by electrophoresis. Interestingly, ultracentrifugal analysis of the patient's serum some seven years later revealed the presence of faster-sedimenting components (29 S and 38 S) (Figure 1). This would be anticipated if the patient had Waldenström macroglobulinaemia in view of the observed increase in the level of the 19 S component to 2g/100 ml. Earlier studies (Ratcliff et al., 1963), to be referred to in more detail later (see p. 197), had shown that the faster-sedimenting components characteristic of this form of paraproteinaemia are apparent in the serum when a minimal level of the 19 S component (IgM monomer) is reached. When the patient eventually died from bronchopneumonia, necropsy revealed, in addition to the effects of malnutrition such as atrophic tongue, fatty liver, and osteoporosis, an enlargement of the spleen and extensive hyperplasia of the bone marrow. Furthermore, histological examination showed a widespread lymphocytic infiltration of all organs including the alimentary tract, resembling a reticulosis such as lymphosarcoma. However, features characteristic of Waldenström macroglobulinaemia were not apparent, despite the patient having latterly shown clinical evidence of this condition.

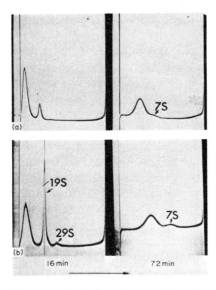

Figure 1 Analytical ultracentrifugation pattern of serum (dilution × 5): (*a*) of supposed early case of Waldenström macroglobulinaemia and (*b*) of sample of serum from same patient 6·5 years later. 59 000 rpm, 20°C, photographs taken at 16 and 72 minutes. (reproduced from Bradley *et al.* (1968)

In this connection, it is also interesting to note that a progressive rise in total serum IgA has been observed in the small number of adult patients with coeliac disease who develop a gastrointestinal lymphoma (Asquith *et al.*, 1969), but the patients apparently show no clinical evidence of myelomatosis. However, the type of pathological condition with which paraproteinaemia has been observed is by no means restricted to malabsorption syndromes; for example, 10 cases of Paget's disease with co-existing multiple myeloma have been reported recently (Srivastava and Kohn, 1974).

2.1.2 Clinical Features

The two major classes of monoclonal gammopathy, multiple myeloma and primary (Waldenström) macroglobulinaemia, are distinguishable at both clinical and cytological levels.

Clinically, cases of multiple myeloma present with bone pain, osteolytic lesions (including the characteristic 'punched-out' effect), and plasma-cell infiltration of the bone marrow. Typical clinical features of the latter disease are a tendency to haemorrhage (particularly in the gums and the retina), discrete lymphadenopathy, splenomegaly, and lymphocytic plasma cell infiltration of the bone marrow. In contrast to the bone picture in multiple myeloma, X-ray examination does not reveal multiple or focal skeletal lesions in patients with primary macroglobulinaemia.

At the cellular (i.e. immunocyte) level there are also distinctions between multiple myeloma and primary macroglobulinaemia, although cytologists continue to argue about the precise origin and morphology of the neoplastic 'lympho-plasma' cells involved. According to Fudenberg (1972), many haematologists feel capable of making a differential diagnosis between the two conditions by morphological examinations. He points out, however, that a macroglobulinaemiac patient occasionally presents with what appears to be a classical myeloma bone-marrow picture; but the marrow of such patients apparently often contains tissue mast cells, a frequent feature of macroglobulinaemia which Waldenström first drew attention to some years ago. In contrast to the plasma cells found throughout the bone marrow of myeloma patients, and which sometimes accumulate as plasmacytomas, the prominent cell type in primary macroglobulinaemia is classified less readily. In his description of macroglobulinaemia, Waldenström (1944) observed that this 'lymphocytoid' cell (sometimes referred to now as lymphocytic plasmacyte) is sessile, like the plasma cell in multiple myeloma and also occurs in the bone marrow where it rarely agglomerates into a lymphosarcoma.

Leukaemia is not seen in primary macroglobulinaemia, and has been found to be rare in multiple myeloma. For instance, of the 87 patients with myeloma seen at one group of American hospitals over a 10-year period, only three showed more than 1 per cent typical plasma cells in the peripheral smears at time of diagnosis (Ogawa and McIntyre, unpublished results, quoted by Ogawa et al., 1969). Plasma-cell leukaemia also has been seen only occasionally in the rarer form of IgD myeloma. It was of particular interest, therefore, when the first two cases of IgE myeloma to be described were reported to possess substantial plasma-cell leukaemias (see Table 2). This haematological feature, which is held generally to indicate a poor prognosis (Pruzanski et al., 1969), has not been uniformly observed in the few reported cases of IgE myeloma.

IgD myeloma shows some clinically different features to those manifest by myelomatoses involving cells producing the IgG and IgA classes, suggesting that the onset and course of the disease may be related to the structure of the M component.

Heavy-chain disease would appear to be another clinical variant of plasma-cell neoplasia. Its manifestations are primarily those of a malignant lymphoma, with little or no bone involvement. The associated abnormality in immunoglobulin metabolism involves excessive production and appearance in the serum and urine of part of a heavy chain devoid of light chains which the immunochemical aspects of this will be considered later (see Section 2.1.4.5.2).

Since Franklin and his associates (1963) described the first patient with γ heavy-chain disease, other cases have been reported involving the overproduction of α or μ, rather than γ, heavy chains. The incidence of these heavy-chain diseases is rare, with only about 100 cases having been reported in the literature since Franklin's first description. Approximately 35 of these cases were of the γ-

Table 6 Summary of seven cases of μ heavy-chain disease*

Case/Sex/ Age (years)	Chronic lymphocytic leukaemia duration (years)	Vacuolated plasma cells	Serum		Urine		Hepatosplenomegaly	Marked peripheral lympha- denopathy	Bone lesions	Amyloid
			Hypo γ	μ chain band*	Bence-Jones Protein	μ chain				
1/M/58	6	+++	+		κ		+		+	++
2/M/6	9	+++	+				+			
3/F/52	20	++	+		κ		+		?	
4/M/43	1	++	(−)		κ		+			
5/M/79	9	+	+		κ		+	+		
6/M/45	(−)	(−)	(−)	α_2		0·4 g/l	+			
7/F/48	1	?	+		κ		+			

* μ-Chain reactive protein devoid of light chains detected in all sera on immunoelectrophoresis
Reproduced from Franklin (1975)

chain type, 50 of the α type, and 10 of the μ type (Franklin and Frangione, 1975). α-Chain disease (Seligman *et al.*, 1968) was first recognized in what had been known previously in the Middle East as Arabian lymphoma of the small gut. The tumour, however, may spread later to other organs and to the bone marrow. The clinical and laboratory features of seven reported cases of μ heavy-chain disease are summarized in Table 6. The patients' ages ranged from 43–79 years and all but one had chronic lymphocytic leukaemia. It has been pointed out by Franklin (1975), however, that this abnormality of immunoglobulin synthesis is rare in chronic lymphocytic leukaemia; a careful examination of over 180 patients failing to uncover any additional cases of μ heavy-chain disease. Not unexpectedly in view of their supposed low incidence, δ and ε heavy-chain gammopathies have not yet been reported.

Other forms of imbalance between the synthesis of heavy and light immunoglobulin chains involve the excessive production of light chains, which are excreted as Bence–Jones protein and are usually of the same antigenic type—κ or λ—as the intact M component. It is also interesting to note that in some cases of Bence–Jones proteinuria, which are seen most frequently in myelomatosis (30–40 per cent), half light-chains comprising the V_L or C_L region are found in the urine (Cioli and Baglioni, 1966; Solomon *et al.*, 1966). An incomplete half light-chain, related to but clearly distinguishable from C_L has been detected in the urine of four myeloma patients treated with corticosteroids. In other pathological situations, referred to as light-chain disease or Bence–Jones myeloma, the synthesis of heavy polypeptide chains appears to be blocked resulting in the secretion only of light chain of the κ or λ type. An electrophoretically and antigenically similar light-chain fraction is frequently detectable in the serum of such cases.

Even in the absence of whole paraproteins, and even when these light-chain fractions are present in extremely low levels, their presence is considered (Hobbs, personal communication) to be an early criterion of malignancy.

2.1.3 Cellular Studies

Immunofluorescence studies of immunocytes within the bone marrow of paraproteinopathy patients not surprisingly demonstrate a predominance of cells secreting the monoclonal protein found in the patient's serum. In contrast, there is a marked reduction in the number of cells synthesizing other immunoglobulin components. This accounts for the low serum levels of the other globulins observed in the terminal stages of the disease and could, it has been suggested by Ballieux *et al.* (1968), explain the high incidence of infections in the skin, and the respiratory, and urinary tracts. Apart from studies of the frequency of distribution of bone-marrow cells producing different types of monoclonal immunoglobulin, attempts have been made to establish a relationship between the morphological characteristics of the abnormal plasma cells and the actual class of immunoglobulin being synthesized by these cells. Thus, on the basis of cytological examination of marrow smears from 72 patients with myeloma, macroglobulinaemia, or related paraproteinopathies, certain cell types ('flare cells' and 'thesaurocytes') were observed only in the 13 cases of IgA myeloma (Paraskewas *et al.*, 1961).

It has been suggested by Bessis *et al.* (1963) that the high incidence of IgA myeloma cells with large intracytoplasmic paraprotein aggregates may result from a tendency for this immunoglobulin to form high molecular weight polymers in free solution. This proposition leads to the possible clinical significance of the different polymerization patterns displayed by the monoclonal serum IgAs of different myeloma patients. This question will be considered later (see Section 4.1.4.2 and 4.1.4.3), along with the significance of other physicochemical features of serum paraproteins, such as cryoglobulinaemia and hyperviscosity manifestations.

It is interesting to note that intracytoplasmic immunoglobulin crystals also

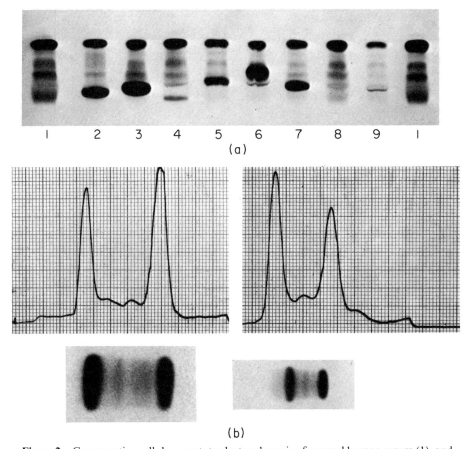

Figure 2 Comparative cellulose acetate electrophoresis of normal human serum (1), and of myeloma sera of IgG1 (2), IgG2 (3), IgG3 (4), IgG4 (5), IgA (6), IgD (8), and IgE (9), and a Waldenström macroglobulinaemic serum (7). (*b*) Densitometric scans of cellulose acetate electrophoretic strips of IgG1 (1) and IgG4 (2) myeloma sera

have been observed in a small percentage of normal and neoplastic plasma cells (Bessis *et al.*, 1963), presumably mirroring the capacity of some immunoglobulin molecules to form ordered structures in free solution.

2.1.4 Immunochemical Aspects

2.1.4.1 Detection and Characterization of Paraproteins. The occurrence of a monoclonal constituent at elevated levels in the serum and/or urine is, of course, the striking immunochemical feature of classical paraproteinopathies. As is indicated by Figure 2 these are readily demonstrable in the serum by electrophoresis on cellulose acetate, although the M-component bands are usually not as pronounced in IgD or IgE myeloma sera. Immunoelectrophoretic analysis of the patient's serum often reveals a 'bowing' of the immunoglobulin precipitin line, caused by the monoclonal component, as will be seen from the examples given in Figure 3. Another frequently observed biochemical characteristic is Bence–Jones proteinuria seen in a high proportion of patients with primary macroglobulinaemia and myeloma; in particular, in those myelomas of the IgD class (Table 5), where the incidence is over 90 per cent. It is also of interest that the light chain of the M component in IgD myeloma patients is predominantly of the λ type, in contrast to the 2:1 ratio of $\kappa:\lambda$ light-chain M components seen in cases of myeloma of the other main immunoglobulin classes and in Waldenström macroglobulinaemia. In this connection, it is worth noting that it has been suggested that the clinical picture and course of multiple myeloma may be related to the class and type of M component. Certainly, it would seem of relevance that of a group of 262 cases of myeloma studied only three showed no abnormality in the serum or urine on electrophoresis or immunoelectrophoresis (Osserman and Takatsuki, 1963).

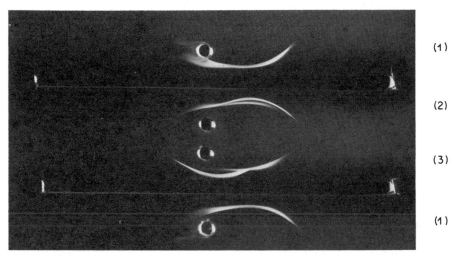

(1)

(2)

(3)

(1)

Figure 3 Immunoelectrophoretic patterns of normal human serum (1) and IgG1 (2), and IgG4 (3) myeloma sera. Antiserum: sheep anti-whole human IgG.

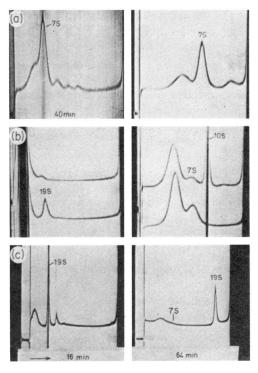

Figure 4 Analytical ultracentrifugation patterns of (a and b) various forms of IgA myeloma sera (dilution × 5) and (c) a typical Waldenström macroglobulinaemic serum (dilution × 20). 59 000 rpm, 20°C. Reproduced from Stanworth (1973a).

Ultracentrifugation is the other basic physicochemical procedure that has thrown light on the nature of paraproteins, and this technique is important in their classification and quantification. As far as myelomatosis is concerned, the approach is of most value in the analysis of IgA gammopathy. In this case, the most frequently observed pattern comprises a marked increase in IgA monomer (7 S) with the appearance of a range of abnormal components (dimer, trimer, etc.) sedimenting between 7 S and 19 S as is illustrated in Figure 4a. A less frequently seen pattern involves only a gross increase in 10 S (dimer) IgA (Figure 4b), whilst a much rarer one comprises an increase in 7 S and 19 S components without the appearance of any intermediate sedimenting forms (Figure 4c). The significance of the polymerized forms, which are observed in the sera of certain cases of IgA myelomatosis, and which appear to arise from inter Fc-region disulphide bridging, is not yet understood. There is preliminary evidence (Roberts-Thomson *et al.*, 1976) which suggests that the patients showing the various types of polymer pattern are not readily distinguishable on clinical grounds. Obviously, it is necessary to exclude the possibility that any additional sedimenting peaks observed in the ultracentrifugation patterns of IgA myeloma sera are not due to complexing with one of the many serum protein constituents (such as albumin, lipoprotein, or α_1-antitrypsin) with which IgA is known to react.

Ultracentrifugation also has proved of some value in the identification of IgE myeloma. The observation that the sedimentation coefficient of the first such reported case by Bennich and Johansson (1967) was closer to 8 S than 7 S provided an early clue that it may correspond to the then unclassified reaginic antibodies found in the sera of patients with allergies of the immediate type. This suspicion was confirmed subsequently by the observation that transfer of reagin-mediated sensitivity to normal individuals' skin was blocked by prior injection of excess IgE myeloma protein (Stanworth et al., 1967). It is interesting, therefore, that myeloma IgE paraproteins isolated from cases reported more recently in Russia and Britain have proved to have lower sedimentation coefficients ($S_{20, \omega}^{\circ}$) of 7·2 S (Stefani et al., 1973) and of 7·28 S (Johns, unpublished results), respectively.

The most frequent application of ultracentrifugation has been in the identification and study of primary (Waldenström) macroglobulinaemia, in which the serum shows a characteristic ultracentrifugal pattern (Figure 4c). This comprises a greatly elevated 19 S peak which often appears as a 'concentration bar' in

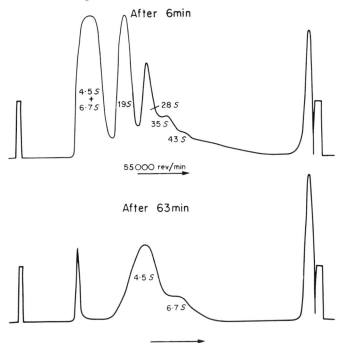

Figure 5 Ultracentrifugation of a typical Waldenström macroglobulinaemia serum (diluted 1 in 5) obtained in a MSE Centriscan 75 machine

the serum Schlieren pattern. There are also faster-sedimenting components (29 S and 38 S) which appear to be polymerized forms of IgM covalently linked by disulphide bridges probably through the C-terminal cysteine residues. In a study of 14 cases of Waldenström macroglobulinaemia (Ratcliff *et al.*, 1963) it was shown that the appearance of the fast-sedimenting polymerized forms of IgM can be expected to be seen in the patient's serum ultracentrifugation pattern when the monomer concentration exceeds about 400 mg/100 ml for the 29 S component, and 1·3 g/100 ml for the 38 S component (Figure 5). This has been confirmed by repeat analysis of the patient's serum depicted in Figure 1, after an interval of several years, by which time the concentration of the 19 S component had risen to above the critical level for the appearance of polymer forms. Recent, more accurate, sedimentation studies of Waldenström macroglobulinaemic sera (Johns, unpublished results) have suggested that the $S_{20,\omega}^{\circ}$ values of the detectable polymerized forms of IgM are 28, 35 and 43 S (representing dimer, trimer, and tetramer respectively).

2.1.4.2 Hyperviscosity Effects. An advantage of ultracentrifugal analysis is that it provides basic information about the physicochemical state of the patient's serum to which can be related other parameters, such as viscosity, and ultimately the clinical consequences. For instance, the increase in plasma viscosity brought about by high levels of paraprotein can lead to a state of hyperviscosity, with interference with essential haemostatic mechanisms. The status of the patient's circulatory system is thought to be a decisive factor in the manifestation of the typical haematological features of Waldenström macroglobulinaemia and

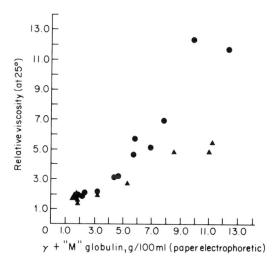

Figure 6 Relationship of relative viscosity to paraprotein concentration of sera from patients with myelomatosis (▲) and Waldenström macroglobulinaemia (●). Reproduced from Ratcliff *et al.* (1963)

some other monoclonal gammopathies. Not unexpectedly, therefore, the hyperviscosity syndrome is observed much more frequently in those cases in which high molecular weight forms of monoclonal immunoglobulin are prominent—IgA myelomatosis and Waldenström macroglobulinaemia. For example, a study of the sera of 34 macroglobulinaemic patients revealed viscosity values in the symptoms range in 38 per cent, these high viscosities being associated usually with serum IgM levels in excess of 5 g/100 ml (McKenzie et al., 1970). Likewise, hyperviscosity effects occur relatively frequently in patients with IgA myelomatosis, where they have been associated with high levels of a paraprotein (presumably an IgA dimer) with a high sedimentation coefficient of around 9 S (Freel et al., 1972). A more recent study (Roberts-Thomson et al., 1976) employed sodium dodecyl sulphate-polyacrylamide gel electrophoresis and gel filtration through Sepharose 6B to show that a high proportion (45 per cent) of 11 IgA myeloma patients, who had more than 50 per cent polymerized paraprotein in their sera, developed the hyperviscosity syndrome; in contrast to another group of 14 patients whose paraprotein was predominantly in the monomeric form, who did not display the effect.

By comparison, the incidence of the hyperviscosity syndrome is much lower in cases of IgG myelomatosis. For example, 4·2 per cent of 238 myeloma patients investigated demonstrated this feature (Pruzanski and Watt, 1972), and these represented 22 per cent of the 46 patients who had serum component levels greater than 5 g/100 ml. As will be seen from Figure 6, it is above this critical immunoglobulin level of 5 g/100 ml that the curves of serum viscosity against M component concentration for Waldenström macroglobulinaemia and IgG myeloma sera begin to part (Ratcliff et al., 1963). Possibly, therefore, the

Table 7 Clinical features of myeloma observed by a number of groups investigating large numbers of cases

	IgG1	IgG2	IgG3	IgG4	Reference
Mean age at diagnosis (years)	62	60	66	66	Schur et al. (1972)
Bence–Jones protein	46/132	17/24	5/14	2/3	
Serum Ca^{2+} > 10·5 mg/100 ml	25/149	4/29	3/15	1/2	
BUN ~ 30 mg/100 ml	26/151	4/27	3/15	0/4	
Osteolytic lesions	61/81	10/15	5/8	2/3	
Hematocrit	32	27	28	26	
Hyperviscosity	14/121	2/121	1/121	1/121	Virella and Hobbs (1971)
Hyperviscosity	5	0	4	0	Capra and Kunkel (1970) McKenzie et al. (1970)
Cryoglobulins	4/121	6/121	4/121	0/121	Virella and Hobbs (1971)
Survival (months)	26	28	20	16	Schur et al. (1972)

From Schur (1972)

hyperviscosity effects shown by certain IgG myeloma sera when the paraprotein concentration exceeds this level can be attributed to the formation of asymmetrical IgG polymers. Indeed, two IgG myelomatosis patients with the hyperviscosity syndrome and paraprotein concentrations between 5–6 g/100 ml serum were reported to have IgG aggregates of 11 and 14 S in their sera (Smith *et al.*, 1965). But it should be mentioned that the paraprotein was stated to be in non-polymerized form in other cases of IgG myelomatosis with hyperviscosity syndrome reported in the literature. Nevertheless, it is interesting that in three myeloma patients with hyperviscosity syndrome associated with the IgG3 subclass (Capra and Kunkel, 1970) the paraprotein showed a concentration-dependent aggregation. Furthermore, the concentration of paraprotein present in the sera of these patients was considerably less than that in a case of hyperviscosity associated with IgG1 paraproteinaemia, presumably because the IgG3 molecule is the more asymmetric. Admittedly, a higher incidence of hyperviscosity syndrome has been observed associated with IgG1 than IgG3 paraproteins (as will be seen from Table 7). But, as Schur (1972) has pointed out, this is probably due to an extremely high serum monomer level, which incidentally might itself be expected to favour polymerization not detected by ultracentrifugation which is of necessity carried out at lower solute concentrations.

2.1.4.3 Cryoglobulinaemia. Although cryoglobulins have been observed to precipitate from the sera of patients with a wide range of conditions, including rheumatoid arthritis and other connective tissue disorders, on lowering the temperature below 37°C, they are most frequently seen on cooling the sera of patients with multiple myeloma and Waldenström macroglobulinaemia. It is important not to confuse cryoglobulin with cryofibrinogen which precipitates or gels when blood is withdrawn into non-siliconized syringes containing anticoagulant and kept at 4° overnight. In contrast, cryoglobulin precipitates or gels when the blood is drawn into 'dry' plastic syringes and maintained at 4° (for preferably more than 24 hours). The resultant precipitate will normally redissolve on restoring the temperature of the serum to 30° in contrast to isolated cryoglobulins, which tend not to redissolve readily in physiological buffers. Examples of the effect of temperature, pH, and ionic strength on the solubility of cryoglobulin preparations are provided in Figure 7 which, in addition, indicates the influence of protein concentration.

The composition of cryoglobulins, and why they tend to come out of solution at low temperatures, has prompted considerable interest among immunochemists. In this connection, it is significant that cryoprecipitates have been found usually to comprise immunoglobulins of different classes (IgG and IgM) or subclasses (for example, of IgG), which has led to the suggestion that they represent antibody–antigen like complexes. There also have been occasional reports of cryoglobulins comprising monoclonal immunoglobulins as, for instance, in some cases of lymphoid malignancy associated with paraproteinaemia (Stone and Metzger, 1967), and the human IgG3 protein (Cra) to which Figure 7a refers.

200

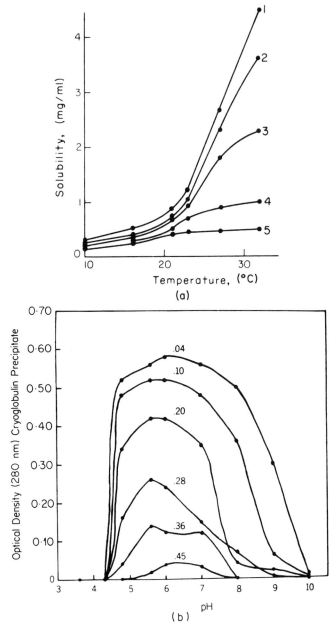

Figure 7 Effect on cryoglobulin precipitation of: (a) temperature using cryoglobulin Cra (human IgG3 myeloma protein); curves 1, 2, 3, 4 and 5 refer to cryoglobulin concentrations of: 9·40, 6·20, 3·10, 1·24, and 0·62 mg/ml, respectively; reproduced from Saluk and Clem (1975); and (b) ionic strength and pH on a cryoglobulin (human IgG myeloma protein); reproduced from Meltzer and Franklin 1966, with permission

In a preliminary study by Meltzer and Franklin (1966) of 29 patients with cryoglobulinaemia, IgG was found in the cryoprecipitate from the sera of eight cases (usually from those with multiple myeloma or idiopathic cryoglobulinaemia), IgM in nine cases, and what were described as 'unusual cryoglobulins with rheumatoid factor-like activity' in the remaining cases. Of this last group, which presented with various clinical symptoms, 11 were found to be mixed cryoglobulins containing both IgG and IgM (Meltzer *et al.*, 1966). Occasionally, cryoglobulin of the IgA class has been reported (see for example, Auscher and Guinand, 1964), but cold-precipitable globulin generally comprises IgG and/or IgM. Immunoglobulin subunits, such as Bence–Jones proteins of either light-chain type (Alper, 1966; Kiss *et al.*, 1967) and α heavy-chain disease protein (Florin-Christensen *et al.*, 1972), also have been reported to possess cryoprecipitation properties.

Important information about the mechanism of temperature-dependent gel formation has been obtained from studies on the proteolytic cleavage fragments of a single-component (6·5 S) human cryoglobulin (γ_1, λ, Gm4) from a patient with idiopathic cryoglobulinaemia (Saha *et al.*, 1970). Although papain Fc and Fab fragments of the cryoglobulin failed to form a gel at reduced temperature, the Fab fragments did exhibit a dimer–monomer equilibrium which was pH-dependent. In contrast, disulphide-bridged pepsin fragments (Fab)$_2$ formed gels in neutral and alkaline buffers at 3°. This suggests that some structural characteristic within the Fab region, probably on the Fd segment, is responsible for IgG monomer association, and ultimately for the cryogel formation. Spectrofluorescence studies have provided evidence of localized conformational change within the Fab region during the polymerization process.

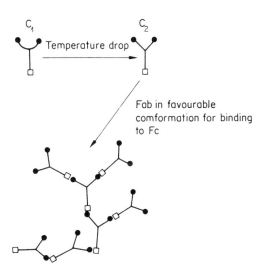

Figure 8 Postulated mechanism of cryoprecipitation of cryoglobulin Cra. Reproduced from Saluk and Clem (1975), with permission

More recent studies by Saluk and Clem (1975) on proteolytic cleavage fragments of Cra, with specificity for IgG1 and IgG3 subclasses, have prompted the proposed mechanism for cryoprecipitation (at least as far as this cryoglobulin is concerned) depicted in Figure 8. This is based on the striking correlation observed between the temperature dependence of cryoprecipitation and Fab–Fc binding, both being relatively temperature-insensitive between 10 and 21°C, but strongly temperature-dependent above 24°C. Moreover, a break in the van't Hoff binding curves at about 25°C, and the demonstration by sedimentation velocity and viscosity studies of temperature-induced conformational alteration in isolated cryoglobulin Fab fragments, suggests that a reduction in temperature below this point changes the conformational state of the Fab region to a more favourable one for the maintenance of the optimal antibody combining site conformation. When in this state, the cryoglobulin builds up large, insoluble complexes by a 'head-to-tail' combination (as is illustrated in Figure 8). The alternative possibility of Fc–Fc interaction during the original high-temperature conformational state is theoretically possible but unlikely.

It should be recognized, however, that the mechanism of cryoprecipitation may be different for cryoglobulins of different immunoglobulin compositions, even when only a single subclass is involved. For instance, in this connection, an interesting suggestion has been made by Saluk and Clem (1975), that the possession of certain allotypic (Gm) antigenic determinants by IgG molecules of the same subclass could possibly influence their functional valency of interaction with cryoglobulin IgG. In contrast to the mechanism proposed above, evidence has been obtained that the cryoprecipitation properties demonstrated by a mixed (IgM–IgG) cryoglobulin reflect the sensitivity of the solubility of the complex (between, for example, IgM antibody and effectively univalent IgG 'antigen' molecules) to changes in environmental temperature (Stone and Metzger, 1968). It has been observed that this IgM antibody, obtained from a case of Waldenström macroglobulinaemia with an atypical lymphoma, possessed functionally univalent and equivalent subunits (IgMs), and that it reacted with single determinant on IgG molecules. More recent studies on the influence of changes in temperature, ionic strength, and pH on the precipitation of a mixed Waldenström macroglobulin antibody–antigen (IgMSie–IgG) complex have indicated that the cryoprecipitation is explicable by the finite size and limited solubility of the IgM–IgG complexes (Stone and Fedak, 1974).

The mechanism whereby cryoglobulins exert their clinical significance is not understood clearly yet, although it can be supposed that in some cases immune-complex formation with concomitant complement activation plays a role in the observed vascular and tissue lesions. Meltzer and Franklin (1966) believe that the temperature at which precipitation begins is more important than the total serum cryoglobulin content. Many patients were observed to be asymptomatic with levels at $1 \cdot 5$–$1 \cdot 8$ g/100 ml, while others with as little as $0 \cdot 1$–$0 \cdot 6$ g/100 ml showed symptoms attributable to the cryoglobulin. It seems conceivable that the precise composition of the cryoprecipitate could be critical as far as the possibility of activating Fc-located effector sites is concerned.

Apparently when the serum cryoglobulin concentration exceeds 2 g/100 ml, it becomes difficult to separate the problems secondary to the increase in serum viscosity from those primarily due to cold precipitation. Indeed it has been suggested by Florin-Christensen (1974) that when serum levels of cryoglobulin rise above 1–2 g/100 ml in a symptomatic patient daily plasmaphoresis in a 37° circuit should be performed. An alternative form of treatment has involved a relatively long course of oral D-penicillamine, a thiol compound which has also been used occasionally in the treatment of Waldenström macroglobulinaemia to prevent the build up of high levels of circulating macroglobulins but which is used more widely in the treatment of Wilson's disease and rheumatoid arthritis. In one such report, a marked reduction in the cryoprecipitation shown by a patient with essential (IgG–IgM) cryoglobulinaemia was observed, but this was not accompanied by any clinical improvement (Goldberg and Barnett, 1970).

Obviously, further physicochemical and immunochemical studies are required on human cryoglobulins of differing composition and specificity. Moreover, valuable information about factors influencing the synthesis of cryoglobulins and the structural basis of their precipitability in the cold should be forthcoming from studying experimentally-induced cryoglobulinaemias in animals. Such a model has been established, in New Zealand Red rabbits immunized with streptococcal Group B/C vaccines (Herd, 1973a, b). Cryoglobulins begin to appear in the serum about three weeks after the commencement of immunization, and reach maximal levels ranging from less than 0·1 to greater than 6 mg/ml. The isolated cryoglobulins thus produced have been shown to comprise IgM and IgG antiglobulins (mainly of the IgM class), and homogeneous IgG antibodies against streptococcal antigens and DNA.

2.1.4.4 Paraproteins with Antibody Activity. The occurrence of circulating monoclonal immunoglobulins with antibody activity in some patients with hyperimmunoglobulinopathies is now well established. Apart from the anti-γ-globulin (rheumatoid factor-like) activity often manifested by cryoprecipitation (as discussed in Section 2.1.4.3), cold-agglutinin (anti-I and anti-i) activity is probably the most frequently observed. Sometimes even both reduced temperature effects are expressed in the same case of Waldenström macroglobulinaemia. Naturally occurring cold agglutinins, like those that develop during infections, are usually polyclonal immunoglobulins of the IgM class possessing both κ and λ light-chain types (Harboe and Lind, 1966). In contrast, the cold agglutinins found in the sera of patients with lymphoproliferative disorders are monoclonal IgM proteins, which were thought originally to be exclusively of the κ type (Harboe *et al.*, 1965), but which have been shown more recently to be sometimes of the λ light-chain type. Feizi (1967), for example, has reported a disorder of the latter type in three patients with chronic haemolytic anaemia.

Another widely investigated aspect is the hapten-binding activity of monoclonal immunoglobulins occurring in the sera of patients with multiple myelomatosis, Waldenström macroglobulinaemia, and related disorders. Indeed, such paraproteins have been employed widely by immunochemists as model 'antibodies' in the study of kinetic and structural aspects of antigen–(hapten)-binding interactions. Apart from the academic value of this approach, it would seem to be of some practical significance. This is indicated by the interesting observation of Bauer (1974) that three Waldenström macroglobulins have been found which precipitated derivatives of triiodoaminobenzoic acid present in the contrast media used for cholecystography. Intravenous injection of a derivative resulted in a fatal immunological reaction in one Waldenström macroglobulinaemic patient, whose IgM was shown to have 'hapten'-binding activity localized within the Fab regions. Another 'antibody'-like Waldenström macroglobulin, which has been studied in some depth, possesses specificity against phosphorylcholine (Reisen, 1975).

It is imperative in the identification of paraproteins with antibody activity to demonstrate that the presumptive ligand is bound to the monoclonal immunoglobulin *via* its Fab region. This applies particularly to suspected cases of specific binding by paraprotein of lipoprotein, which has been reported in cases of myeloma with accompanying hyperlipaemia and xanthomatosis, and of other plasma protein constituents such as albumin. Some immunoglobulins (for example, IgA) have been observed to bind these plasma proteins non-specifically.

Other instances of monoclonal immunoglobulins with antibody activity include anti-tissue antibodies, such as those directed against microsomes, mitochondria, smooth muscle, and foetoproteins in acute and chronic liver disease (Florin-Christensen and Roux, 1974). Membrane-bound monoclonal immunoglobulins with anti-IgG, anti-Forsmann, and cold-agglutin activity also have been reported (Seligman and Feizi, 1974). Interestingly, the membrane-bound IgM of a variable proportion of small lymphocytes in peripheral blood of such patients has been shown to possess the same antibody specificity and idiotype as the monoclonal IgM in the serum—where detectable. This has prompted the suggestion by Harboe and Feizi (1974) that monoclonal populations of lymphocytes from patients with chronic lymphatic leukaemia may prove to be as useful in cellular immunological studies as monoclonal immunoglobulins isolated from the serum of patients with myelomatosis and Waldenström's macroglobulinaemia have been in the delineation of immunoglobulin structure.

Important information about the nature of paraproteins with antibody activity is being obtained also from studies on immunoglobulins with restricted heterogeneity induced experimentally by immunization of animals such as rabbits. This aspect will be discussed later when considering experimental models (Section 4.1.1).

2.1.4.5 Depleted Paraproteins

2.1.4.5.1 Heavy-chain disease proteins. The fore-runner of the increasingly available 'library' of spontaneously occurring depleted paraproteins was the heavy chain-like protein first reported by Franklin (1964). This protein was detected in the serum and urine of a 43-years old male patient who was admitted to hospital initially with generalized lymph node enlargement, but who showed evidence of a malignant lymphoma eventually. A large, abnormal homogeneous peak of fast γ mobility (8·4 g/100 ml) was observed on electrophoresis of the patient's serum. A similar dominant electrophoretic peak was observed, along with lesser amounts of albumin and globulin in the urine, approximately 12 g/day being excreted. Preliminary analyses showed it to possess a sedimentation coefficient ($S_{20,\omega}^{\circ}$) of 3·7 S, a molecular weight of 53 000 when determined by the Archibald method, and conjugated carbohydrate. It was found also to possess Gm-genotype specificity, but to lack light-chain InV specificity.

This initial observation was followed soon after by a report by Osserman and Takatsuki (1964) of four further cases of this so-called heavy-chain disease in the U.S.A. with many clinical and biochemical features similar to the original case. Many further examples of this condition, as well as of the production of defective α and μ heavy chains, have been recorded since. For instance, a survey of the literature reported 35 cases of γ; 50 of α, and 10 of μ heavy-chain disease (Franklin and Frangione, 1971). A subdivision of heavy-chain diseases, on the basis of immunological studies, has revealed 68 per cent to be of the γ_1 subclass, 7 per cent of the γ_2, 21 per cent of the γ_3, and only 4 per cent of the γ_4 (Frangione and Franklin, unpublished results). The reason for the unexpectedly high incidence of γ_3 heavy-chain disease proteins is not understood yet.

Table 8 Major types of abnormal heavy chains observed so far in heavy-chain diseases

	Variants	Species*	
Heavy chain	Heavy-chain disease proteins (γ, α, μ)—altered heavy chains—usually no light chains		
	Internal deletion	H	?M
	Degradation	H	
	Intact heavy chain and probable degradation	H	M
	Free heavy and light chains—unassembled	H	
	Whole molecule with altered heavy chain		
	Internal deletion like heavy-chain disease		M
	Missing hinge	H	
	Missing C_H3 domain	H	M
	Missing Fc μ fragment	H	
	Half molecules with deletion missing plus an additional change		M
	Degradation of N-terminal domain	H	
	Hybrid molecules and longer heavy chains	H	M
Light chain	Myelomas with altered light chains		
	Internal deletion	H	
	Elongated light chain	H	M
	Light-chain deletions or fragments		
	Internal deletion and carbohydrate	H	
	C-region only		M
	Amyloid—immunoglobulin related	H	

* H = human, M = murine

From Franklin and Fraugione (1973)

Subsequent immunochemical analyses have shown that while the original heavy-chain disease provides the most striking abnormality in immunoglobulin synthesis, a series of other more subtly altered molecules is produced under certain pathological conditions, or experimentally in mice. The major types of abnormality of immunoglobulin chains so far observed are listed in Table 8.

Although initial immunochemical studies suggested that heavy-chain proteins were essentially Fc fragments, detailed amino acid sequential analyses have revealed (as illustrated in Figure 9) a wide variety of structural abnormalities. Such abnormalities range from apparently intact free heavy chains in one instance to proteins with internal deletions of part, or most, of the V region as well as the C_H1 domain up to, and sometimes including, the hinge region. A number of molecules has been found to lack the whole of the variable region and the C_H1 domain (Franklin and Frangione, 1971). Moreover, the discovery of a γ_3 heavy-chain disease protein (OMM) existing in two forms, namely the intact heavy chain as well as the Fc fragment including the hinge region (Aldersberg *et al.*,

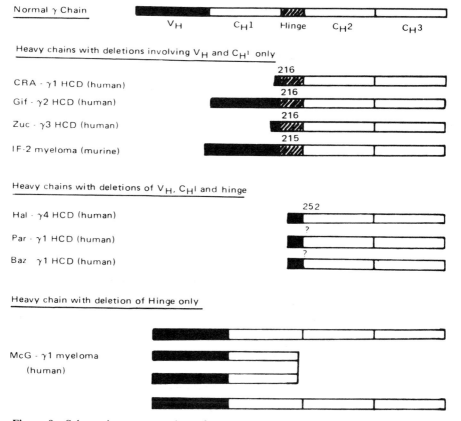

Figure 9 Schematic representation of various types of deletion seen in heavy-chain disease and myeloma proteins with internal deletions, compared to normal heavy chain. Reproduced from Franklin and Frangione (1975), with permission

unpublished results), has led to the suggestion that such structures probably result from proteolytic degradation of a larger precursor molecule.

Two major types of deleted heavy-chain disease proteins are now recognizable (see Figure 9): (*i*) those with internal deletion of part of the V region and the C_H1 domain, with resumption of normal sequences at glutamate 216; and (*ii*) those with internal deletion of the V region, the C_H1 domain, and the hinge region. In addition, other γ heavy-chain disease proteins have been found to be deleted only at the hinge region. Others begin at the hinge region and comprise the whole of C_H2 and C_H3 domains, thus appearing to be degradation products. Biosynthetic studies by, for example, Buxbaum (1973), employing tissue culture of cells from patients with heavy-chain (γ, α, or μ) disease, have failed to produce evidence of post-ribosomal degradation, thereby suggesting a synthetic origin for the abnormal proteins. Moreover, the results of the study of the immunoglobulin products of spontaneously arising structural gene mutants in a cultured cell line of the mouse myeloma MOPC 21 strain would seem to be consistent with this possibility. Such proteins display an internal heavy-chain deletion in a position (residue 215) homologous to the one (residue 216) implicated in the majority of internal deletions observed in human heavy-chain disease (Milstein *et al.*, 1974).

α and μ heavy-chain disease proteins are not yet as well characterized as the γ heavy-chain immunoglobulins, but an essentially similar picture is beginning to emerge (see Table 9). For instance, the α heavy-chain disease proteins resemble the γ proteins in the size of the monomer form (35 000–42 000), in comprising primarily the C-terminal half of the heavy polypeptide chain, and in being rich in carbohydrate. Furthermore, all proteins so far studied lack heavy-light chain disulphide bridges, while retaining part or all of the heavy–heavy disulphide bridges and possessing a normal C-terminus (Seligmann *et al.*, 1971). Interestingly, all are of the major $\alpha1$ subclass. They also seem to contain J chain, as is indicated in Table 9. A quite different IgA abnormality seen in three generations

Table 9   Properties of γ, α, and μ heavy-chain disease proteins

Property	γ	α	μ
Mobility	Fast γ-β	β	$\alpha1$
Sedimentation rate	2·8–4 S	4–11 S	10·8–11 S
Molecular weight of monomer	25 000–58 000 (most 35 000)	35 000–42 000	35 000–55 000
Carbohydrate	Rich–up to 20 per cent	Rich	Rich
Present in urine	Usually	Sometimes	Never
Light-chain production	Not yet observed	Not yet observed	5/7
J chain	No	Often	In some
Approximate number of cases	35	50	10
Subclass	$\gamma1$ 19/28 $\gamma2$ 2/28 $\gamma3$ 6/28 $\gamma4$ 1/28	All $\alpha1$	—

From Franklin and Frangione (1973)

of a family in which the propositus suffered from recurrent infections (Moroz *et al.*, 1971) would seem to represent a familial defect of IgA1 heavy and light polypeptide chain assembly.

A smaller number of μ heavy-chain disease proteins have been studied so far. It is noteworthy (see Table 6) that six out of seven were found to have chronic lymphocytic leukaemia (Franklin, 1975) and that two features common to all were the presence of κ type Bence–Jones proteins and vacuolated plasma cells in the marrow. The μ chain protein with a molecular weight of around 55 000, compared with about 6000 for the normal, is a synthetic not a degradation product (Franklin, 1975). The cells appear to synthesize an incomplete μ chain and a light chain, which may be due to a mutation giving rise to an internal deletion of the μ chain so that it cannot be joined into a complete macroglobulin molecule.

Other types of altered chain seen in myeloma proteins of human and murine origin include: deletions of the C-terminal end of the heavy chain (in a human IgA myeloma); the omission of the whole Fc region of μ (that is C_H3 and C_H4 domains); half molecules (for example of IGA) with deletion; internal deletion of light chain with loss of the V region of the heavy chain (for example in an IgG myeloma protein); and molecules which appear to be hybrids of two different subclasses, as in the case of murine IgG2a and IgG2b. An example of the last abnormality was the report by Kunkel and associates (1969) of human IgG molecules in normal individuals comprising γ_3 Fab and γ_1 Fc fragments. Reports of other, even more subtle examples of hybridized normal and myeloma human IgG molecules are beginning to appear in the literature.

2.1.4.5.2 Light-chain variants. Apart from the synthesis and secretion of free light chains in hyperimmunoglobulinopathic conditions, similar abnormalities to those outlined above have been encountered involving both structural deletions and alterations. These too are listed in Table 8.

Minor internal deletions are, of course, often revealed in comparisons of the primary amino acid sequences of different light-chain proteins by the necessity of leaving short gaps to permit proper alignment. Of greater interest, however, are reports of omission of whole V and C regions for synthetic or degradative reasons, the resultant product being sometimes distinguishable by antigenic analysis and peptide mapping from a normal light-chain domain. An example of such a protein is the newly recognized form of light chain in four cases of myelomatosis treated with intermittent corticosteroids (Solomon *et al.*, 1966). This was associated with a marked but transient decrease in the 'complete' Bence–Jones proteinuria along with the transitory appearance of the new protein (designated C*). Similar light-chain products have been shown to be produced by mouse myeloma cell lines, and should throw important light eventually on the genetic control of light-chain synthesis and the reasons for the appearance of the aberrant forms in human disease states.

Other types of light-chain variants include elongated light chains, and myeloma proteins with internally deleted light and heavy chains, such as the human IgG myeloma protein (SM) which has been found to possess deletions of similar magnitude (molecular weights of approximately 10 000) in both V regions (Isobe and Osserman, 1974). This abnormal protein with a molecular weight of around 110 000) was detectable at levels of 5–6 g/100 ml in the sera along with the free Fc fragment. The latter also was seen in the urine together with a daily urinary secretion of 10–20 g of deleted light chains with molecular weight of about 15 000.

It would seem obvious that the types of immunoglobulin variants described here will prove of increasing value as 'structural tools' besides providing further clues about the factors controlling immunoglobulin synthesis. Hopefully, their further study will throw more light on the influence of plasma cell proliferative and lymphoproliferative disorders on normal antibody production.

2.1.5 Amyloidosis

The nature of amyloid is dealt with in detail by Pras and Gafni (Chapter 14): Nevertheless, a brief account is included here for completeness.

Although amyloid deposits have been observed in the tissues in a variety of conditions, they are seen frequently in association with Bence–Jones proteinuria in patients with multiple myeloma. Initially, they were thought to consist mainly of carbohydrates (hence the term amyloid—meaning starch-like) but were found later to be of a proteinaceous nature. More recent studies (summarized by Glenner et al., 1972) provided convincing evidence that amyloid comprises, at least in part, deposits of light-chain related immunoglobulin fragments. But non-immunoglobulin components, including polysaccharide, appear to be present in many if not all 'secondary' amyloid deposits and in certain 'primary' and macroglobulinaemia-related amyloids.

Biophysical and chemical analyses have revealed amyloid to be fibrillar, with typical Congo red staining and polarization birefringence, and an X-ray diffraction pattern characteristic of a β-pleated sheet conformation. Recent detailed X-ray diffraction studies of immunoglobulin subunits have demonstrated a similar conformation in certain parts of the structural domains, including the V_L and C_L domains (see Chapter 8, by Feinstein and Beale). It would seem to be highly significant, therefore, that some amyloid has been shown by immunochemical studies (Glenner et al., 1970) to resemble immunoglobulins in possessing both C and V idiotypic regions (see Pras and Gafni, Chapter 14). Moreover, a comparison of the primary structures of two purified amyloid proteins with those of a well-defined κ Bence–Jones protein (Ker) has provided convincing evidence that the amyloid fibrils are derived from κ light chains (Glenner et al., 1971a), and in particular from the V regions of the latter. But, since amyloid proteins have been found to possess somewhat higher molecular weights than those V_L regions, it has been concluded that they also contain some C-region material or non-immunoglobulin constituents.

The light-chain origin of amyloid deposits is supported also by observations of Glenner and associates (1971b) that precipitates with similar Congo red staining and conformational characteristics are formed when some Bence–Jones proteins are subjected to proteolytic cleavage using pepsin under nearly physiological conditions (0·05 M glycine HCl at pH 3·5). Moreover, there are reasons to suppose that certain light chains, particularly of the λ subtype, are prone more structurally to form amyloid fibrils. For, the ratio of $\kappa : \lambda$ chains in paraproteins associated with amyloidosis is 1 : 2 (Pick and Osserman, 1968); and Bence–Jones proteins from patients with amyloidosis have been reported to show a greater tendency to bind to certain normal tissues than do the Bence–Jones proteins from patients with plasma-cell dyscrasias in which amyloidosis has not been observed (Osserman *et al.*, 1964).

Further elucidation of the pathogenesis of amyloidosis could well provide important new information about the aetiology of those paraproteinaemias with which the characteristic deposit formation is particularly associated. Possible origins of amyloid which have been considered so far (see Glenner *et al.*, 1972) include: (*i*) an aberration of a normal light-chain synthetic process, which as suggested by Franklin and Frangione (1971) might involve deletions in the light-chain gene resulting in the production of light-chain fragments analogous to the heavy-chain disease fragments discussed in Section 2.1.4.5.2; and (*ii*) a product of antigen–antibody complex breakdown by macrophages (Waldmann and Strober, 1969).

It is conceivable that further information on the mode of production of amyloid will be provided by studying animal models. In this connection, it should be noted that the susceptibility of mice to amyloidosis correlates neither with the H-2 histocompatibility locus nor with immune traits (Franklin and Clerici, 1974). Current studies on cellular immunological aspects of amyloidogenesis in mice receiving repeated injections of casein should prove rewarding. One noteworthy observation from this approach has been that amyloid and anti-casein antibody production can be elicited in 'nude mice', implying that T cells do not play a prominent role in the genesis of the disease.

2.2 Other Forms of Gammopathy

As mentioned earlier (see Section 1), immunoglobulinopathies have been observed in a whole range of conditions other than malignant immunoproliferative diseases (such as myelomatosis and Waldenström macroglobulinaemia), but usually at relatively lower levels and often in polyclonal forms. Apart from the benign monoclonal gammopathies seen particularly in normal individuals of advancing age (where the level of abnormal protein in the serum is usually less than 2 g/100 ml), gammopathies are also observed in chronic infective states.

These include: (*i*) liver disease, where a particular immunoglobulin class is seen to be predominant in the serum in different forms; for example IgM occurs in primary biliary cirrhosis; IgG in the macronodular chronic aggressive hepatitis; IgA in the micronodular type of Laennec type of cirrhosis (Hobbs, 1971); and IgE in a high incidence of patients with acute or chronic liver disease of widely differing aetiology; (ii) Malabsorption states such as active Crohn's disease and ulcerative colitis associated with a raised IgA; (iii) skin diseases such as dermatitis herpetiformis, dermatomyositis, and erythema nodosum, in which raised IgA levels are observed; in addition, atopic dermatitis (eczema) is often associated with extremely high levels of serum IgE.

It also should be mentioned that transient paraproteins are observed sometimes (see Young, 1969), which increase rapidly to a peak serum level and disappear spontaneously within a matter of weeks or months. It has been suggested by Hobbs (1971) that such a transient production of paraprotein represents a weak recognition of antigen, but that eventually 'antibody' is produced with a high enough affinity for combination to occur and to switch off the response.

In the context of the present discussions, however, monoclonal gammopathies would seem to be of greater significance. These have been observed, for instance, in a rare chronic skin disease, lichen myxoedematosus; where they always are associated with IgG and, with the absence of Bence–Jones proteinuria (James et al., 1967), and where they are considered to be of benign nature. There is also the possibility that polyclonal gammopathies can, under certain circumstances, convert to monoclonal gammopathy (Osserman and Takatsuki, 1963). This has been observed in animal studies and, possibly, in a young child whose polyclonal pattern turned into a monoclonal one with accompanying Bence–Jones proteinuria (Stoop et al., 1968).

3 IMMUNE DEFICIENCY STATES

3.1 Primary Hypogammaglobulinaemia

The originally recognized immune deficiency state was referred to as agammaglobulinaemia (Bruton, 1952), but later studies employing more sensitive techniques revealed that it was possible to detect some circulating γ-globulin in virtually every case. Hence, the term hypogammaglobulinaemia was adopted. In England, a Medical Research Council Working Party set up to study this condition chose a γ-globulin level of 200 mg/100 ml (100 mg/100 ml for children of less than one year) as the arbitrary level below which such a diagnosis would apply (Soothill, 1962). Immunodeficiency has proved, however, to be considerably more complex than was anticipated at that time.

At the cellular level, primary immunodeficiencies can involve a B-cell defect (as in, for example, infantile sex-linked hypogammaglobulinaemia) or a T-cell defect (as in Di George's syndrome), where there is a congenital absence of the thymus due to defective embryogenesis. In other conditions, both B and T-cell defects occur, as will be seen from Table 10.

Reduced synthesis and secretion of immunoglobulins (IgG, IgA, and IgM) by peripheral blood lymphocytes of patients with common variable hypogammaglobulinaemia were demonstrated when the cells were cultured for several days in the presence of pokeweed mitogen (Waldmann et al., 1974). This has led to the suggestion that this form of immunodeficiency may be attributable

Table 10   Classification of primary immunodeficiency disorders*

Type	Suggested cellular defect		
	B-cells	T-cells	Stem cells
Infantile X-linked agammaglobulinaemia	+		
Selective immunoglobulin deficiency (IgA)	+ (some)		
Transient hypogammaglobulinaemia of infancy	+		
X-linked immunodeficiency with hyper-IgM	+	?	
Thymic hypoplasia (pharyngeal pouch syndrome, Di George's syndrome)		+	
Episodic lymphopaenia with lymphocytotoxin		+	
Immunodeficiency with or without hyperimmunoglobulinaemia	+	+ (sometimes)	
Immunodeficiency with ataxia telangiectasia	+	+	
Immunodeficiency with thrombocytopaenia and eczema (Wiskott–Aldrich syndrome)	+	+	
Immunodeficiency with thymoma	+	+	
Immunodeficiency with short-limbed dwarfism	+	+	
Immunodeficiency with generalized haematopoietic hypoplasia	+	+	+
Severe combined immunodeficiency			
autosomal recessive	+	+	+
X-linked	+	+	+
sporadic	+	+	+
Variable immunodeficiency (common, largely unclassified)	+	+ (sometimes)	

* References to disorders not mentioned above appear in an earlier classification; see *Wld Hlth Org. techn. Rep. Ser.* (1968), No. 402, p. 27
From Bull. Wld Hlth Org. (1971), **45**, 125

to an abnormality of regulatory T cells, which act to suppress B-cell maturation and antibody production. The emphasis in this section will be placed, however, on deficiencies in circulating immunoglobulins.

The first indication of an immunoglobulin deficiency is provided usually by serum electrophoresis, or preferably immunoelectrophoretic analysis (see Figure 10), which is confirmed and measured by a quantitative procedure, using antisera specific for the main immunoglobulin classes and subclasses. In some conditions, such as infantile sex-linked hypogammaglobulinaemia with thymoma and autosomal recessive alymphocytic hypogammaglobulinaemia, all classes of immunoglobulin are extremely deficient. At the other end of the scale, some deficiency states, such as autosomal recessive lymphopenia and thymic aplasia, are characterized by entirely normal circulating immunoglobulin levels. Probably the most interesting cases from the immunochemist's point of view are

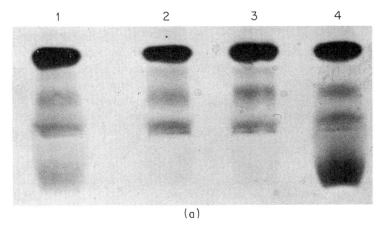

(a)

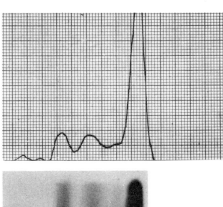

(b)

Figure 10 (a) Cellulose acetate electrophoretic patterns of sera from two patients with primary hypogammaglobulinaemia (2 and 3) compared with normal serum patterns (1 and 4). (b) Densitomeric scan of cellulose acetate electrophoretic strip of hypogammaglobulinaemic serum. (c) Immunoelectrophoretic patterns of hypogammaglobulinaemic serum (1) and normal human serum (2) developed against anti-whole human serum (3) and anti-human IgG (4)

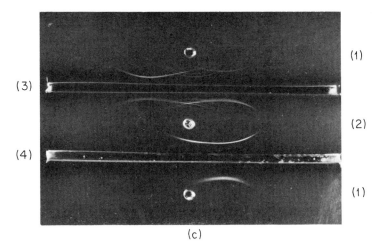

(c)

those showing a selective deficiency of a particular immunoglobin class or subclass. For example some apparently normal individuals have been shown to be deficient in IgA as measured by quantitative immunodiffusion (Rockey *et al.*, 1964). One such case showed classical symptoms of immediate-type hypersensitivity (hayfever). Where such serum IgA deficiency occurs, the two subclasses IgA1 and IgA2 usually are reduced in equal proportions, and there is often a deficiency in the IgA secretions too. Occasionally, however, patients have been encountered with normal levels of circulating IgA but low levels of IgA in secretions and *viceversa* (Goldberg *et al.*, 1969).

There have been reports of selective IgM deficiency in children dying of fulminating meningococcal septicaemia (Hobbs *et al.*, 1967) and in an infant with recurrent *Pseudomomas* infections who possessed IgG and IgA-staining immunofluorescence—but not IgM-staining—plasma cells in the spleen (Faulk *et al.*, 1971). Low levels of IgM have been reported also to be associated with both meningitis and disseminated non-progressive vaccinia (Hobbs *et al.*, 1967).

Selective IgG deficiencies have been observed in patients with recurrent pyogenic infections (Schur *et al.*, 1970), and in some cases deficiencies of particular subclasses have been found to occur. This possibility was suggested originally by the observation of Golebiowska and Rowe (1967) that sera from patients with hypogammaglobulinaemia were sometimes deficient in either slow or fast γ-globulins on immunoelectrophoresis. Since then, various examples of selective IgG deficiency have been reported. For example, IgG2 and IgG3 deficiencies have been observed to be associated with infection in a child (Terry, 1968), and chronic infection has been reported in a family with hereditary deficiency of IgG2 and IgG4 (Oxelius, 1974). Of 59 patients with various immune disorders studied by Yount *et al.* (1970), 11 out of 13 with IgG imbalance showed relative increases in IgG3, especially of the Gm(b) type, and decreases in immunoglobulin with the Gm(g) marker. It is significant, however, that most cases of IgG deficiency so far studied have displayed accompanying deficiencies in other immunoglobulin classes (IgM and IgA), and it has been suggested (Schur, 1970) that the IgG subclasses are linked so closely genetically that it might be impossible to see a deficiency in one subclass which does not affect other subclasses severely and even other classes of immunoglobulin. Indeed, in a recent study of the IgG subclasses in a group of 35 patients with primary hypogammaglobulinaemia all subclasses were found to be depressed in the majority of cases (Shakib, 1976). But an overall comparison of the mean IgG subclass levels of the group, compared with those of normal individuals, revealed that the IgG1 and IgG3 subclasses were least depressed. This finding is consistent with the observed high capacity of the immune system to produce these subclasses not only in young adults, but also in early infancy (Morell *et al.*, 1972; Van der Giessen *et al.*, 1975) and in very old age, that is in individuals over 95-years old (Radl *et al.*, 1975).

It is interesting to note that a patient with ataxia telangectasia with IgA deficiency was found also to be deficient in IgG2, whereas his father was deficient in IgG1 (Rivat *et al.*, 1969). But a potentially more significant association has been suggested between IgA and IgE, on the basis of the observation by Amman and coworkers (1969) of IgE deficiency, as demonstrated by reverse cutaneous anaphylaxis testing with anti-IgE, in 11 out of 16 patients with ataxia telangectasia and IgA deficiency; nine of whom had recurrent sinopulmonary infections of varying degrees. Such observations have been interpreted as evidence that the production of IgA and IgE are linked in some important way. Other findings of IgE deficiency associated with chronic sinopulmonary infection (Cain *et al.*, 1969) have led to the idea that one of the normal functions of IgE is the protection of the respiratory mucosa from infection. A more recent finding of Polmar *et al.* (1972), that 11 out of 25 individuals with isolated IgA deficiency also lacked circulating IgE (as measured by radioimmunosorbent test), and yet were uniformly asymptomatic, fails to support the concept of a protective role for IgE in respiratory tract immunity. Moreover, a case has been reported (Levy and Chen, 1970) of a healthy individual, with increased incidence of infection, but with no history of allergic disease, who was deficient in circulating IgE; her serum contained less than $0.01 \ \mu g/ml$, although her leucocytes did release histamine on incubation with anti-IgE.

Nevertheless, as pointed out by Amman *et al.* (1970), the immune system is extremely complex in nature and has the ability to compensate for imbalances, so that the absence of any single factor in an apparently normal healthy individual does not necessarily mean that the factor is without a role in defence. Moreover, the high incidence of autoimmune disease and phenomena seen in individuals with selective IgA deficiency (Amman and Hong, 1970) suggests that deficiency of this immunoglobulin class, at least, cannot always be considered to be benign. Other investigators (for example, Koistinen and Sarna, 1975) have made the point that the high incidence of immunological abnormalities in a group of blood donors suggests that IgA deficiency is not a mere laboratory finding.

Another interesting aspect of the question of an interrelationship between IgE and IgA synthesis is the provocative suggestion of Soothill that the onset of atopy of the immediate-type in early life is attributable to a transient IgA deficiency. This is based on the observation by Taylor *et al.* (1973) that the development of atopy, as indicated by eczema and direct positive skin-test responses to common allergens, in three-month old infants is associated with a serum IgA deficiency when measured by quantitative immunodiffusion. In this connection, it is of possible relevance that approximately one in 700 of a population of mostly healthy individuals have been shown to have a selective IgA deficiency (Bachmann, 1965), and that a familial cluster of such a selective IgA deficiency in a healthy population of blood donors has been reported (Koistinen, 1976). The findings of another study on the serum of IgA levels of 64 588 new blood donors (Koistinen, 1975) bring out the important point that the degree of deficiency of a particular immunoglobulin observed will depend on the accuracy of the assay. For the incidence of IgA deficiency in this large normal population was found to be one in 396 by Ouchterlony analysis (sensitivity: $10 \ \mu g/ml$), one in 507 by haemagglutination-inhibition testing (sensitivity: $0.5 \ \mu g/ml$), and one in 821 by radioimmunoassay (sensitivity: $0.015 \ \mu g/ml$).

The reliability and comparability of the immunoglobulin assays employed is of particular importance in studies of IgE-deficiency states, where it is essential to adopt some radioimmunosorbent procedure. Application of a radiolabelled, modified Mancini method as used by Spitz *et al.* (1972) has failed to detect any measurable IgE (30 ng/ml or more) in the sera of the majority of patients with common variable and sex-linked hypogammaglobulinaemia. Another study (Waldmann *et al.*, 1972) reported that the IgE levels, which had been estimated by using a double-antibody radioimmunoassay were below the limit of detection (4 ng/ml) in nine out of 10 patients with common variable immune deficiency and in seven out of eight patients with thymoma and hypogammaglobulinaemia. On the other hand, a recent study (McLaughlan *et al.*, 1974) has revealed that most patients with common variable and sex-linked hypogammaglobulinaemia had detectable serum IgE (using the radioimmunosorbent procedure). It was also observed that there appeared to be no relationship between the level of IgE in the patients' sera and their reactivity to injected γ-globulin or drugs, or with the occurrence of eczema.

Certain other disorders often are associated with immune deficiency states. For instance, malignancies are particularly frequent in ataxia telangiectasia and in the Wiscott–Aldrich syndrome, where they are responsible for about 10 per cent deaths. There is also a high incidence of autoantibodies, with or without autoimmune disease, in patients with immunodeficiency (as already mentioned see p. 215. In one such example of eight patients with primary hypo-gammaglobulinaemia who developed a severe polyarthritis with some features in common with rheumatoid arthritis, the disease improved dramatically as a result of treatment with γ-globulin (Webster *et al.*, 1976). As classical rheumatoid arthritis does not respond to such treatment, it has been suggested that the arthritis of hypogammaglobulinaemia is due to an organism or toxin which is neutralized by antibody within the injected IgG. In this connection, it is worth noting that an IgA deficiency has been seen to develop occasionally in rheumatoid arthritic patients treated with oral D-penicillamine over relatively long periods. Several such cases have been followed in the author's laboratory (Stanworth *et al.*, 1977). In one the drug was withdrawn immediately when it was realized that the serum level was falling dramatically but it was thought that the subject would have become IgA deficient anyway. Nevertheless, the possibility of drug-induced hypogammopathies of this type in certain genetically predisposed individuals should be recognized.

Conditions which have been reported in association with selective IgA deficiency include recurrent respiratory tract infections, intestinal disorders, juvenile rheumatoid arthritis, and other autoimmune diseases. But, as with the association of polyarthritis referred to above, it would seem more likely that these associated immunological abnormalities are a consequence of the immune deficiency rather than of the genetic defects themselves. As has been pointed out by Good and Yunis (1974) in the primary immune deficiency which develops during ageing in man, and is accompanied by various autoimmune conditions and a high frequency of amyloidosis; antigens and organisms gain access to normally forbidden areas of the body where they persist and abnormally stimulate the residual immunological systems to an excessive degree.

3.2 Secondary Hypogammaglobulinaemia

Hypogammaglobulinaemia can occur sometimes secondary to another disorder, particularly those involving the loss of abnormal amounts of immunoglobulin by excretion (such as occurs in the nephrotic syndrome) or by an aberration of metabolism (such as protein-losing enteropathies like coeliac disease and ulcerative colitis, familial idiopathic hypercatabolic lipoproteinaemia, and myotonic dystrophy). Secondary hypogammaglobulinaemia is substantially more common than the primary form. For instance, secondary deficiency as defined by a serum IgG level of below 200 mg/100 ml, was seen in 0·5 per cent of a group of patients screened at the Hammersmith Hospital, compared with the 10 (0·05 per cent) who proved to be suffering from a primary deficiency (Hobbs, 1968).

It is also interesting to note that polyclonal immunoglobulin of one or other class was found to be reduced significantly in 82 per cent of patients with lymphoproliferative and plasma-cell proliferative disease (Cwynarski and Cohen, 1971), thus accounting for the infection that is frequently the terminal event in such cases. Immunoglobulin deficiency was found to be equally prevalent in all classes of monoclonal gammopathy, but was considerably more common in myelomatosis than in benign monoclonal gammopathy. Moreover, evidence has been obtained from cell culture experiments, which suggests that the observed deficiencies in circulating polyclonal immunoglobulins in these conditions are attributable to a failure of synthesis. Polyclonal deficiency in macroglobulinaemia is ascribed to the peripheral spread of neoplastic cells, a process which apparently does not account for the immunoglobulin deficiencies observed in typical cases of myelomatosis.

With regard to the association of hypogammaglobulinaemia with renal disease, it is interesting to note that an asymmetric depression has been observed in the serum levels of certain IgG subclasses in some patients with 'minimal-change' nephrotic syndrome, focal glomerulosclerosis, and proliferative glomerulonephritis (Shakib et al., 1976). This suggests that the urinary loss of IgG alone cannot account for the low blood levels of this immunoglobulin class encountered in these conditions.

4 EXPERIMENTAL MODELS

4.1 Experimental Paraproteinopathies

4.1.1 Induction of Hypergammaglobulinaemia in Animals

Although, as far as is known, naturally occurring or experimentally induced plasma-cell neoplasms have not been reported in rabbits, as they have in other species such as mice, the experimental immunization of this species with

218

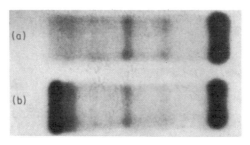

Figure 11 Zone electrophoretic patterns of serum from a rabbit taken (a) before and (b) after immunization with group A streptococcal vaccine. Reproduced from Osterland *et al.* (1966), with permission

streptococcal carbohydrates has led *in some animals* to the production of an electrophoretically uniform γ-globulin at an elevated serum concentration of the order of 20–50 mg/ml. This, in many ways, resembles the monoclonal paraproteins seen in the sera of patients with multiple myeloma (Osterland *et al.*, 1966). Figure 11 shows microzone electrophoretic patterns of the serum of rabbits before and four weeks after intravenous immunization with group A-variant *Streptococcus*. Similar homogeneous antibody responses have been observed in some rabbits immunized with types III and VIII pneumococcal capsular polysaccharide (Pincus *et al.*, 1970*a*, *b*).

Apart from the zone electrophoretic homogeneity, evidence for restricted heterogeneity of such antibodies has been indicated by: (*i*) the monodisperse distribution of their light chains on disc electrophoresis, (*ii*) allotype exclusion, and (*iii*) the identical amino acid sequences of the N-terminal regions (residues 1–41) of their light chains (Braun *et al.*, 1975). In all respects, therefore, the rabbit antibodies appear to be as homogeneous as human myeloma immunoglobulin.

Hopefully, the study of this animal model will provide important information about those malignant processes in humans that lead to the production of monoclonal immunoglobulins. It is interesting to note, therefore, that of the various factors which have been found to influence the production of paraproteinaemia in rabbits, the most important appears to be the choice of animal with the appropriate genetic background and the repeated intravenous immunization with a vaccine composed of whole bacteria, with intact surface carbohydrate (Braun *et al.*, 1969). It has been found, for instance, that immunization with vaccine *via* the intraperitoneal route is much less effective, as is the use of purified soluble bacterial carbohydrates alone as immunogens. In addition, the selective breeding of high and low-responding rabbits has provided data which suggest that the magnitude of the immune response is transmitted genetically.

Histological examination of rabbits sacrificed at the time of maximal serum paraprotein level has revealed intensive proliferation of plasma cells in the spleen, lungs, and lymph nodes (Braun and Krause, 1969). Immunofluorescence studies showed that the majority of plasma cells in the spleens of rabbits immunized with type VII *Pneumoccocus* species were indeed synthesizing antibodies to this antigen. It has been suggested by Krause (1970) that the intense immunization by repeated intravenous injections of vaccine over a prolonged period selects a restricted population of cells which undergoes proliferation. Attention has been drawn to an interesting parallelism with the development of a myeloma-like condition in mink with Aleutian disease. Late in the course of this condition some mink show a transition from a heterogeneous hypergammaglobulinaemia to a homogeneous myeloma-like disease, suggesting the ascendancy of a few predominant clones of plasma cells (Porter *et al.*, 1965). As mentioned earlier, it is conceivable that a similar transition sometimes occurs in those humans who initially exhibit a benign polyclonal hypergammaglobulinaemia which ultimately develops into a malignant monoclonal form.

As in the human condition, certain rabbits in which paraproteinaemia has been induced experimentally by immunization with bacterial vaccines exhibit cryoglobulinaemia. For instance, cryoglobulin production in New Zealand Red rabbits immunized with streptococcal (group B/C) vaccines began around three weeks after the start of immunization and reached maximal serum levels ranging from less than 0·1 mg/ml to greater than 6 mg/ml (Herd, 1973b). It should be noted that these experimentally induced cryoglobulins were shown to comprise IgM and IgG—including IgM anti-γ-globulin and homogeneous IgG anti-streptococcal antibodies—as well as DNA. Hence, they resemble closely the composition of the spontaneously occurring human counterparts and, for this reason, would seem to offer a useful model. In this connection, Herd (1973b) has postulated, on the basis of her studies using the experimental rabbit system, that cryoglobulins are formed in two stages, the first involving structural modification of IgG followed by its precipitation with anti-γ-globulin. She has also suggested (Herd 1973a) that anti-γ-globulins might be operative in the experimental production of paraproteinaemia in rabbits, in suppressing immunoglobulin synthesis by heterogeneous clones of antibody-forming cell precursors while stimulating proliferation of selected clones which secrete the homogeneous antibodies. Evidence in support of this idea has been provided from recent studies of antibody production in rabbits immunized with streptococcal group A and C carbohydrate antigens (Aasted, 1974), which have revealed that the appearance of an antibody response of restricted heterogeneity is accompanied by the production of anti-antibody (IgG) as measured by the latex fixation test. It is possible that such anti-antibodies are directed against previously secluded determinants within the Fc region of the original anti-streptococcal IgG antibody, which are revealed because of a conformational change brought about by combination with the bacterial antigen. This probably occurs in a manner similar to that postulated to explain the production of anti-γ antibodies in rabbits immunized with preformed antigen–antibody (rabbit IgG) complexes (Henney and Stanworth, 1966). In this connection, it is significant that 7 S anti-IgG antibodies have been isolated by immunosorption from the sera of rabbits immunized against streptococcal carbohydrates which have specificity for the Fc region of rabbit IgG (Bokisch *et al.*, 1973), and which are themselves also of restricted heterogeneity, besides possessing idiotypic specificity.

4.1.2 *Spontaneous or Experimentally Induced Plasma-Cell Tumours*

The study of hyperimmunoglobulinopathy has also been facilitated by the availability of spontaneously occurring or experimentally induced plasma-cell tumours in species such as rats and mice. For instance, the inbred C3H (Potter *et al.*, 1957) and the F_1 hybrids of CBA × DBA/2 mice (Rask-Neilsen *et al.*, 1959) show a unique predilection to develop 'spontaneous' plasma-cell tumours. Consequently, these animals have been used widely in the study of genetic and other factors relevant to the pathogenesis of plasma-cell neoplasia. Another example of a highly valuable experimental model is the spontaneously occurring ileocoecal immunocytoma frequently found in the inbred LOU/WS1 strain of rat, whose secreting properties are maintained over many passages in histocompatible animals (Bazin *et al.*, 1974). Such tumours have been shown to secrete monoclonal immunoglobulin which possesses immunological, chemical, and biological properties characteristic of rat IgE.

Alternatively, immunoglobulin-secreting tumours have been induced experimentally in various species by transplantation, or by injection, of some suitable irritant. For example, one transplantation line of leukaemia in the (CBA × DBA/2) F_1 murine strain is characterized by the appearance of a macroglobulin component in the serum, and a histological pattern resembling human macroglobulinaemia (Clausen *et al.*, 1960). Another, a transplanted plasma-cell tumour of ileococcal origin (× 5563) in the C3H strain, has been shown to be histologically similar to the neoplasms of human multiple myeloma and to be accompanied by a similar development of osteolytic bone lesions and the production of an abnormal serum protein of γ electrophoretic mobility, which is also extractable from the tumours (Potter *et al.*, 1957).

Plasma-cell neoplasms also have been induced experimentally in strain BALB/c mice by intraperitoneal injection of a mineral oil–*Staphylococcus* mixture, or even mineral oil alone. The highest incidence of tumours was observed in mice receiving three injections (0·5 ml) of the latter at two-months intervals (Potter and Boyce, 1962). Similar intraperitoneal plasma-cell neoplasms have been induced in this mouse strain by implantation of a Millipore diffusion chamber (Merwin and Algire, 1959); it being concluded that, like mineral oil, this is only mildly irritating and therefore tolerated well by most mice, and is not removable by host defence mechanisms but can cause a reactive tissue on the peritoneal surfaces.

As mentioned earlier, a marked hypergammaglobulinaemia is a regular feature of virus-inducible Aleutian disease in mink (see Section 4.1.1); which shows histological features in common with human plasma-cell dyscrasias, such as a parallelism between the severity of the disease and the rise in serum levels of 7 S γ-globulin (Henson *et al.*, 1963). Moreover, the hypergammaglobulinaemia as revealed by paper electrophoretic analysis of serum in some cases transforms into a homogeneous myeloma-like disease with time, resulting in the appearance of Bence–Jones protein in the urine (Porter *et al.*, 1965). This has been interpreted as being due to the transition from a hyperplastic state, where the viral agent is assumed to be affecting a number of clones of plasma cells, to a neoplastic one involving monoclonal plasma-cell proliferation.

4.1.3 In Vitro *Culture of Paraprotein-Producing Cell Lines*

The *in vitro* synthesis and secretion of immunoglobulins by myeloma and lymphoblastoid-cultured cell lines is now well established (Table 11), and has already provided valuable information about the factors influencing paraprotein production in the patient, besides offering an alternative source of monoclonal immunoglobulin. For instance, the immunoglobulin produced by established cell lines of human multiple myeloma origin derived from buffy coat material was of a single light-chain type and showed well-defined electrophoretic mobility (Matsuoka *et al.*, 1968). Thus, one cell line (RPMI 8235) produced only κ-type IgG, another line (RPMI 4666) produced κ-type IgA and free κ light chains, while a third (RPMI 8226) produced only λ light chains. Moreover, the time course of immunoglobulin accumulation and cell proliferation indicates that the cells were able to synthesize and secrete immunoglobulin actively only while they were able to proliferate.

One of these cell lines (RPMI 8226) has been cultured continuously over a number of years, and been shown to continue to grow well and to produce only λ-

Table 11   Ig-secreting cell lines of human haemapoietic origin

Number	Source	Characteristics of Ig product(s)	Secretion rate	Reference
RPMI 8235	Buffy coat of patients with chronic myelogeneous leukaemia	IgG (κ) only	3 mg Ig/10^6 cells day^{-1}*	Matsuoka *et al.* (1968)
RPMI 4666	,,	IgA (κ); free κ light chains (inbalance of heavy and light-chain synthesis)	,,	
RPMI 8226	Buffy coat of patient with multiple myeloma	Free light chains only	+ 220 ng light chains/10^6 cells day^{-1}*	
266 B1,	Bone marrow from patient with multiple myeloma	IgE	$8 \cdot 1 \times 10^{-12}$ g†/ cell hr^{-1}	Nilsson (1971)

* In most active phases of synthesis and secretion   † Max. rate of synthesis.

type light chains (Matsuoka *et al.*, 1969). Moreover, many of the cells were seen to resemble morphologically immature plasma cells with well-developed endoplasmic reticula and numerous ribosomes. Furthermore, the light-chain material isolated from these cultures was shown to possess physical and chemical features characteristic of λ-type Bence–Jones proteins, sedimenting as a dimer ($S^{\circ}_{20, \omega}$ = 3·6 at 12·5 mg/ml) at neutral pH in the ultracentrifuge (Matsuoka *et al.*, 1969).

IgE-producing cell lines (266B1 and 268 Bm) also have been established *in vitro* from the first case of human myeloma of this type, reported in Sweden (Nilsson *et al.*, 1970; Nilsson, 1971). From this work it was concluded that myeloma cells are unusually exacting in their metabolic requirements, and only if media rich in vitamins and amino acids (for example F10 and RPM1 1640) are conditioned by the presence of growing cells will the *in vitro* IgE production be optimal. It will then approach the secretion rate obtained in fresh explants of human myeloma cells, which is presumed to reflect the *in vivo* synthetic rate of immunoglobulins. Indeed, the average rate of synthesis of IgG by myeloma cells *in vitro* has been used, together with a quantitative measurement of the total body rate of IgG synthesis *in vivo*, to estimate the numbers of tumour cells in patients with IgG myeloma (Salmon and Smith, 1970) by substitution in the equation:

$$ MCT_{\mathrm{B}} = \frac{RT_{\mathrm{B}}}{R_{\mathrm{M}}} \times MC \ i.v. $$

where MCT_{B} = total body myeloma-cell number, $MC \ i.v.$ = number of myeloma cells *in vitro*, RT_{B} = rate of total body IgG synthesis (g/24 hr) *in vivo* R_{M} = rate of total myeloma IgG synthesis (g/24 hr) *in vitro*. The tumour cell number thus determined was then used in the clinical evaluation of the extent of the disease, being employed to estimate the average rate of growth of this particular malignancy.

Average molecular synthetic rates in different patients have been found to range from 12 500 to 81 000 molecules IgG/myeloma cell min^{-1}; and the total body myeloma-cell number was found to range from $0·5 \times 10^{12}$ to $3·1 \times 10^{12}$ myeloma cells, and could be correlated with the degree of skeletal damage observed on radiographs. Likewise, a patient with IgE myelomatosis (P.S in Table 2) was shown to synthesize IgE molecules at a comparable rate of 26 000 molecules/myeloma cell min^{-1}, despite a concomitant plasma-cell leukaemia (Salmon *et al.*, 1971). However, autoradiographic studies demonstrated a significantly greater labelling of DNA in this patient's bone marrow cells than is seen in cells from IgG-myeloma patients.

The IgE-producing cell line 266B1 has continuously produced, over a long period, immunoglobulin molecules identical to those synthesized by the patient *in vivo* at an optimal rate over a 48-hour period of $1·7 \times 10^{-13}$ g IgE/cell hr^{-1}. The maximal rate of synthesis ($8·1 \times 10^{-12}$ g IgE/cell hr^{-1}) was correlated with rapid cell growth (at $10^6/30$ ml cell densities), and with the presence of feeder human skin fibroblasts or glia-like cells, or with the use of conditioned media harvested from such cells.

The study of *in vitro* systems is providing valuable information about the regulation of synthesis and secretion of immunoglobulins by myeloma cells. An *in vitro* approach, which is potentially even more powerful is based initially on the isolation of mutant mouse myeloma cell lines obtained by selecting single cells from a continuous culture of mouse MOPC 21 myeloma cells (Cotton *et al.*, 1973; Secher *et al.*, 1973). Four immunoglobulin structural mutants produced spontaneously by such cell lines have been characterized using amino acid sequencing, cell-free synthesis, and studies on the isolated mRNA, and have been shown to arise due to defects in the heavy-chain cistron (Milstein *et al.*, 1977). Thus, mutant proteins (IF1 and IF3) involve deletions of the C_H3 domain (see Figure 12), due to early termination and to a frame shift, respectively. IF2 has an internal deletion resembling the heavy-chain disease of humans and IF4 (not illustrated in Figure 12) shows an amino acid substitution due to point mutation.

An even more exciting advance in this area, however, has been the development by cell fusion of new lines capable of antibody synthesis. This has been accomplished by, for example, fusing mouse myeloma cells with spleen cells from normal mice which have been immunized with sheep erythrocytes or hapten-carrier antigens, using TNP as the hapten. The resultant hybrids express both the parental myeloma polypeptide chains and, in addition, a light and heavy chain responsible for antibody specificity. Methods for the specific detection of clonal variants have been devised, and it has been shown that such clonal lines can be grown as tumours in mice, from whose sera specific antibody can be isolated.

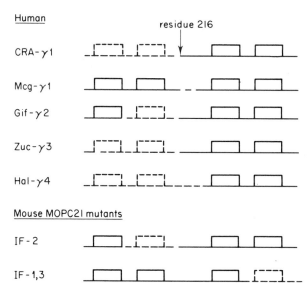

Figure 12 Comparison of deletions observed in human heavy chains and in mouse mutants. Reproduced from Milstein *et al.* (1974) with permission

4.2 Experimental Hypogammaglobulinaemia

As in the experimental study of hypergammaglobulinaemia (see Sections 4.1.1 and 4.1.2), the growing use of animal models is providing a valuable insight into the various factors influencing the induction and perpetuation of immunodeficiency states in humans, as well as pointing to possible means of clinical treatment. It is thus possible to investigate both the cellular and immune elements of immunodeficiency states, and their underlying genetic defects.

The three main approaches which have been adopted concern: (*i*) congenital, and surgically or chemically induced defects, involving the thymus, or the bursa of Fabricius in chickens, (*ii*) infectious unresponsiveness, and (*iii*) allotypic suppression. Examples of each will be considered.

The study of congenitally thymus-lacking so-called 'nude' (nu/nu) mice offers a means of determining the influence of T cells on immunoglobulin synthesis. For instance, by this approach it has been shown that the establishment of normal serum concentrations of IgA, IgG2a, and especially IgG1, in this species requires a viable thymus; whereas IgM production shows no such T-cell dependency (Pritchard *et al.*, 1973). On the other hand, studies in chickens which have been 'bursectomized' hormonally suggest that impaired J-chain synthesis may constitute a limiting process in IgM production by B cells in this species (Ivanyi, 1975). Other congenital deficiencies in animals, such as the fatal one seen in arab foals, involve a combined B and T-lymphocyte impairment (McGuire *et al.*, 1974).

Loss of bursal function also can arise in chickens as a result of naturally occurring viral infections. An example of such a situation is infectious bursal disease, formerly known as Gumboro disease, which is characterized by the destruction of the lymphoid tissue in the bursa without repopulation (Cheville, 1967). The observed reduction in haemagglutinating antibody (IgG) response to Newcastle disease vaccine and in the serum IgG levels of such birds has been interpreted as providing further evidence that the switch over from IgM to IgG antibody production takes place within the bursa (Faragher *et al.*, 1972). The observation is also consistent with an earlier report that bursectomy in late embryonic life has no influence on IgM antibody responses in chickens, but prevents an IgG response.

The third experimental approach to the induction of immunodeficiency states in animals involves the suppression of synthesis of immunoglobulin molecules carrying particular allotypic markers by treatment with anti-allotype antiserum. Long-lasting suppression can be achieved with relative ease and regularity in the rabbit in this way. In the mouse suppression is obtained only with certain strain combinations and tends to be sporadic (Adler, 1975). Although the type of allotype suppression first described in the rabbit by Dray (1962) was brought about by maternal transmission of the anti-allotype (isoantibody), suppression is achieved most conveniently in experimental models by neonatal injection of antiserum (Mage and Dray, 1965). Suppression thus induced can be directed selectively and specifically against alleles of the two genetic loci used by cells in the synthesis of all classes of rabbit immunoglobulin: the a locus (on the Fd region of the heavy chain) and the b locus (on κ light chains). Possible mechanisms of this form of allotypic suppression have been proposed recently by Catty *et al.* (1975). Cultured spleen cells from rabbits which have been chronically suppressed in this way provide a useful *in vitro* model. Adler (1975) has shown that treatment of these cells with anti-allotypic serum specific for the non-suppressed allotype will abrogate the experimentally induced suppression. This has provided a valuable means of learning more about the suppression mechanism, by studying those conditions under which such reversal of suppression occurs.

5 PARAPROTEINS AS TOOLS IN IMMUNOGLOBULIN CHARACTERIZATION

The availability of monoclonal paraproteins representative of the various classes and subclasses has advanced the structural elucidation of human immunoglobulins. This is particularly the case, of course, with regard to IgE and IgD, which normally are found at such low levels in the sera of non-neoplastic individuals that their isolation in sufficient amounts for full characterization has presented a most formidable task. Heavy polypeptide chains of paraproteins of each human class and subclass have been or have are being sequenced, following the primary structural elucidation of light-chain (including Bence–Jones protein) preparations. Where crystalline forms are available, tertiary structural studies are also in progress. Moreover, the paraproteins produced by experimental animals such as those of ileococcal origin in the rat (mentioned in Section 4.1.2), likewise offer the key to the structural characterization of immunoglobulins of these species; as do the highly homogeneous antibodies produced by some rabbits immunized with streptococcal vaccines (see Section 4.1.1).

Such paraproteins are also proving valuable tools in functional studies of their normal immunoglobulin counterparts. For instance, proteolytic and chemical-cleaved fragments of the first described myeloma IgE protein were used in inhibition of Prausnitz-Küstner (PK) (Stanworth *et al.*, 1967, 1968) and inhibition of passive cutaneous anaphylaxis (PCA) (Stanworth, 1973*b*) tests to provide convincing evidence that reaginic antibodies belong to this new class of immunoglobulin and that they bind to target mast cells through sites within their Fc regions. Likewise studies with the rat myeloma IgE protein (Bazin *et al.*, 1974), mentioned in Section 4.1.2, have confirmed that rat reaginic antibody molecules are also of this class. To quote another example of this type, chemical cleavage fragments of the mouse myeloma protein IgG2a MOPC 173 have been employed in investigations aimed at locating the position of complement-activating sites (Kehoe *et al.*, 1969). Similarly, inhibition studies with human myeloma proteins have demonstrated the association of certain biological activities with particular IgG subclass; for example this approach has been employed in studies of the inhibition of monocyte phagocytosis of erythrocytes coated with anti-Rh antibodies to show that monocyte binding is restricted to the IgG1 and IgG3 subclasses (Huber and Fudenberg, 1968). There are many analogous examples, involving studies of the inhibition of other Fc-located biological activities by certain myeloma immunoglobulin subclasses and their cleavage fragments (see Stanworth and Turner, 1973; Stanworth, 1974; Stanworth and Stewart, 1975).

An alternative, but parallel, approach has involved the use of incomplete or deleted paraproteins in these sort of tests for Fc-located immunoglobulin functions. An example of this approach is the demonstration of the failure of IgG proteins lacking a C_H3 domain (IF1, IF3), obtained from mutant cell lines of MOPC/2 mice, to inhibit rosette formation by mouse lymphocytes, in contrast to another mutant protein (IF2) which lacks the C_H1 domain. This provides further evidence that the C_H3 region is essential for the binding of IgG to Fc receptors on lymph-node cells (Ramasamy et al., 1975). The further study of paraproteins with more limited deletions could well help to pinpoint more precisely the location of various cell-binding and other Fc-located effector sites.

Conversely, the studies of hapten-binding paraproteins (referred to earlier in Section 2.1.4.4) have provided important information about the nature of the Fab-located antigen-binding sites of antibody molecules. Thus, the gammopathies, whether occurring spontaneously or induced experimentally, have presented and will continue to present a rich source of material for the immunochemist interested in the nature and role of immunoglobulins in health and disease.

ACKNOWLEDGEMENTS

The author is most grateful to his colleagues Philip Johns and Helen Evans for providing the illustrations reproduced in Figures 2, 3, 5 and 10; and to the other people who have permitted him to reproduce their data.

REFERENCES

Aasted, B. (1974). *Scand. J. Immunol.*, **3**, 553.
Adler, L. T. (1975). Transplant. Rev., **27**, 3.
Alper, C. A. (1966). *Acta med. scand.*, **Suppl. 445**, 200.
Amman, A. J., Cain, W. P., Ishizika, K., Hong, R., and Good, R. A. (1969). *New Eng. J. Med.*, **281**, 469.
Amman, A. J., and Hong, R. (1970). *Clin. Exp. Immunol.*, **7**, 883.
Amman, A. J. (1970). *New Eng. J. Med.*, **283**, 542.
Apitz, K. (1940). *Virchows Archs Path. Anat.*, **306**, 631.
Asquith, P., Thompson, R. A., and Cooke, W. T. (1969). *Lancet*, **ii**, 129.
Auscher, C., and Guinand, S. (1964). *Clin. Chim. Acta*, **9**, 40.
Axelsson, U., and Bachmann, R., and Hällén, J. (1966). *Acta med. scand.*, **179**, 235.

Bachmann, R. (1965). *Scand. J. Clin. Lab. Invest.*, **17**, 316.
Ballieux, R. E., Imhof, J. W., Mul, N. A. J., Zegers, B. J. M., and Stoop, J. W. (1968). *Clin. Chim. Acta*, **22**, 7.
Bauer, K. (1974). In *Progress in Immunology II*, Vol. 3, (Brent, L., and Holborow, J., eds.), North Holland Publishing Co., Amsterdam, p. 390.
Bazin, H., Querinjean, P., Becker, S. A., Heremans, J. F., and Dessy, F. (1974). *Immunology*, **26**, 713.

Bennich, H., and Johansson, S. G. O. (1967). *Immunology*, **13**, 381.
Bernier, G. M., Ballieux, R. E., Tominaga, K., and Putnam, F. E. (1967). *J. Exp. Med.*, **125**, 303.
Bessis, M., Briton-Gorius, J., and Binet, J. L. (1963). *Nouv. Rev. Franc. Hematol.*, **3**, 159.
Bokisch, V. A., Chia, O. J. W., and Bernstein, D. (1973). *J. Exp. Med.*, **137**, 1354.
Bradley, J., Hawkins, C. F., Rowe, D. S., and Stanworth, D. R. (1968). *Gut*, **9**, 564.
Braun, D. G., Eichmann, K., and Krause, R. M. (1969). *J. Exp. Med.*, **129**, 809.
Braun, D. G., Huser, H., and Jaton, J.-C. (1975). *Nature, (Lond.)*, **258**, 363.
Braun, D. G., and Krause, R. M. (1969). *Z. Immun. Forsch.*, **139**, 104.
Bruton, O. C. (1952). *Pediatrics*, **9**, 722.
Buxbaum, J. (1973). *Semin. Hematol.*, **10**, 33.

Cain, W. A., Ammann, A. J., Hong, R., Ishizaka, K., and Good, R. A. (1969). *J. Clin. Invest.*, **48**, 120.
Capra, J. D., and Kunkel, H. G. (1970). *J. Clin. Invest.*, **49**, 610.
Catty, D., Lowe, J. A., and Gell, P. G. H. (1975). *Transplant. Rev.*, **27**, 157.
Cheville, N. F. (1967). *Am. J. Pathol.*, **51**, 527.
Cioli, D., and Baglioni, C. (1966). *J. Mol. Biol.*, **15**, 385.
Clausen, J., Rask-Nielsen, R., Christiensen, H. E., Lontie, R., and Herremans, J. (1960). *Proc. Soc. Exp. Biol. Med.*, **103**, 802.
Cotton, R. G. H., Secher, D. S., and Milstein, C. (1973). *Eur. J. Immunol.*, **3**, 135.
Cwynarski, M. T., and Cohen, S. (1971). *Clin. Exp. Immunol.*, **8**, 237.

Dray, S. (1962). *Nature, (Lond.)*, **195**, 677.

Faragher, J. T., Alan, W. H., and Cullen, G. A. (1972). *Nature, New Biol.*, **237**, 118.
Faulk, W. P., Kiyasu, W. S., Cooper, M. D., and Fudenberg, H. H. (1971). *Pediatrics*, **47**, 399.
Feizi, T. (1967). *Science, N.Y.*, **156**, 1111.
Fishkin, B. G., Orloff, N., Scaduto, L. E., Borucki, D. T., and Spiegelberg, H. L. (1972). *Blood*, **39**, 361.
Florin-Christensen, A. (1974). *Curr. Titles*, **2**, (11), p. 275.
Florin-Christensen, A., Donaich, D., and Newcomb, P. J. (1972). *Brit. Med. J.*, **ii**, 413.
Florin-Christensen, A., and Roux, R. (1974). In *Progress in Immunology II*, Vol. I, (Brent, L., and Holborow, J., eds.), North Holland Publishing Co., Amsterdam, p. 285.
Frangione, B., and Franklin, E. C. (1973). *Semin. Hematol.*, **10**, 53.
Franklin, E. C. (1964). *J. Exp. Med.*, **120**, 691.
Franklin, E. C. (1975). *Archs Int. Med.*, **135**, 71.
Franklin, E. C., and Clerici, E. (1974). In *Progress in Immunology II*, Vol. 4, (Brent, L., and Holborow, J., eds.), North Holland Publishing Co., Amsterdam, p. 381.
Franklin, E. C., and Frangione, B. (1971). *Proc. Nat. Acad. Sci., U.S.A.*, **68**, 187.
Franklin, E. C., and Frangione, B. (1975). *Contemp. Top. Mol. Biol.*, **4**, 89.
Franklin, E. C., Meltzer, M., Guggenheim, F., and Lowenstein, J. (1963). *Fed. Proc.*, **22**, 264.
Freel, R. J., Maldonado, J. E., and Gleich, G. J. (1972). *Am. J. Med.*, **264**, 117.
Fudenberg, H. H. (1972). In *Cancer Chemotherapy II* (Brodsy, I., Kahn, S. B., and Moyer, J. H., eds.), Grune and Stratton Inc., New York, p. 393.

Glenner, G. G., Ein, D., Eanes, E. D., Bladon, H. A., Terry, W., and Page, D. (1971*b*). *Science, N.Y.*, **174**, 712.
Glenner, G. G., Ein, D., and Terry, W. D. (1972). *Am. J. Med.*, **52**, 141.
Glenner, G. G., Harada, M., Isersky, C., Cuatrecasas, C., Page, D., and Keiser, H. R. (1970). *Biochem. Biophys. Res. Commun.*, **41**, 1013.

228

Glenner, G. G., Terry, W., Harada, M., Isersky, C., and Page, D. (1971a). *Science, N.Y.*, **171**, 1150.

Goldberg, L. S., and Barnett, E. V. (1970). *Ann. Int. Med.*, **125**, 145.

Goldberg, L. S., Douglas, S. S., and Fudenberg, H. H. (1969). *Clin. Exp. Immunol.*, **4**, 579.

Golebiowska, H., and Rowe, D. S. (1967). *Clin. Exp. Immunol.*, **2**, 275.

Good, R. A., and Yunis, E. (1974). *Fed. Proc.*, **33**, 2040.

Grey, H. M., and Kunkel, H. G. (1964). *J. Exp. Med.*, **120**, 253.

Hallén, J. (1963). *Acta med. scand.*, **173**, 737.

Harboe, M., and Feizi, T. (1974). In *Progress in Immunology II*, Vol. 3, (Brent, L., and Holborow, J., eds.), North Holland Publishing Co., Amsterdam, p. 390.

Harboe, M., and Lind, K. (1966). *Scand. J. Haematol.*, **3**, 269.

Harboe, M., van Furth, R., Schubothe, H., Lind, K., and Evans, R. S. (1965). *Scand. J. Haematol.*, **2**, 259.

Henney, C. S., and Stanworth, D. R. (1966). *Nature, (Lond.)*, **210**, 1071.

Henson, J. B., Gorham, J. R., and Leader, R. W. (1963). *Nature, (Lond.)*, **197**, 206.

Herd, Z. L. (1973a). *Immunology*, **25**, 923.

Herd, Z. L. (1973b). *Immunology*, **25**, 931.

Hobbs, J. R. (1968). *Proc. Roy. Soc. Med.*, **61**, 883.

Hobbs, J. R. (1969). *Brit. J. Haematol.*, **16**, 599.

Hobbs, J. R. (1971). *Adv. Clin. Chem.*, **14**, 219.

Hobbs, J. R., Milner, R. D. G., and Watt, P. J. (1967). *Brit. Med. J.*, **iv**, 583.

Huber, H., and Fudenberg, H. H. (1968). *Int. Archs Allergy*, **34**, 18.

Isobe, T., and Osserman, E. F. (1974). *Blood*, **43**, 505.

Ivanyi, I. (1975). *Immunology*, **28**, 1015.

James, K., Fudenberg, H., Epstein, W. L., and Schuster, J. (1967). *Clin. Exp. Immunol.*, **2**, 153.

Jancelwicz, Z., Takatuski, K., Sugai, S., and Pruzanski, W. (1975). *Archs Int. Med.*, **135**, 87.

Kehoe, J. M., Fougereau, M., and Bourgois, A. (1969). *Nature, (Lond.)*, **224**, 1212.

Kiss, M., Fudenberg, H. H., and Kritzman, J. (1967). *Clin. Exp. Immunol.*, **2**, 467.

Knedel, M., Fateh-Moghadam, A., Edel, H., Bartl, R., and Neumeier, D. (1975). *Dtsch. Med. Woch.*, **101**, 496.

Koistinen, J. (1975). *Vox. Sang.*, **29**, 192.

Koistinen, J. (1976). *Vox. Sang.*, **30**, 181.

Koistinen, J., and Sarna, S. (1975). *Vox. Sang.*, **29**, 203.

Krause, R. M. (1970). *Adv. Immunol.*, **12**, 1.

Kunkel, H. G., Natvig, J. B., and Joslin, F. G. (1969). *Proc. Nat. Acad. Sci., U.S.A.*, **62**, 144.

Leddy, J. P., Deitchman, J., and Bakemeier, R. F. (1970). *Arth. Rheumat.*, **13**, 331.

Levy, D. A., and Chen, J. (1970). *New Engl. J. Med.*, **283**, 541.

Mage, R. G., and Dray, S. (1965). *J. Immunol.*, **95**, 525.

Martin, N. H. (1970). *Brit. J. Hosp. Med.*, **3**, 662.

Matsuoka, Y., Takahashi, M., Yagi, Y., Moore, G. E., and Pressman, D. (1968). *J. Immunol.*, **101**, 1111.

Matusoka, Y., Yagi, Y., Moore, G. E., and Pressman, D. (1969). *J. Immunol.*, **102**, 1136.

McGuire, T. C. *et al.* (1974). *J. Am. Vet. Med. Ass.*, **164**, 70.

McKenzie, M. R., Fudenberg, H. H., and O'Reilly, R. A. (1970). *J. Clin. Invest.*, **49**, 15.

McLaughlan, P., Stanworth, D. R., Webster, A. D. A., and Asherson, G. L. (1974). *Clin. Exp. Immunol.*, **16**, 375.

Meltzer, M., and Franklin, E. C. (1966). *Am. J. Med.*, **40**, 828.

Meltzer, M., Franklin, E. C., Elias, K., McCluskey, R. T., and Cooper, N. (1966). *Am. J. Med.*, **40**, 837.

Merwin, R. M., and Algire, G. H. (1959). *Proc. Soc. Exp. Biol. Med.*, **101**, 437.

Mills, R. J., Fahie-Wilson, M. N., Carter, P. M., and Hobbs, J. R. (1976). *Clin. Exp. Immunol.*, **23**, 228.

Milstein, C., Adetugbo, K., Cowan, N. J., Köhler, G., Secher, D. S., and Wilde, C. D. (1977). *Cold Spring Harbor Symposium on Quantitative Biology*, **41**, 793.

Milstein, C., Adetugbo, K., Cowan, N. J., and Secher, D. S. (1974). In *Progress in Immunology II*, Vol. I, (Brent, L., and Holborow, J., eds.), North Holland Publishing Co., Amsterdam, p. 157.

Morell, A., Skvaril, F., Hitzig, W. H., and Barandum, S. (1972). *J. Pediatrics*, **80**, 960.

Moroz, C., Amir, J., and de Vries, A. (1971). *J. Clin. Invest.*, **50**, 2726.

Natvig, J. B., Kunkel, H. G., and Litwin, S. D. (1967). *Cold Spring Harbor Symp. Quant. Biol.*, **32**, 173.

Nilsson, K. (1971). *Int. J. Cancer*, **7**, 380.

Nilsson, K., Bennich, H., Johansson, S. G. O., and Pontén, J. (1970). *Clin. Exp. Immunol.*, **7**, 477.

Ogawa, M., Kochwa, S., Smith, C., Ishizaka, K., and McIntyre, O. R. (1969). *New Engl. J. Med.*, **281**, 1217.

Osserman, E. F., and Kohn, J. (1974). In *Progress in Immunology II*, Vol. 3, (Brent, L., and Holborow, I., eds.), North Holland Publishing Co., Amsterdam, p. 390.

Osserman, E. F., and Takatsuki, K. (1963). *Medicine*, **42**, 357.

Osserman, E. F., and Takatsuki, K. (1964). *Am. J. Med.*, **37**, 351.

Osserman, E. F., Takatsuki, K., and Talal, N. (1964). *Semin. Hematol.*, **1**, 3.

Osterland, C. K., Miller, E. J., Karakawa, W., and Krause, R. M. (1966). *J. Exp. Med.*, **123**, 599.

Oxelius, V. A. (1974). *Clin. Exp. Immunol.*, **17**, 19.

Paraskewas, F., Heremans, J., and Waldenström, J. (1961). *Acta med. scand.*, **170**, 575.

Pick, A. L., and Osserman, E. F. (1968). In *Amyloidosis* (Mandema, E., Ruinen, L., Scholter, J. H., and Cohen, A. S., Excerpta), Medica, Amsterdam, p. 1.

Pincus, J. H., Jaton, J. C., Bloch, K. J., and Harboe, E. (1970a). *J. Immunol.*, **104**, 143.

Pincus, J. H., Jaton, J. C., Bloch, K. J., and Harboe, E. J. (1970b). *J. Immunol.*, **104**, 1149.

Polmar, S. H., Waldmann, T. A., Balestra, S. T., Jost, M. C., Terry, W. D. (1972). *J. Clin. Invest.*, **51**, 326.

Porter, D. D., Dixon, F. J., and Larsen, A. E. (1965). *Blood*, **25**, 736.

Potter, M., and Boyce, C. R. (1962). *Nature, (Lond.)*, **193**, 1086.

Potter, M., Fahey, J. L., and Pilgrim, H. I. (1957). *Proc. Soc. Exp. Biol. Med.*, **94**, 372.

Pritchard, H., Riddaway, J., and Micklem, H. S. (1973). *Clin. Exp. Immunol.*, **13**, 125.

Pruzanski, W., and Watt, F. (1972). *Ann. Intern. Med.*, **77**, 813.

Pruzanski, W., Platts, E., and Ogryzlo, M. A. (1969). *Am. J. Med.*, **47**, 60.

Radl, J. (1974). In *Progress in Immunology II*, Vol. 3, (Brent, L., and Holborow, J., eds.), North Holland Publishing Co., Amsterdam, p. 390.

Radl, J., Sepers, J. M., Skvaril, F., Morell, A., Hijmans, W. (1975). *Clin. Exp. Immunol.*, **22**, 84.

Ramasamy, R., Secher, D. S., and Adetugbo, K. (1975). *Nature, (Lond.)*, **253**, 656.

Rask-Nielsen, R., Gormsen, H., and Clausen, J. (1959). *J. Nat. Cancer Inst.*, **22**, 509.

Ratcliff, P., Soothill, J. F., and Stanworth, D. R. (1963). *Clin. Chim. Acta*, **8**, 91.

Reisen, W. (1975). *Biochemistry*, **14**, 1052.

Rivat, L., Ropartz, C., Burtin, P., and Karitzky, D. (1969). *Vox Sang.*, **17**, 5.

Roberts-Thompson, P. J., Mason, D., and MacLennan, I. C. M. (1976). *Brit. J. Haematol.*, **33**, 117.

Rockey, J. H., Hanson, L. A., and Heremans, J. F. (1964). *J. Lab. Clin. Med.*, **63**, 205.

Saha, A., Chowdhury, P., Sambury, S., Smart, K., and Rose, B. (1970). *J. Biol. Chem.*, **245**, 2730.

Salmon, S. E., McIntyre, D. R., and Ogawa, M. (1971). *Blood*, **37**, 696.

Salmon, S. E., and Smith, B. A. (1970. *J. Clin. Invest.*, **49**, 1114.

Saluk, P. H., and Clem, W. (1975). *Immunochemistry*, **12**, 29.

Schur, P. H. (1972). *Prog. Clin. Immunol.*, **1**, 71.

Schur, P. H., Borel, H., Gelfand, E. W., Alper, C. A., and Rosen, F. C. (1970). *New Engl. J. Med.*, **283**, 631.

Scrivastava and Kohn, J. (1974). In *Progress in Immunology II*, Vol. 3, (Brent, L., and Holborow, J., eds.), North Holland Publishing Co., Amsterdam, p. 390.

Secher, D. S., Cotton, R. G. H., and Milstein, C. (1973). *FEBS Letters*, **33**, 311.

Seligmann, M., Danon, F., Hurez, D. M., Haesco, E., and Preud'homme, J. L. (1968). *Science, N.Y.*, **162**, 1396.

Seligmann, M., and Feizi, T. (1974). *Progress in Immunology II*, Vol. I, (Brent, L., and Holborow, J., eds.), North Holland Publishing Co., Amsterdam, p. 285.

Seligmann, M., Mihaesco, E., and Frangione, B. (1971). *Ann. N.Y. Acad. Sci.*, **190**, 4871.

Shakib, F. (1976). Ph.D. Thesis, University of Birmingham.

Shakib, F., Stanworth, D R., Drew, R., and Catty, D. (1975). *J. Immunol. Methods*, **8**, 17.

Shakib, F., Stanworth, D. R., Hardwicke, J., and White, R. H. R. (1977). *Clin. Exp. Immunol.*, **28**, 506.

Smith, E., Kochwa, S., and Wasserman, L. R. (1965). *Am. J. Med.*, **39**, 35.

Solomon, A., Killander, J., Grey, H. M., and Kunkel, H. G. (1966). *Science, N.Y.*, **151**, 1237.

Soothill, J. F. (1962). *Proc. Roy. Soc. Med.*, **55**, 395.

Spitz, E., Gelfand, E. W., Sheffer, A. L., and Austen, K. F. (1972). *J. Allergy Clin. Immunol.*, **49**, 337.

Stanworth, D. R. (1973*a*). In *Handbook of Experimental Immunology*, (Weir, D. M., ed.) 2nd edn. Blackwell, Oxford, p. 9.1.

Stanworth, D. R. (1973*b*). In *Frontiers of Biology*, Vol. 28, North Holland Publishing Co., Amsterdam.

Stanworth, D. R. (1974). *Haematologia*, **8**, 299.

Stanworth, D. R., Humphrey, J., Bennich, H., and Johansson, S. G. O. (1967). *Lancet*, **ii**, 330.

Stanworth, D. R., Humphrey, J., Bennich, H., and Johansson, S. G. O. (1968). *Lancet*, **ii**, 17.

Stanworth, D. R., Johns, P., Williamson, N., Shadforth, M., Felix-Davies, D. D., and Thompson, R. A. (1977). *Lancet*, **i**, 1001.

Stanworth, D. R., and Stewart, G. A. (1975). In *Maternofoetal Transmission of Immunoglobulins*, (Hemmings, W. A., ed.), Cambridge University Press, Cambridge, p. 7.

Stanworth, D. R., and Turner, M. W. (1973). In *Handbook of Experimental Immunology*, (Weir, D. M., ed.), 2nd edn., Blackwell, Oxford, p. 10.1.

Stefani, D. V. Guser, A. I. and Mokeeva, R. A. (1973. *Immunochemistry*, **10**, 559.

Stone, M. J., and Fedak, J. E. (1974). *J. Immunology*, **113**, 1377.

Stone, M. J., and Metzger, H. (1967). *Cold Spring Harbor Symp. Quant. Biol.*, **32**, 83.

Stone, M. J., and Metzger, H. (1968). *J. Biol. Chem.*, **243**, 5977.

Stoop, J. W., Zegers, B. J. M., van der Heiden, C., and Ballieux, R. E. (1968). *Blood*, **32**, 774.

Taylor, B., Norman, A. P., Orgel, H. A., Stokes, C. R., Turner, M. W., and Soothill, J. F. (1973). *Lancet*, **ii**, 111.

Terry, W. D. (1968). In *Immunologic Deficiency Diseases in Man*, Vol. 4, (Bergsma, D., ed.), The National Foundation, New York, p. 357.

Terry, W. D., Fahey, J. L., and Steinberg, A. G. (1965). *J Exp. Med.*, **122**, 1087.

Van der Giessen, M., Rossouw, E., Algra Van-Veen, T., Van Loghern, E., Segers, B. J. M., and Sander, P. C. (1975). *Clin. Exp. Immunol.*, **21**, 501.

Virella, G., and Hobbs, J. R. (1971). *Clin. Exp. Immunol.*, **9**, 973.

Waldenström, J. (1944). *Acta med. scand.*, **117**, 216.

Waldenström, J. (1961). *Harvey Lecture Series*, **56**, 211.

Waldmann, T. A., and Strober, W. (1969). *Prog. Allergy*, **13**, 1.

Waldmann, R., Durm, M., and Broder, S. (1974). *Lancet*, **ii**, 609.

Waldmann, T. A., Polmar, S. H., Balestra, S. T., Jost, M. C., Bruce, R. M., and Terry, W. D. (1972). *J. Immunol.*, **109**, 304.

Webster, A. D. B., Loewi, G., Dourmashkin, R. D., Golding, D. N., Ward, D. J., and Asherson, G. L. (1976). *Brit. Med. J.*, **i**, 1314.

Young, V. H. (1969). *Proc. Roy. Soc. Med.*, **62**, 778.

Yount, W. J., Hong, R., Seligman, M., Good, R. A., and Kunkel, H. G. (1970). *J. Clin. Invest.*, **49**, 1957.

CHAPTER 7

Affinity of the Antibody—Antigen Reaction and its Biological Significance

M. W. Steward

1 INTRODUCTION

The interaction of antibody and antigen has been studied widely at both the qualitative and quantitative levels. Qualitative analysis of the antibody–antigen reaction in kinetic and thermodynamic terms has provided considerable information as to the nature of this reaction. It is clear from these observations that for an understanding of the antibody–antigen reaction and its functional significance in biology an appreciation of the importance of antibody affinity is essential. Karush (1970) has expressed this view in the following way: 'the measurement of antibody affinity and the recognition of its decisive role in the biological activities of the antibody molecule have brought a new dimension to our understanding and exploration of the immune response'. In this discussion of the antibody–antigen reaction, particular emphasis will be given to a consideration of antibody affinity and its biological significance.

2 FORCES INVOLVED IN THE ANTIBODY–ANTIGEN REACTION

The interaction of antibody and antigen at equilibrium may be expressed in the following way

$$Ab + Ag \underset{k_d}{\overset{k_a}{\rightleftharpoons}} Ab\text{–}Ag \tag{1}$$

where Ab represents free antibody; Ag, free antigen; Ab–Ag, the antibody–antigen complex; k_a and k_d, the association and dissociation constants, respectively.

Applying the law of mass action to this interaction,

$$k_a[Ab][Ag] = k_d[Ab\text{–}Ag] \tag{2}$$

thus the equilibrium constant or affinity (K) may be calculated

$$\frac{k_a}{k_d} = K = \frac{[Ab\text{–}Ag]}{[Ab][Ag]}$$

The intermolecular forces which contribute to the stabilization of the complex are the same as those involved in the stabilization of the specific configuration of proteins and other macromolecules. Antibody affinity may be considered therefore as the summation of attractive and repulsive non-covalent intermolecular forces resulting from the interaction of the antibody binding site and the homologous antigenic determinant.

2.1 Hydrogen Bonding

Hydrogen bonds result from the interaction of an hydrogen atom covalently linked to an electronegative atom with the unshared electron pair of a second electronegative atom. The hydrogen donor and acceptor atoms are usually strongly electronegative, and in antibody–antigen reactions, amino and hydroxyl groups are involved predominantly. The contribution of this type of bond for the stabilization of the antibody–antigen complex is small, particularly in view of the competitive effect of an aqueous polar solvent environment.

2.2 Apolar or Hydrophobic Bonding

The interaction of apolar or hydrophobic molecules with an aqueous environment is of particular importance in antibody–antigen reactions. Apolar or hydrophobic bonding occurs as a result of the preference of such groups for self-association so that their extent of contact with water decreases. In this way, a lower energy state is achieved with a concomitant increase in entropy, resulting in a net attractive force. Hydrophobic bonding is an entropy driven, endothermic process, and the strength of such interactions increases with temperature.

2.3 Ionic or Coulombic Interaction

This attractive force is the result of the interaction of oppositely charged ionic groups such as an ionized amino group (NH_3^+) and an ionized carboxyl group (COO^-). While it is clear that an inverse relationship exists between the charge on an immunogen and the charge on the antibody it induces, these coulombic interactions do not appear to play a prominent role in the stabilization of the antibody–antigen complex.

2.4 Van der Waals Interactions

These forces result from the interaction of the electron clouds of polar groups. This interaction involves the induction of oscillating dipoles in the two molecules concerned and results in an attractive force. The greater the complementarity of the electron clouds of the two groups concerned, the closer will be the association of the two molecules, resulting in an increased attractive force.

2.5 Steric Repulsive Forces

The attractive forces discussed so far all increase as the distance between the interacting groups decreases. The coulombic forces are inversely proportional to the square of this distance and Van der Waals forces are inversely proportional to the sixth power of this distance. Steric repulsion, on the other hand, is more sensitive to distance and varies inversely with the twelfth power of the distance between the interacting groups. The repulsive force between non-bonded atoms arises from the interpenetration of their respective electron clouds and therefore the closer the complementarity of the electron cloud shapes, the lower will be the repulsive force. In the antibody–antigen reaction this force therefore governs the degree to which an antigenic determinant can fit into the binding site of the antibody. A non-homologous antigenic determinant will not have an electron cloud which is complementary to that of the various groups defining the antibody binding site and thus the repulsive force will be high and the attractive forces will be minimized. In this way, the antibody will exhibit a low affinity for the particular antigenic determinant. Conversely, where the electron clouds of the antigenic determinant and antibody combining site are complementary, steric repulsion will be minimized and the attractive forces maximized resulting in a high affinity antibody–antigen interaction. Steric repulsive forces may be viewed, therefore, as providing the basis for antibody specificity in its selective interaction with a specific antigenic determinant.

3 THERMODYNAMIC ASPECTS OF THE ANTIBODY–ANTIGEN REACTION

The law of mass action plays a central role in the derivation of equations for thermodynamic affinity measurement. This subject has been reviewed recently in detail by Day (1972), thus only a brief discussion will be included here.

For thermodynamic measurement of antibody affinity, it is necessary for the reactants, both antibody and antigen, to be pure and in solution. In addition, the reactants should be homogeneous with regard to antigenic determinants and antibody binding sites for ideal affinity measurement. In practice, however, such ideal situations do not exist; antibodies are notoriously heterogeneous, particularly with regard to their structure, and also exhibit multivalence for antigen. However, in spite of these limitations, reasonably precise affinity measurements can be made using purified antibodies to defined monovalent haptens. The experimental determination of antibody-bound hapten and free hapten at equilibrium over a range of free hapten concentrations, followed by the analysis of the data by the equation presented below form the basis of affinity measurements.

From the application of the law of mass action to the antibody–antigen reaction (Equation (2)) a form of the Langmuir Adsorption isotherm may be derived

$$\frac{[\text{Ab–Ag}]}{[\text{Ab}]} = r = \frac{nK[\text{Ag}]}{1 + K[\text{Ag}]} \tag{3}$$

where r is the moles of antigen (hapten) bound per mole of antibody; [Ab–Ag], bound antibody concentration; [Ab], free antibody concentration; [Ag], free hapten concentration; n, antibody valence; and K, equilibrium constant or affinity.

From Equation (3)

$$\frac{r}{[\text{Ag}]} = nK - rK \tag{4}$$

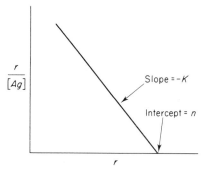

Figure 1 Scatchard plot of ideal antibody–antigen binding

Therefore a plot of $r/[\text{Ag}]$ *versus* r over a range of free hapten concentrations (Scatchard, 1949) allows values of antibody affinity (K) and antibody valence to be derived (see Figure 1). For divalent anti-hapten antibody (where $n = 2$) Equation (4) can be used to calculate the average intrinsic association constant K_0 of the antibody for the hapten. When half the antibody binding sites are bound ($r = 1$), then

$$\frac{r}{[\text{Ag}]} = nK - rK$$

becomes

$$\frac{1}{[Ag]} = 2K - K = K_0$$

Therefore K_0 is equal to the reciprocal of the free hapten concentration at equilibrium when half the antibody sites are hapten-bound.

Antibody affinity also may be calculated by the Langmuir plot (Figure 2) using the following equation derived from Equations (3) or (4):

$$\frac{1}{r} = \frac{1}{n} \cdot \frac{1}{[Ag]} \cdot \frac{1}{K} + \frac{1}{n} \tag{5}$$

For ideal antibody–antigen binding both Scatchard and Langmuir equations should give rise to linear plots. However, even when using isolated and purified anti-hapten antibody, their plots deviate from linearity. The reason for this deviation has been ascribed to the existence of heterogeneity of antibody affinities within an antibody population. The existence of such heterogeneity has been known for many years, Pauling *et al.* (1944), Karush (1956) and Heidelberger and Kendall (1935), have shown that the distribution of affinities in an antibody population can be described in terms of a Gaussian error function. Similarly, Nisonoff and Pressman (1958) have shown that affinity distribution can be described by the closely related Sipsian distribution function (Sips, 1948)

$$\frac{r}{n} = \frac{[K_0\text{Ag}]^a}{1 + [K_0\text{Ag}]^a}$$

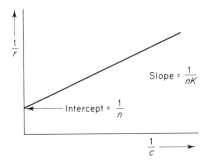

Figure 2 Langmuir plot of ideal antibody–antigen binding

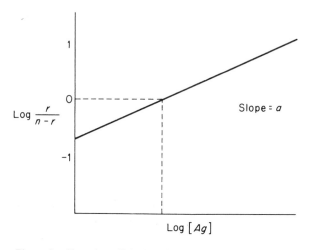

Figure 3 Sips plot of ideal antibody–antigen binding. The graphical determination of average intrinsic association constant (K_0) and heterogeneity index (a)

Karush (1962), utilizing the logarithmic transformation of the Sips' equation

$$\log \frac{r}{n - r} = a \log K_0 + a \log [\text{Ag}]$$

has demonstrated that a plot of $\log r/(n - r)$ *versus* $\log$ Ag yields a straight line where the index of heterogeneity (a) is given by the slope (Figure 3). As the heterogeneity index approaches 1·0 the antibody population approaches homogeneity with regard to association constants. Furthermore, K_0, the average intrinsic association constant, is given by $1/[\text{Ag}]$ where $\log r/(n - r) = 0$ and is thus the peak of the presumed normal distribution (Figure 3). While this type of analysis of antibody–hapten binding data represents a convenient approximation of the true situation, Pressman *et al.* (1970) have challenged the assumption that there is a continuous heterogenous population of antibodies with affinities following a Gaussian distribution. They have suggested the existence of limited heterogeneity, in which the majority of the antibody population is composed of a limited number of types of antibody with different affinities. Medof and Aladjem (1971) also have reported that the distribution of affinities could not be approximated to a Gaussian or Sipsian distribution. Werblin and Siskind (1972) demonstrated that DNP–anti-DNP binding data plotted according to the Sips' equation are not linear, suggesting that the distribution of affinities is actually asymmetric. These authors confirmed the existence of an asymmetrical distribution of affinities by the use of iterative computational techniques to generate approximate affinity distributions from the experimental binding data. In this way, it was shown that only in rabbit anti-DNP serum obtained seven days after immunization with DNP–BGG in Freund's complete adjuvant was the distribution of affinities approximately symmetrical. In serum obtained at intervals for up to one year after immunization, the distribution of affinities became progressively more asymmetrical.

The non-linearity of Sipsian binding curves and the asymmetrical distribution of affinities therefore challenges the assumption that K_0 (average intrinsic affinity) precisely describes the affinity characteristics of a given antibody population. The non-linearity of binding curves clearly means that the slope will differ at various parts of the curve. Accordingly, values of K_0 and a, calculated with the assumption of linearity, will differ depending on the portion of the binding curve used. The conclusion to be drawn from these studies is that while average affinity values calculated by the assumption of a Gaussian or Sipsian distribution of affinities are relatively easy to obtain, and are satisfactory for many purposes, the handling of binding data by more complex methods, such as described by Werblin and Siskind (1972), is required for a more precise description of the distribution of affinity. More recently, Mukkur et al. (1974) have described a simpler, graphical method for determining the *total* affinity constant, K_t which represents the sum of the weighted affinities of the antibody subpopulations in an antibody preparation. K_t values obtained graphically are in close agreement to those determined by computer calculation.

It will be clear from the preceding discussion that measurement of K_0 requires a precise knowledge of the total amount of antibody present in the system. This poses several difficulties, particularly since there is no completely suitable method for determining the amount of antibody. The traditional method of precipitin analysis has the obvious limitation that non-precipitating antibody will not be detected. Furthermore, there is evidence that antibodies of differing affinities have different precipitating characteristics (Morgan et al., unpublished observations). Antibody purification procedures involving adsorption onto and elution from antigen immunoadsorbents provide 'pure' antibody preparations, but the possibility of selection for antibodies of a particular affinity cannot be ruled out. Thus, for many purposes, this type of procedure is not suitable. In situations where isolation and purification of antibody is not possible or is not desirable, the calculation of affinity can be made with respect to total antibody binding sites (Ab_t) rather than to antibody concentration and valence (Nisonoff and Pressman, 1958). Equation (5) is thus rewritten as

$$\frac{1}{b} = \frac{1}{Ab_t} \cdot \frac{1}{[Ag]} \cdot \frac{1}{K} + \frac{1}{Ab_t}$$

where b is bound antigen and Ab_t the total antibody binding sites. Therefore, in this procedure, the antibody binding site concentration is determined by saturation of the total sites by high concentrations of free antigen. Thus, in a plot $1/b$ *versus* $1/[Ag]$, when $1/[Ag] = 0$, then $1/b = 1/Ab_t$. The value for Ab_t is obtained graphically by extrapolation of the binding curve to infinite free antigen concentration. This method also is not without its serious limitations. Firstly, saturation of low-affinity antibody binding sites requires high concentrations of antigen. In addition, graphical extrapolation to infinite free antigen concentration is a particularly uncertain procedure when heterogeneous antibody populations are being studied. Relatively small errrors in the estimation of Ab_t can give rise to considerable errors in the subsequent calculation of an affinity value. Therefore, the measurement of antibody binding sites is an operationally defined concept and at best gives an arbitrary definition of the amount of antibody. It still remains as an important limitation to a fuller understanding of the thermodynamics of the antibody–antigen reaction.

Alternative approaches to the measurement of the affinity of antibody populations, which do not involve direct estimation of antibody level, have been proposed. Celada *et al.* (1969) described an empirical relationship between antibody dilution and antigen concentration which provides an estimate of an index of avidity* of the antiserum

$$\log \mu l \text{ antiserum} = m + s \log \mu g \text{ Ag}$$

where μl antiserum is the volume of antiserum required to bind 50 per cent of the antigen added, Ag; s is the slope and represents the index of avidity; and m is the intercept on the ordinate when $\log \mu g$ Ag $= 0$. The slope (s) of the plot of log volume of antiserum required to bind half the added antigen *versus* log amount of antigen added varies between 0 and 1, and has been shown to correlate with affinity values determined by other methods (Schirrmacher, 1972; Steward and Petty, 1972*a*; Ahlstedt *et al.*, 1973). Taylor (1975), in a detailed mathematical appraisal of this method, has suggested that while for biological reasons, s is generally correlated with affinity K_0, it is not mathematically dependent upon K_0 but depends on the distribution of antibody subpopulations of different affinity within the antiserum.

Recently, Paul and Elfenbein (1975) have reported a technique for the determination of affinity which is independent of a measurement of total antibody, based on the antigen capacity method of Farr (1958). The following expression was derived

$$K = \frac{R(B/F)_x \cdot B_i - (B/F)_i \cdot B_x}{(1 - R)B_i \cdot B_x}$$

in which $R = ABC_x/ABC_i$ where ABC_i and ABC_x refer to the antigen binding capacity (concentration of antigen bound × serum dilution) with the index concentration i of antigen and a lower concentration of antigen x, respectively. B_i and B_x refer to bound antigen at the two antigen concentrations. These authors demonstrated that for myeloma anti-DNP antibody, this method yields unambiguous values for K_t which compare well with those determined by equilibrium dialysis. They pointed out that for heterogeneous antibody populations, the estimated value for K varies according to the value of R—that is K

---

* In the literature, *affinity* and *avidity* commonly are used synonymously. However, it is now accepted generally that the term *affinity* is a thermodynamic expression of the primary binding energy of an antibody binding site for an antigenic determinant. Experimentally, this term has its most precise application in monovalent hapten–anti-hapten systems. *Avidity*, on the other hand, although it is dependent on affinity, also involves other contributing factors such as antibody valence, antigenic valence, and factors associated with binding, but not concerned directly with the primary antibody–antigen interaction.

increases as the fraction of antibody binding sites bound falls. These observations are consistent with those of Werblin and Siskind (1972) using anti-hapten antibody and of Steward and Petty (1972a) using anti-protein antibody, illustrating that because of antibody heterogeneity, affinity values obtained depend upon the region of the binding curve employed for calculation. Thus, although this procedure overcomes the problem of antibody site determination, the problem of heterogeneity of antibody affinities remains and the value of K obtained is not an average intrinsic association constant.

Antibody heterogeneity and the adequate measurement of the level of the antibody are two problems which have put considerable constraint on the understanding of the thermodynamics of the antibody–antigen reaction. Nevertheless, using the methods described above, workers in several laboratories have been able to make significant contributions to the available knowledge of this aspect of the immune response.

4 KINETIC ASPECTS OF THE ANTIBODY–ANTIGEN REACTION

It has been known for many years that antibody–antigen reactions occur rapidly (Hooker and Boyd, 1935), and it is this speed of reaction which has made kinetic studies difficult when traditional kinetic methods are employed. Utilizing concentrations of reactants necessary for efficient measurement, the time of mixing is the rate-limiting step and equilibration occurs before any changes in concentration can be determined as a function of time. Furthermore, kinetic data obtained with complex antigens proved to be difficult to interpret (Goldberg and Campbell, 1951). However, the application of more sophisticated techniques and instrumentation to the study not of a complex antigen–antibody system but rather of the simple hapten–anti-hapten reaction

$$Ab + H \underset{k_{2,1}}{\overset{k_{1,2}}{\rightleftharpoons}} Ab\text{–}H$$

has broadened our knowledge of the kinetics of this reaction. The use of techniques for the study of fast reactions such as the temperature-jump relaxation method (Eigen and DeMaeyer, 1963) and the stopped-flow technique (Chance, 1963), in combination with sensitive spectrophotometric methods for the measurement of hapten binding has provided an opportunity to make meaningful kinetic measurements of the antibody–antigen reaction.

A concise account of the principle and application of both the stopped-flow and the temperature-jump relaxation techniques has been given recently by Froese and Sehon (1971, 1975). In brief, the stopped-flow technique consists of forcing the reactants at high volocity into a reaction chamber and monitoring spectrophotometric changes with time using an oscilloscope. In this way, data for the calculation of the association rate constant $k_{1,2}$ are obtained. In the temperature-jump technique, the antigen–antibody system under study is allowed to reach equilibrium. The equilibrium is then disturbed by a sudden change in temperature of five to 10°C achieved by the discharge of a high-voltage

Table 1 Hapten–antihapten rate constants

Antibody	Hapten	$k_{1,2}$ $(M^{-1} sec^{-1})$	$k_{2,1}$ (sec^{-1})	K_0† (M^{-1})	Reference
Rabbit anti-DNP	DNP–lysine (i)	8.4×10^7	11‡	7.7×10^7	Day et al. (1963)
Mouse anti-DNP*	DNP–lysine (ii)	1.1×10^7	0.5‡	2.2×10^7	Kelly et al. (1971)
Rabbit anti-DNP	DNP–lysine (iii)	1.3×10^8	53	2.0×10^6	Pecht et al. (1972a)
"	DNP–glycine	1.9×10^8	1300	—	Pecht et al. (1972b)
"	DNP–aminocaproate	9.7×10^7	1.1‡	9.1×10^7	Day et al. (1963)
"	DNP–aminocaproate	8.0×10^7	8.7		Barisas et al. (1975)
"	TNP–aminocaproate	4.0×10^7	27.0		Barisas et al. (1975)
"	1N-3,6S-2–DNP	8.0×10^7	1.4‡	5.9×10^7	Day et al. (1963)
"	1N-2,5S-4–DNP*	9.5×10^6	76	1.5×10^5	Kelly et al. (1971)
"	1N-2,5S-4–DNP†	1.6×10^7	80	1.5×10^5	Froese (1968)
"	1N-2,5S-4–pNP	1.4×10^7	410	1.0×10^4	Froese (1968)
Rabbit anti-TNP	TNP–aminocaproate	9.0×10^7	1.6		Barisas et al. (1975)
"	DNP–aminocaproate	7.5×10^7	6.7		Barisas et al. (1975)
Rabbit anti-p-nitrophenyl	DHNDS–NP	1.8×10^8	760	5.8×10^5	Froese and Sehon (1965)
Rabbit anti-p-azobenzenearsonate	N–R′	2.0×10^7	50		Froese et al. (1962)
	DMP–R′	1.1×10^7	1.4×10^{-3}		Ferber (1965)
Bovine anti-ADHB†	ADHB	6.2×10^8	6000		Haustein (1971)
Rabbit anti-fluorescein	Fluorescein	4.0×10^8	5.0×10^{-3}	6.5×10^{10}	Levison (1971)
Sheep anti-digoxin	Digoxin	1.7×10^7	3.4×10^{-4}	1.9×10^{10}	Smith and Skubitz (1975)
Rabbit anti-ouabain	Ouabain	1.3×10^7	6.4×10^{-3}	3.5×10^9	Smith and Skubitz (1975)
"	"	8.0×10^6	1.5×10^{-3}	3.5×10^9	Skubitz and Smith (1975)

DNP, 2,4-dinitrophenyl: TNP, 2,4,6-trinitrophenyl: 1N-3,6S-2–DNP, 1-hydroxy-2-(2,4-dinitrophenylazo)-3,6 naphthalene disulphonate: 1N-2,5S-4–DNP, 1-hydroxy-4-(2,4-dinitrophenylazo)-2,5-naphthalene disulphonate; 1N-2,5S-4–pNP, 1-hydroxy-4-(p-nitrophenylazo)-2,5-naphthalene disulphonate; DHNDS–NP, 4,5-dihydroxy-3-(p-nitrophenylazo)-2,7-naphthalene disulphonate; N–R′, 1-naphthol-4-[4-(4′-azobenzeneazo) phenylarsonate]; DMP–R′, p-dimethyl-aminophenylazo)-benzenearsonate; ADHB, 4-(3-aminophenyl)-2,6-diphenyl-pyridinium-N-(4-hydroxyphenyl)-betaine

* Mouse myeloma (MOPC 315) IgA protein with anti-DNP activity

† Determined by equilibrium measurement

‡ Calculated from $k_{2,1} = k_{1,2}/K_0$

Data, in part, from Froese and Sehon (1975), with permission

condenser. The re-equilibration of the system is followed as a function of time using an oscilloscope. From the trace, the relaxation time τ may be determined. The relationship between relaxation time and the rate constants of the new equilibrium is given by the expression

$$\frac{1}{\tau} = k_{2,1} + k_{1,2} \left[(Ab) + (H) \right]$$

where (Ab) and (H) are the equilibrium concentrations of antibody sites and hapten, respectively. The slope and intercept of a plot of $1/\tau$ *versus* $[(Ab) + (H)]$ give the values for $k_{1,2}$ and $k_{2,1}$, respectively. Recently, Skubitz and Smith (1975) have described a simplified technique for the determination of $k_{1,2}$ and $k_{2,1}$, using dextran-coated charcoal to determine antibody-bound and free hapten. The specific activity of the hapten is sufficiently high to allow the use of concentrations of reactants (10^{-10}–10^{-9} M) well below those at which mixing is the rate-limiting step. The data are analysed by first-order and pseudo-second-order treatments.

The work of several authors using the stopped-flow and temperature-jump techniques has shown that the value for $k_{1,2}$ is approximately the same for all antibody–hapten systems tested; all the values obtained are within one order of magnitude of 10^8 M^{-1} sec^{-1}. On the other hand, a great variation in the dissociation rate constants k_{21} has been observed (Table 1). Froese (1968) demonstrated that a 10-fold difference in the average association constant k_0 of anti-DNP antibody for two cross-reacting haptens is due to differences in $k_{2,1}$ rather than to $k_{1,2}$ (Table 2) and suggested that the stability of the antibody–hapten complex was governed by the dissociation rate constant. These results plus those of others (Haselkorn *et al.*, 1971; Pecht *et al.*, 1972a, b; Barisas *et al.*, 1975; Skubitz and Smith, 1975; Smith and Skubitz, 1975) have confirmed that it is $k_{2,1}$ that determines the affinity of antibody for hapten.

Table 2 Kinetic and equilibrium measurements of anti-DNP antibody reacting with two cross-reacting haptens

Hapten	$k_{1,2}$(M^{-1} sec^{-1})	$k_{2,1}$(sec^{-1})	$K = k_{1,2}/k_{2,1}$ (M^{-1})	K_0(M^{-1})‡
1N–2,5S–4–DNP*	1.6×10^7	80	2.0×10^5	1.5×10^5
1N–2,5S–4–pNP†	1.4×10^7	410	3.4×10^4	1×10^4

* hydroxy-4-(2,4-dinitrophenylazo)-2,5-naphthalene disulphonate
† 1-hydroxy-4-(p-nitrophenylazo)-2-5-naphthalene disulphonate
‡ From equilibrium data
Data from Froese (1968). Reproduced by permission of Pergamon Press and the author

5 EXPERIMENTAL PROCEDURES FOR DETERMINING ANTIBODY AFFINITY

Several techniques are currently available for estimating the affinity and avidity of antibodies. Thermodynamic estimations of affinity essentially involve

Table 3 Methods for the measurement of the affinity and kinetics of the antibody–antigen reaction

Method	Principal applicable antigens	Parameter measured	Reference
Equilibrium dialysis	Haptens, dialysable antigens	Affinity	Eisen (1964)
Fluorescence quenching	Haptens and antigens with specific fluorescence properties	Affinity	Velick et al. (1960)
Fluorescence enhancement			Parker et al. (1967)
Fluorescence polarization	Haptens, proteins	Affinity / Avidity	Dandliker et al. (1964)
Ammonium sulphate globulin precipitation	Haptens, antigens soluble in 50 per cent saturated ammonium sulphate	Affinity / Avidity	Stupp et al. (1969); Steward and Petty (1972b); Gaze et al. (1973)
Dextra-coated charcoal	Protein antigens	Avidity index	Celada et al. (1969)
Antiglobulin precipitation	Haptens	Affinity	Herbert et al. (1965)
	Haptens, proteins, carbohydrates	Affinity / Avidity	Steward and Petty (1972b)
Equilibrium molecular sieving	Haptens, proteins, carbohydrates	Affinity / Avidity	Stone and Metzger (1968)
Ultracentrifugation	Proteins	Avidity	Normansell (1970)
Phage neutralization	Haptens	Avidity	Mäkelä (1966)
Equilibrium filtration	Viruses	Avidity	Fazekas de St. Groth (1961)
Haemolysin transfer	Erythrocytes	Relative avidity	Taliaferro et al. (1959)
Plaque-forming cell avidity	Haptens, proteins	Avidity	Andersson (1970)
Association and dissociation rate measurement			
Ammonium sulphate	Antigens soluble in 50 per cent saturated ammonium sulphate	$k_{1,2}$ / $k_{2,1}$	Talmage (1960)
Dextran-coated charcoal	Haptens with high specific radioactivity	$k_{1,2}$ / $k_{2,1}$	Skubitz and Smith (1975)
Stopped-flow technique	Haptens	$k_{1,2}$	Chance (1963)
Temperature-jump relaxation technique	Haptens	$k_{1,2}$ / $k_{2,1}$	Eigen and De Meyer (1963)

the determination of the concentration of free and bound antigen under equilibrium conditions using techniques that do not disturb the equilibrium. In general, the separation of antibody-bound and free antigen is achieved either by dialysis, selective precipitation, or gel filtration, or by utilizing changes in the properties of the antigen or antibody, such as fluorescence, occurring as a result of binding. The kinetic approaches to the measurement of affinity have been described above. Other techniques applicable to avidity measurement at the antibody-forming cell level and to highly complex antigens such as erythrocytes also have been described. The various techniques are listed in Table 3, together with pertinent references.

6 THE BIOLOGICAL SIGNIFICANCE OF ANTIBODY AFFINITY

6.1 The Role of Antibody Polyvalence

The average intrinsic association constant, K_0, for the interaction of an antibody binding site with a monovalent antigen (intrinsic affinity) is clearly of both conceptual and experimental importance. However, in view of the polyvalence of antibody molecules, it is obvious that in biological terms it is unlikely that intrinsic affinity adequately describes the interaction of antibody and polyvalent antigen.

The term 'functional affinity' has been used to describe the energy of interaction of the antibody combining sites with the antigenic determinants on a polyvalent antigen—(avidity, see p. 240). Since naturally occurring antigens such as viruses and bacteria have repeating antigenic structures on their surfaces, it is clear that in immune responses to infection in vivo it is the functional rather than intrinsic infinity of the antibody which is important. Several years ago, Burnet et al. (1937) speculated that bivalent attachment of antibody to a viral particle would be energetically more advantageous than monovalent binding. Recent theoretical considerations (Crothers and Metzger, 1972) and experimental observations (reviewed by Hornick and Karush, 1972) have confirmed the validity of this early prediction concerning the advantage of multivalence in energetic terms, to the immune system.

The study of viral neutralization has provided much information relevant to the role of antibody multivalence in biological systems and there are several reports which show the reduction in neutralization of both animal viruses (Lafferty, 1963; Vogt et al., 1964; Keller, 1966) and bacteriophages (Goodman and Donch, 1964; Klinman et al., 1967; Stemke, 1969) when univalent antibodies have been used. However, a significant advance in this type of study was provided by the observation by Mäkelä (1966) that hapten-conjugated bacteriophage can be neutralized by anti-hapten antibody. Using 3-iodo-4-hydroxy-5-nitrophenyl acetyl (NIP)-conjugated T2 bacteriophage, Sarvas and Mäkelä (1970) obtained evidence for the superiority of IgM over IgG anti-NIP antibodies in neutralizing the phage and ascribed this superiority to the polyvalence of IgM. Hornick and Karush (1972) in a study of the neutralization of DNP-conjugated bacteriophage

ϕx174 by anti-DNP antibody have provided convincing evidence for the energetic advantage of polyvalent over monovalent antibody interaction with this polyvalent antigen. In these studies, IgG anti-DNP antibodies wish intrinsic affinity for the DNP group of 10^7 M^{-1} showed a functional affinity for DNP–ϕx174 of 10^{10} M^{-1}, which represents an enhancement due to divalent attachment of 1000-fold. In addition, degradation of IgG antibody to monovalent fragments resulted in a 100-fold reduction in functional affinity with no reduction in intrinsic affinity. On the other hand, IgM anti-DNP antibodies with an intrinsic affinity of 10^4–10^5 M^{-1} exhibited a functional affinity of 10^{11} M^{-1} which represents an enhancement due to multivalency of 10^6-fold. These authors suggest that this represents multivalent attachment of IgM–DNP to the conjugated phage *via* at least three of its binding sites.

Multivalent antibody binding has clear functional and biological advantages over monovalent binding. The most obvious advantage is the far lower concentration of multivalent antibody required for effective humoral immunity compared with the level of monovalent antibody which would be required for a similar degree of immunity.

Multivalence is of considerable importance in the binding of antigen by receptors on antigen-sensitive cells. Davie and Paul (1972a), and Bystryn *et al.* (1973) have demonstrated the enhanced binding of multivalent compared to monovalent ligands to cell-surface bound antibody. The latter authors showed that a multivalent DNP–conjugate bound to cells with an avidity which was 100–300-fold greater than that with a univalent DNP hapten. The high functional affinity of receptors on cells for multivalent antigens may render these interactions essentially irreversible, and viewed in the light of recent suggestions (Ramseier, 1971) that prolonged contact of antigen with antigen-sensitive cells is necessary for stimulation, points to an important role of polyvalent attachment in the initiation of the immune response. Evidence is available supporting a major assumption in the clonal selection theory (Burnet, 1959) that the affinity of cell receptors for antigen is the same as that of antibodies produced by progeny plasma cells (Siskind and Benacerraf, 1969; Mäkelä, 1970; Julius and Herzenberg, 1974). Cells with receptors of low intrinsic affinity for single antigenic determinants may, by virtue of polyvalent binding, bind antigen sufficiently well to be stimulated. Thus, the progeny of cells with receptors of high functional affinity—IgM—may produce low intrinsic affinity antibody. Polyvalent binding of antigen by cell-bound receptors may therefore be important in the production of low-affinity antibody and may explain why IgM antibodies often have lower K_0 values for hapten than IgG antibodies present in the serum at the same time (Mäkelä *et al.*, 1970).

In any discussion of the role of polyvalence in antibody affinity, the controversy concerning the valence of IgM must be considered (reviewed by Metzger, 1970). On the basis of its pentameric structure, it would be expected that IgM would exhibit decavalence for antigen. However, there are reports that IgM is pentavalent (Onoue *et al.*, 1965; Voss and Eisen, 1968), while there are others that the molecule is indeed decavalent (Cooper, 1967; Merler *et al.*, 1968;

Ashman and Metzger, 1969). Further controversy has been generated by the suggestion (Onoue *et al.*, 1968; Oriol and Rousset, 1974*a*, *b*) that there are five high and five low affinity antibody binding sites on a single molecule. However, Ashman and Metzger (1969) have suggested that an alternative explanation of the data of Onoue *et al.*, (1968) was the existence of heterogeneity among different molecules in the IgM population. It is clear that the valence of IgM is very much influenced by the size of the antigen used. Thus the observed valence of IgM anti-dextran antibody varied from 10 for dextran of molecular weight 342 to five for dextrans of molecular weights 7000–237 000; while with dextran of molecular weight of $1·87 \times 10^6$ the observed IgM antibody valence was 2·3 (Edberg *et al.*, 1972). Steric factors presumably play a role in the observations of reduced IgM valencies for certain antigens but cannot be invoked to explain reduced valencies for haptenic antigens.

6.2 Temporal Changes in Antibody Affinity

Progressive changes in the affinity or avidity of antibody with increasing time after immunization with a variety of antigens (toxins, viruses, or purified proteins) have been acknowledged for several years. Studies of the temporal changes in the affinity of antibodies to defined haptenic determinants (such as DNP) have confirmed the progressive increase in K_0 with time (Eisen and Siskind, 1964) and this phenomenon has been termed the 'maturation of the immune response' (Siskind and Benacerraf, 1969). That affinity maturation is the result of changes in the cell population producing antibody rather than the selective removal of high affinity antibody by the excess antigen present early in the response was demonstrated *in vitro* (Steiner and Eisen, 1967). The affinity of antibody produced *in vitro* by lymphoid cells taken from immunized rabbits early in the immune response is lower than that produced by cells taken late in the response.

Siskind and Benacerraf (1969) have expanded the clonal selection theory of Burnet (1959) to accommodate these observed variations in antibody affinity by suggesting that precursors of antibody-forming cells bind antigens *via* receptors having the same specificity and affinity as the antibody secreted by progeny cells. Thus, the maturation of the immune response is viewed as a progressive, antigen-driven preferential selection and stimulation of cells with the highest affinity receptors. Immunization with large doses of antigen in Freund's complete adjuvant results in a reduction in the rate of maturation of affinity compared to immunization with small doses (Eisen and Siskind, 1964), and this effect on affinity is consistent with this hypothesis and has been ascribed to the stimulation of even low affinity cells in the presence of excess antigen. Furthermore, under such situations it is possible that the high affinity cells may be rendered tolerant. Further evidence consistent with this hypothesis has been obtained at the serum level indicating progressive changes in the affinity distribution of antibody (Werblin and Siskind, 1972; Werblin *et al.*, 1973). If cells with high affinity receptors are indeed being selected preferentially by antigen, then during an

248

immune response these cells should be the most rapidly proliferating ones. Thus the use of cytotoxic drugs such as cyclophosphamide, which inhibit rapidly dividing cells, should preferentially inhibit high affinity antibody-producing cells, and antibody of low affinity would be produced. This indeed has been shown to be the case in groups of mice immunized with human serum albumin (HSA) in Freund's Complete Adjuvant and treated with increasing amounts of cyclophosphamide. In this case both levels and affinity of anti-HSA are reduced in treated compared to control mice. The levels and affinity of antibody decrease with increasing doses of cyclophosphamide (Steward *et al.*, 1973a).

The cell selection by antigen hypothesis also requires that the specificity and affinity of antigen receptors be correlated directly with the affinity and specificity of the antibody produced by progeny antibody-producing cells. Evidence consistent with this hypothesis has been obtained from recent studies in several laboratories (Andersson, 1970, 1972; Davie and Paul, 1972a, b, 1973; Claflin *et al.*, 1973; Claflin and Merchant, 1973; Julius and Herzenberg, 1974) in which

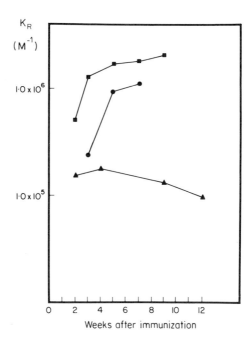

Figure 4 The effect of immunization of mice with human serum transferrin in Freund's complete adjuvant or with *Bordetella pertussis* on the increase in K_R with time compared to mice immunized with antigen in saline. ■, Freund's complete adjuvant; ●, *Bordetella pertussis*; ▲, saline. From Petty and Steward (1977a), reproduced by permission of Blackwell Scientific Publications Ltd

both the affinity of serum antibody and the avidity of antigen receptors on antigen-binding cells have been correlated with the avidity of antibody secreted at the plaque-forming cell level. There is clearly abundant evidence consistent with the concept of cell selection by antigen, resulting in a progressive increase in the affinity of serum antibody. However, observations of temporal changes in affinity, which cannot be interpreted readily on the basis of this concept, have been made. For example, Petty et al. (1972), Kimball (1972), and Urbain et al. (1972) have reported a fall in antibody affinity late in the immune response following the expected early rise.

The results of Petty et al. (1972) and Urbain et al. (1972) were obtained using mice and rabbits, respectively, which had been immunized with antigen in saline. The observations showing maturation of affinity with time and upon which the cell selection by antigen theory was based were obtained only following immunization in Freund's complete adjuvant. Mice showing a fall in affinity late in the immune response to antigen when injected in saline produce a long-lasting high-affinity response to the same antigen injected in Freund's complete and other adjuvants (Soothill and Steward, 1971; Petty and Steward, 1977a) (Figure 4). It is clear that the pattern of temporal changes in the affinity of serum antibody is affected markedly by the nature of the immunogenic stimulus. The antigen-depot effect produced by immunization in Freund's complete adjuvant with the resulting slow release of antigen over long periods results in sustained maturation of affinity. Immunization in saline results in the relatively rapid elimination of the antigen and subsequent termination of antigen stimulation. The fall in average affinity of serum antibody in this situation may be attributed to the death of short-lived high affinity antibody-producing cells. It is interesting to note that maturation of antibody affinity occurs with both Freund's complete adjuvant and *Bordetella pertussis* (see Figure 4). This observation suggests that affinity maturation is not restricted necessarily to adjuvants producing an antigen depot.

Other adjuvants, such as Freund's incomplete adjuvant, lipopolysaccharide B, BCG, alum precipitates, oestradiol, carbon, and latex also are able to enhance both level and affinity of anti-protein antibody. However, all these adjuvants vary in the degree to which they augment the parameters of the immune response. Some—Freund's complete and incomplete adjuvants, and carbon—induce the production of high levels of high affinity antibody, whereas the others elicit lower levels of high affinity antibody. The possibility therefore exists that adjuvants exert their influence on the antibody response at two stages: (i) at the level of antigen selection of cells for proliferation; and (ii) at the level of proliferation of antibody-forming cells (Petty and Steward, 1977a).

The observations of Kimball (1972) showing maturation and late fall in the affinity of antibody to type III pneumococcal antigen—which is not eliminated readily by mammals—indicate that competition for decreasing amounts of circulating antigen is not the only selective force for affinity maturation. Siskind et al. (1968) and Heller and Siskind (1973) have shown that passively administered antibody suppresses low affinity antibody-forming cells more readily than the high affinity cells, and results in an increase in the affinity of the antibody synthesized. It is, therefore, possible that the increase in affinity of anti-type III antibody is a consequence of the competition of antigen-sensitive cells and circulating antibody for antigen.

Other time-related variations in antibody affinity also have been reported in which there is an alteration of high and low affinity antibody during the immune response *in vivo* (Doria *et al.*, 1972; Kim and Karush, 1973) and *in vitro* (Macario and Conway de Macario, 1973). Furthermore, antibody responses have been described in which there is no demonstrable maturation of affinity during the immune response (Haber and Stone, 1969).

In view of the complex temporal changes in antibody affinity observed *in vivo* and *in vitro*, the concept of antigen-driven cell selection during the maturation of the immune response is perhaps an over-simplification. It has been suggested that there are at least four factors which are involved in the control of antibody affinity: (*i*) preferential selection of high affinity cells by antigen; (*ii*) tolerance induction in high affinity cells; (*iii*) the presence of circulating antibody; and (*iv*) the extent of cell proliferation during the response (Mond *et al.*, 1974).

6.3 Factors Affecting Antibody Affinity

In addition to the nature of the immunogenic stimulus, it is possible that several other variables determine the affinity of antibody in the circulation. These include genetic factors, reticuloendothelial system function, dietary factors, quantitative and qualitative aspects of lymphocyte function, and the effects of free antibody, antigen, or immune complexes.

6.3.1 Genetic Factors

The ability to respond to a range of natural and synthetic antigens by the production of specific immune responses is under autosomal-dominant genetic control and is, in many instances, associated with the histocompatibility antigens of the species concerned (McDevitt and Benacerraf, 1969; Benacerraf and McDevitt, 1972). Although strain-related variations in the specificity of anti-bodies to a variety of antigens in the mouse, guinea-pig, and rat have been demonstrated by several laboratories, conflicting evidence has been obtained by others. The existence of such variations in the affinity of antibody has only been reported by one laboratory using mice (Soothill and Steward, 1971; Petty *et al.*, 1972) and one using rats (Ruscetti *et al.*, 1974). The failure by many investigators to obtain evidence consistent with the genetic control of affinity may be due, in part, to the use of adjuvants in the immunization procedure (see p. 248–249).

Soothill and Steward (1971), and Petty *et al.* (1972) have demonstrated consistent strain-related differences in the affinity of antibodies produced in response to human serum albumin and human serum transferrin injected in saline (Figure 5). Similar, but less marked, differences were observed for antibody to the DNP hapten. Immunization with antigen Freund's complete adjuvant eliminates

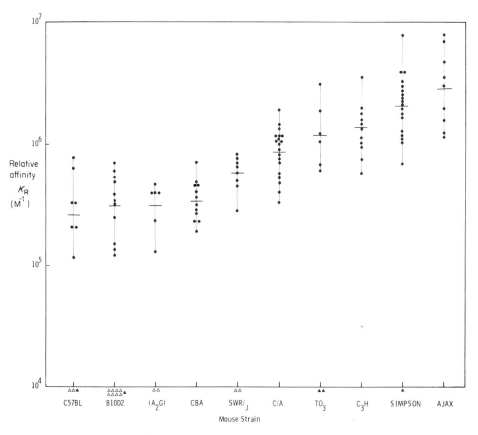

Figure 5 The relative affinity values K_R, of antibody to human serum albumin in 10 mouse strains. ▲, animals producing antibody but K_R values incalculable; △, animals not producing detectable antibody. From Petty *et al.*, 1972, reproduced by permission of Blackwell Scientific Publications Ltd.

these strain differences; all strains produce antibody of similar affinity of greater than $10^6 \ M^{-1}$. Steward and Petty (1976) have measured the amount and affinity of antibody produced in response to protein antigens injected in saline in parents, F_1 hybrids, and backcross offspring of inbred mice that produce high ($> 10^6 \ M^{-1}$) and low affinity ($< 10^6 \ M^{-1}$) antibody to these antigens. The F_1 hybrids of the cross between a high-affinity strain (A/JAX) and a low-affinity strain (B10D 2 NEW) produced anti-human serum transferrin antibodies with a mean affinity between that of the two parents. When the F_1 hybrids were backcrossed to the high and low affinity parents, segregation of affinity values was observed which is consistent with some form of genetic control. Thus, the distribution of antibody affinity values in the ($F_1 \times$ high affinity parent) backcrosses are not significantly different from that of the high affinity parent strain. Similarly, the antibody produced by the ($F_1 \times$ low affinity parent) backcross have a distribution similar to the low affinity parents (Figure 6a).

252

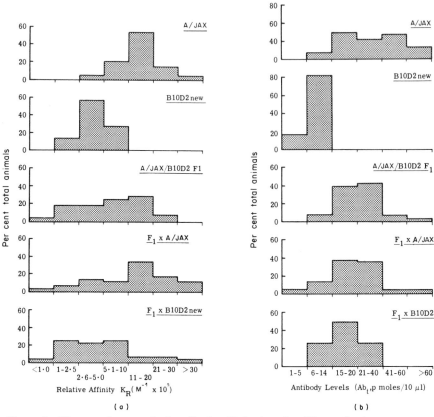

Figure 6 The genetic control of antibody affinity in mice. The antibody response to human serum transferrin in A/JAX and B10D2 new line mice, their F_1 hybrids, and backcross offspring. (a) Relative affinity K_R of antibody, and (b) antibody levels, Ab_t. From Steward and Petty (1976), reproduced by permission of Blackwell Scientific Publications Ltd.

Antibody levels, however, do not show the same trend as that observed for affinity (Figure 6b) and are not correlated with affinity. The results confirm the suggestion of genetic control of antibody affinity indicated in Figure 5, and furthermore indicate that antibody levels and affinity are two parameters of the immune response which are under independent genetic control.

Ruscetti *et al.* (1974) have reported that the affinity of antibodies to poly (Glu$_{52}$, Lys$_{33}$, Tyr$_{15}$) injected in Freund's complete adjuvant into rats is under genetic control. These workers demonstrated that high-responding strains produce higher affinity antibody than do the low-responding strains. They also reported that the use of aggregated antigen increases both the level and affinity of antibody in the low-responder strains, but decreased both parameters in the high-responding ones. These data thus underline the importance of the nature of the immunogenic stimulus in the affinity of antibody.

Further evidence confirming the genetic control of antibody affinity has been obtained by Katz and Steward (1975). Mice from an initial random-bred

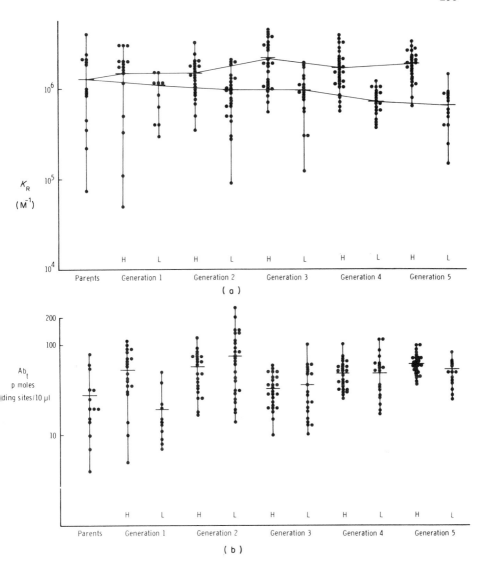

Figure 7 The genetic control of antibody affinity in mice. The antibody response to protein antigens in TO mice selectively bred on the basis of antibody affinity (K_R) into two lines; H, high affinity line; L, low affinity line. (a) Relative affinity values, K_R; and (b) antibody levels, Ab_t. After Katz and Steward (1975)

population were bred selectively on the basis of the affinity the antibody produced to protein antigens injected in saline. At each generation of selective breeding, mice producing antibody (with affinity greater than 10^6 M^{-1}) were mated. Similarly mice producing antibody with affinity lower than 10^6 M^{-1} were mated. After five generations of selective breeding, differences on affinity between the two lines were highly significant ($p < 0.0005$), whereas antibody levels were not significantly different ($p < 0.2$). This breeding programme has resulted in a progressive separation of the two lines with regard to antibody affinity, but has not produced a corresponding separation of antibody levels (Figure 7a, b). These results suggest that antibody affinity is under polygenic control and that it is exerted independently of that controlling antibody levels.

6.3.2 The Role of the Reticuloendothelial System

It is clear that macrophages play an important part in the afferent limb of the immune response. Transfer experiments have demonstrated that macrophages co-operate with T and B lymphocytes in initiating and achieving an optimal antibody response (Unanue and Cerrottini, 1970; Feldman, 1972), and antigen that has been processed by macrophages shows increased immunogenicity compared to the unprocessed antigen (Unanue, 1972). Furthermore, the use of agents affecting macrophage function, such as adjuvants (Spitznagel and Allison, 1970) and carbon (Sabet et al., 1969; Souhami, 1972) can either enhance or decrease antibody titres. In view of this central role of macrophages in the immune response, the possibility exists that differences in macrophage function could result in variations in antibody affinity as well as in antibody levels. This suggestion is supported by the observation that adjuvants increase both levels and affinity of antibody in inbred strains of mice (Soothill and Steward, 1971), whereas blockade of macrophages by carbon reduces antibody affinity but does not alter antibody levels (Passwell et al., 1974a). Inbred strains of mice differ in the affinity of antibody they produce to antigens injected in saline (see Figure 5). Using the clearance of colloidal carbon as a measure of macrophage function, Passwell et al. (1974a) have shown that the production of low affinity antibody corresponds to either poor carbon clearance or slow recovery from carbon blockade. However, Morgan and Soothill (1975) have utilized the clearance of [^{125}I] polyvinyl pyrolidone as a measure of macrophage function and have demonstrated a more precise correlation between antibody affinity and macrophage function. The ranking orders of of the mouse strains for both K_{PVP} (the constant for the clearance of PVP) and for K_R (antibody affinity) correlate significantly. These authors suggested that the more precise correlation of PVP clearance with affinity compared to that of carbon clearance with affinity may be because PVP is more similar in size to immunogenic microaggregates of soluble proteins than the carbon particles are, and that partial macrophage blockade may have occurred with the dose of carbon used.

These *in vivo* correlations of macrophage function with antibody affinity have been confirmed recently by *in vitro* experiments. The uptake of radiolabelled immune complexes by cultured peritoneal macrophages from several inbred mouse strains have been found to correlate with the affinity of serum antibody (Wiener and Steward, unpublished data).

The importance of macrophage function in determining the affinity of antibody is further supported by the observations that other factors affecting macrophage activity also result in a corresponding effect on antibody affinity. (*i*)

Oestrogens, which stimulate macrophage function (Flemming, 1967), produce an increased carbon clearance and high-affinity production in mice normally producing low affinity antibody (Passwell *et al.*, 1974*a*). (*ii*) Protein deprivation suppresses macrophage function and results in the production of low affinity antibody in mice normally producing high affinity (Passwell *et al.*, 1974*b*). (*iii*) Infection with malaria leads to macrophage blockade, and mice normally producing high affinity antibody synthesize low affinity antibody following the infection (Steward and Voller, 1973).

The observations cited here serve to illustrate the possible role of macrophages in determining the affinity of serum antibody. The precise way in which 'poor' macrophage function leads to low affinity antibody synthesis and 'good' macrophage function to high affinity antibody production is not known. However, it is possible that poor function leads to inefficient processing of antigen and presentation to immunocompetent cells. Spitznagel and Allison (1970) have suggested that macrophages prevent tolerance by limiting the access of antigen to B cells. The possibility, therefore, exists that in animals with poor macrophage function, antigen (perhaps 'unprocessed') reaches the B cells and preferentially induces tolerance in high affinity cells which are more susceptible to this induction (Theis and Siskind, 1968). Data in support of this hypothesis have been obtained from experiments with mouse strains producing either high or low affinity antibody when injected with antigen in saline (Steward *et al.*, 1974). 'High affinity' and 'low affinity' mice were preimmunized with antigen in saline and then challenged with antigen in Freund's complete adjuvant. Both preimmunized and non-preimmunized high affinity mice produced high affinity antibody on challenge. However, preimmunized low affinity mice produced low affinity antibody on challenge, whereas non-preimmunized low affinity mice produced the high affinity antibody. These results suggest that the preimmunization of low affinity mice results in some form of immunological tolerance—because of a possible macrophage defect—in which high affinity cells are unable to respond to the challenge of antigen in adjuvant.

6.3.3 Other Factors

It is very probable that several other factors affect the affinity of antibody produced by an animal. It is particularly likely that qualitative and quantitative variations in lymphocyte function play an important role in this regard. Indeed, Gershon and Paul (1971) have shown that T cells are required for the production of high-affinity anti-hapten antibody and that the affinity of the antibody produced is in part determined by the number of T cells present in the immunized animal. However, Taniguchi and Tada (1974) have obtained contradictory evidence showing the augmentation of antibody affinity in rabbits following thymectomy of adults. This observation was confirmed and extended in mice by Takemori and Tada (1974), who demonstrated that adoptive transfer of thymus or spleen cells from carrier-primed donors results in a significant decrease in the avidity of anti-DNP plaque-forming cell antibodies (in both primary and secondary responses) produced by syngeneic recipients following immunization with DNP–carrier.

The New Zealand mice show a progressive loss in T-cell helper function with age (Denman and Denman, 1970), and a similar age-related loss of suppressor function precedes the loss of helper function (Gerber *et al.*, 1974). It is therefore possible that the fall in affinity of anti-protein antibody with increasing age (Petty and Steward, 1977*b*) may be related to the loss of T cells. A similar fall in the avidity of antibody to DNA in NZB/W F_1 hybrid mice with increasing age (Steward *et al.*, 1975) may also be a result of T-cell deficiencies. Furthermore, these mice show a progressive fall in macrophage function as assessed by PVP clearance (Morgan and Steward, 1976). This fall in macrophage function with increasing age may be an age-related defect in the macrophages themselves or alternatively may be a consequence of reticuloendothial system fatigue arising from the excess of circulating DNA–anti-DNA complexes in these mice. In older mice, the affinity of antibody therefore may be affected as a result of impaired antigen processing by the fatigued reticuloendothelial system. The fall in the avidity of circulating anti-DNA antibody in NZB/W F_1 hybrid mice may arise from yet another factor which affects antibody affinity—circulating antigen. In the presence of excess circulating antigen, high affinity antibody may be removed in a complexed form leaving predominantly low affinity antibody in the circulation. This argument also applies to any situation in which antigen is likely to be present in excess. Rheumatoid factors have been shown to be of low affinity (Normansell, 1970; Steward *et al.*, 1975), but since the corresponding antigen (autologous IgG) is present in excess, the low affinity serum antibody may be that remaining after elimination of the high affinity antibody in immune complex form.

A further factor that may affect the affinity of antibody produced is circulating antibody. Such antibody may compete with antigen-sensitive cells for antigen and increase the affinity of the antibody subsequently produced. Furthermore, it has been shown that low affinity antibody-forming cells are suppressed more readily by passively transferred antibody than are high affinity cells, and that low affinity is less efficient at such suppression than is high affinity antibody (Siskind *et al.*, 1968; Walker and Siskind, 1969). Finally, Werblin *et al.* (1973) have shown that in a genetically diverse population of rabbits, the a1 allotype is associated with the production of high affinity antibody and the a6 allotype with low affinity antibody to the DNP hapten. These observations therefore suggest that structural variations in the V_H region of the molecule may influence antibody affinity.

6.4 The Biological and Immunopathological Significance of Antibody Affinity

Since experimental evidence supports the concept of a progressive selection of cells capable of producing the highest affinity antibody and that antibody multivalence provides an enormous amplification in energetic terms in the antibody–antigen reaction, it would seem that it is biologically important for an

Table 4 Biological reactions in which high affinity antibody is more effective than low affinity antibody

Reaction	Reference
Destruction of D-positive erythrocytes	Hughes-Jones (1967)
Passive haemagglutination	Levine and Levytska (1967)
Complement fixation	Fauci *et al.* (1970)
	Warner and Ovary (1970)
Passive cutaneous anaphylaxis	Fauci *et al.* (1970)
	Warner and Ovary (1970)
Haemolysis	Warner and Ovary (1970)
Immune elimination	Alpers *et al.* (1972)
Virus neutralization	Blank *et al.* (1972)
Membrane damage	Six *et al.* (1973)
Enzyme inactivation	Erickson (1974)
Protective capacity against bacteria	Ahlstedt *et al.* (1974)

animal to develop high affinity antibody in response to an immunological challenge. Furthermore, data are available which demonstrate the superiority of high affinity compared with low affinity antibodies in biological reactions, including several which are of importance in providing effective immunity in the host. Some of the biological reactions in which high affinity antibody is more effective are listed in Table 4.

Aside from the perhaps obvious advantage of high affinity antibody in forming potentially more stable bonds with antigen, the superiority of high affinity antibody in reactions such as complement fixation, may arise from the more efficient induction of essential conformational changes in the antibody molecule occurring as a result of high affinity reactions with the antigen. The evidence for conformational changes in antibody structure following interaction with antigen is discussed elsewhere in this volume (see Feinstein, Chapter 8).

When reading the literature on the subject of antibody affinity, one can gain the impression that the role of low affinity antibody in the immune response is merely as an intermediate in the pathway towards high affinity antibody production, and that cells producing the former are eliminated somehow during affinity maturation. However, recent work by, for example, Werblin and Siskind (1972) has illustrated that low affinity antibodies persist throughout the immune response, even though they are perhaps of secondary importance to high affinity antibodies. The possibility exists that, since cells with low affinity receptors are less readily susceptible to tolerance induction by antigen than cells with high affinity receptors (Theis and Siskind, 1968), the persistence of low affinity cells may provide a useful first-line defence against antigenic insult by the production of antibody (particularly IgM) having low intrinsic affinity but high functional affinity (or avidity). It is possible that low affinity antibody may also be of value in amplifying complement-fixation reactions by binding first to one site on a cell membrane, fixing complement, and, then because of its low affinity, dissociating from the first site, thus becoming free to bind a second site and to activate the complement system again.

Quite apart from the difficulty in adequately assigning a positive role to low-affinity antibody, there has been interest in the possibility that a predominantly low affinity antibody response may be viewed as an expression of immuno-deficiency (Soothill and Steward, 1971 *et al.*, 1972). As discussed in Section 6.3, the affinity of an antibody response can be influenced by a variety of factors including genetic and environmental ones, abnormalities in macrophage and T-cell helper function, and other lymphocyte abnormalities such as increased susceptibility to tolerance induction of high affinity antigen-sensitive cells (Steward *et al.*, 1974). Such a genetically determined low affinity antibody response to viral or microbial infections may have serious immunopathological consequences in the host as the antibody would be likely to fail to eliminate the antigen (Alpers *et al.*, 1972), thus favouring the production and persistence of antigen-excess immune complexes in the circulation. These complexes could either be formed with the low affinity antibody itself or with any high affinity antibody produced by the host; complement-mediated damage would follow their subsequent deposition in tissues. This hypothesis is being investigated currently in both human and murine immune complex diseases (Steward, 1976) and is outlined schematically in Figure 8.

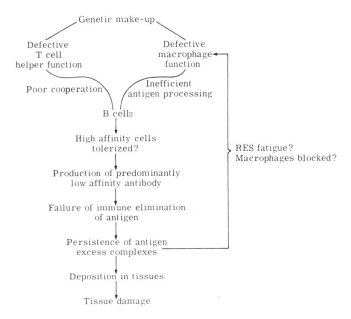

Figure 8 Schematic representation of the possible role of low affinity antibody in immune complex disease. From Steward (1976), reproduced by permission of Blackwell Scientific Publications Ltd.

ACKNOWLEDGEMENTS

Work in the author's laboratory cited here was aided by a grant from the Medical Research Council. Financial support from the Arthritis and Rheumatism Council also is acknowledged gratefully.

The author thanks Miss J. S. Linfield for help in the preparation of the manuscript.

REFERENCES

Ahlstedt, S., Holmgren, J., and Hanson, L. A. (1973. *Immunology*, **25**, 917.
Ahlstedt, S., Holmgren, J., and Hanson, L. A. (1974). *Int. Archs. Allergy appl. Immunol.*, **46**, 470.
Alpers, J. H., Steward, M. W., and Soothill, J. F. (1972). *Clin. Exp. Immunol.*, **12**, 21.
Andersson, B. (1970). *J. Exp. Med.*, **132**, 77.
Andersson, B. (1972). *J. Exp. Med.*, **135**, 312.
Ashman, R. F., and Metzger, H. (1969). *J. Biol. Chem.*, **244**, 3405

Barisas, B. G., Singer, S. J., and Sturtevant, J. M. (1975. *Immunochemistry*, **12**, 411.
Benacerraf, B., and McDevitt, H. O. (1972). *Science, N.Y.*, **175**, 273.
Blank, S. E., Leslie, G. A., and Clem, L. W. (1972). *J. Immunol.*, **108**, 665.
Burnet, F. M. (1959). *The Clonal Selection Theory of Acquired Immunity*, Cambridge University Press, Cambridge.
Burnet, F. M., Keogh, E. V., and Lush, D. (1937). *Aust. J. Exp. Biol. Med. Sci.*, **15**, 226.
Bystryn, J. C., Siskind, G. W., and Uhr, J. W. (1973). *J. Exp. Med.*, **137**, 301.

Celada, F., Schmidt, D., and Strom, R. (1969). *Immunology*, **17**, 189.
Chance, B. (1963). In *Technique of Organic Chemistry* Vol. 8, part II, Interscience, New York.
Claflin, L., Merchant, B., and Inman, J. (1973). *J. Immunol.*, **110**, 241.
Claflin, L., and Merchant, B. (1973). *J. Immunol.*, **110**, 252.
Cooper, A. G. (1967). *Science, N.Y.*, **157**, 933.
Crothers, D. M., and Metzger, U. (1972). *Immunochemistry*, **9**, 341.

Dandliker, W. B., Schapio, H. C., Meduski, J. W., Alonso, R., Feigen, G. A., and Hamrick, J. R., Jr. (1964). *Immunochemistry*, **1**, 165.
Davie, J. M., and Paul, W. E. (1972*a*). *J. Exp. Med.*, **135**, 643.
Davie, J. M., and Paul, W. E. (1972*b*). *J. Exp. Med.*, **135**, 660.
Davie, J. M., and Paul, W. E. (1973). *J. Exp. Med.*, **137**, 201.
Day, E. D. (1972). *Advanced Immunochemistry*, Williams and Wilkins, Baltimore, p. 181.
Day, L. A., Sturtevant, J. M., and Singer, S. T. (1963). *Ann. N.Y. Acad. Sci.*, **103**, 611.
Denman, A. M., and Denman, E. J. (1970). *Clin. Exp. Immunol.*, **6**, 457.
Doria, G., Schiaffini, G., Garavini, M., and Mancini, C. (1972). *J. Immunol.*, **109**, 1245.

Edberg, D., Bronson, P., and Van Oss, C. J. (1972). *Immunochemistry*, **9**, 273.
Eigen, M., and DeMaeyer, L. (1963). In *Techniques of Organic Chemistry* Vol. 8, part II, Interscience, New York.
Eisen, H. N. (1964). *Methods Med. Res.*, **10**, 106.
Eisen, H. N., and Siskind, G. W. (1964). *Biochemistry*, **3**, 996.
Erickson, R. P. (1974). *Immunochemistry*, **11**, 41.

Farr, R. S. (1958). *J. infect. Dis.*, **103**, 239.

260

Fauci, A. S., Frank, M. M., and Johnson, J. S. (1970). *J. Immunol.*, **105**, 215.
Fazekas de St. Groth, S. (1961). *Aust. J. Exp. Biol. Med. Sci.*, **39**, 563.
Feldman, M. (1972). *J. Exp. Med.*, **135**, 1049.
Ferber, J. M. (1965). M.S. Thesis, MIT, Cambridge, Mass.
Fleming, K. B. P. (1967). *Adv. Exp. Med. Biol.*, **1**, 188.
Froese, A. (1968). *Immunochemistry*, **5**, 253.
Froese, A., and Sehon, A. H. (1965). *Immunochemistry*, **2**, 135.
Froese, A. and Sehon, A. H. (1971). In *Methods in Immunology and Immunochemistry*, Vol. III, (Chase, M., and Williams, C., Eds) Academic Press, New York and London, p. 412.
Froese, A., and Sehon, A. H. (1975). *Contemp. Top. Mol. Immunol.*, **4**, p. 23.
Froese, A., Sehon, A. H., and Eigen, M. (1962). *Can. J. Chem.*, **40**, 1786.

Gaze S. E., West, N. J., and Steward, M. W. (1973). *J. Immunol. Methods*, **3**, 357.
Gerber, N. L., Hardin, J. A., Chused, T. M., and Steinberg, A. D. (1974). *J. Immunol.*, **113**, 1618.
Gershon, R. K., and Paul, W. E. (1971). *J. Immunol.*, **106**, 872.
Goldberg, R. J., and Campbell, D. M. (1951). *J. Immunol.*, **66**, 79.
Goodman, J. W., and Donch, J. J. (1964). *J. Immunol.*, **93**, 96.

Haber, E., and Stone, M. (1969). *Israel J. Med. Sci.*, **5**, 332.
Haselkorn, D., Pecht, I., Friedman, S., Yaron, A., Givol, D., and Sela, M. (1971). *Israel J. Chem.*, **9**, 53.
Haustein, D. (1971). Doctoral Dissertation, Universitat Freiberg, Germany.
Heidelberger, M., and Kendall, F. E. (1935). *J. Exp. Med.*, **61**, 563.
Heller, K. S., and Siskind, G. W. (1973). *Cell. Immunol.*, **6**, 59.
Herbert, V., Lau, K. S., Gottlieb, C. W., and Bleicher, S. J. J. (1965). *Clin. Endocrinol. Metab.*, **25**, 1375.
Hooker, S. B., and Boyd, W. C. (1935). *J. Gen. Physiol.*, **19**, 373.
Hornick, C. L., and Karush, F. (1972). *Immunochemistry*, **9**, 325.
Hughes-Jones, N. C. (1967). *Immunology*, **12**, 565.

Julius, M. H., and Herzenberg, L. A. (1974). *J. Exp. Med.*, **140**, 904.

Karush, F. (1956). *J. Am. Chem. Soc.*, **78**, 5519.
Karush, F. (1962). *Adv. Immunol.*, **2**, 1.
Karush, F. (1970). *Ann. N.Y. Acad. Sci.*, **169**, 56.
Katz, F. E., and Steward, M. W. (1975). *Immunology*, **29**, 543.
Keller, R. (1966). *J. Immunol.*, **96**, 96.
Kelly, K. A., Sehon, A. H., and Froese, A. (1971). *Immunochemistry*, **8**, 613.
Kim, Y. D., and Karush, F. (1973). *Immunochemistry*, **10**, 365.
Kimball, J. W. (1972). *Immunochemistry*, **9**, 1169.
Klinman, N. R., Long, C., and Karush, F. (1967). *J. Immunol.*, **99**, 1128.

Lafferty, K. J. (1963). *Virology*, **21**, 61.
Levine, B. B., and Levytska, V. (1967). *J. Immunol.*, **98**, 648.
Levison, S. A., Portman, A. J., Kierszenbaum, F., and Dandliker, W. B. (1971). *Biochem. Biophys. Res. Commun.*, **43**, 258.

Macario, A. J. L., and Conway de Macario, E. (1973). *Nature, (Lond.)*, **245**, 263.
Mäkelä, O. (1966). *Immunology*, **10**, 81.
Mäkelä, O. (1970). *Transplant. Rev.*, **5**, 3.
Mäkelä, O., Ruoslahati, E., and Seppälä, I. J. T. (1970). *Immunochemistry*, **7**, 917.

McDevitt, H. O., and Benacerraf, B. (1969). *Adv. Immunol.*, **11**, 31.
Medof, M. E., and Aladjem, F. (1971). *Fed. Proc.*, **30**, 657.
Merler, E., Karlin, L., and Matsumoto, S. (1968). *J. Biol. Chem.*, **243**, 386.
Metzger, H. (1970). *Adv. Immunol.*, **12**, 57.
Mond, J., Kim, Y. T., and Siskind, G. W. (1974). *J. Immunol.*, **112**, 1255.
Morgan, A. G., and Soothill, J. F. (1975). *Nature (Lond.)*, **254**, 711.
Morgan, A. G., and Steward, M. W. (1976). *Clin. Exp. Immunol.*, **26**, 133.
Mukkur, T. K. S., Szewczuk, M. R., and Schmidt, D. E., Jr. (1974). *Immunochemistry*, **11**, 9.

Nisonoff, A., and Pressman, D. (1958). *J. Immunol.*, **80**, 417.
Normansell, D. E. (1970). *Immunochemistry*, **7**, 787.

Onoue, K., Yagi, Y., Grossberg, A. L., and Pressman, D. (1965). *Immunochemistry*, **2**, 401.
Onoue, K., Yagi, Y., Grossberg, A. L., and Pressman, D. (1968). *Science, N.Y.*, **162**, 574.
Oriol, R., and Rousset, M. (1974a). *J. Immunol.*, **112**, 2227.
Oriol, R., and Rousset, M. (1974b). *J. Immunol.*, **112**, 2235.

Parker, C. W., Yoo, T. J., Johnson, M. C., and Godt, S. M. (1967). *Biochemistry*, **6**, 3408.
Passwell, J. H., Steward, M. W., and Soothill, J. F. (1974a). *Clin. Exp. Immunol.*, **17**, 159.
Passwell, J. H., Steward, M. W., and Soothill, J. F. (1974b). *Clin. Exp. Immunol.*, **17**, 491.
Paul, W. E., and Elfenbein, G. J. (1975). *J. Immunol.*, **114**, 261.
Pauling, L., Pressman, D., and Grossberg, A. L. (1944). *J. Am. Chem. Soc.*, **66**, 784.
Pecht, I., Givol, D., and Sela, M. (1972a). *J. Mol. Biol.*, **68**, 241.
Pecht, I., Haselkorn, D., and Friedman, S. (1972b). *FEBS Letters*, **24**, 331.
Petty, R. E., and Steward, M. W. (1977a). *Immunology*, **32**, 49.
Petty, R. E., and Steward, M. W. (1977b). *Ann. Rheumat. Dis.*, **36**, 39.
Petty, R. E., Steward, M. W., and Soothill, J. F. (1972). *Clin. Exp. Immunol.*, **12**, 231.
Pressman, D., Roholt, O. A., and Grossberg, A. L. (1970). *Ann. N.Y. Acad. Sci.*, **169**, 65.
Ramseier, H. (1971). *Eur. J. Immunol.*, **1**, 171.
Ruscetti, S. K., Kunz, H. W., and Gill, T. J. (1974). *J. Immunol.*, **113**, 1468.

Sabet, T., Newlin, L., and Friedman, H. (1969). *Immunology*, **16**, 433.
Sarvas, H., and Mäkelä, O. (1970). *Immunochemistry*, **7**, 933.
Scatchard, G. (1949). *Ann. N.Y. Acad. Sci.*, **51**, 660.
Schirrmacher, V. (1972). *Eur. J. Immunol.*, **2**, 430.
Sips, R. (1948). *J. Chem. Phys.*, **16**, 490.
Siskind, G. W., and Benacerraf, B. (1969). *Adv. Immunol.*, **10**, 1.
Siskind, G. W., Dunn, P., and Walker, J. G. (1968). *J. Exp. Med.*, **127**, 55.
Six, H. R., Uemura, K., and Kinsky, S. C. (1973). *Biochemistry*, **12**, 4003.
Skubitz, K. M., and Smith, T. W. (1975). *J. Immunol.*, **114**, 1369.
Smith, T. W., and Skubitz, K. M. (1975). *Biochemistry*, **14**, 1496.
Soothill, J. F., and Steward, M. W. (1971). *Clin. Exp. Immunol.*, **9**, 193.
Souhami, R. L. (1972). *Immunology*, **22**, 685.
Spitznagel, J. K., and Allison, A. C. (1970). *J. Immunol.*, **104**, 128.
Steiner, L. A., and Eisen, H. N. (1967). *J. Exp. Med.*, **126**, 1161.
Stemke, E. W. (1969). *J. Immunol.*, **103**, 596.
Steward, M. W. (1976). In *Infection and Immunology in the Rheumatic Diseases* (Dumonde, D. C., ed.), Blackwell, Oxford, p. 439.
Steward, M. W., Alpers, J. H., and Soothill, J. F. (1973a). *Proc. Roy. Soc. Med.*, **66**, 808.
Steward, M. W., Gaze, S. E., and Petty, R. E. (1974). *Eur. J. Immunol.*, **4**, 751.
Steward, M. W., Katz, F. E., and West, N. J. (1975). *Clin. Exp. Immunol.*, **21**, 121.
Steward, M. W., and Petty, R. E. (1972a). *Immunology*, **23**, 881.

Steward, M. W., and Petty, R. E. (1972b). *Immunology*, **22**, 747.

Steward, M. W., and Petty, R. E. (1976). *Immunology*, **30**, 789.

Steward, M. W., Turner, M. W., Natvig, J. B., and Gaarder, P. I. (1973b). *Clin. Exp. Immunol.*, **15**, 145.

Steward, M. W., and Voller, A. (1973). *Brit. J. Exp. Pathol.*, **54**, 198.

Stupp, V., Yoshida, T., and Paul, W. E. (1969). *J. Immunol.*, **103**, 625.

Takemori, T., and Tada, T. (1974). *J. Exp. Med.*, **140**, 253.

Taliaferro, W. H., Taliaferro, L. G., and Pizzi, A. K. (1959). *J. Infect. Dis.*, **105**, 197.

Taniguchi, M., and Tada, T. (1974). *J. Exp. Med.*, **139**, 108.

Talmage, D. W. (1960). *J. Infect. Dis.*, **107**, 115.

Taylor, R. B. (1975). *Immunology*, **29**, 989.

Theis, G. A., and Siskind, G. W. (1968). *J. Immunol.*, **100**, 138.

Unanue, E. R. (1972). *Adv. Immunol.*, **15**, 95.

Unanue, E. R., and Cerrottini, J. C. (1970). *Semin. Hematol.*, **7**, 225.

Urbain, J., van Acker, A., De Vos-Cloetens, C. H., and Urbain-Vansanten, G. (1972). *Immunochemistry*, **9**, 121.

Velick, S. F., Parker, C. W., and Eisen, H. N. (1960). *Proc. Nat. Acad. Sci., U.S.A.*, **46**, 1470.

Vogt, A., Kopp, R., Mass, G., and Reich, L. (1964). *Science, N.Y.*, **145**, 144.

Voss, E. W., and Eisen, H. N. (1968) *Fed. Proc.*, **27**, 2361.

Walker, J. G., and Siskind, G. W. (1969). *J. Exp. Med.*, **127**, 55.

Warner, N. L., and Ovary, Z. (1970). *J. Immunol.*, **105**, 812.

Werblin, T. P., Kim, Y. T., Mage, R., Benacerraf, B., and Siskind, G. W. (1973). *Immunology*, **25**, 17.

Werblin, T. P., and Siskind, G. W. (1972). *Immunochemistry*, **9**, 987.

CHAPTER 8

Models of Immunoglobulins and Antigen–Antibody Complexes

A. Feinstein and D. Beale

1 INTRODUCTION

In this chapter an account will be given of the structural background needed for the consideration of changes that might take place in antibodies when they bind to antigen.

The recognition of amino acid sequence homology regions in the polypeptide chains of IgG (Hill *et al.*, 1967; Edelman *et al.*, 1969) led to the development of the domain hypothesis (Edelman and Gall, 1969). This hypothesis postulated that each immunoglobulin chain is folded into several globular regions with different biological functions.

Several groups of X-ray crystallographers have confirmed the domain hypothesis; their work has been reviewed by Poljak (1975*a*, *b*) and by Davies *et al.* (1975*a*, *b*). It has become possible to speculate on the biological functions of

264

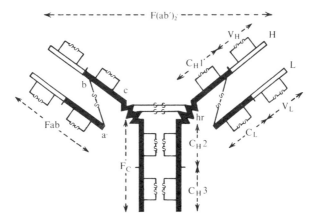

Figure 1 Chemical structure of human IgG4. L, light
chain; H, heavy chain; hr, extra-domain hinge region; and
–S–S–, cystine disulphide bridge. Light and heavy chains
are represented as extended structures by lines, which are
shaded for C regions and unshaded for V regions. Each
chain has been divided into domains and each domain has
an intra-chain disulphide bridge. Fab, F(ab')$_2$, and Fc
indicate proteolytic fragments

immunoglobulins in three-dimensional terms and such an approach has been
made by Beale and Feinstein (1976).

2 BASIC IMMUNOGLOBULIN STRUCTURE

Numerous laboratories, but particularly those of Porter and of Edelman,
contributed to the early studies of immunoglobulin structure. This work has been
reviewed extensively by Cohen and Porter (1964), Cohen and Milstein (1967) and
Turner in Chapter I of this book. In addition, Porter (1973) has given a general
account of the structure of immunoglobulins, hence only a brief outline will be
included in this chapter.

Immunoglobulins can be regarded as being based on a common structure of
two light and two heavy polypeptide chains linked by the disulphide bridges of
cystine residues. The structure of human IgG4 is shown in Figure 1. Light chains

Table 1 Polypeptide chain composition of
immunoglobulins

Immunoglobulin	Polypeptide chains
IgG1	$(L-\gamma_1)_2$
IgG4	$(L-\gamma_4)_2$
IgM	$[(L-\mu)_2]_5J$
IgA	$(L-\alpha)_2$ or $[(L-\alpha)_2]_2J$
IgE	$(L-\varepsilon)_2$
IgD	$(L-\delta)_2$

occur as two types (κ or λ) and are common to all normal immunoglobulins. They consist of a domain (V_L) of variable amino acid sequence, involved in antigen binding, and a domain (C_L) of constant amino acid sequence. Each domain has an essential intra-chain disulphide bridge. Heavy chains of different primary structure determine the class and subclass of immunoglobulins (Table 1). Different classes of H chain differ in their number of domains and non-domain regions. These variations are summarized in Table 2.

Table 2 Domain composition of immuno-globulin chains

Chain	Composition				
Light chain					
λ	V_λ	C_λ			
κ	V_κ	C_κ			
Heavy chain					
γ	V_H	$C_\gamma 1$ hr	$C_\gamma 2$	$C_\gamma 3$	
μ	V_H	$C_\mu 1$ $C_\mu 3$	$C_\mu 3$	$C_\mu 4$ tp	
α	V_H	$C_\alpha 1$ hr	$C_\alpha 2$	$C_\alpha 3$ tp	
ε	V_H	$C_\varepsilon 1$	$C_\varepsilon 2$	$C_\varepsilon 3$	$C_\varepsilon 4$

hr, hinge region; tp, tail piece

Amino acid sequence studies of IgG predicted that the γ chain has four domains (V_γ, $C_\gamma 1$, $C_\gamma 2$, $C_\gamma 3$) (Edelman et al., 1969) with a short 'hinge' region lying between the $C_\gamma 1$ and $C_\gamma 2$ domains (see Figure 1). It is within this region that flexibility between the two Fab units and Fc occurs.

In human and mouse IgG1 the light-heavy disulphide bridge joins a to c rather than a to b in IgG4 (Figure 1). In rabbit IgG there is an additional intra-chain bridge joining b to c. Due to the three-dimensional folding of a domain (see Figure 4) a, b, and c are really close together in space. The hinge region differs in the number of residues and disulphide bridges depending on the species and subclass of IgG. Fab and Fc fragments are produced by proteolytic cleavage between the $C_H 1$ domain and the hinge region. $F(ab')_2$ fragment is formed by cleavage between the hinge region and $C_H 2$ domain. IgG3 and IgA have extended hinge regions. IgA has an extra-domain tail piece immediately following the $C_H 3$ domain. IgA can form dimers and tetramers.

Similar studies of IgM indicate that the μ chain has five domains (V_H, $C_\mu 1$, $C_\mu 2$, $C_\mu 3$, $C_\mu 4$) (Putnam et al., 1973; Watanabe et al., 1973) with an additional non-domain 'tail' piece of 19 residues immediately following the $C_\mu 4$ domain (Figure 2). J Chain is found linked by disulphide bonds to the tail piece (Mestecky and Schrohenloher, 1974) and probably regulates intra-cellular polymerization (see reviews by Inman and Mestecky, 1975; Koshland, 1975; and Parkhouse, Chapter 3 of this volume). The μ chain has no sequence analogous to the hinge region of the γ chain. The genetic information for this region probably replaces that for a domain deleted from the ancestral gene. Thus, immunoglobulins have either a non-domain hinge region or an additional domain.

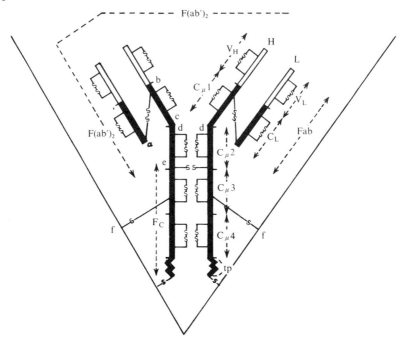

Figure 2 The human IgM 7S subunit. L, light chain; H, heavy chain (μ); tp, extra-domain tail piece; –S–S–, cystine disulphide bridge. In the cyclic 19 S molecule five subunits are disulphide bridged with a J chain. Fab fragment is formed by proteolytic cleavage between the $C_\mu 1$ and $C_\mu 2$ domains. $F(ab')_2$ is formed by cleavage just below, and $(Fc)_5$ just above, bridge e

Sequence studies on the α chain (Putnam, 1974; Kratzin *et al.*, 1975; Low *et al.*, 1976) have revealed the presence of four domains (V_H, $C_\alpha 1$, $C_\alpha 2$, $C_\alpha 3$). There is a non-domain region lying between the $C_\alpha 1$ and $C_\alpha 2$ domains which is analogous to but different from the hinge regions of the γ chains. An additional tail piece follows the $C_\alpha 3$ domain and is homologous with that of the μ chain.

Homologies in the primary structure of the ε chain indicate that there are five domains (Bennich and Bahr-Lindström, 1974), but no non-domain regions related to the hinge region of the γ chain or to the tail piece of the μ chain.

IgG and IgE are found only as monomers, but IgA can be monomeric, dimeric, or tetrameric, while IgM is usually pentameric. These polymeric immunoglobulins generally have one J chain per molecule. Only immunoglobulins that have the additional tail piece exist as polymers.

Proteolytic enzymes such as pepsin, papain, and trypsin when used under carefully controlled conditions tend to cleave immunoglobulins between domains rather than within domains, although extensive degradation will occur if the digestion is prolonged. In the case of IgG, the hinge region is particularly susceptible, with Fab, $F(ab')_2$, and Fc fragments being produced (see Figure 1). IgM can be cleaved between the $C_\mu 1$ and $C_\mu 2$ domains preferentially, and between the $C_\mu 2$ and $C_\mu 3$ domains to give Fab, $F(ab')_2$, and $(Fc)_5$ fragments (Figure 2).

3 CRYSTALLOGRAPHIC EVIDENCE FOR DOMAINS

Several groups of X-ray crystallographers have obtained striking confirmation of the domain hypothesis. Poljak *et al.* (1972) analysed crystals of human IgG (NEW) Fab' fragment to a resolution of 0·6 nm and interpreted the results in terms of four domains. Almost simultaneously, Edmundson *et al.* (1972) analysed crystals of Bence–Jones λ chain dimer (McG) to a resolution of 0·6 nm and also interpreted their results in terms of four domains. Resolution to 0·35 nm (Schiffer *et al.*, 1973) clearly showed four globular domains and eventually a 0·23 nm model was realized (Edmundson *et al.*, 1974; Edmundson *et al.*, 1975). Higher resolution of Fab' (NEW) to 0·28 nm (Poljak *et al.*, 1973) clearly showed four globular regions (Figure 3), and further resolution provided a 0·2 nm model (Poljak *et al.*, 1974).

The four domains (V_λ, C_λ, V_H, and $C_\lambda 1$) of Fab' (NEW) and the four domains (V_λ, C_λ, V_λ, C_λ) of dimer (Mcg) have a distorted tetrahedral arrangement in both cases. The angle between the pseudo two-fold axis of rotation of the V and C domains is approximately 130°. All the domains have a similar peptide chain folding, although V domains have extra folds relative to C domains formed from additional amino acid sequences (Figure 4).

Analysis of a mouse IgA (k) Fab fragment by Padlan *et al.* (1973) to a resolution of 0·45 nm showed four globular domains and the binding region for

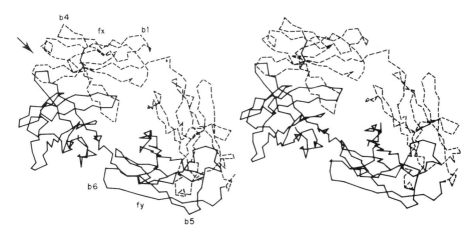

Figure 3 Stereo drawing of the 0·28 nm model of Fab' fragment of human IgG (NEW) (from Poljak *et al.*, 1973). The thin line traces the α-carbon backbone of the V_L domain (left) and the C_L domain (right). The thick line traces the α-carbon backbone of the V_H domain (left) and the $C_\gamma 1$ domain (right). Note that the C_λ and $C_\gamma 1$ domains have almost identical folding, and interact at their x faces. The V domains are interacting at their y faces and the antigen-binding site is indicated by an arrow. The overall dimensions of the Fab' molecule are $8 \times 5 \times 4$ nm and those of a domain are $4 \times 2·5 \times 2·5$ nm

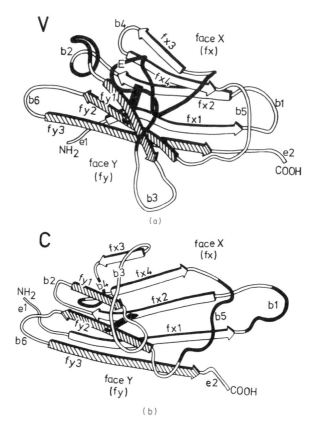

Figure 4 Peptide chain folding of (a) V domain and (b) C domain (adapted from Edmundson *et al.* 1975). The chain is folded to form seven roughly linear segments in the order fx1, fx2, fy1, fx3, fx4, fy2, and fy3. Segments fx1–4 (unshaded) and fy1–3 (shaded) form two roughly parallel faces, of anti-parallel β-pleated sheet, linked by the domain intra-chain disulphide bridge (filled rectangle). Between the β-pleated segments are other segments (b1–6) which form bends, helices, and other structure. Because of the three-dimensional tilt segments fx3, fx4, fy1, and b4 are fore-shortened considerably. The V domain and the C domain differ in some of the segments b1–6 (filled in areas), in particular, V domains have an extra loop (E). The x and y faces of the V domain are more distorted than those of the C domain. The $C_\gamma 1$ domain is orientated to approximately the same position as the C domain shown in Figure 3.

phosphorylcholine. Subsequent resolution to 0·31 nm (Figure 5) by Segal *et al.* (1974) demonstrated that all four domains (V_κ, C_κ, V_H, $C_\alpha 1$) had a similar peptide chain folding to those of Fab' (NEW) and dimer (Mcg). Again a distorted tetrahedral arrangement of domains was observed with an angle of 135° between the pseudo two-fold axis of rotation of the V and C domains.

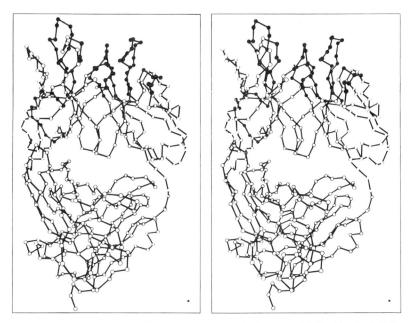

Figure 5 Stereo drawing of the 0·31 nm model of mouse (McPc 603) IgA Fab fragment (from Davies *et al.*, 1975*b*). The α-carbon backbone, –0–; hypervariable regions, –•–. The V_κ domain is top right, C_κ is bottom right, V_H is top left, and $C_\alpha 1$ is bottom left. Filled circles indicate the hypervariable regions. The orientation is about 80° clockwise to that of Figure 3. Note that the C_κ and $C_\alpha 1$ domains have almost identical folding which is the same as that of the C_λ and $C_\gamma 1$ domains of Figure 3. The C domains are again in contact at their x faces whereas the V domains interact at their y faces

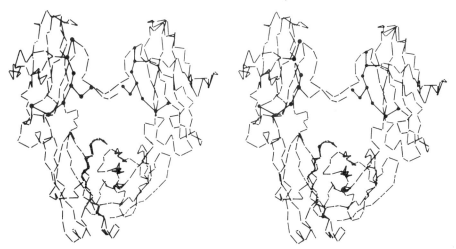

Figure 6 Stereo drawing of the α-carbon backbone of the Fc fragment from human IgG (from Deisenhofer *et al.*, 1976). The $C_\gamma 2$ domains are at the top and do not interact. Approximate centres of carbohydrate units (•).

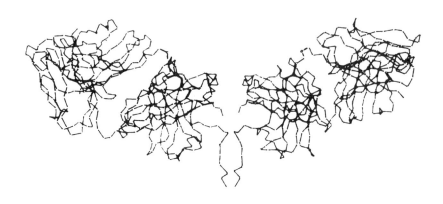

Figure 7   Tracing of the α-carbon backbone of the F(ab′)$_2$ region from IgG1 (Kol). From Colman *et al.*, 1976

Epp *et al.* (1974) analysed a V-region dimer to a resolution of 0·28 nm and revealed that the peptide chains fold into two globular domains. Subsequent resolution to 0·2 nm (Epp *et al.*, 1975) indicated that the two domains (V_κ, V_κ) have a similar peptide-chain folding to that of other crystallographic domains.

Analysis at 0·35 nm resolution of a human IgG Fc fragment has been reported by Deisenhofer *et al.* (1976). Four globular domains ($C_\gamma 2$, $C_\gamma 3$)$_2$ could be distinguished. These domains display a similar chain folding to those of other crystallographic models. However, $C_\gamma 2$ shows some characteristic differences from other C domains (Figure 6).

X-ray crystallographic studies of whole IgG molecules generally have yielded only low resolution results which at best indicate only gross structure (Edmundson *et al.*, 1970; Sarma *et al.*, 1971). Recently, however, Colman *et al.* (1976) and Huber *et al.* (1976) have reported analysis at 0·4 nm resolution for crystals of IgG (Kol). They obtained an α carbon interpretation of the F(ab′)$_2$ region (Figure 7), but could not resolve the Fc region which appeared to be disordered. Two points of interest to emerge were that there is no contact between the Fab arms and that the angle between the pseudo two-fold axes of rotation of V and C domains is nearly 180°, in contrast to the angle of 130° seen in Fab crystals.

4 DOMAIN STRUCTURE

Detailed comparisons of high resolution crystallographic results have been made (Davies *et al.* (1975a, b); Epp *et al* (1975); Padlan and Davies (1975); Poljak (1975a, b); Deisenhofer *et al.* (1976); Huber *et al.* (1976). In all immunoglobulin domains studied, the peptide chain is folded to form two roughly parallel, rather distorted, anti-parallel β-pleated sheets linked by the essential domain intra-chain disulphide bridge (see Figure 4). The space between the two β-pleated sheets is filled with the hydrophobic amino acid side chains, resulting in the domain interior being inaccessible to water. The two β-pleated sheets also provide the domain with two external, somewhat curved, faces (x and y in Figure 4) which are responsible for the main contacts between domains.

V Domains generally have an extra amino acid sequence, relative to C domains, which can produce various kinks or folds of different size and orientation from one V domain to another (see Davies *et al.* 1975*b*). These extra kinks or folds generally involve one of the hypervariable regions that contribute to the antigen-binding site. V_L domains have three hypervariable regions (corresponding approximately to b2, E, and b6 in Figure 4) but V_H domains have a fourth hypervariable region which is remote from the binding site (Figure 5) (see reviews by Kabat and Wu, 1971; Capra and Kehoe, 1975; Davies *et al.*, 1975*a*; Poljak, 1975*a*). The crystallographic structures of binding sites have been compared by Davies *et al.* (1975*a, b*), and Edmundson *et al.* (1975) have discussed the divergence of V and C domains.

The high resolution crystallographic data indicate that the C_λ, C_κ, $C_\gamma 1$, $C_\gamma 3$, and $C_\alpha 1$ domains have remarkably similar tertiary structures (Poljak *et al.*, 1973; Schiffer *et al.*, 1973; Segal *et al.*, 1974; Deisenhofer *et al.*, 1976) (compare Figures 3, 5, and 6) and the $C_\gamma 2$ domain has a closely related structure as shown in Figure 6 (Deisenhofer *et al.*, 1976; Huber *et al.*, 1976). Since the space between the two β-pleated sheets of a domain is filled with hydrophobic amino acid side chains, hydrophobic residues will tend to occur at alternating positions along those segments of peptide which form β-pleated sheets (fx1, 2, 3, and 4 and fy1, 2, and 3 in Figure 4). Other segments (b1, 2, 3, 4, 5, and 6) which are involved in bends, helices, and other non pleated structures do not appear to have this characteristic. Beale and Feinstein (1976) have examined the available amino acid sequences of C domains. They found that all sequences have the pattern of amino acid residues seen in the crystallographic models. This is shown in Figure 8.

It will be seen from Figure 8 (rows 1–4) that although the β-pleated and non-β-pleated segments of the V and C domains fall into approximately the same positions there are some pronounced differences. Thus in V domains, segment b1 forms a hair-pin bend, and fx1 and fx2 are displaced somewhat relative to the analogous segments of the C domains. In V domains, an extra loop occurs after b3, and fx3 is displaced relative to the analogous C domain segments. Segment b4 of V domains is considerably shorter than that of the C domains.

It will be seen from Figure 8 (columns 5–32) that in C domains the best regions of overall homology correspond to the β-pleated segments of Fab′ (NEW), although it is poor in fx3 and fy3, particularly with regard to the μ and ε domains. In most of these regions, short runs of alternating hydrophobic residues tend to occur (see columns 6, 8, 10, 26, 28, 30, 32, 42, 45, 47, 66, 83, 85, 89, 91, 104, 106, 108, 119, and 124) and correspond to those with side chains pointing into the interior of the crystallographic domains.

Some of these conserved hydrophobic side chains form interesting clusters in the C_L and $C_\gamma 1$ domains of Fab′ (NEW). Thus the side chains of residues in

Sample	Domain	No.					e1				fx1	10		
Human (New) IgG₁	V_L	1					Z	S	V	L	~~T~~	Q	~~P~~	~~P~~
	V_H	2					Z	V	~~Q~~	L	~~P~~	E	~~S~~	G
	C_L	3	Q	P	K	A	A	P	~~S~~	V	~~T~~	L	~~F~~	P
	C_γ1	4	A	S	T	~~K~~	G	P	~~S~~	V	~~F~~	P	~~L~~	A
								▼			▼	▼		
Human (Eu) IgG₁	C_γ2	5	E	L	L	G	G	P	S	V	F	L	F	P
	C_γ3	6	Q	P	—	R	E	P	Q	V	Y	T	L	P
Human (Vin) IgG₄	C_γ1	7	A	S	T	K	G	P	S	V	F	P	L	A
	C_γ2	8	E	F	L	G	G	P	S	V	F	L	F	P
	C_γ3	9	Q	P	—	R	E	P	Q	V	Y	T	L	P
Mouse (MOPC 21) IgG₁	C_γ1	10	A	K	T	T	P	P	T	V	Y	P	L	A
	C_γ2	11	E	V	—	—	—	S	S	V	F	I	F	P
	C_γ3	12	—	K	P	R	A	P	Q	V	Y	T	I	P
Mouse (MOPC 173) IgG₂ₐ	C_γ1	13	A	K	T	T	A	P	S	V	Y	P	L	A
	C_γ2	14	N	L	L	G	G	P	S	V	F	I	F	P
	C_γ3	15	—	S	V	R	A	P	Q	V	Y	V	L	P
Guinea pig IgG₂	C_γ1	16	A	S	T	T	A	P	S	V	F	P	L	A
	C_γ2	17	E	N	L	G	G	P	S	V	F	I	F	P
	C_γ3	18	—	A	P)	R	M	P	D	V	Y	T	L	P
Rabbit IgG	C_γ1	19	S	G	T	K	A	P	S	V	F	P	L	A
	C_γ2	20	E	L	L	G	G	P	S	V	F	I	F	K
	C_γ3	21	E	P	L	—	E	P	K	V	Y	T	M	G
Human (Gal) IgM	C_μ1	22	G	S	A	S	A	P	T	L	F	P	L	V
	C_μ2	23	Z	L	P	P	K	V	S	V	F	V	P	P
	C_μ3	24	D	Z	B	T	A	I	R	V	F	A	I	P
	C_μ4	25	V	A	L	H	R	P	D	V	Y	L	L	P
Human (ND) IgE	C_ε1	26	G	S	T	T	G	P	T	V	F)	P	L	T
	C_ε2	27	R	B	F	T	P	P	T	V	K	I	L	Z
	C_ε3	28	A	D	S	D	P	R	G	V	S	A	Y	L
	C_ε4	29	G	P	R	A	A	P	E	V	Y	A	F	A
Human IgA₁	C_α1	30	A	S	P	T	S	P	K	V	F	P	L	S
	C_α2	31	P	S	C	C	H	P	R	L	S	L	H	R
	C_α3	32	—	N	T	F	H	P	E	V	R	L	L	R
								▲			▲	▲		
Human (Mcg)	C_L	33	Q	P	K	A	N	P	T	V	T	L	F	P
	V_L	34					Z	S	A	L	T	Q	P	P
β-microglob'		35	—	I	Q	R	T	P	K	I	Q	V	Y	S

Single-letter

A	alanine (n)	G	glycine (n)
B	aspartic-acid or asparagine	H	histidine
C	cysteine	I	isoleucine (h)
D	aspartic acid	K	lysine
E	glutamic acid	L	leucine (h)
F	phenylalanine (h)	M	methionine(h)
		N	asparagine

Figure 8 Alignment of amino acid sequences in terms of crystallographic models. In rows 1–4 the amino acid sequences of the four domains of Fab′ (NEW) are aligned by the method of Poljak *et al.* (1974) with residues occupying equivalent positions in the 0·2 nm model placed in the same column. Hydrogen-bonded residues are indicated by cancelled

						b1										fx2		
S	V	S	G	A	P	—	—	—	—	G	Q	R	V	T	I	S	C	T
P	E	L	V	S	P	—	—	—	—	G	Z	T	L	S	L	T	C	T
P	S	S	E	E	L	Q	—	—	—	A	N	K	A	T	L	V	C	L
P	S	S	K	S	T	S	—	—	—	G	G	T	A	A	L	G	C	L
▼																▼	▼	

							20									30		
P	K	P	K	D	T	—	L	M	I	S	R	T	P	E	V	T	C	V
P	S	R	E	E	—	—	—	M	T	K	N	Q	V	S	L	T	C	L
P	C	S	R	S	T	S	—	—	—	E	S	T	A	A	L	G	C	L
P	K	P	K	D	T	—	L	M	I	S	R	T	P	E	V	T	C	V
P	S	Q	E	E	—	—	—	M	T	K	N	Q	V	S	L	T	C	L
P	G	S	N	A	A	S	—	—	—	Q	S	M	V	T	L	G	C	L
P	K	P	K	D	T	—	L	L	I	T	V	T	P	K	V	T	C	V
P	P	K	E	Q	—	—	—	M	A	K	D	K	V	S	L	T	C	M
P	V	C	G	D	T	T	—	—	—	G	S	S	V	T	L	G	C	L
V	K	I	K	N	P	—	L	M	I	S	L	S	P	I	V	T	C	V
P	P	Z	S	—	—	—	—	M	T	K	K	E	V	T	L	T	C	M
A	S	C	V	D	T	S	—	—	—	G	S	M	**M**	T	L	G	C	L
P	K	P	K	D	T	—	L	M	I	S	L	T	P	R	V	T	C	V
P	S	R	D	E	—	—	—	L	S	K	S	K	V	S	V	T	C	L
P	C	C	G	D	T	P	—	—	—	S	S	T	V	T	L	G	C	L
P	P	P	K	D	T	—	L	M	I	S	R	T	P	E	V	T	C	V
P	P	R	E	Q	—	—	—	L	S	S	R	S	V	S	L	T	C	M
S	C	E	N	S	B	P	—	—	—	S	S	T	V	A	V	G	C	L
R	D	G	F	F	G	N	—	—	—	P	R	K	S	K	L	I	C	Q
P	S	F	A	S	—	—	I	F	L	T	K	S	T	K	L	T	C	L
P	A	R	E	Q	—	—	L	N	L	R	E	S	A	T	I	T	C	L
R	C	C	K	B	I	P	—	S	*N*	A	T	S	V	T	L	G	C	L
S	S	C	B	G	L	—	—	G	H	F	P	P	T	I	Z	L	C	L
S	R	P	S	P	F	D	L	F	I	R	K	S	P	T	I	T	C	L
T	P	E	W	P	G	S	—	—	—	R	D	K	**R**	T	L	A	C	L
L	C	S	T	Z	P	—	—	—	—	B	G	B	V	V	I	A	C	L
P	A	L	Q	D	—	—	L	L	L	G	S	E	A	*N*	L	T	C	T
P	P	S	Q	Q	—	—	L	A	L	N	Q	L	V	T	L	T	C	L
▲												▲		▲		▲		
P	S	S	E	E	L	Q	—	—	—	A	N	K	A	T	L	V	C	L
S	A	S	G	S	L	—	—	—	—	G	Q	S	V	T	I	S	C	T
R	H	P	A	E	N	—	—	—	—	G	K	S	N	F	L	N	C	Y

amino acid code:

P	proline (h)	W	tryptophan
Q	glutamine	Y	tyrosine
R	arginine	Z	glutamic acid
S	serine		or glutamine
T	threonine		
V	valine (h)	(n)	non-polar
		(h)	hydrophobic

letters. Segments participating in pleated sheets are underlined and labelled fx1–4 and fy1–3, in accordance with Figure 4. Segments forming bends, helices, or other structure are labelled b1–6. Residues of other structure at the ends of the domain are e1 and e2. C_y1. Residues whose side chains point to the interior of the domain have a filled triangle

	1	2	3	4	5	6	7	8	b2 (9)	10	11	12	fyl (13)	14	15
Human (New) IgG₁	~~G~~	~~S~~	S	S	N	I	—	—	G	A	G	N	~~H~~	V	~~K~~
	~~G~~	~~S~~	T	V	S	T	—	—	F	A	V	—	~~Y~~	~~I~~	~~V~~
	~~I~~	~~S~~	~~D~~	F	Y	P	—	—	G	A	V	—	~~T~~	V	~~A~~
	~~V~~	~~K~~	~~D~~	Y	~~F~~	P	—	—	E	P	~~V~~	—	~~T~~	V	~~S~~
	▼			▼									▼		▼

(40)

	1	2	3	4	5	6	7	8	9	10	11	12	13	14	15
Human (Eu) IgG₁	V	V	D	V	S	H	E	D	P	Q	V	—	K	F	N
	V	K	G	F	Y	P	—	—	S	D	I	—	A	V	E
Human (Vin) IgG₄	V	K	.	.	.	.	.	.	.	.	.	.	.	.	.
	V	V	D	V	S	Q	E	D	P	Z	(V	—	Z	F)	N
	V	K	G	F	Y	P	—	—	S	D	I	—	A	V	E
Mouse (MOPC 21) IgG₁	V	K	G	Y	F	P	—	—	E	P	V	—	T	V	T
	V	V	D	I	S	K	D	D	P	E	V	—	Q	F	S
	I	T	D	F	F	P	—	—	E	D	I	—	T	V	E
Mouse (MOPC 173) IgG₂ₐ	V	K	G	Y	F	P	—	—	E	P	V	—	T	L	S
	V	V	D	V	S	E	D	D	P	D	V	—	Q	I	S
	V	T	N	F	M	P	—	—	E	D	I	—	Y	V	E
Guinea pig IgG₂	V	K	G	Y	F	P	—	—	E	P	V	—	T	V	K
	V	V	D	V	S	Q	D	E	P	E	V	—	Q	F	T
	L	I	N	F	F	P	—	—	A	D	I	—	H	V	E
Rabbit IgG	V	K	G	Y	L	P	—	—	E	P	V	—	T	V	T
	V	V	D	V	S	Z	B	(D	P	Z	V	—	Z)	F	T
	I	D	G	F	Y	P	—	—	S	D	I	—	S	V	G
Human (Gal) IgM	A	Z	D	F	L	P	—	—	D	S	I	—	T	F	S
	A	T	G	F	S	P	—	—	R	Q	I	—	Q	V	S
	V	T	D	L	T	Y	—	—	D	S	V	—	T	I	S
	V	T	G	F	S	P	—	—	A	D	V	—	F	V	Q
Human (ND) IgE	A	T	G	Y	F	P	—	—	E	P	V	—	M	V	T
	V	S	G	Y	T	P	—	—	G	T	I	—	𝒩	I	T
	V	V	B	L	A	P	S	K	G	T	V	—	𝒩	L	T
	I	Q	N	F	M	P	—	—	E	D	I	—	S	V	Q
Human IgA₁	V	Q	G	F	F	P	—	Q	Q	P	L	—	S	V	T
	L	T	G	L	R	D	—	A	S	G	V	—	T	F	T
	A	R	G	F	S	P	—	—	K	D	V	—	L	V	R
	▲			▲									▲		▲
Human (Mcg)	I	S	D	F	Y	P	—	—	G	A	V	—	T	V	A
	G	T	S	S	D	V	—	—	G	G	Y	N	Y	V	S
β-microglob'	V	S	G	F	H	P	—	—	S	D	I	—	E	V	D

Single-letter

A	alanine (n)	G	glycine (n)
B	aspartic-acid or asparagine	H	histidine
		I	isoleucine (h)
C	cysteine	K	lysine
D	aspartic acid	L	leucine (h)
E	glutamic acid	M	methionine (h)
F	phenylalanine (h)	N	asparagine

underneath. Rows 5–32, available amino acid sequences of C_H domains aligned by homology, which has been maximized by leaving gaps (–). The numbering between rows 4 and 5 refers to columns not to residues. C, Cysteine residues; 𝒩, sites for complex N-linked oligosaccharide; S, sites for O-linked carbohydrate. Columns which tend to conserve

			50			b3							60			
~~W~~	~~Y~~	Q	Q	~~L~~	P	G	~~T~~	extra loop				P	L	R	S	~~R~~
~~W~~	~~V~~	~~R~~	~~Q~~	P	P	G	~~R~~					P	L	R	S	~~R~~
~~W~~	~~K~~	—	—	~~A~~	D	S	~~S~~	—	—	—	—	P	V	K	A	—
~~W~~	~~N~~	—	—	—	S	G	—	—	—	—	—	A	L	T	S	—
▼																
W	Y	—	—	V	D	G	—	—	—	—	—	V	Q	V	H	—
W	E	—	—	S	N	D	—	—	—	—	—	G	E	P	E	—
.	.	.	.	.	.	.	.	.	.	.	.	.	.	.	.	.
W	Y	—	—	V	D	G	—	—	—	—	—	V	E	V	H	—
W	Z	—	—	S	(B	B	—	—	—	—	—	G	Z	P	Z	—
W	N	—	—	—	S	G	—	—	—	—	—	S	L	S	S	—
W	F	—	—	V	D	N	—	—	—	—	—	V	E	V	H	—
W	E	—	—	S	N	G	—	—	—	—	—	Q	A	P	E	—
W	T	—	—	—	L	G	—	—	—	—	—	B	S	S	S	—
W	F	—	—	V	D	N	—	—	—	—	—	V	E	V	H	—
W	T	—	—	N	N	G	—	—	—	—	—	K	T	E	L	—
W	N	—	—	—	S	G	—	—	—	—	—	A	L	T	S	—
W	F	—	—	V	D	N	—	—	—	—	—	K	P	V	G	—
W	A	—	—	S	N	R	—	—	—	V	P	V	S	E	K	—
W	N	—	—	—	S	G	—	—	—	—	—	T	L	T	D	—
W	Y	—	—	I	B	B	—	—	—	—	—	Z	Q	V	R	—
W	E	—	—	K	D	G	—	—	—	—	—	K	A	E	D	—
W	K	—	—	Y	K	*N*	—	—	—	—	N	S	D	I	S	—
W	L	—	—	R	E	G	—	—	—	—	K	Q	V	G	S	—
W	T	—	—	R	Q	D	—	—	—	—	—	G	E	—	—	—
W	Q.	—	—	M	Q	R	—	—	—	G	Q	P	L	S	P	E
W	B	—	—	—	T	G	—	—	—	—	—	S	L	*N*	—	—
W	L	—	—	Z	B	G	—	—	—	—	—	Z	V	M	—	—
W	S	—	—	R	A	S	—	—	—	—	—	G	K	—	—	—
W	L	—	—	H	N	E	—	—	—	—	—	V	Q	L	P	—
W	S	—	—	—	Z	S	—	—	—	—	—	G	Z	G	V	—
W	T	—	—	—	P	S	—	—	—	—	—	S	G	K	S	—
W	L	—	—	Q	G	S	—	—	—	—	Q	E	L	P	R	E
▲					▲											
W	K	—	—	A	D	G	S	—	—	—	—	P	V	K	—	—
W	Y	Q	Q	H	A	G	K	—	—	—	—	—	—	—	—	R
L	L	—	—	K	D	G	—	—	—	—	—	E	R	I	—	—

amino acid code:

P	proline (h)		W	tryptophan
Q	glutamine		Y	tyrosine
R	arginine		Z	glutamic acid
S	serine			or glutamine
T	threonine			
V	valine (h)		(n)	non-polar
			(h)	hydrophobic

hydrophobic residues at alternating positions are shown by sans serif letters. A column in which serine residues are largely conserved is similarly shown. Rows 33 and 34, the domains of Bence–Jones dimer (Mcg) have been aligned using the results of Edmundson *et al.* (1975). Residues having extended structure, mainly involved in β-pleated sheets are

			fx3											b4
Human (New) IgG₁	F	S	V	S	K	S	G	—	—	—	—	—	—	—	—
	V	T	M	L	V	N	T	—	S	—	—	—	—	—	—
	—	G	V	E	T	T	T	P	S	K	Q	—	—	S	N
	—	G	V	H	T	F	P	A	V	L	Q	—	—	S	S

(filled triangles ▼ below columns 3 and 5)

							70								
Human (Eu) IgG₁	—	N	A	K	T	K	P	R	E	Q	Q	—	—	Y	*N*
	—	N	Y	K	T	T	P	P	V	L	D	—	—	S	D
Human (Vin) IgG₄	—	N	A	K	T	K	P	R	E	E	Q	—	—	F	*N*
	—	B	Y)	K	T	T	P	P	V	L	D	—	—	S	D
Mouse (MOPC 21) IgG₁	—	G	V	H	T	F	P	A	V	L	Q	—	—	S	D
	—	T	A	Q	T	Q	P	R	E	E	Q	—	—	F	*N*
	—	N	Y	K	N	T	Q	P	I	M	D	—	—	T	D
Mouse (MOPC 173) IgG₂ₐ	—	G	V	H	T	F	P	A	V	L	Q	—	—	S	D
	—	Q	A	Q	T	T	H	T	R	Q	N	—	—	Y	*N*
	—	N	Y	K	N	T	Q	P	V	L	D	—	—	S	D
Guinea pig IgG₂	—	G	V	H	T	F	P	A	V	L	Q	—	—	S	G
	—	N	A	E	T	K	P	R	V	E	Q	—	—	Y	*N*
	—	E	Y	K	N	T	P	P	I	E	D	—	—	A	D
Rabbit IgG	—	G	V	R	T	F	P	S	V	R	Q	—	—	S	S
	—	T	A	R	P	P	L	R	E	Q	Q	—	—	F	*N*
	—	D	Y	K	T	T	P	A	V	L	D	—	—	S	D
Human (Gal) IgM	—	S	T	R	G	F	P	S	V	L	R	—	—	G	G
	—	G	V	T	T	N	E	V	Z	A	Z	A	K	E	S
	—	A	V	K	T	H	T	*N*	I	S	Z	S	H	P	*N*
	—	K	Y	V	T	S	A	P	M	P	E	P	Q	A	P
Human (ND) IgE	—	G	T	T	L	P	A	T	T	L	T	—	—	L	S
	—	D	V	D	L	S	T	A	S	T	E	—	—	S	E
	—	P	V	B	H	S	T	R	K	E	E	K	Q	R	*N*
	—	D	A	R	H	S	T	T	Q	P	R	K	T	K	G
Human IgA₁	—	T	A	R	B	F	P	P	S	Z	B	—	—	A	S
	—	A	V	Q	G	P	P	B	R	D	L	—	—	C	G
	—	K	Y	L	T	W	A	S	R	Q	Q	P	S	Q	G

(open triangles ▲ above columns 3, 5 and 8)

Human (Mcg)	A	G	V	E	T	T	K	P	S	K	Q	—	—	S	N
	F	S	G	S	K	S	G	—	—	—	—	—	—	—	—
β-microglob'	E	K	V	E	H	S	D	L	S	F	—	—	—	S	K

Single-letter

A	alanine (n)	G	glycine (n)
B	aspartic-acid or	H	histidine
	asparagine	I	isoleucine (h)
C	cysteine	K	lysine
D	aspartic acid	L	leucine (h)
E	glutamic acid	M	methionine (h)
F	phenylalanine (h)	N	asparagine

underlined. Residue whose side chains point to the interior of the C_L domain are marked at the top by a filled triangle. hr, hinge region. tp, extra-domain tail piece. Amino acid sequences were obtained from: human IgG1 (NEW)—Poljak *et al.* (1974); human IgG1 (Eu), human IgG4 (Vin), and rabbit IgG—Dayhoff (1972), Croft (1974); mouse IgG1—

```
                        fx4                                    b5
— — — — — — — S  S  A  T  L  A  I  T  G  L  Q  — —
— — — — — K   N  Q  F  S  L  R  L  S  S  V  T  — —
N — — K Y A   S  S  Y  L  S  L  T  P  E  Q  — —
G — — L Y S L S  S  V  V  T  V  P  S  S  S  — —
          ▼        ▼        ▼        ▼

    80                              90
S — — T Y R V V S V L T V L H Q N — —
G — — S F F L Y S K L T V D K S R — —
.     .   .   .   .   .   .   .   .   .   .   .   .   .   .   .   .
S — — T Y R V (V S V L T V L H Z B — —
G — — S F F L Y S R L T V D K S R — —

— — — L Y T L S S S V S V P T S P — —
S — — T F R V V S A L P I M H Q D — —
G — — S Y F V Y S K L N V Q K S N — —

— — — L Y S S S V T V T V T S S S T —
S — — T L R V V S A L P I Q H Q N — —
G — — S Y F M Y S K L R V E K K N — —

— — — L Y S L T S M V T V P S S Q — —
T — — T F R V E S V L P I Q H Q D — —
G — — S Y F L Y S K L T V D K S A — —

G — — L Y S V P S T V S V S Z P — —
S — — T I R V V S T L P I A H E D — —
G — — S W F L Y S K L S V P T S E — —

— — — K Y A A T S Q V L L P S K D V M
G P T T Y K V T S T L T I K E S B — —
A — — T F S A V G E A S I C E B B — —
G — — R Y F A H S I L T V S E E E — —

G — — H Y A T I S L L T V S G A — —
G E — L A S T E S E L T L S Q K H — —
G — — T L T V T S T L P V G T R B — —
S — — G F F V F S R L E V T R A E — —

G B — L Y T T S S Q L T L P A T Z C —
C — — — Y S V S S V L P G C A Q P — —
T E — T F A V T S I L R V A A E D — —
          ▲        ▲        ▲        ▲
N — — K Y A A S S Y L S L T P E Q — —
— — — — — N T A S L T V S G L Q — —
N W — S F Y L L L Y S Y T E F T P T — —
```

amino acid code:

P	proline (h)	W	tryptophan
Q	glutamine	Y	tyrosine
R	arginine	Z	glutamic acid
S	serine		or glutamine
T	threonine		
V	valine (h)	(n)	non-polar
		(h)	hydrophobic

Milstein *et al.* (1974), Adetugbo *et al.* (1975); mouse IgG2a—Bourgois *et al.* (1974), Rocca-Serra *et al.* (1975); guinea-pig IgG2—Tracy and Cebra (1974), Trischmann and Cebra (1974); human IgM (Gal)—Watanabe *et al.* (1973); human IgE (ND)—Bennich and Bahr-Lindström (1974); human IgA1—Kratzin *et al.* (1976); Bence–Jones dimer (Mcg)—Edmundson *et al.* (1975); β-microglobulin—Cunningham (1974)

							fy2							b6
Human (New)	A	E	D	E	A	D	Y	Y	C	Q	S	Y	D	R	S
IgG₁	A	A	D	T	A	V	Y	Y	C	A	R	B	L	I	A
	W	K	S	H	K	S	Y	S	C	Q	V	T	H	—	—
	—	L	G	T	Q	T	Y	I	C	N	V	N	H	K	P
				▼			▼			▼			▼		

Position markers: **100** (over 3rd column), **110** (over 13th column)

Human (Eu)	W	L	D	G	K	E	Y	K	C	K	V	S	N	K	A
IgG₁	W	Q	Q	G	N	V	F	S	C	S	V	M	H	E	A
Human (Vin)	.	.	.	.	.	T	Y	T	C	N	V	D	H	K	P
IgG₄	W	L	B	G)	K	E	Y	K	C	K	V	S	N	K	G
	(W	Z	Z	G	B	V	F	S	C	S	V	M	(H	Z	A
Mouse (MOPC	—	—	—	—	E	T	V	T	C	N	V	A	H	A	P
21) IgG₁	W	L	N	G	K	E	F	K	C	R	V	N	S	A	A
	W	Q	A	G	N	T	F	T	C	S	V	L	H	E	G
Mouse (MOPC	W	P	S	Q	S	I	T	N	C	N	V	A	H	P	A
173) IgG₂ₐ	W	M	S	G	K	E	F	K	C	K	V	N	N	K	D
	W	V	E	R	N	S	F	S	C	S	V	V	H	Q	G
Guinea pig	—	—	—	—	—	K	A	T	C	N	V	A	H	P	A
IgG₂	W	L	R	G	K	E	F	K	C	K	V	Y	N	K	A
	W	D	Q	G	T	V	Y	T	C	S	V	M	H	E	A
Rabbit IgG	—	—	—	—	—	(P	S)	T	C	B	V	A	H	A	(T
	W	L	R	G	K	E	F	K	C	K	V	H	D	K	A
	W	Q	R	G	D	V	F	T	C	S	V	M	H	E	A
Human (Gal)	Q	G	T	N	E	H	V	V	C	K	V	Z	H	P	B
IgM	W	L	S	Q	S	M	F	T	C	R	V	D	H	R	G
	W	N	S	G	E	R	F	T	C	T	V	T	H	T	D
	W	N	T	G	E	T	Y	T	C	V	V	A	H	E	A
Human (ND)	W	A	K	—	Q	M	F	T	C	R	V	A	H	—	—
IgE	W	L	S	D	R	T	Y	Z	C	E	V	T	Y	—	—
	W	I	E	G	E	T	Y	Z	C	R	V	T	H	P	H
	W	Q	E	K	D	E	F	I	C	R	A	V	H	E	A
Human IgA₁	—	L	A	G	K	S	V	T	C	H	V	K	H	—	—
	W	N	H	G	K	T	F	T	C	T	A	A	Y	P	E
	W	K	K	G	D	T	F	S	C	M	V	G	H	E	A
	▲						▲		▲			▲		▲	
Human (Mcg)	W	K	S	H	R	S	Y	S	C	Q	V	T	H	—	—
	A	E	D	E	A	D	Y	Y	C	S	S	Y	E	G	S
β-microglob'	—	E	K	—	D	E	Y	A	C	R	V	N	H	—	—

Single-letter

A	alanine (n)	G	glycine (n)
B	aspartic-acid or asparagine	H	histidine
C	cysteine	I	isoleucine (h)
D	aspartic acid	K	lysine
E	glutamic acid	L	leucine (h)
F	phenylalanine (h)	M	methionine (h)
		N	asparagine

```
                    fy3                                      e2
— — —   L̶  R   —  V̶  F   G̶  G   G̶ T̶  K̶  L̶  T̶  V  L̶  R   1  V_L
G — —   C̶  I   B̶ V̶  W   G̶  Q   G̶ S̶  L  V̶  T̶  V  S̶  S   2  V_H
E G —   S̶  T   —  V̶  B   K̶  T   —  V̶  A  P   T   E  C   S   3  C_L
S N —   T̶  K   —  V̶  D   K   R   —  V̶  E  P   K   S  C   hr  4  C_γ1
                    ▼                        ▼
                    120
L P —   A  P   —  I   E   K   T   —  I   S  K   A   K  G       5  C_γ2
L H N   H  Y   —  T   Q   K   S   —  L   S  L   S   P  G       6  C_γ3
S N —   T  K   —  V   D   K   R   —  V   E  S   K   Y  G   hr  7  C_γ1
L P —   S  S   —  I   E   K   T   —  I   S  K   A   K  G       8  C_γ2
L H B   H  Y)  —  T   Q   K   S   —  L   S  L   S   L  G       9  C_γ3
S S —   T  K   —  V   D   K   K   —  I   V  P   R   D  C   hr 10  C_γ1
F P —   A  P   —  I   E   K   T   —  I   S  K   T   K  G      11  C_γ2
L H N   H  H   —  T   E   K   S   —  L   S  H   S   P  G      12  C_γ3
S S —   T  K   —  V   D   K   K   —  I   E  P   R   G  P   hr 13  C_γ1
L P —   A  P   —  I   E   R   T   —  I   S  K   P   K  G      14  C_γ2
L H N   H  V   —  S   T   K   S   —  F   S  R   T   P  G      15  C_γ3
S S —   T  K   —  V   D   K   T   —  V   E  P   I   R  T   hr 16  C_γ1
L P —   A  P   —  I   E   K   T   —  I   S  K   T   K  G      17  C_γ2
L H N   H  V   —  T   Q   K   A   —  I   S  R   S   P  G      18  C_γ3
B) — —  T  K   —  V   D   K   T   —  V   A  P   S   T  C   hr 19  C_γ1
L P —   A  P   —  I   E   K   T   —  I   S  K   A   R  G      20  C_γ2
L H N   H  Y   —  T   Q   K   S   —  I   S  R   S   P  G      21  C_γ3
G B —   K  E   —  K   D   V   P   —  L   P  V   I   A  —      22  C_μ1
— — —   L  T   —  F   Q   Q   N'  —  A   S  S   M   C  V   P  23  C_μ2
L P —   S  P   —  L   K   Q   T   —  I   S  R   P   K  G      24  C_μ3
L P N   R  V   —  T   E   R   T   —  V   D  K   S   T  G   tp 25  C_μ4
T P —   S  S   —  T   B   N'  V   —  K   T  F   S   V  C   S  26  C_ε1
Z G ←   H  T   —  F   Z   B   S   —  T   K  K   C   —  —      27  C_ε2
L P —   R  A   —  L   M   R   S   —  T   T  K   T   S  —      28  C_ε3
A S P   S  Q   —  T   V   Q   R   A  V   S  V   N   P  G   K  29  C_ε4
Y T —   B  P   —  S   Z   B   V   —  T   V  P   C   —  —   hr 30  C_α1
— — —   S  K   —  T   P   L   T   A  T   L  S   K   S  G      31  C_α2
L P L   A  F   —  T   Q   K   T   —  I   D  R   L   A  G   tp 32  C_α3
                    ▲                        ▲
E G —   S  T   —  V   E   K   —   T  V   A  P   T   E  C   S  33  C_L
D — —   N  F   —  V   F   G   T   G  T   K  V   T   V  L   G  34  V_L
V T —   L  S   —  Q   P   K   I   —  V   K  W   D   R  D   M  35
```

amino acid code:

P	proline (h)	W	tryptophan
Q	glutamine	Y	tyrosine
R	arginine	Z	glutamic acid
S	serine		or glutamine
T	threonine		
V	valine (h)	(n)	non-polar
		(h)	hydrophobic

columns 8, 32, 108, and 119 in Figure 8 are in close proximity in the three-dimensional model and involve segments fx1, fx2, fy2, and fy3. Similarly, the side chains of residues in columns 28, 66, and 89 are near to each other and involve segments fx2, fx3, and fx4. The tendency to form such hydrophobic clusters probably influences the pattern of folding of the domains. Regions of the C-domain sequences which correspond to non-β-pleated segments of the crystallographic models have very little overall homology.

Examination of V-domain sequences (Dayhoff, 1972) shows that some of the conserved hydrophobic sites found in C domains also occur in V domains (see columns 6, 8, 26, 28, 30, 45, 47, 89, 91, 104, and 106), but others do not. On the other hand, V domains tend to conserve hydrophobic residues at some positions where C domains do not (columns 14, 16, 64, 87, 94, 126, and 128). Different hydrophobic clusters are produced therefore. For example, in V_L (NEW) the side chains of residues in columns 14, 26, 91, 94, 126, and 128 are in close proximity. Another cluster involves side chains from residues in columns 28, 47, 66, 89, and 104, and two sites in the loop which C domains do not have. Such differences in hydrophobic clustering probably influence the differences in chain-folding between V and C domains.

From this discussion, it appears highly probable that the C domains shown in rows 5–32 of Figure 8 would have the same basic immunoglobulin fold as that seen in high-resolution crystallographic models. Also, it is likely that these C domains would have more of the characteristics of the crystallographic C domains than of the V domains.

Some C domains appear to have conserved certain sequence features, thus suggesting the possibility of specialized folding in localized regions of the domain. From Figure 8 it will be seen that $C_\gamma 2$, $C_\mu 3$, and $C_\varepsilon 3$ have three consecutive hydrophobic residues in segment b1 (columns 20–22). Furthermore, most C domains have a noticeably conserved triplet of residues in columns 35–37 consisting of an aromatic, a hydrophobic and proline residue. $C_\gamma 2$, $C_\mu 3$, and $C_\alpha 2$ clearly lack this feature of segment b2. $C_\gamma 2$, $C_\alpha 2$ and $C_\mu 2$ domains do not have a histidine residue (H) in column 110 as do other C domains.

Regions where homology is very poor, such as columns 58–81 in Figure 8 may have undergone specialized folding, particularly in C_μ and C_ε domains. Even when homology is good there can be some unexpected differences in peptide chain folding. Thus, Deisenhofer et al. (1976) and Huber et al. (1976) have reported that, although most of the $C_\gamma 2$ domain has a remarkably similar folding to that of $C_\gamma 3$ and $C_\gamma 1$, there are significant variations in two of the bends and two of the β-pleated segments. In Figures 4 and 8, these differences would involve b3, fx3, b4, and fx4. Although homology between $C_\gamma 2$ and $C_\gamma 3$ is very good from columns 65 to 70 of Figure 8, the peptide-chain folding is significantly different. In $C_\gamma 3$, these residues form part of the β-pleated segment fx3 as in $C_\gamma 1$ and C_L, whereas in $C_\gamma 2$, they form an extension to b3 to give an extra kink somewhat reminiscent of V domains. Segment fx3 consequently is shortened and displaced in $C_\gamma 2$ relative to the analogous segment in $C_\gamma 3$, $C_\gamma 1$, and C_L. Accompanying displacements of b4 and fx4 also occur. Huber et al. (1976) have pointed out that the differences result in these segments showing some resemblance to V-domain folding.

5 DISULPHIDE BRIDGES

Each domain has an intra-domain disulphide bridge. It lies in the hydrophobic space between the domain faces and is therefore inaccessible to thiol-reducing agents in aqueous solution. The light-chain cysteine residue which participates in the light–heavy disulphide bridge is situated at the C-terminal end of the C_L domain (segment e2 of Figure 4; rows 3, 33 of Figure 8). In human and mouse IgG1, the heavy-chain cysteine residue completing this light–heavy disulphide bridge lies at the C-terminal end of the $C_\gamma 1$ domain (segment e2 of Figure 4; rows 4 and 10 of Figure 8). In all other immunoglobulins shown in Figure 8, the light–heavy bridge is completed by a cysteine residue lying in segment b1 of the $C_\gamma 1$, $C_\mu 1$, $C_\varepsilon 1$, or $C_\alpha 1$ domains (columns 14 or 15, Figure 8). Examination of the crystallographic models shows that e2 and b1 are in close spatial proximity (Figure 9). Rabbit IgG and human IgE have an additional intra-chain disulphide bridge. This bond is accessible to thiol reagents in aqueous solution. In both cases, the cysteine residues which form this bridge lie in segments b1 and e2 (rows 19 and 26, columns 14 or 15 and 129; Figure 8) which are in close proximity (Figure 9). IgA probably has additional intra-chain disulphide bridges, which are accessible to reducing agents, linking b5 and e2 in the $C_\alpha 1$ domain (row 30, columns 14 and 127, Figure 8; Figure 9) and linking b4 to e1 in the $C_\alpha 2$ domain (row 31, columns 4 and 27, Figure 8; Figure 9).

The inter-heavy chain disulphide bridges of IgG lie in the non-domain hinge region (see Figure 10). IgM has no such region but has a symmetrical bridge at the C-terminal end of the $C_\mu 2$ domain in segment e2 (row 23, column 128, Figure 8; Figure 10). There is also a μ bridge between μ chains at b5 in the $C_\mu 3$ domain of human IgM, and this was thought to act as the only inter-subunit bridge (Beale and Feinstein, 1969, 1970; Miekka and Deutsch, 1970). In contrast the inter-μ-chain bridge in the extra-domain tail piece (Figure 10) was thought to be intra-subunit; however more recent evidence (Feinstein *et al.*, 1976) has shown that this extra-domain bridge is also inter-subunit, as in Figure 2. The $C_\mu 3$ bridge has not been detected in mouse IgM (Milstein *et al.*, 1975). IgE also has no hinge region analogous to that of IgG. There are, however, two inter-ε chain bridges in segments b1 and b2 of the $C_\varepsilon 2$ domain (row 27, columns 15 and 127, Figure 8; Figure 10). IgA possibly has inter-heavy chain bridges at e1 or b4 of the $C_\alpha 2$ domains (row 31, Figure 8; Figure 9). Cysteine residues in b5 of the $C_\alpha 2$ domain and in the non-domain tail piece also probably from inter-α-chain bridges one of which may be involved in polymerization (row 31, Figure 8; Figure 9).

6 OLIGOSACCHARIDE SITES

All immunoglobulin heavy chains contain N-linked oligosaccharide and there appears to be an homologous site in segment b4 of $C_\gamma 2$, $C_\mu 3$, and $C_\varepsilon 3$ domains,

282

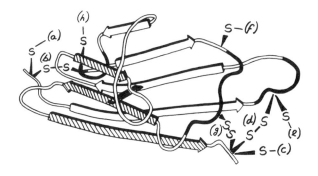

Figure 9 Location of disulphide bridges on the three-dimensional model of the C domain (adapted from Edmundson *et al.*, 1975). Light–heavy bridge links position (c) of the C_L domain to position (e) in the C_H1 domain of all immunoglobulins shown in Figure 8, except human and mouse IgG1, which have the L chain attached to position (c) of the C_H1 domain. IgG has inter-γ-chain bridges in the extra-domain region (Figure 10). Rabbit IgG has an additional intra-chain bridge (d) in the C_H1 domain. IgM has an inter-μ-chain bridge at position (c) in the $C_\mu2$ domain. A bridge at (f) in the $C_\mu3$ domain of human IgM is probably inter-subunit but absent in mouse IgM. IgE has an additional intra-chain bridge at (d) in the $C_\varepsilon1$ domain, and inter-ε-chain bridges at (c) and (e) in the $C_\varepsilon2$ domain. IgA has several bridges in the hinge region (Figure 10). In the $C_\alpha1$ domain there is an additional intra-chain bridge at (g). In the $C_\alpha2$ domain there are probably inter-α-chain bridges at positions (a, f, and h) and an additional intra-chain bridge at (b)

but not in the $C_\alpha2$ domain (column 78, Figure 8; Figure 11). There are also sites in b3/$C_\mu1$, fy3/$C_\mu2$, fx3/$C_\mu3$, b1/$C_\varepsilon1$, b3/$C_\varepsilon1$, fy3/$C_\varepsilon1$, fy1/$C_\varepsilon2$, fy1/$C_\varepsilon3$, and fx2/$C_\alpha2$ (Figure 11). All these sites are at positions analogous to those which point away from the domain interior in the model of Fab' (NEW). This provides further support for the concept that all C domains have similar peptide-chain folding since oligosaccharide would be excluded from the essentially hydrophobic interior of the domain. The role of this oligosaccharide is uncertain but some of it may influence domain interaction as discussed in the next section. It should be noted that IgA is unique in having *O*-linked carbohydrate in a non-domain region analogous to the hinge region of IgG (see Figure 10).

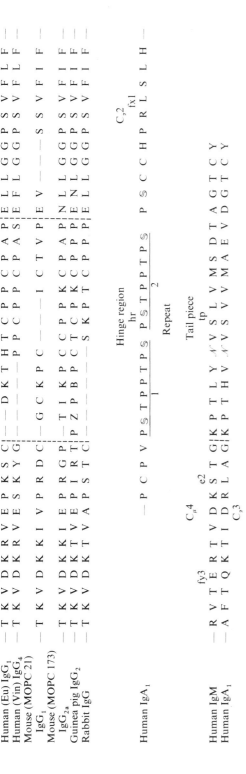

Figure 10 sequence alignment (Extra-domain regions):

```
                                  fy3                 e2                                      hr            el           fx1
Human (Eu) IgG₁       — T K V D K R V E P K S C — — — D K T H T C P P C P A P E L L G G P S V F L F —
Human (Vin) IgG₄      — T K V D K R V E S K Y G — — — —   P P C P S C E F L G G P S V F L F —
Mouse (MOPC 21)
  IgG₁                — T K V D K K I V P R D C — — — G C K P C — — I C T V P E V — — S S V F I F —
Mouse (MOPC 173)
  IgG₂ₐ               — T K V D K K I E P R G P — T I K P C C P P K C P A P N L L G G P S V F I F —
Guinea pig IgG₂       — T K V D K T V E P I R T P Z P B P C T C P P P E N L G G P S V F I F —
Rabbit IgG            — T K V D K T V A P S T C — — — — S K P T C P P P E L L G G P S V F I F —
```

Hinge region
hr
C_γ2
fx1

```
Human IgA₁   — P C P V P S T P P P T S   P S T P P P T S   P S C C H P R L S L H —
                       1                  2
```

Repeat

Tail piece
tp

C_μ4   e2
fy3   C_γ3

```
Human IgM     — R V T E R T V D K S T G K P T L Y N V S L V M S D T A G T C Y
Human IgA₁    — A F T Q K T I D R L A G K P T H V V S V V M A E V D G T C Y
```

Figure 10 Extra-domain regions. The top part of the figure shows the hinge regions of the immunoglobulins given in Figure 8. Probable end of the C_γ1 domain and the most probable beginning of the C_γ2 domain are indicated by vertical broken lines. The centre of the figure gives the hinge region of IgA1. The first cysteine (C_γ2) residue most probably lies at the end of the C_α1 domain. The unique nature of this hinge region makes the location of the beginning of the C_γ2 domain uncertain. However, the first β-pleated segment (fx1) probably starts at the last proline (P) residue shown. S sites for simple O-linked carbohydrate. The bottom of the figure shows the extra tail piece which is found only in μ and α chains. In IgM pentamers, and IgA dimers and tetramers one J chain per polymer is attached to the cyteine residue of a tail piece. N, Sites of N-linked oligosaccharide

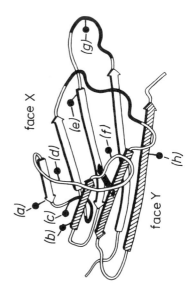

face X

face Y

(a) (b) (c) (d) (e) (f) (g) (h)

Figure 11 Sites of attachment of oligosaccharide on the three-dimensional model (adapted from Edmundson et al., 1975) of the C domain (see also Figure 6). IgG has site (c) in the C_γ2 domain. IgM has site (f) in the C_μ1 domain; (h) in C_μ2; (a) and (c) in C_μ3. IgE has sites (g), (d), and (h) in C_ε1; (b) in C_ε2; (b) and (c) in C_ε3. IgA has site (e) in C_α2 and also sites in the hinge region

7 DOMAIN INTERACTIONS

7.1 Pairing

The high resolution crystallographic results for Fab' (NEW) (Poljak *et al.*, 1973), Bence–Jones dimer (Schiffer *et al.*, 1973), mouse Fab (Segal *et al.*, 1974), and V-region dimer (Epp *et al.*, 1974) have revealed that V domains and C domains pair at different faces (Figures 3 and 5). Contact between V domains involves segments fy1, fy2, fy3, and part of the extra loop, whereas contact between C domains involves segments fx1, fx2, and fx3. Some of the residues most likely to provide contacts between C_L and $C_\gamma 1$ domains lie in columns 9, 11, 29, 31, and 69 of C_L, and columns 7, 9, 11, 31, 69, and 72 of $C_\gamma 1$ (Figure 8). Residues in columns 11, 29, 31, 69, 86, and 88 of provide important contacts between the C_L domains in the λ dimer (Edmundson *et al.*, 1975).

It will be seen from Figure 8 that many of the columns containing the contact residues for the $C_\gamma 1$ and C_L domains display noticeably conserved features, such as an aromatic residue in column 9, phenylalanine (F) or leucine (L) residues in column 11, and valine (V) or leucine (L) residues in column 31. Although this suggests that other C domains interact in a similar manner to that of the $C_\gamma 1$ and C_L domains of Fab' (NEW) (Fab–C-like pairing), Beale and Feinstein (1976) have pointed out that $C_\gamma 2$, $C_\alpha 2$, $C_\mu 3$, and $C_\varepsilon 3$ domains are highly unlikely to undergo such pairing. In Fab–C-type pairing, domains are crossed in such a way as to allow their C-terminal regions to come relatively close together, often linked by a disulphide bridge, but their N-terminal regions are more remote from each other. The restriction imposed by the disulphide-bridged hinge region at the N-terminus of $C_\gamma 2$ domains makes Fab–C-like pairing virtually impossible. $C_\alpha 2$ domains probably have an inter-α-chain bridge at their N-terminal ends again making Fab–C-like pairing of these domains impossible. Similarly, the inter-chain disulphide bridge at the C-terminal ends of the $C_\mu 2$ domains (almost certainly paired Fab–C-like) means that the N-termini of the $C_\mu 3$ domains must be held too close together to allow similar pairing of these domains. Likewise, the inter-chain disulphide bridge at the C-terminal ends of the $C_\varepsilon 2$ domain would not allow such pairing of $C_\varepsilon 3$ domains.

Beale and Feinstein (1976) have further pointed out that, since $C_\gamma 2$, $C_\alpha 2$, $C_\mu 3$, and $C_\varepsilon 3$ are much more closely related to other C domains than to V domains, V-like pairing of these C domains is as unlikely as Fab–C-like pairing. They also suggest that there is no apparent reason why $C_\gamma 3$, $C_\alpha 3$, $C_\mu 4$, and $C_\varepsilon 4$ domains should not pair in a Fab–C-like manner.

The crystallographic results for a human IgG Fc fragment obtained by Deisenhofer *et al.*, (1976) and discussed by Huber *et al.*, (1976) support the above predictions concerning domain pairing. The results show that $C_\gamma 3$ domains pair in a similar manner to the C_L and $C_H 1$ domains of Fab' (NEW) and mouse Fab, whereas the $C_\gamma 2$ domains are not in contact with each other (see Figures 6 and 14).

Deisenhofer *et al.* (1976) and Huber *et al.* (1976) have reported the introduction of a polar group in the $C_\gamma 2$ domain at a site which carries a hydrophobic contact residue in $C_\gamma 1$ and $C_\gamma 3$ domains. Such a modification could prevent Fab–C-like pairing of $C_\gamma 2$ domains. These authors also state that the oligosaccharide of the $C_\gamma 2$ domain appears to obscure some of the residues that might be expected to make inter-domain contact (columns 9, 11, 31, and 33, Figure 8). It is intriguing to speculate whether the role of this oligosaccharide is to prevent the formation of such contacts during chain assembly. The homologous oligosaccharide in $C_\mu 3$ and $C_\varepsilon 3$ domains may indicate a similar arrangement of these domains to that of the $C_\gamma 2$ domains, although the $C_\alpha 2$ domain does not have this homologous oligosaccharide site (c), but has a unique site (e) at which the oligosaccharide could play a similar role (see Figure 11).

7.2 Longitudinal Contact

The high resolution crystallographic results of Fab' (NEW), Bence–Jones dimer and mouse Fab (Poljak *et al.*, 1973; Schiffer *et al.*, 1973; Segal *et al.*, 1974) show that there is limited longitudinal contact between V_L and C_L, and between V_H and $C_H 1$. In the model of Fab' (NEW) (Poljak *et al.*, 1973, 1974) only segment b4 of the C_L domain is near the V_L domain (see Figure 4) and only segments b2 and b6 of $C_H 1$ approach the V_H domain. Due to the angle between the pseudo two-fold axes of rotation for the V-domain pair and the C-domain pair, V_L and C_L are more separated than are V_H and $C_H 1$. In crystals of IgG (Kol), the domains of the Fab region are arranged more symmetrically than in Fab' (NEW) and mouse Fab, and neither V domain is in close contact with a C domain (Colman *et al.*, 1976; Huber *et al.*, 1976).

In the crystallographic Fc fragment (Deisenhofer *et al.*, 1976; Huber *et al.*, 1976), segments b1 and b5 of $C_\gamma 2$, and b2/fy1 and b6 of $C_\gamma 3$ provide longitudinal contacts. Huber *et al.* (1976) have pointed out that the $C_\gamma 2$–$C_\gamma 3$ contact is homologous to the V_H–$C_H 1$ contact in Fab crystals. In Fc crystals, there is a true axis of two-fold rotational symmetry so that these contacts are identical in both chains.

Such longitudinal contacts are important to any theory of immunoglobulin function involving changes in domain interactions and this aspect will be discussed more fully in a later section (see Section 9).

8 MODEL BUILDING

It has been shown, in the case of IgM, that data of the type discussed so far together with electron micrographs of IgM molecules free and attached to particulate antigens can be used to build a satisfactory model of this immunoglobulin (Feinstein, 1974; Beale and Feinstein, 1976; Feinstein *et al.*, 1976). The general principles which have been used are equally applicable to other immunoglobulin classes, and can be briefly summarized.

(*i*) As has been seen, on the basis of sequence homologies shown in Figure 8, it is reasonable to assume that the positions of cysteine residues may be mapped spacially onto the immunoglobulin fold (Figure 9). Inter-domain disulphide bridges then provide useful clues to the spacial relationship of the domains involved, and will stabilize weak specific interactions. Where crystallographic data reveal adaptations in the folding of a particular domain, these should, of course, be incorporated when considering that of any evidently homologous domain in other immunoglobulin classes or subclasses.

(*ii*) The assumption has been made that longitudinal interactions between heavy chain domains, approximating to those seen in crystals of Fab fragments, would be conserved and used elsewhere along heavy chains, resulting in a zig-zag or helical arrangement of domains along the chain. Deisenhofer *et al.* (1976) have since shown that there is indeed such a homologous longitudinal interaction

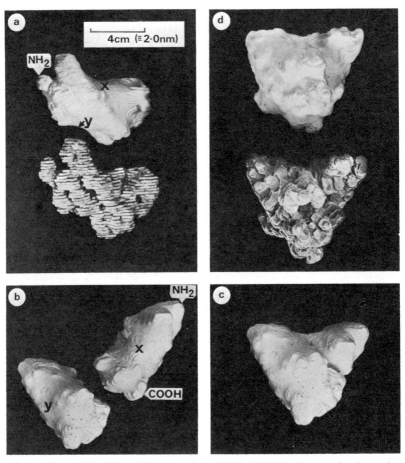

Figure 12 (a) Models of $C_\gamma 1$ domains of Fab' (NEW). *Bottom* glued wooden sections representing density at 0·1 nm intervals. *Top* plaster of Paris cast of the wooden model. (b) Two $C_\gamma 1$ domain casts orientated to give an 'exploded view' of a Fab–C-like pair. (c) Model showing Fab–C-like pairing of two $C_\gamma 1$ domains. (d) Models of C_L–$C_\gamma 1$ pairs of Fab' (NEW). *Bottom* glued wooden sections representing density at 0·1 mn intervals. *Top* plaster of Paris cast of the wooden model (seen from a slightly different aspect to that in c)

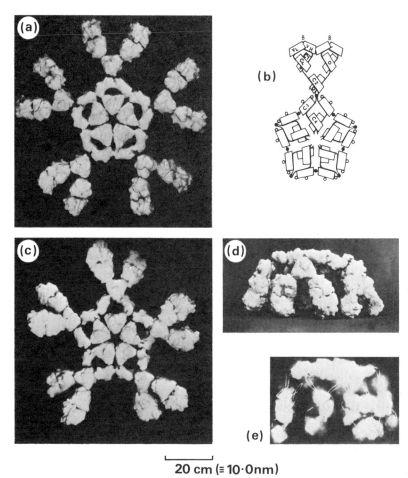

20 cm (≡ 10·0nm)

Figure 13 IgM models. (a) Model made from cast domains showing all five F(ab')₂ arms; (b) model showing only one of the five F(ab')₂ arms (from Feinstein, 1974). •, interchain disulphide bridge; 0, site of attachment of oligosaccharide; □, regions of polypeptide chains folded into domains. $C_\mu2$ and $C_\mu4$ each form Fab–C-like pairs. (c) the arrangement of the $C_\mu3$ domains modified to resemble the arrangement of $C_\gamma2$ domains of the Fc of IgG as described by Deisenhofer *et al.* (1976) and Huber *et al.* (1976). (d) 'Table' form of the IgM model corresponding to the 'staple' in electron micrographs (see Figure 16). (e) X-ray photograph in the 'table' form to simulate the 'staple' in electron micrographs

between the $C_\gamma2$ and $C_\gamma3$ domains in human IgG Fc crystals (see Figures 6 and 14).

(*iii*) Where the contact residues permit it, it has been assumed that corresponding C domains along adjacent heavy chains will pair off laterally in a Fab–C-like manner. Two such pairs cannot occur sequentially along the chains without disrupting the longitudinal interactions, and moreover would require additional sequences between domains.

In the case of IgM, the model must be consistent with the electron micrographs. These will be discussed later (Figure 16). As previously described (Beale and Feinstein, 1976; Feinstein *et al.*, 1976) wooden models based on α-carbon co-ordinates provided by Dr. R. Poljak, were constructed of a single $C_\gamma 1$ domain (Figure 12a), a $C_L-C_\gamma 1$ pair (Figure 12d), and a V_L-V_H pair, then moulds were prepared, and multiple identical plaster of Paris casts were made. Regions representing the few residues at the end of domains were replaced by appropriate lengths of wire. Figure 13a shows the assembled IgM model. As indicated in the corresponding diagram (Figure 13b), it was assumed that the $C_\mu 2$ and $C_\mu 4$ domains each form Fab–C-like pairs. The similarity of the arrangement of domains $C_\mu 3$ and $C_\mu 4$ arrived at in each subunit to those found by Huber *et al.* (1976) in the Fc of IgG was encouraging, and in Figure 13c the $C_\mu 3$ domains have been rearranged slightly to resemble the corresponding $C_\gamma 2$ arrangement more closely.

The Fab–C-like pairing of $C_\mu 2$ domains is in accordance with the frequent appearance of a compact region lying between a pair of Fab arms and the central Fc disc in electron micrographs. Although there is no stable interaction between the $C_\mu 2$ domain in isolated Fab′ fragments a weak interaction may be stabilized by the disulphide bridge linking the C-terminal ends of these domains, and possibly by longitudinal interactions between the $C_\mu 2$ and $C_\mu 3$ domains. Evidence for such interaction in human IgM is provided by the failure to observe non-covalent interactions in reduced Fc_μ preparations (Hester *et al.*, 1975) whereas the two halves of a reduced IgM subunit continue to interact non-covalently.

The arrangement of the Fab arms also was chosen to conform to the appearance in electron micrographs, where there is a considerable degree of uniformity in the angle between pairs of Fab units (see for example Figure 16; Parkhouse *et al.*, 1970; Feinstein *et al.*, 1971). This suggests a longitudinal interaction, and once again the relation of the $C_\mu 1$ to $C_\mu 2$ domains chosen to fit electron micrographs was found to resemble that between $C_\gamma 2$ and $C_\gamma 3$ domains (Deisenhofer *et al.*, 1976; Huber *et al.* 1976). Thus, homologous longitudinal interactions are used in the IgM model throughout the μ chains.

The inter-subunit bridges linking the $C_\mu 3$ domains in human IgM (Beale and Feinstein, 1969, 1970; Miekka and Deutsch, 1970) are incorporated into the model, and presumably stabilize a weak specific interaction between $C_\mu 3$ domains in neighbouring subunits. These inter-subunit bridges have not been detected in mouse IgM (Milstein *et al.*, 1975).

The situation may vary in the case of the other immunoglobulins. The same units may be used to build the $F(ab')_2$ and Fc models discussed earlier, which were arrived at from crystallographic studies of human IgG1 and an IgG Fc fragment (Colman *et al.*, 1976; Deisenhofer *et al.*, 1976; Huber *et al.*, 1976). Although the conformation of the IgG molecule in solution is not known, a possible arrangement of the units and the hinge region is shown in Figure 14. The sequence and disulphide bridges in IgE are compatible with the domains in this immunoglobulin having an arrangement which resembles a subunit in the IgM pentamer. This has been discussed more fully by Beale and Feinstein (1976).

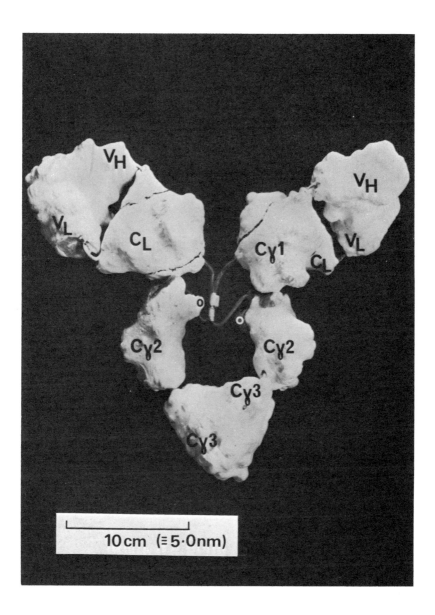

Figure 14 Plaster of Paris model of human IgG1, based on the data of Colman *et al.* (1976) and Deisenhofer *et al.* (1976) In the right-hand Fab the pseudo two-fold axes of rotation for the V domains and C domains have been aligned in the manner seen by Colman *et al.* (1976). in an IgG (Kol) crystal. In crystals of Fab fragments, the pseudo axes are at approximately 130° to each other so that the longitudinal contact between V_H and C_H1 is different from that between V_L and C_L. $\bigcirc$, sites of attachment of oligosaccharide to segment b4 of $C_\gamma2$ domains (see Figures 6 and 11)

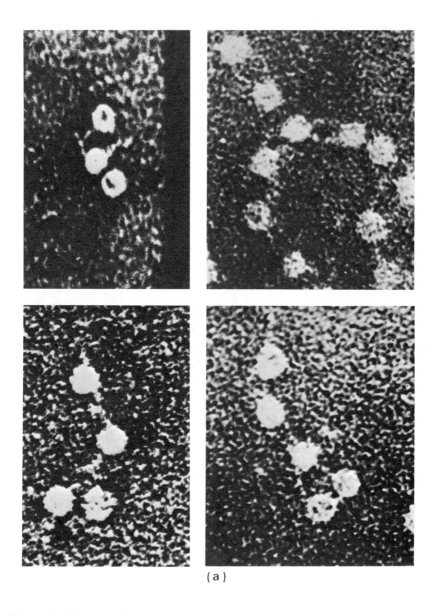

(a)

Figure 15 Electron micrographs of IgG antibody. (a) Complexes of IgG and F(ab′)$_2$ antibody and ferritin. The angle between the Fab arms is variable. The Fc can be distinguished in the IgG complexes (left hand pictures). Note cyclic oligomers. (b) The various, almost symmetrical shapes formed by polymers of IgG complexed with a divalent hapten. A, dimers; B, trimers; C, tetramers; and D, pentamer. The Fc can be seen as a projection on most of the corners. Reproduced from Valentine (1967)

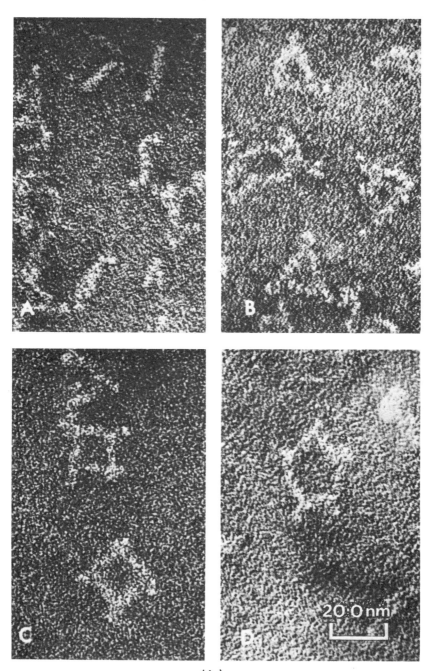

(b)

There are many explanations for IgA forming dimers in preference to larger cyclic oligomers (see Figure 19). Disulphide bridges link the $C_\alpha 2$ domains just below the hinge region, which would bring these domains together in a manner quite unlike the $C_\gamma 2$ domains. The $C_\alpha 2$ domains lack the oligosaccharide found in segment b4 of other immunoglobulins (see Figure 11) which might prevent them from approaching each other. It may be that this different arrangement of the $C_\alpha 2$ domains prevents any interaction between $C_\alpha 2$ domains of neighbouring subunits of the type suggested in the IgM model for the $C_\mu 3$ domains. Alternatively, the sequence differences, or the oligosaccharide attached to $C_\alpha 2$ domains, but not to $C_\mu 3$, near the region forming the inter-$C_\mu 3$ contact (Figure 11) may not permit such interactions.

9 ELECTRON MICROSCOPY OF ANTIBODIES LINKED TO ANTIGENS

Crystallographic studies have established the general nature of the binding site formed by the hypervariable regions of the variable domains of immunoglobulins (Davies et al., 1975a, b; Poljak, 1975a, b). There is no direct evidence in favour of a change in shape of this region of the antibody on binding with antigen (Metzger, 1974). Electron microscopy has proved of some value in studying the gross conformation of immunoglobulins; early work in this field has been reviewed by Green (1969). The types of structure, seen using electron microscopy, usually using negative staining, will be examined below when antibodies are complexed with antigen in such a manner so as to form cyclic, cross-linked, or lattice structures. How these structures may be explained in terms of antibody models formed from domains linked in the manner described in Section 8 of this chapter will also be considered.

9.1 Immunoglobulin G

Electron microscopy of IgG anti-ferritin–ferritin complexes (Figure 15a) shows that there is a marked tendency to form cyclic structures (Feinstein and Rowe, 1965). In the presence of a mild excess of antigen, not only are two ferritin molecules observed linked by two or more IgG molecules, but also larger cyclic structures have been noted which show a variable angle between the Fab arms of the antibody molecules. At approximately equivalence, in larger complexes, many more IgG molecules are observed whose overall length and appearance suggest angles approaching 180°. Exact angles have not been calculated since the orientation of the antibody molecules is unknown. Valentine and Green (1967) used a bivalent hapten to obtain cyclic antibody–hapten complexes (Figure 15b). Polygonal rings containing any number from three to 10, or more, of distinct IgG molecules were seen. Some dimers and linear polymers also were formed. The angle between the Fab arms varied from 10° in dimers to 180° in some of the large rings and open-chain polymers. However, the rings were seen lying flat on the substrate and it is not known how they are folded in solution.

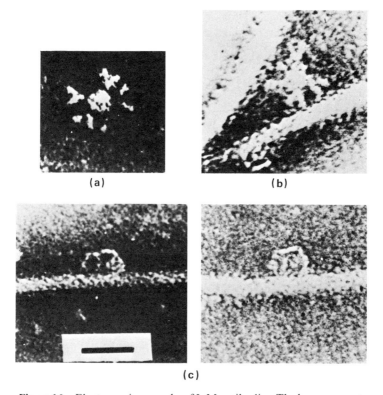

(a)   (b)

(c)

Figure 16 Electron micrographs of IgM antibodies. The bar represents 25 nm. (a) Unbound IgM; (b) IgM cross-linking two bacterial flagella; and (c) two examples of IgM, seen in profile as a 'staple', bound to a single flagellum

These electron micrographs are all interpretable in terms of the domain model of IgG (Figure 14). They indicate that there is flexibility at the hinge region of the IgG molecule, but they do not reveal if there is some flexibility or longitudinal interaction within Fab or Fc units.

9.2 Immunoglobulin M

Electron micrographs of IgM agglutinating *Salmonella* (Feinstein and Munn, 1969; Feinstein *et al.*, 1971) can be interpreted as indicating only a change in spatial relationship between relatively rigid $F(ab')_2$ and $(Fc)_5$ units which are not altered visibly. In Figure 16b, an IgM molecule may be seen cross-linking flagella, or attached, with Fab arms folded down, to a single flagellum (Figure 16c) giving a characteristic 'staple' appearance. The interpretation of these pictures is that the central $(Fc)_5$ discs of the IgM molecules are seen in profile and parallel to the flagellar surface. The negative staining techniques used in these experiments do not permit face-on views of attached IgM to be visualized.

Micrographs which can be interpreted as showing similar structures have been obtained for IgM attached to fragments of erythrocyte membrane (Humphrey and Dourmashkin, 1965). Similar views of IgM attached to T2 bacteriophage sheaths also have been observed.

Electron micrographs of $(Fc)_5$ preparations (Figure 17) reveal the presence of discs and rods. The latter structures are presumably the disc-like fragment seen in profile (Feinstein *et al.*, 1976).

Using the spray-freeze technique of Bachmann and Schmitt (1971) and of Bachmann and Schmitt-Fumian (1973) it has been possible to examine in face-view IgM molecules attached to flagella (Figure 18) (Feinstein *et al.*, 1976). Such micrographs can be interpreted as showing discs, parallel to the flagellum surface, attached through upright legs.

In many pictures of IgM, the $F(ab')_2$ arms appear to maintain a fixed inter-Fab angle and behave as one unit. Frequently, it is clear that only one of the component Fab units is attached to a flagellum. Various workers have shown that the pentameric molecule has an apparent valency of only five with large antigens, but has the expected value of 10 with smaller antigens, or when subunits or Fab fragments of IgM are examined. These results have been reviewed by Edberg *et al.* (1972), who showed that the apparant valency of IgM anti-dextran varied with the increasing molecular weight of the antigen from 10 through five to as low as 2·3. Values of less than 10 clearly are due to steric hindrance, which implies restricted relative movement between pairs of Fab arms in each subunit. This is in accordance with the authors' interpretation of the electron microscopic obser-

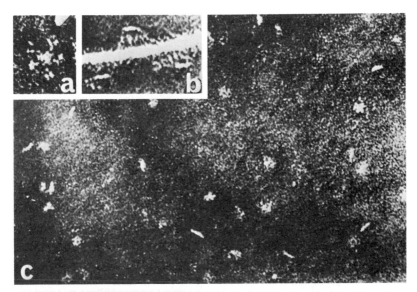

Figure 17 A comparison of electron micrographs of intact IgM and $(Fc)_5$ fragment. (a) Intact human IgM lying flat in the stain; (b) intact rabbit IgM seen edge on attached to bacterial flagellum; and (c) $(Fc)_5$ from pepsin-digested pig IgM. Similar fields have been obtained of $(Fc)_5$ from hot tryptic digests of pig IgM and from papain digests of human IgM

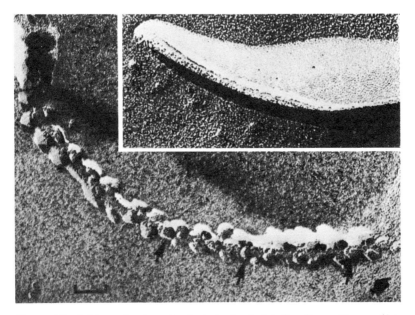

Figure 18 IgM molecules attached to bacterial flagellum. Preparations obtained by the spray-freeze etching technique were etched for 2 minutes at −100°, shadowed with platinum–carbon (in the direction of the large arrow, the shadows are white) and then backed with carbon. Some molecules seen in top view are arrowed. *Inset*, part of flagellum from control preparation without antibodies. The scale bar represents 50 nm

vations. The electron micrographs suggest a tendency for flexion to occur between $C_\mu 2$ and $C_\mu 3$ domains, although there is no amino acid sequence in this region which corresponds to that of the hinge region of IgG. A strained conformation might, however, be involved. On the basis of their studies of the depolarization of fluorescence in the nanosecond range, Holowka and Cathou (1976) claimed that, in shark IgM, the $(Fab')_2$ segments do move as a unit in this way. In horse IgM however, they believe that hindered rotation of Fab or Fab' units independently can also occur. As stated earlier the authors believe that electron micrographs suggest little or no relative movement of Fab arms in mouse and human as well as in dogfish IgM.

When the arms of the IgM model, described in the previous section, are folded down (see Figure 13d) and examined by X-radiography, the resulting picture, when reversed (Figure 13e), simulates closely the staple appearance of attached IgM in negatively stained images (see Figure 16c).

9.3 Immunoglobulin A

Electron micrographs of IgA complexes have been the most difficult to interpret. Although primary structural information has become available

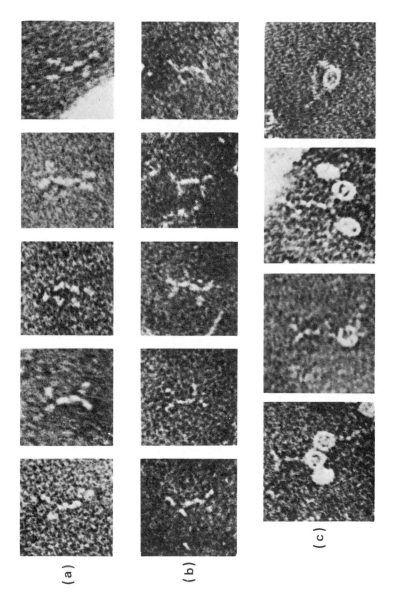

Figure 19 Electron micrographs of IgA dimer molecules. (a) Selected individual molecules of human IgA. (b) Selected molecules prepared from serum of mice carrying the plasma cell tumour MOPC 315. (c) Mouse IgA dimer attached to DNP-ferritin

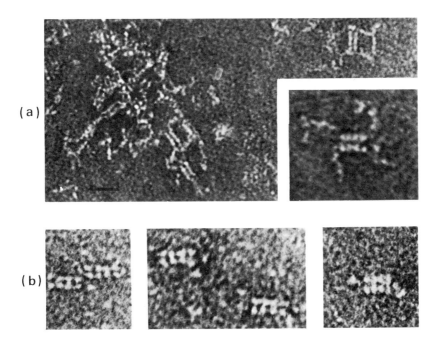

Figure 20 Electron micrographs of mouse IgA reacted with bifunctional hapten bis-DNP–glycyl-lysine. (a) Lattices of characteristic ladder-like structures made with dimer and hapten. Inset shows an individual ladder with material projecting from each of its four corners; (b) Selected individual ladders formed from IgA monomer–hapten complexes

recently, only very tentative IgA models can be devised. Unattached murine and human IgA dimers appear in double Y-forms (see Figure 19a, b).

When dimers of murine IgA anti-DNP were added to DNP–ferritin in the resulting precipitates (Figure 19c) the cross-linking double Y-shaped units appeared to be unaltered (Feinstein *et al.*, 1971; Munn *et al.*, 1971). However, using the bifunctional hapten bis-DNP–glycyl-lysine remarkable cyclic complexes of units having a ladder-like appearance were formed (Figure 20a). Monomer IgA–anti-DNP–bis-DNP hapten complexes appeared as individual ladders (Figure 20b) or as propeller-shaped structures.

Virtually identical observations have been made by Dourmashkin *et al.* (1971) who also observed double-Y shaped structures with IgA dimers, and Green *et el.* (1971), using bis-(DNP–β-alanyl)- diaminosuccinate, who obtained double bar and propeller-like images. These structures were interpreted as tetramers formed by side-by-side aggregation of two cyclic dimers of a repeating double-Y unit or, which is less likely, as a hapten-linked tetramer of four double-Y units. It was proposed that each of the four subunits seen along each bar corresponds to a pair of domains. If this is so the two Fab units in each IgA monomer have been able to interact laterally at a very low angle to each other, emphasizing their freedom of movement relative to each other.

10 POSSIBLE MECHANISMS OF COMPLEMENT FIXATION

Activation of the complement system by the classical pathway is the effector phenomenon which has been responsible mainly for speculation concerning a possible change in shape in antibodies after combination with antigens. Reid and Porter (1975) have reviewed the first steps of this process in which the C1q component is bound to the antibody molecules of an antigen–antibody complex, thereby leading to activation of protease–esterase activity in the C1s component. A feature of great interest is that different domains are involved in antigen binding and complement fixation. Antigen, as has been seen (Section 9), is bound to the V domains, thus involving the domain at the N-terminus of the heavy chain. However, complement is fixed at sites which, in both IgG and IgM molecules, lie in the C-terminal Fc region of the heavy chain.

10.1 Immunoglobulin G

There is convincing evidence that the complement-fixing site of IgG lies in the $C_\gamma 2$ domains (see Colomb and Porter, 1975; Reid and Porter, 1975; Ovary et al., 1976; Yasmeen et al., 1976). The C1q component is polymeric (Reid and Porter, 1975) and in free solution is bound weakly to several molecules of monomeric IgG with affinity constants ranging from 0.9×10^4 to 7×10^4 M^{-1}, depending on the subclass (Sledge and Bing, 1973; Müller-Eberhard, 1975; Hughes-Jones, 1976). Binding is much stronger (0.5×10^8—3×10^8 M^{-1} to aggregated IgG or to IgG antibody–antigen complexes (Hughes-Jones, 1976).

The attachment of at least two neighbouring IgG molecules to an erythrocyte membrane appears to be required for the activation of complement-mediated lysis (Borsos and Rapp, 1965a, b; Humphrey and Dourmashkin, 1965). Cohen (1968) found a similar requirement for the activation by IgG anti-ovalbumin–ovalbumin complexes. A possible explanation for this is that a polyvalent attachment of C1q is necessary. This could simply increase the association constant or could satisfy an activation mechanism which requires multiple attachment to sites that are relatively fixed in spatial relation to each other. No shape change of IgG antibody on binding to antigen need be involved.

After carefully reviewing the relevant data, Metzger (1974) considered that in the absence of any conclusive evidence for such shape changes, it was wisest *not* to propose mechanisms involving them. Although the authors agree with this advice, it is difficult to rule out completely the possibility of at least the partial involvement of shape changes. It is therefore worthwhile to discuss possible mechanisms in relation to immunoglobulin structure and in the light of recent crystallographic and spectroscopic results.

Feinstein and Rowe (1965) reported a variety of angles between the Fab arms in small soluble complexes of excess ferritin with rabbit anti-ferritin, when viewed using electron microscopy. They suggested flexibility about a hinge region. However, in larger insoluble complexes, formed near equivalence, the angle between the Fab arms approached 180° most frequently; it seems unlikely that the angle in these large, highly cross-linked lattices could change during their preparation for electron microscopy. Since complexes formed in antigen excess do not fix complement whereas those formed at, or near, equivalence do, it was suggested that the larger angle between the Fab arms in complexes formed near equivalence might correlate with the presence of complement-fixing sites, possibly arising from an alteration in the relationship between Fab and Fc (Feinstein and Rowe, 1965; Feinstein et al., 1971). It is, however, perfectly possible the the requirement for aggregation accounts for the difference in the complement-fixing activity of such complexes.

Hyslop et al. (1970) prepared cyclic complexes (Figure 15b) by means of a divalent hapten, and fractionated them into different sizes. They found that monomers and dimers did not fix C1 but maximal activity occurred with rings of four to eight IgG molecules. In the inactive complexes, the angle between the Fab arms was less than 60° whereas in active ones, the angle was between 90° and 180°. The shape of the rings in solution is unknown, and again the requirement for aggregation could explain the results.

It is possible to pose a question in the negative form, and to ask if there are positions of the Fab arms that do *not* permit complement fixation? The answer appears to be that there are. Isenman et al. (1975) have shown that although intact IgG4 does not fix C1, the Fc fragment does so with an affinity similar to that of IgG1. They suggested that the Fab arms in IgG4 modulate the complement-fixing sites. Beale and Feinstein (1976) have pointed out that human IgG4 has fewer residues between the end of the $C_\gamma 1$ domain and the first disulphide bridge of the hinge region (Figure 9) than do complement-fixing immunoglobulins. Mouse IgG1 is also non-complement-fixing and again has an unusually short hinge region (Figure 9).

A related point of interest is the effect of reduction of the inter-heavy-chain disulphide bridges in the hinge region. In rabbit IgG (Isenman et al., 1975; Press, 1975) and human IgG (Isenman et al., 1975), it has been shown that such reduction lowers C1 binding activity suggesting that the hinge region might be involved in the complement-fixing mechanism. However, Isenman et al. (1975) have found that reduction of the hinge disulphide bridges of Fc fragment does not affect its C1 fixing activity. These authors proposed that reduction of the hinge bridges in IgG might allow an interaction with Fab arms to modulate the C1-binding site. They pointed out that the possibility of IgG4 fixing the complement after interaction with antigen has never been tested, and could prove to be a genuine case of Fab arms being moved away from the modulation position.

There are two reports of complement fixation by IgG antibody—antigen complexes in which no aggregation of IgG could be detected. Goers et al. (1975) used the monovalent hapten nonadeca-lysyl-ε-DNP–lysine and rabbit anti-DNP antibody to form monomeric complexes. These complexes efficiently fix complement by the classical pathway. The authors suggested that although the complexes were monomeric, the amino groups of the bound antigen might function as C1 acceptor sites in addition to the site on the IgG molecule and thereby might satisfy aggregation requirements. However, these authors did not rule out the possibility of a conformational change upon binding such a large, positively charged hapten.

Pecht (1976) has reported that monomeric IgG antibody complexed to two monovalent lysozyme loops joined by a 3·5 nm spacer (bis-loop) can fix complement. Complexes with single loops (mono-loop), however, do not fix complement. Pecht (1976) suggested that in the bis-loop complexes the angle between the Fab arms of the IgG could be different from that in the mono-loop complexes.

Pecht (1976) and Schlessinger et al. (1975) used circular polarization of luminescence to look for conformational changes in IgG antibody when complexed to these loops. Circular polarization of luminescence is the emission analogue of the more widely used circular dichroism and is an expression of the asymmetry of the chromophore in its excited state. In immunoglobulin, the emission is due mainly to tryptophan residues, and the method is capable of detecting small changes in their asymmetry. Unfortunately such data give no indication of the nature or scale of the movements involved in these changes, but the method may be so sensitive as to detect very small changes indeed.

Spectroscopic differences were observed between Fab–mono-loop complexes and IgG–mono-loop complexes which suggests that antigen binding induces conformational changes in the Fc region. Further spectroscopic differences were observed when IgG was complexed to bis-loop suggesting additional changes in the Fc region. Reduction of inter-heavy-chain disulphide bridges removed the spectroscopic changes that had been attributed to the Fc region. Pecht (1976) argued that these results favour an allosteric change in the IgG molecule when it binds a suitably large and stable antigen, and further, that such an allosteric change may not be sufficient to trigger complement fixation which probably requires an accompanying angle change between Fab and Fc. However, the authors believe that there is no logical need to invoke allosterism, since the observed complement fixing may have been brought about by angle change alone. The circular polarization of luminescence changes observed with mono-loop binding may be irrelevant. It is important to confirm that no aggregates were present in these experiments.

In closely related studies, Jaton et al. (1975, 1976) used rabbit IgG anti-pneumococcal polysaccharide and a series of oligosaccharide antigens of increasing size. With oligosaccharide of up to 16 units, the complexes with antibody consist of monomers and dimers, with possibly a few trimers. These complexes do not fix complement, but luminescence measurements reveal spectroscopic differences which could be attributed to conformational changes in the Fc region of the IgG antibody. Complexes with oligosaccharide of 21 or more units contain appreciable amounts of polymer. Such complexes fix complement and show additional spectroscopic changes. Reduction of inter-heavy-chain bridges removes the changes attributed to the Fc region. These authors argue that binding of suitable antigen will induce an allosteric change in the IgG molecule but that this alone is insufficient to induce complement fixation and appropriate aggregation might be a requirement. It is felt that in this study the system is too complex to interpret usefully.

On the basis of the crystallographic results of IgG and its proteolytic fragments, discussed earlier in this chapter (see Section 3), Huber et al. (1976) have proposed a speculative model for an allosteric change in IgG when it binds antigen. They suggest that the molecule becomes more rigid after reaction with antigen. This is brought about through the formation of specific longitudinal contacts between domains, which are assumed to be absent in the unreacted molecule. As has been pointed out already (Section 7.2), the crystallographic results of Colman et al. (1976) and of Huber et al. (1976) show that such contacts are lacking in the Fab arms of IgG Kol, but other crystallographic results show the presence of these contacts in Fab fragments (Poljak et al., 1973; Davies et al., 1975a, b), Bence-Jones λ-chain dimer (Schiffer et al., 1973), and Fc fragment (Deisenhofer et al., 1976; Huber et al., 1976).

It is thought that the allosteric mechanism proposed by Huber et al. (1976) as a possible requirement for complement fixation is unlikely for the following reasons.

(i) It is difficult to visualize how a single mechanism can be activated by a large variety of ways of fitting antigenic determinants into binding sites. (Richards et al., 1975 and Chapter 2 this volume).

(ii) It is difficult to devise a mechanism for transmitting the proposed rigidification down individual Fab arms to the $C_\gamma 2$ domains.

(iii) There are particularly strong reasons why it would be disadvantageous for IgG molecules bound to particulate antigens to be converted into a single specific rigid form. In cases where IgG molecules are bound to erythrocytes (Greenbury et al., 1965), tobacco mosaic virus (Regenmortel and Hardie, 1976), or bacteriophage (Klinman and Karush, 1967), most of the molecules are attached to a single particle by both binding sites. A flexible IgG molecule would be essential for such double binding since the repeating antigenic determinants in different cases would be fixed in space very differently in relation to each other. On the other hand, a specifically rigid IgG molecule would have to maintain a fixed identical distance between its binding sites regardless of the antigen and would have a single fixed two-fold rotational symmetry relationship between its two binding sites. Any ancestral organism whose surface determinants fitted such rigid requirements would surely have evolved so as to evade them.

(iv) The polarity of repeating determinants along a particulate antigen such as bacterial flaggellum or tobacco mosaic virus particle also would be incompatible with the ability to bind doubly a symmetrically rigidified IgG molecule whose binding sites would be anti-parallel.

The specific rigidified shape chosen by Huber et al. (1976) is a T-shaped molecule which could not attach doubly to a surface. It would be satisfactory for lattice formation with soluble antigens and under these circumstances electron microscopy has revealed the presence of such shapes (Feinstein and Rowe, 1965; Valentine and Green, 1967). However, IgG molecules in small complexes or seen doubly attached to flagella are Y-shaped with varying angles between the Fab arms (Feinstein and Rowe, 1965; Valentine, 1967; Green, 1969).

For the above reasons, if there is a requirement for a shape change in IgG in order to fix complement, the authors would favour a non-allosteric dislocation mechanism. This could arise through the stabilization of a variety of possible final active forms of IgG differing from the inactive form.

10.2 Immunoglobulin M

It has already been pointed out that most cases of complement fixation by IgG–antigen complexes could be brought about conceivably purely by aggregation of the IgG. This cannot be so in the case of the pentameric IgM molecule, since it is known that a single attached molecule can activate the complement system (Borsos and Rapp, 1965a, b; Ishizaka et al., 1968). The IgM molecule therefore must be altered in some way when binding to the appropriate antigen.

Ishizaka et al. (1968) found that complement is not fixed by complexes of IgM with soluble blood group substances formed in the presence of excess antigen. Optimal fixation was obtained in antibody excess for IgM, but at equivalence in the case of IgG. These workers point out that their results strongly suggest that combination of IgM antibody molecules through multiple combining sites to antigenic sites on a particle or in a lattice is essential for IgM to fix complement. The formation of such complexes, of course, would involve almost certainly dislocation of Fab or $F(ab)_2$ arms. In studies which will be discussed below Pecht (1976) also showed a considerably depressed complement fixation by IgM in antigen excess.

In contrast to these results, Brown and Koshland (1975), using mono-Lac-ribonuclease and anti-Lac IgM, have reported the formation of non-aggregated antigen–antibody complexes which efficiently fix complement. Similarly, Pecht (1976), using the lysozyme loop as a monovalent antigen, has reported complement fixation by non-aggregated IgM anti-loop–mono-loop complexes. Circular polarization of luminescence studies on these complexes were interpreted as indicating a conformational change in the Fc region. Pecht (1976) argued that an allosteric change in the IgM antibody molecule is probably all that is necessary to induce complement fixation. However, he obtained a considerably lowered complement fixation in antigen excess. This observation contradicts the suggestion of an allosteric mechanism, instead it suggests that possibly aggregation of antigen is responsible for the activity observed at lower antigen levels.

It is difficult to imagine how binding of monovalent antigens by IgM can transmit a change from the V domains, through the $C_\mu 1$ and $C_\mu 2$ domains to the Fc region, unless the antigen aggregates, before or (possibly within a single IgM molecule) after binding, leading to the distortion of the molecule. It is thought that any more subtle effect normally would be disrupted completely by the gross dislocation of $F(ab')_2$ arms when IgM is multiply bound to particulate antigens, as seen in electron micrographs (Feinstein and Munn, 1969; Feinstein et al., 1971) (Figures 16c and 18). Indeed, there are cases which indicate that not every type of combination between IgM antibody and antigen is sufficient to induce complement fixation. For example, IgM anti-Rh D will agglutinate erythrocytes without fixing or activating complement (Mollison, 1972). Also, Ishizaka *et al.* (1968) and Pecht (1976) obtained little or no fixation by IgM antibody in antigen excess.

It might be thought that studies comparing the complement-fixing properties of IgM and its $(Fc)_5$ fragment could help to distinguish between mechanisms of activation of IgM involving merely the folding of Fab arms away from the Fc disc to expose sites preexisting in the Fc, and mechanisms whereby specific changes are brought about within the Fc region. Human $(Fc)_5$ preparations isolated after IgM cleavage with trypsin at or near 60° (Plaut and Tomasi, 1970) have failed consistently to fix C1 (Hurst *et al.*, 1974; Füst *et al.*, 1976; Reid, Herbert and Feinstein, unpublished observations) or C1q (Sledge and Bing, 1973) any more effectively than intact IgM. This does not rule out necessarily that IgM is inactive merely due to hindrance of sites by $(Fab')_2$ segments, since the treatment could inactivate the Fc. Moreover, a stretch of each $C_\mu 2$ domain carrying an oligosaccharide moiety which could continue to block C1 fixing sites remains on the $(Fc)_5$ disc. It is of considerable interest that $(Fc)_5$ isolated after papain cleavage of human IgM fixes C1 much more efficiently than does the original IgM (Reid, Herbert and Feinstein, unpublished observations). It is not known where in the IgM molecule the papain cleavage occurs.

In conclusion, it should be stressed that in the case of IgM, as for IgG, the authors believe that any change in antibody conformation required to induce complement fixation is brought about by dislocation of an inactive form to an active form. Such a dislocation must be compatible with a large number of ways of arranging Fab or $F(ab')_2$ arms in relation to each other and to the Fc, not to one specific conformation. The reason for making this a requirement is that each antigen will have a different spatial pattern of determinants, so that no single final arrangement of Fab or $F(ab')_2$ arms can be involved.

REFERENCES

Adetugbo, K., Poskus, E., Svasti, J., and Milstein, C. (1975). *Eur. J. Biochem.*, **56**, 503.

Bachmann, L., and Schmitt, W. W. (1971). *Proc. Nat. Acad. Sci., U.S.A.*, **68**, 2149.
Bachmann, L., and Schmitt-Fumian, W. W. (1973) In *Freeze-Etching Techniques and Applications* (Benedetti, E. L., and Favard, B., eds.), Société Francaise de Micros-copie Electronique, Paris, p. 73.
Beale, D., and Feinstein, A. (1969). *Biochem. J.*, **112**, 187.
Beale, D., and Feinstein, A. (1970). *FEBS Letters*, 7, 175.
Beale, D., and Feinstein, A. (1976). *Quart. Rev. Biophys.*, **9**, 135.
Bennich, H., and Bahr-Lindstrom, H. von (1974). *Progress in Immunology II*, Vol. X (Brent, L., and Holborow, J., eds.), North Holland Publishing Co., Amsterdam, p. 49.
Borsos, T., and Rapp, H. J. (1965a). *J. Immunol.*, **95**, 559.
Borsos, T., and Rapp, H. J. (1965b) *Science, N.Y.*, **150**, 505.
Bourgois, A., Fougereau, M., and Rocca-Serra, J. (1974). *Eur. J. Biochem.*, **43**, 423.

Brown, J. C., and Koshland, M. E. (1975). *Proc. Nat. Acad. Sci., U.S.A.*, **72**, 5111.

Capra, J. D., and Kehoe, M. J. (1975). *Adv. Immunol.* **20**, 1.
Cathou, R. E., Holowka, D. A., and Chan, L. M. (1974). In *Progress in Immunology II*, Vol. 1 (Brent, L., and Holborow, J., eds.), North Holland Publishing Co., p. 63.
Cohen, S. (1968). *J Immunol.*, **100**, 407.
Cohen, S., and Milstein, C. (1967). *Adv. Immunol.*, **7**, 1.
Cohen, S., and Porter, R. R. (1964). *Adv. Immunol.*, **4**, 287.
Colman, P. M., Deisenhofer, J., Huber, R., and Palm, W. (1976). *J. Mol. Biol.*, **100**, 257.
Colomb, M., and Porter, R. R. (1975). *Biochem. J.*, **145**, 177.
Croft, L. R. (1964). *Handbook of Protein Sequences*. Joynson-Bruvvers, Oxford.
Cunningham, B. A. (1974). In *Progress in Immunology II*, Vol. 1 (Brent, L., and Holborow, J., eds.), North Holland Publishing Co., Amsterdam, p. 5.

Davies, R. D., Padlan, E. A., and Segal, D. M. (1975a). *Ann. Rev. Biochem.*, **44**, 639.
Davies, R. D., Padlan, E. A., and Segal, D. M. (1975b). In *Contemporary Topics in Molecular Immunology*, Vol. 4 (*Inman, F. P., and Mandy, W. J., eds.*), Plenum Press, New York, p. 127.
Dayhoff, M. O. (1972). *Atlas of Protein Sequence and Structure*, Vol. 5, National Biomedial Research Foundation, Silver Spring.
Deisenhofer, J., Colman, P. M., Huber, R., Haupt, H., and Schwick, G. (1976). *Hoppe-Seyler's Z. Physiol. Chem.*, **357**, 435.
Dourmashkin, R. R., Virella, G., and Parkhouse, R. M. E. (1971). *J. Mol. Biol.*, **56**, 207.

Edberg, C. S., Bronson, P.-M., and Van Oss, C. J. (1972). *Immunochemistry*, **9**, 273.
Edelman, G. M., Cunningham, B. A., Gall, W. E., Gottlieb, P. D., Rutishauser, U., and Waxdal, M. J. (1969). *Proc. Nat. Acad. Sci., U.S.A.*, **63**, 78.
Edelman, G. M., and Gall, W. E. (1969). *Ann. Rev. Biochem.*, **38**, 415.
Edmundson, A. B., Ely, K. R., Abola, E. E., Schiffer, M., and Panagiotopoulos, N. (1975). *Biochemistry*, **14**, 3953.
Edmundson, A. B., Ely, K. R., Girling, R. L., Abola, E. E., Schiffer, M., and Westholm, F. A. (1974). In *Progress in Immunology II*, Vol. 1 (Brent, L., and Holborow, J., eds.), North Holland Publishing Co., Amsterdam, p. 103.
Edmundson, A. B., Schiffer, M., Ely, K. R., and Wood, M. K. (1972). *Biochemistry*, **11**, 1822.
Edmundson, A. B., Wood, M. K., Schiffer, M., Hardman, K. D., Ainsworth, C. F., Ely, K. R., and Deutsch, H. F. (1970). *J. Biol. Chem.*, **245**, 2763.
Epp, O., Colman, P., Fehlhammer, H., Bode, W. W., Schiffer, M., Huber, R., and Palm, W. (1974). *Eur. J. Biochem.*, **45**, 513.
Epp, O., Lattman, E. E., Schiffer, M., Huber, K., and Palm, W. (1975). *Biochemistry*, **14**, 4943.

Feinstein, A. (1974). In *Progress in Immunology II*, Vol. X (Brent, L., and Holborow, J., eds.), North Holland Publishing Co., Amsterdam, p. 115.
Feinstein, A., and Munn, E. A. (1969). *Nature, N.Y.*, **224**, 1307.
Feinstein, A., Munn, E. A., and Richardson, N. E. (1971). *Ann. N.Y. Acad. Sci.*, **190**, 104.
Feinstein, A., Richardson, N. E., and Munn, E. A. (1976). *Proceedings 3rd John Innes Symposium* (Markham, R. and Horne, R. W., eds.), Elsevier/North Holland Publishing Company, Amsterdam, p. 111.
Feinstein, A., and Rowe, A. J. (1965). *Nature (Lond.)*, **205**, 147.
Füst, G., Csecsi-Nagy, M., Medgyesi, G. A., Kulics, J., and Gergly, J. (1976). *Immunochemistry*, **13**, 793.

Green, N. M. (1969). *Adv. Immunol.*, **11**, 1.
Green, N. M., Dourmashkin, R. R., and Parkhouse, R. M. E. (1971). *J. Mol. Biol.*, **56**, 203.
Greenbury, C. L., Moore, D. H. and Nunn, L. A. C. (1965). *Immunology*, **8**, 420.
Goers, J. W., Schumaker, V. N., Glovsky, M. M., Rebek, J., and Müller-Eberhard, H. J. (1975). *J. Biol. Chem.*, **250**, 4918.

Hester, R. B., Mole, J. E., Schrohenloher, R. E. (1975). *J. Immunol.*, **114**, 486.
Hill, R. L., Lebovitz, H. E., Fellows, R. E., and Delaney, R. (1967). In *Gamma Globulins: Structure and Biosynthesis* (Killander, J., ed.), John Wiley and Sons, New York and London, p. 109.
Holowka, D. A., and Cathou, R. E. (1976). *Biochemistry*, **15**, 3379.
Huber, R., Deisenhofer, J., Colman, P. M., Matsushima, M., and Palm, W. (1976). *Das Immunsystem.* (Melchers, F., and Rajewsky, K., eds.). Springer Verlag, Berlin.
Hughes-Jones, N. C. (1977). *Immunology*, **32**, 191.
Humphrey, J. H. and Dourmashkin, R. R. (1965). In *Complement* (Wolstenholme, G. E. W., and Knight, J., eds.), Churchill, London, p. 175.
Hurst, M. M., Volanakis, J. E., Hester, R. B., Stroud, R. M., and Bennett, J. C. (1974). *J. Exp. Med.*, **140**, 1117.
Hyslop, N. E., Dourmashkin, R. R., Green, N. M., and Porter, R. R. (1970). *J. Exp. Med.*, **131**, 783.

Inman, F. P., and Mestecky, J. (1975). In *Contemporary Topics in Immunology*, Vol. 3 (Inman, F. P., and Mandy, W. J., eds.), Plenum Press, New York, p. 111.
Isenman, D. E., Dorrington, K. J., and Painter, R. H. (1975). *J. Immunol.*, **114**, 1726.
Ishizaka, T., Tada, T., and Ishizaka, K. (1968). *J. Immunol.*, **100**, 1145.

Jaton, J.-C., Huser, H., Braun, D. G., Givol, D., Pecht, I., and Schlessinger, J. (1975). *Biochem.*, **14**, 5312.
Jaton, J.-C., Huser, H., Riesen, W. F., Schlessinger, J., and Givol, D. (1976). *J. Immunol.*, **116**, 1363.

Kabat, E. A., and Wu, T. T. (1971). *Ann. N.Y. Acad. Sci.*, **190**, 382.
Klinman, N. R., and Karush, F. (1967). *Immunochemistry*, **4**, 387.
Koshland, M. E. (1975). *Adv. Immunol.*, **20**, 41.
Kratzin, H., Altevogt, P., Ruban, E., Kortt, A., Staroscik, K., and Hilschmann, N. (1976). *Hoppe-Seyler's Z. Physiol. Chem.*, **356**, 1337.

Low, T. L. K., Liu, V. Y., and Putnam, F. W. (1976). *Science, N.Y.*, **191**, 390.

Mestecky, J., and Schrohenloher, R. E. (1974). *Nature (Lond.)*, **249**, 650.
Metzger, H. (1974). *Adv. Immunol.*, **12**, 57.
Miekka, S. I., and Deutsch, H. F. (1970). *J. Biol. Chem.*, **245**, 5534.
Milstein, C., Adetugbo, K., Cowan, N. J., and Secher, D. S. (1974). In *Progress in Immunology II*, Vol. 1 (Brent, L., and Holborrow, J., eds.), North Holland Publishing Co., Amsterdam, p. 157.
Milstein, C. P., Richardson, N. E., Deverson, E. V., and Feinstein, A. (1975). *Biochem. J.*, **151**, 615.
Mollison, P. L. (1972). *Blood Transfusion in Clinical Medicine*, 5th ed. Blackwell, Oxford.
Müller-Eberhard, H. A. (1975). *Ann. Rev. Biochem.*, **44**, 697.
Munn, E. A., Feinstein, A., and Munro, A. J. (1971). *Nature (Lond.)*, **331**, 527.

Ovary, Z., Saluk, P. H., Quijada, L., and Lamm, M. E. (1976). *J. Immunol.*, **116**, 1265.

Padlan, E. O., and Davies, D. R. (1975). *Proc. Nat. Acad. Sci.*, *U.S.A.*, **72**, 819.

Padlan, E. O., Segal, D. M., Rudikoff, S., Potter, M., Spande, T., and Davies, D. R. (1973). *Nature, New Biol.*, **245**, 165.

Parkhouse, R. M. E., Askonas, B. A., and Dourmashkin, R. R. (1970). *Immunology*, **18**, 575.

Pecht, I. (1976). In *Des Immunsystem.* (Melchers, F., and Rajewsky, K., eds.), Springer Verlag, Berlin.

Plaut, A. G., and Tomasi, T. B. (1970). *Proc. Nat. Acad. Sci.*, *U.S.A.*, **65**, 318.

Poljak, R. J. (1975a). *Nature* (*Lond.*), **256**, 373.

Poljak, R. J. (1975b). *Adv. Immunol.*, **21**, 1.

Poljak, R. J., Amzel, L. M., Avey, H. P., Becka, L. N., and Nisonoff, A. (1972). *Nature, New Biol.*, **235**, 137.

Poljak, R. J., Amzel, L. M., Avey, H. P., Chen, B. L., Phizackerley, R. P., and Saul, F. (1973). *Proc. Nat. Acad. Sci.*, *U.S.A.*, **70**, 3305.

Poljak, R. J., Amzel, L. M., Chen, B. L., Phizackerley, R. P., and Saul, F. (1974). *Proc. Nat. Acad. Sci.*, *U.S.A.*, **71**, 3440.

Porter, R. R. (1973). In *MTP International Review of Science, Biochemistry, Series One*, Vol. 10 (Kornberg, H. L., and Phillips, D. C., eds.), Butterworths, London, p. 159.

Press, E. M. (1975). *Biochem. J.*, **149**, 285.

Putman, F. W. (1974). In *Progress in Immunology II* Vol. 1 (Brent, L., and Holborow, J., eds.), North Holland Publishing Co., Amsterdam, p. 25.

Putman, F. W., Florent, G., Paul, C., Shinoda, T., and Shimizu, A. (1973). *Science, N.Y.*, **182**, 287.

Reid, K. B. M., and Porter, R. R. (1975). In *Contemporary Topics in Molecular Immunology*, Vol. 4 (Inman, F. P., and Mandy, W. J., eds.), Plenum Press, New York, p. 1.

Regenmortel, M. H. V. Van, and Hardie, G., (1976). *Immunochemistry*, **13**, 503.

Richards, F. F., Konigsberg, W. H., Rosenstein, R. W., and Varga, J. M. (1975). *Science, N.Y.*, **187**, 130.

Rocca-Serra, J., Milili, M., and Fougereau, M. (1975). *Eur. J. Biochem.*, **59**, 511.

Sarma, V. R., Silverton, E. W., Davies, D. R., and Terry, W. D. (1971). *J. Biol. Chem.*, **246**, 3753.

Schiffer, M., Girling, R. L., Ely, K. R., and Edmundson, A. B. (1973). *Biochemistry*, **23**, 4620.

Schlessinger, J., Steinberg, I. Z., Givol, D., Hochman, J., and Pecht, I. (1975). *Proc. Nat. Acad. Sci.*, *U.S.A.*, **72**, 2775.

Segal, D. M., Padlan, E. A., Cohen, G. H., Rudikoff, S., Potter, M., and Davies, D. R. (1974) *Proc. Nat. Acad. Sci.*, *U.S.A.*, **71**, 4298.

Sledge, C. R., and Bing, D. H. (1973). *J. Biol. Chem.*, **248**, 2818.

Tracy, D. E., and Cebra, J. J. (1974). *Biochemistry*, **13**, 4796.

Trischmann, T. M., and Cebra, J. J. (1974). *Biochemistry*, **13**, 4804.

Valentine, R. C. (1967). In *Gamma Globulins: Structure and Biosynthesis* (Killander, J., ed.), John Wiley & Sons, New York and London, p. 251.

Valentine, R. C., and Green, N. M. (1967). *J. Mol. Biol.* **27**, 615.

Watanabe, S., Barnikol, H. U., Horn, J., Bertram, J., and Hilschmann, N. (1973). *Hoppe-Seyler's Z. Physiol. Chem.*, **354**, 1505.

Yasmeen, D., Ellerson, J. R., Dorrington, K. J., and Painter, R. H. (1976). *J. Immunol.*, **116**, 518.

CHAPTER 9

Molecular Basis of Immunogenicity and Antigenicity

R. Arnon and B. Geiger

1 INTRODUCTION

Immunology covers a variety of topics and phenomena of which the common denominator is the immune response, elicited by substances, usually foreign to the host, defined as antigens. In order to gain a better understanding of immunological phenomena at a molecular level, more information is needed about the structure of these antigens. The two features most characteristic of the immune response are its huge diversity, and its exquisite specificity; two features which do not always correlate. Most naturally-occurring materials, including proteins and polysaccharides, as well as synthetic molecules, when injected into vertebrates to which the materials are foreign, induce an immune response, leading to biosynthesis of antibodies. These antibodies, in turn, are capable of interacting specifically with distinct areas of the antigen, called antigenic determinants, and those dictate the antigenic specificity. The distinction between these two entities will be defined and discussed in detail in Section 2.

In this chapter, the various parameters influencing antigenicity and immunogenicity will be discussed. In view of the scope of antigenic substances, the subject will be limited to protein and protein-like antigens, including the naturally occurring proteins, their artificial derivatives, and synthetic polypeptides. Data on other classes of antigens, such as polysaccharides, lipids and nucleic acids, are available in recent reviews (see Stollar, 1973; Hakomori and Kobata, 1974; Niedieck, 1975; Alving, 1976), as well as in other chapters in this book.

All proteins are probably immunogenic, that is they evoke an immune response and antibody production, although individual proteins may differ markedly in the extent of their antigenicity. Such differences, as well as variations in the induction of cell-mediated immunity *versus* antibody production, are dependent on the molecular structure of the protein involved. This aspect will be discussed in Section 6.

To investigate the contribution of the various structural parameters to the antigenic properties of proteins two main approaches may be adopted. The first uses as starting material an immunogenic protein, which is subjected to enzymic or chemical degradation, and the resulting fragments are screened for their capacity to elicit an immune response or to interact with antibodies induced by the original protein. In this manner, information is obtained about the size and the nature of fragments possessing antigenic properties. This method of elucidating the molecular requirements for antigenicity may be termed analytical as it is based on the dismembering of a natural antigen. An alternative method is the synthetic one using amino acids, which by themselves have no antigenic properties. The amino acids are used for the synthesis of polypeptides, which are investigated for their immunogenicity or antigenicity. The synthetic approach offers the advantage that, once the antigenicity of one synthetic material has been established unequivocally many analogues may be prepared and tested. Since the chemistry of the polypeptides is known, it should be feasible through a systematic study of such polymers, which show only limited variations in their chemical formulae and structure, to determine the role of various structural features in their antigenic function. This chapter will be concerned with these approaches.

This chapter will not deal at all with immunological tolerance and its relationship to antigenic structure, but it will discuss the implication of the antigenic properties on several immunological phenomena such as genetic control of the immune response, and the cellular recognition of antigen *versus* humoral antibody production. In the case of the latter, experimental evidence strongly suggests that the induction of humoral and of cell-mediated immunity depends largely on the molecular structure of the protein, but that these two responses manifest different structural requirements. A case in point is the relationship between native proteins and their denatured derivatives, which will be discussed in detail in Sections 4 and 6 of this chapter. The availability of antigens of limited structural complexity, such as the synthetic polypeptides, along with the existence of inbred strains of mice, whose genetics are well documented and whose major histocompatibility locus is recognized, has made possible the study of the genetic control of the immune response to a single antigenic determinant. This has been the subject of several recent reviews (see Benacerraf and Katz, 1975; Mozes 1975), but the essence of this subject and, in particular, the role of the molecular structure of the antigens in this important immunological feature, will be discussed in Section 7.

2 IMMUNOGENICITY AND ANTIGENIC SPECIFICITY

In the course of an immune response, antigens exhibit two distinct reactivities, which may not necessarily coincide. The first is *immunogenicity*, that is the capacity of the antigenic substance to elicit an immune response, which is manifested either by production of antibodies (in the humoral response) or by proliferation of committed lymphocytes (in a cell-mediated immune response). The second characteristic, *antigenic specificity*, refers to the antigens' capacity to interact in a specific manner with antibodies or with immune lymphocytes, regardless of how these have been raised. The region in the antigen molecule which directly comes into contact with the active site of the antibodies, or with a cell-surface receptor is defined as an antigenic determinant.

Proteins and large polypeptides may carry a large number and variety of possible antigenic determinants which dictate the antigenic specificity of that particular macromolecule. However, only a limited number of the potential antigenic sites is immunogenic or immunopotent, whereas the rest (also referred to as non-immunogenic or immunosilent) cannot evoke a response. In some cases, an entire molecule is not immunogenic by itself, but can react with antibodies elicited by a related molecule, thus demonstrating antigenic specificity. Some examples will be given to illustrate the distinction between immunogenicity and antigenic specificity.

Animals injected with *Bacillus anthracis* produce antibodies that react specifically with poly-γ-D-glutamic acid, which constitutes a specific component of the cell wall of these bacteria. The antigen (poly-γ-D-glutamic acid), when injected, cannot elicit any immune response, and is, therefore, non-immunogenic, even though it carries the antigenic specificity of the intact *Bacillus* (Roelants and Goodman, 1968).

Gelatin is an example of a similar phenomenon. Although it is a very poor immunogen and hardly provokes any antibody production (Haurowitz, 1950), gelatin is capable of reacting readily with antibodies elicited by a mildly tyrosylated derivative (Arnon and Sela, 1960). Thus, the tyrosylation brings about a marked enhancement of the immunogenicity of gelatin, while retaining its original antigenic specificity.

The most clear-cut demonstration of the distinction between immunogenicity and antigenicity is offered by low molecular weight fragments of immunogenic macromolecules. Many such fragments, including a peptide of flagellin with a molecular weight of less than 4000 (Ichiki and Parish, 1972), a fragment of lysozyme containing the N and C-terminal peptide (Fujio *et al.*, 1968*a,b*), and some fragments of silk fibroin (Cebra, 1961*a,b*), encompass defined antigenic determinants of the proteins. As such they are reactive with the antibodies elicited by the intact respective protein. However, they are unable by themselves to evoke any immune response and are thus non-immunogenic.

As a result of accumulated information on antigenicity *versus* immunogenicity, it is now possible to assign several molecular requirements which are associated apparently with the manifestation of immunogenic capacity. Some of these molecular parameters will be discussed below.

2.1 Molecular Size of Immunogens

It has been long recognized that small molecules are not, by themselves, immunogenic and cannot stimulate the immune system unless they are coupled to large, complex (usually immunogenic) carriers (Landsteiner, 1945; Eisen, 1960). Thus, a protein molecule can be regarded as a carrier with various single antigenic determinants of different sizes that are not necessarily immunogenic by themselves as haptenic groups. However, the assumption that a minimal size is a prerequisite for immunogenicity is not borne out by the experimental results, since it has been found that small proteins and peptides with molecular weights in the range of 4000–5000 sometimes are able to elicit an immune humoral or cellular response (Maurer, 1963, 1964; Sela, 1966, 1969; de Weck, 1974).

Insulin and peptides derived from it have been shown to be immunogenic in a variety of species (Yagi *et al.*, 1965) in spite of their low molecular weight (6000 or less). Native peptides with relatively low molecular weight such as glucagon (Unger *et al.*, 1959) and gastrin (Schneider *et al.*, 1967) have been reported also to bring about immune response. Similarly, it has been found that an isolated antigenic fragment of lysozyme, the 'loop' peptide with a molecular weight of around 2000, can evoke by itself a low but significant immune response in mice (Geiger and Arnon, 1974). This was manifested both at the level of the B cells (presence of antibody-forming cell against the 'loop' region), and the T cells (positive carrier effect to DNP–lysozyme after priming with isolated loop).

In addition, studies with synthetic peptides have shown that a polymer of glutamic acid and tyrosine with a molecular weight of less than 4000 is immunogenic (Sela *et al.*, 1962). Even very small oligopeptides of tyrosine such as tri- to hexa-tyrosine, provided that a *p*-azobenzenearsonate group is attached to them, can elicit antibody production (Borek *et al.*, 1965, 1967). It thus seems that molecular size alone is not a crucial parameter in conferring immunogenicity.

It should be mentioned, however, that all these relatively small antigens are comparatively poor immunogens and may be rendered more immunogenic by coupling them to large carrier molecules. Similarly, proteins of molecular weights of about 10 000 such as flagellin (Nossal *et al.*, 1964) or cytochrome c (Reichlin *et al.*, 1970) also can be rendered more immunogenic when administered in a polymeric form. Molecular size is therefore an auxiliary parameter, but not an absolute factor for conferring immunogenicity.

In the context of antigenic specificity, size requirements concern mainly the size of the individual antigenic determinants. Inhibition of the immune reaction by inhibitors of varying size has been assessed. In the case of antibodies against synthetic polypeptides, raised primarily by immunizing with polypeptide–carrier conjugates, the size of the antigenic determinant is thought to be four to six residues. This is true for either poly-L-lysine system (Arnon *et al.*, 1965), poly-D-lysine system (Van Vunakis *et al.*, 1966), poly-D-alanine (Schechter *et al.*, 1966), or poly-γ-D-glutamic acid (Goodman *et al.*, 1968). Antigenic determinants of some native proteins also were shown by this technique to occupy a similar size—six to seven residues. Thus, several defined determinants of myoglobin comprise regions of six to seven residues (Atassi, 1975), and in the case of tobacco mosaic virus the C-terminal hexapeptide has been shown to interfere with the immunological reactivity of the intact virus (Anderer, 1963*a*).

It is of interest that in studies of polysaccharides the size of the antigenic site is similar to that of polypeptides and proteins. Thus, the interaction of dextran with human anti-dextran is inhibited to varying extents by a series of isomaltose oligomers. The upper limit of inhibition is achieved with the hexasaccharide isomaltohexaose (Kabat, 1960).

Specificity studies with anti-nucleic acid antibodies pointed to the fact that the size of the antigenic determinants is that of four to six nucleotides (Stollar, 1973). It should be mentioned that the size of the various peptidyl determinants ($2.5–3.6 \times 1.1–1.7 \times 0.65$ nm) is similar to the size of the isomaltohexaose molecule ($3.4 \times 1.2 \times 0.7$ nm) and this is probably the size of the antibody combining site (Kabat, 1967).

2.2 Accessibility of Antigenic Determinants at the Surface of the Antigen Molecule

The interactions of individual antigenic determinants with specific receptors of

312

the immunocompetent cell or with the combining site of an antibody molecule
(which are, by definition, the requirements for immunogenicity and antigenic
specificity, respectively), necessitate, the exposure of the receptors on the surface
of the antigenic molecule. This conclusion was reached from a study using
synthetic antigens, which are identical in their overall composition but which
differ in the arrangement of the antigenic groups in the molecule. Both synthetic
antigens contained the random oligopeptide (Tyr-Glu)n as an antigenic determinant (Sela *et al.*, 1962). The first was the branched polymer, poly(L-Tyr-L-
Glu)-poly-DL-Ala-poly-L-lys denoted (T,G)-A–L and the second, denoted A-(T,
G)–L, in which the (Tyr-Glu) oligo-peptide chains are bound directly to the
polylysyl backbone, and the poly-DL-alanine chains are attached at their N-
termini (see Figure 1). It has been shown clearly that whereas the first antigen
elicits a good anti (T,G) response upon injection into experimental animals, the
second antigen lacks this capacity, probably because the antigenic determinants
are buried under the polyalanyl 'coat' and are not exposed.

A similar conclusion has been drawn from studies on several protein antigens
in which antigenic determinants have been identified. For example, detailed
studies on myoglobin have pointed out that the antigenic regions are located in
'corners' of the molecule which are exposed to the outer environment (Crumpton,
1974; Atassi, 1975); this subject will be discussed in further detail in Sections 4
and 5. Another example is lysozyme in which the loop region, which is an
immunodominant determinant in the molecule (Arnon, 1968; Arnon and Sela,
1969; Maron *et al.*, 1971), protrudes from it and is exposed at one of its corners
(Blake *et al.*, 1965).

Similarly, studies on flagellin have suggested that one fragment of the molecule
mainly retains the capacity to inhibit the reaction of the reconstituted flagella
with their antibodies. This region, which can be isolated after cleavage with
cyanogen bromide, is present most probably on the outside surface of the intact
flagella. This is concluded also from its relatively high susceptibility to iodination
(Nossal *et al.*, 1964, 1965; Parish and Ada, 1969). Other regions, which probably

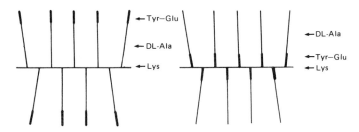

poly(Glu–Tyr)–poly–DL-Ala–poly–Lys   poly–DL-Ala–poly(Glu–Tyr)–poly–Lys

Figure 1   Schematic representation of multichain copolymer in which
L-tyrosine and L-glutamic acid residues are attached to poly-DL-
alanyl–poly-L-lysine, (T,G)-A–L and of one in which L-tyrosine and L-
glutamic acid are attached directly to the lysine backbone and then
elongated with alanine peptides, A-(T,G)–L

form part of the interior of the flagellum cannot be expressed as antigenic determinants.

A similar phenomenon has been observed in the case of tobacco mosaic virus (TMV), where a single determinant of the coat protein has been reported to be capable of considerable inhibition of the TMV–anti-TMV reaction, probably since it is exposed repeatedly on the surface of the intact virus (Anderer, 1963a). (See Section 5).

2.3 Foreignness and Immunogenic Capacity

Under normal circumstances, animals do not show an immune response against self components. The fact that many proteins of phylogenetically related species show considerable structural homology may provide an explanation for the low immune responses obtained when they are used for immunization. Consequently, proteins such as collagen or cytochrome c, which are similar in most animal species, are poor immunogens (Beard et al., Chapter 13; Jonsson and Palens, 1966; Furthmayr and Timple, 1976). Moreover, it is believed that in such related molecules the antigenic determinants which are common to the antigen and to the constituents of the immunized animal are not immunogenic. Such a situation can be exemplified by the antigenic properties of adrenocortico-trophic hormone (ACTH).

ACTH consists of 39 amino acid residues, out of which the 24 N-terminal amino acids and the C-terminal hexapeptide are common to all species tested (Dayhoff and Eck, 1969), whereas the region 25–33 is variable. When coupled to a protein carrier and injected into rabbits, ACTH stimulates the production of antibodies which have been shown by inhibition studies to react predominantly with the variable, C-terminal region (Fleischer et al., 1965; Fleischer et al., 1966; Gelzer, 1968). It should be mentioned, however, that immunization with antigens structurally similar to self components may also induce an immune response to some self determinants. Thus, rabbits immunized with heterologous cytochrome c produced antibodies that also react with the rabbit protein (Nisonoff et al., 1970). Similarly, guinea-pig, after immunization with the triple-helical synthetic antigen, (L-Pro-Gly-L-Pro)n respond in skin reaction to the injection of autologous guinea-pig skin collagen (see Sections 4 and 5).

2.4 Role of Specific Amino Acids in Immunogenicity

Extensive studies on a wide variety of protein antigens do not point to the requirement for specific amino acids, in or outside the antigenic determinants, for the expression of immunogenic capacity. However, attempts to render a protein immunogenic by specific modification with oligopeptides have contributed some information on this subject. Gelatin for example, is a very poor immunogen both in rabbits and in guinea-pigs, but modification by tyrosylation caused a marked enhancement in its immunogenicity (Sela et al., 1956; Arnon and Sela, 1960; Sela and Arnon, 1960a). It was found that even mild modification with as little as 2 per cent tyrosine results in a marked increase in the anti-gelatin response, without changing the antigenic specificity of the gelatin. However, when heavy modification with 10 per cent or more tyrosine is employed, most of the antibodies formed are directed towards the tyrosyl determinants (Arnon and Sela, 1960). The role of specific amino acids in the construction of antigens has been studied systematically with a series of synthetic polypeptide antigens and proteins, the results of which have been summarized in reviews by Sela (1966, 1969) and will not be detailed here.

The participation and major contribution of particular amino acid residues to the antigenic specificity of native proteins also have been demonstrated. In several cases, such as isoleucine 58 in cytochrome c (Margoliash et al., 1967; Nisonoff et al., 1970) or proline 117 in oxidized ribonuclease (Brown and Liu, 1970), these specific residues emerge as the immunodominant part in the respective antigenic determinants. This aspect will be discussed in more detail in following sections which deal with the various protein antigens and their defined antigenic determinants.

3 ANTIGENIC PROPERTIES OF PROTEIN ANTIGENS

Protein molecules are all immunogenic, although not all to the same extent. These complex macromolecules usually contain a large number of antigenic determinants which are responsible for the proteins' antigenic specificity, but also may be immunogenic by themselves. The antigenic complexity of proteins stems both from their primary structure and from the three-dimensional folding of their polypeptide chain(s). Studies on the antigenic properties of proteins have included the elucidation of the role of various molecular parameters in the antigenic functions, as well as attempts to identify specific antigenic determinants in naturally occurring proteins and in protein-like, synthetic molecules. Whereas the detailed description of defined antigenic determinants, which have been identified in several proteins (mostly by analysis of isolated fragments), will appear in Section 5, the present section will consider the general immunological properties of proteins.

The proteins will be discussed according to their classification—fibrous proteins, globular proteins and synthetic protein-like materials—and their antigenic properties will be related mainly to their structural features. Separate discussion will be devoted to proteins with biological activity, since in these molecules inhibition of their function by antibodies may serve as an additional tool for antigenic analysis. In most cases, the information about the antigenic structure has been obtained mainly by two approaches. The first consists of chemically modifying specific amino acid residues and analysing the effect on the antigenic properties. In this way information is obtained on the extent to which these residues contribute to the antigenic specificity. The other approach is to study immunological cross-reaction between homologous proteins, such as molecules of the same protein, obtained from different animal species, or molecules originating from a common ancestor. When detailed information is available on the sequences and structures of such related proteins, it may be possible to localize and identify some antigenic determinants or particular residues which are involved in their antigenic specificity. The information on both sequence analysis and crystallography of a large variety of proteins that has accumulated during the past two decades has made possible this type of investigation, and has forwarded our understanding of the molecular basis of antigenicity of various proteins.

3.1 Fibrous Proteins

This category of proteins includes antigens which, in their intact form, have an elongated, rod shape. It is necessary to distinguish between fibrous protein antigens that are the result of polymerization of many globular subunits, as in the case of polymerized flagellin and microtubules, and proteins that exist in solution as stretched polypeptide chains with only limited tertiary complexity. One characteristic common to most of these antigens is the fact that they are built up of repeated determinants, a feature which may be of importance for antibody induction. Its main influence, however, is on the cellular mechanism of immunogenicity and this aspect will be discussed in Section 6.

3.1.1 Silk Fibroin

One of the typical fibrous proteins is silk fibroin, which forms the main protein constituent of silk. Its molecular structure consists of pleated sheaths, arranged in the β-form, and the protein in its native state is devoid of α-helical or tertiary structure. In an attempt to evaluate the nature of its antigenic determinants (Landsteiner, 1942; Cebra, 1961a,b), it has been shown that the antigenic specificity characteristic of the intact fibroin is retained after tryptic cleavage of the antigenic molecule. This is evident also from the capacity of the chymotryptic digest to inhibit entirely the precipitin reaction between soluble fibroin and rabbit antiserum directed against it. Inhibition was effected by a homologous series of varying size fragments of fibroin, all containing tyrosine as the C-terminal amino acid. Further studies indicated that the extent of the precipitin inhibition by these peptides is proportional to the size of the inhibitory fragment. A C-terminal tyrosine residue in each fragment seems to play a paramount role in the antigenic specificity of this protein, since when cleaved by carboxypeptidase the inhibitory capacity of the antigenic oligopeptides drastically is decreased. This has lead to the conclusion that some specific single residues may play a major role in antigenicity. It also indicates that in a fibrous protein like silk fibroin a limited number of fragments in the molecule of the immunogen, or possibly even a single, repeating fragment, retains most of the original antigenic specificity of the protein.

3.1.2 Collagen

Another characteristic fibrous protein is collagen, which forms the main protein constituent of connective tissue and which is the most abundant protein in animals. Collagen from vertebrates is composed of three polypeptide chains, two of which are identical, and are denoted α1 chains plus one α2 chain. Each chain has a molecular weight of approximately 100 000, and thus the collagen molecule has a total mass of 300 000. Except for the C and N-terminal regions, each of the polypeptide chains of the native collagen forms a left-handed helix which is supercoiled with the other two chains, as a right-handed triple helix (Cowan *et al.*, 1955). The fibrillar nature of the collagen molecule has been shown by Gross (1961), who found that the collagen molecule has the shape of a helical rod with the dimensions of $1·5 \times 300$ nm. Studies on the primary structure of collagen indicate that it has repeating sequences of the triplet Gly-X-Y, in which X is frequently proline or hydroxyproline (Traub and Piez, 1971). No such sequence was detected in the terminal parts of each chain which apparently have a pleated, non-helical structure.

Several immunochemical studies on collagen have been carried out in the last few years (reviewed by Kirrane and Glynn, 1968; O'Dell, 1968; Timpl *et al.*, 1973*a*; Timpl, 1975; Furthmayr and Timpl, 1976; Beard *et al.*, Chapter 13). In this chapter a description of the various aspects of the antigenicity and immunogenicity of collagen will be presented. The well-defined antigenic determinants of collagen, which reside mainly in the C and N-terminal regions, and the peculiar antigenic properties stemming from its triple-helical confor- mation will be dealt with later (see Section 5.4). In this section the overall antigenic properties of collagen, as a fibrous protein, the antigenicity of collagens from different sources, the interrelationships between collagen and procollagen, and data concerning the immunogenicity of this molecule will be discussed.

Collagen, in spite of its large size, is a weak immunogen. This characteristic has been attributed mainly to the fact that collagens of different vertebrate species are structurally similar. Experiments in rabbits have shown that, in native collagens the triple-helical part of the molecule is immunologically silent, whereas the main response is to the heterogeneous C or N-terminal regions, denoted telopeptides (Davidson *et al.*, 1967; Furthmayr *et al.*, 1971; Furthmayr and Timpl, 1972). The antigenic similarity between collagens of various vertebrates is manisfested not only by the weak immunogenicity but also by the similar antigenic specificity among various vertebrate collagens once an immune response is provoked (Borek *et al.*, 1969).

On the other hand, an evolutionary remote and structurally distinct collagen from *Ascaris* cuticle has been found to differ considerably in its antigenic properties from vertebrate collagens. This molecule is composed of triple-helical subunits which are formed by reverse folding of the same chain (molecular weight 62 000). The resultant subunits are interlinked by disulphide bridges, yielding an aggregate with a molecular weight of 900 000 (McBride and Harrington, 1967*a,b*), which is the immunogenic species. The reduction of this collagen, however, does not abolish completely its antigenic specificity, although it destroys many of its immunogenic sites (Fuchs and Harrington, 1970; Maoz *et* *al.*, 1971). This collagen exhibits no antigenic similarity to those from mammals, as indicated by their complete lack of cross-reactivity at the humoral level (Michaeli *et al.*, 1972). However, limited antigenic relationships still exist between these two types of collagen, since a cross-reaction at the level of cell-mediated immunity has been observed between them, and in addition, they both cross-react to some extent with antibodies raised against the synthetic triple-helical polymer (L-Pro-Gly-L-Pro)*n* (Maoz *et al.*, 1973*b*).

Another approach in the immunochemical studies of collagen is its correlation with procollagen. A structural characteristic of the procollagen molecule is that, in addition to the fibrillar moiety, its N-terminal region contains an extra globular region. Immunochemical studies using procollagen or pro-α chains for immunization (Sherr and Goldberg, 1973; Van der Mark *et al.*, 1973; Dehm *et al.*, 1974; Kohn *et al.*, 1974) have indicated that, in contrast to the native collagen, procollagen is a strong immunogen in which the immunodominant moiety is the globular area. The latter moiety, after separation from the collagen fibrils, exhibits antigenic properties which are common to most globular antigens, namely conformation dependency (Timpl *et al.*, 1973*b*; Dehm *et al.*, 1974). However, it can cross-react antigenically with the intact procollagens (Furthmayr and Timpl, 1976).

3.1.3 Flagellin

The last example to be given here to illustrate the antigenic properties of fibrous protein is flagellin, the subunit protein which builds the flagella of the various strains of *Salmonella*. It can be prepared either in the soluble, globular monomeric form, or as a long fibrillar polymer (POL). Nossal and his group studied the antigenic structure of flagellin from *Salmonella adelaide*, and have compared the antigenicity of POL, monomeric flagellin, and the cyanogen bromide cleaved peptides (Nossal *et al.*, 1964, 1965; Parish and Ada, 1969). Their studies have demonstrated that one fragment of the flagellin molecule, denoted peptide A (with a molecular weight of 18 000 compared with 40 000 for the complete flagellin molecule) is responsible for most of the antigenic specificity of the reconstituted flagella. This region is exposed probably in a repeated fashion on the outer surface of the flagella, as indicated by its high rate of iodination and heavy methylation of lysine residues (10 out of 11) during the chemical modifications, as compared to other parts of the molecule. In this respect, the polymerized flagellin is similar to the silk fibroin described previously.

Preparations of POL, monomeric flagellin, and peptide A also differ in their immunogenicity. POL is highly immunogenic in rabbits and elicits the production of antisera with high titres following a single injection in saline. However, the monomer is a weaker immunogen, but still stimulates antibody production, and the peptide is almost non-immunogenic in rats. Moreover, in the primary response to POL, IgM antibodies are formed in the initial response and only later is IgG found in the antiserum, whereas the monomer stimulates the formation of IgG only (Nossal *et al.*, 1964). An important difference between the monomer and the polymer is found also in the cellular mechanism of antigenic stimulation of these two antigens. It has been well established that, in contrast to the monomeric flagellin which is a classical T-dependent antigen, the assembled form does not require T cells (Armstrong *et al.*, 1969; Feldmann and Basten, 1971). This again may be the result of the repeating units being present in the polymeric structure.

As emerges from the cumulative variations in immunity observed between these three antigens, the differences among them do not stem from dissimilarity in size alone, but are due also to the expression of varied antigenic determinants in the overall antigenic specificity of the molecule, due to its fibrillar structure and to the arrangement of the small molecular units in the aggregated form.

3.2 Globular Proteins

Globular proteins are complex molecules in which the various antigenic determinants may include regions in which primary, secondary, tertiary, and quarternary structures are expressed. The specific folding of each individual protein results in the exposure or concealment of different regions or residues, and may bring into juxtaposition regions that are remote from each other on the polypeptide chain, or that are present on different polypeptide chains of the native protein.

In contrast to some fibrillar antigens or denatured proteins in which the polypeptide chain may undergo structural changes easily in solution, globular proteins usually exhibit a rigid overall structure. The precise folding of globular proteins is dictated by their primary structure (Anfinsen, 1973) and is stablized by a variety of inter- or intra-molecular interactions including disulphide bridges, electrostatic forces, hydrogen, and hydrophobic bonds. Each of the determinants on the surface of the molecule involved in the immune system is therefore more uniform in structure and less susceptible to environmental changes than are those in fibrous proteins. However, different globular proteins may differ in their complexity, size, and rigidity.

Attempts to characterize the antigenic properties of globular proteins started in the early 1950s, with gel diffusion and double-diffusion techniques becoming available for comparison of specificity (reviewed by Kaminsky, 1965). Even fragmentation of proteins and examination of the isolated fragments started as early as 1957 with independent studies by Porter and by Lapresle on the antigenic properties of bovine and human serum albumins, respectively. However, these studies made a relatively meagre contribution to the present understanding of the antigenic specificity, since at the time there was almost no information available on the molecular structure of these proteins. Increasing progress in the elucidation of the amino acid sequence and the spatial structure of a large variety of proteins, as well as the development of advanced techniques for fragmentation of proteins and for peptide synthesis, has enabled a more meaningful investigation of the molecular regions participating in immunological activity, and thus has provided a better insight into the structural basis of antigenicity of this category of protein antigens.

There are several approaches to the investigation of the antigenic properties of globular proteins. (*i*) Cross-reactivity between the native protein and its denatured form (obtained by partial or complete reduction or oxidation, or as a result of physical denaturation) may be compared. This approach yields information on the role of molecular folding in conferring the antigenic properties. (*ii*) The molecule may be cleaved enzymically or chemically in order to obtain fragments which may still possess antigenic activity. In the case of proteins with well-defined structure, this approach permits the delineation of the antigenic determinants. (*iii*) Another approach is feasible in the case of proteins which have been conserved structurally and functionally throughout evolution and which can be studied by immunological comparison. The existence of isofunctional enzymes is a general phenomenon, but in certain cases, such as the cytochrome c of various species or the lysozymes, evolution has resulted in very restricted molecular changes. The study of cross-reaction between such related molecules, which have only minimal differences in their amino acid sequence, might enable the localization and identification of residues involved in the antigenic activity.

It should be borne in mind, however, that the results of every such investigation depend not only on the antigen used but on the antiserum as well. The presence of many specificity determinants on the same antigen brings about inevitable heterogeneity in the antibodies, and different individual antisera will, therefore, differ in their potential capacity to react with the various antigenic sites of the molecule. To overcome this difficulty, one should differentiate between antisera which vary in the distribution of antibodies with distinct specificities towards different antigenic determinants of the same multideterminant antigen, or use antisera directed exclusively to defined regions of the molecule.

The detailed description of several globular proteins and their antigenic properties will illustrate the various points mentioned above.

3.2.1 Cytochrome c

Cytochrome c is found in many animal species (Margoliash and Schejter, 1966), and is a globular protein with a molecular weight of about 13 000. Intensive studies on cytochrome c isolated from different species have shown that the similarity in the sequence of amino acids of the different molecules is related generally to the phylogenetic distance between the species (Nolan and Margoliash, 1968; Dayhoff and Eck, 1969). Moreover, the tertiary structure of cytochromes c of various species is almost identical (Margoliash and Schejter, 1966; Dickerson et al., 1968). These finding suggest that this protein may be a useful model for investigating the role of specific structural variations in the antigenic properties.

Early attempts to prepare antibodies against cytochrome c were unsuccessful (Storck et al., 1964; Jonsson and Palens, 1966). This poor immunogenicity may stem from the relatively small size of the antigen, as well as from the structural similarity between the immunogen and the autologous cytochrome of the immunized animal. The latter is corroborated by the finding that the use of an evolutionary-remote cytochrome c for immunization enables production of positive antisera (Okada *et al.*, 1964). Margoliash and coworkers (Reichlin *et al.*, 1968; Margoliash *et al.*, 1970) more recently have succeeded, however, in obtaining an immune response to cytochrome c of man and other species after injection of the protein emulsified in Freund's complete adjuvant into rabbits.

In some instances the antisera obtained have failed to precipitate the proteins used for immunization, but they reacted well with the polymerized form of the homologous immunogens (Reichlin *et al.*, 1970). This rare phenomenon, namely immunogenicity contrasted by lack of antigenicity (as manifest by an inability to form an immune precipitate) of the monomeric antigen, may be due to the low valency of the antigenic molecule. This problem is especially critical in the case of small proteins which possess a high proportion of 'silent' antigenic determinants. The positive effect of polymerization upon the antigenic properties of cytochrome c was shown to operate at the level of immunogenicity as well as at the interaction with antibodies. Thus, the increase in antigenic valence results also in a better stimulation of the immunocompetent cells.

The most valuable results on the antigenicity of cytochrome c were obtained by comparing the cross-reactivity between cytochromes from 25 different species. In these studies (Margoliash *et al.*, 1967, 1970), it was found that cytochromes c from different species which have identical amino acid sequences are immunologically indistinguishable. In those cytochromes which differ by a single

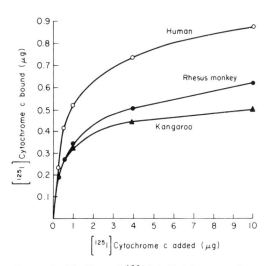

Figure 2 Binding of ^{125}I-labelled human, rhesus monkey, and kangaroo cytochrome c by anti-human cytochrome c. Each tube contained 0·3 ml of diluted anti-serum (1:25). From Nisonoff *et al.* (1970)

amino acid residue, the immunological distinction may vary from a very minor to a major one. When the difference involves several residues, there is a rough correlation between the number of variations in primary structure and the homologous antigen, and the extent of their immunological cross-reactivity. It is anticipated that when minimal differences exist in the amino acid sequences, and those are delineated exactly, the results may be used to identify and to localize some of the antigenic determinants (Nisonoff *et al.*, 1970). In this manner, it has been established that isolenicine 58 is an 'immunodominant' residue in human cytochrome c, and is responsible for the partial cross-reactivity with kangaroo cytochrome c. Its replacement by threonine in rhesus monkey causes a 30 per cent reduction in the immunological reactivity (Figure 2). Interestingly, antibodies to rhesus monkey cytochrome c react identically with the monkey and human proteins, indicating that threonine in this position is 'immunosilent', in contrast to the immunodominant isoleucine.

3.2.2 Sperm Whale Myoglobin

One of the most investigated globular proteins in immunological terms is sperm whale myoglobin, which is also one of the first proteins whose structure has been characterized fully. Kendrew and coworkers (1961) completed the three-dimensional model of myoglobin, and a few years later the complete amino acid sequence was established by Edmundson (1965). This protein has been shown to consist of one polypeptide chain with a molecular weight of 18 400 (153 amino acid residues) with no disulphide bridges, and containing one haem group per molecule. A large proportion of the molecule (about 75 per cent) is arranged in α helix and β structure, which maintain the structural integrity of this protein.

An elaborate immunological investigation has been carried out on myoglobin since the early 1960s. Subjects considered include parameters involved in the immunochemical characterization of the molecule, such as the topography of the antigenic determinants in the intact protein, the role of the haem in the antigenicity, the size of the individual antigenic determinants, and a synthetic approach for their delineation (Atassi, 1975).

The approaches employed in the immunochemical analysis of myoglobin are varied and include fragmentation to obtain antigenically active peptides, chemical modification of the amino acid residues, and physicochemical characterization of the intact met- and apo-myoglobins as compared to their antigenic properties. The cumulative data obtained from all these studies are extensive:

(*i*) In the myoglobin molecule, there are five antigenically active regions separated from each other by silent areas. These antigenic determinants are located mainly in the non-helical corners at the outer surface of the molecule, and are relatively small, consisting of only six or seven residues (Atassi, 1975).

(*ii*) In addition to these antigenic determinants, which consist of sequence stretches of amino acids, it has been suggested (Atassi and Saplin, 1968; Atassi, 1975) that regions with antigenic activity which are remote on the polypeptide chain, but which come into juxtaposition in the native folded molecule (such as sequences 16–21 and 113–119), may also form antigenic reactive sites.

(*iii*) The available data cannot point to those amino acid residues which are essential for the immunogenicity of the various regions of myoglobin. The residues which participate in the antigenic peptides are those which usually appear on the outer surface of proteins.

(*iv*) Alterations in the tertiary structure of myoglobin imposed on the molecule by removal of the haem (Breslow *et al.*, 1965; Harrison and Blout, 1965) have an effect on the overall antigenicity of the molecule (Reichlin *et al.*, 1963; Crumpton and Wilkinson, 1965; Atassi, 1967*b*). The difference cannot be attributed merely to the presence of the haem, since it has been shown that the haem itself is not antigenic (Reichlin *et al.*, 1963). This point will be discussed in Section 4 which deals with the role of molecular conformation in antigenicity. It should be mentioned here, however, that antibodies prepared against apomyoglobin (the haem-free protein) when binding to the intact metmyoglobin, cause the release of the haem group (Crumpton and Wilkinson, 1966). Moreover, these antibodies, when reacted with the homologous apomyoglobin, prevent complete reconstitution of the molecule upon the addition of the haem group, a reaction which takes place readily in the presence of antimetmyoglobin. In this case, therefore, immunological methods are apparently more sensitive than physical techniques in detecting conformational changes between two molecular species.

3.2.3 Hen Egg White Lysozyme

Another globular protein which has been subjected to extensive immunochemical investigation is hen egg white lysozyme. Its immunochemical properties have been discussed in detail in a recent review (Arnon, 1976). This protein consists of one polypeptide chain with 129 amino acids. It is particularly suitable for the investigation of antigenic structure because its amino acid sequence (Canfield, 1963), as well as its three-dimensional structure (Blake *et al.*, 1965), are known in detail and its mode of action has been elucidated also (Phillips, 1967). The information obtained from the immunochemical studies can, therefore, be interpreted in molecular terms. Moreover, lysozymes from many species have been isolated and subjected to analysis, including the determination of their amino acid sequences. Hence, clarification of their immunological relationships may yield information on a molecular level, concerning their detailed antigenic structure, and the changes that the enzyme has undergone during evolution (Wilson and Prager, 1974).

Valuable information on the effect of minor structural variations on the antigenic specificity of lysozyme has been obtained by comparing lysozymes obtained from avian and non-avian species. It has been shown that lysozymes from 16 birds differ in their capacity to react with antibodies against hen egg white lysozyme (Arnheim and Wilson, 1967), and also against lysozymes of turkey, Japanese quail, bobwhite quail, and duck (Prager and Wilson, 1971*a,b*). Using a microcomplement fixation test or phage inactivation it was found that

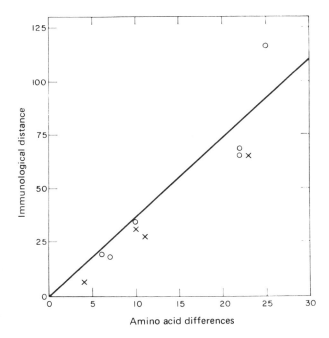

Figure 3 Antigenic differences *versus* number of amino acid differences for bird lysozymes of known sequences (0); Cross reactions involving Bobwhite quail lysoyzme (×). Cross-reactions were measured by complement fixation with anti-sera to every lysozyme. The degree of antigenic difference is expressed as the immunological distance. From Prager *et al.* (1972)

the degree of cross-reactivity is related directly to the sequence homology of the tested enzymes (Figure 3) (Arnheim *et al.*, 1969; Maron *et al.*, 1970; Prager and Wilson 1971*a,b*; Prager *et al.*, 1972). This approach has proved to be a powerful tool since it can discriminate between two closely related lysozymes of duck, which differ only in a limited, defined area of the molecule (Jollés *et al.*, 1967), and at the same time it has detected antigenic cross-reactivity between the lysozymes of birds and the evolutionarily remote human lysozyme obtained from patients with chronic lymphatic leukaemia (Maron *et al.*, 1970; Miller *et al.*, 1971). Comparison of various lysozymes has provided information concerning the contribution of particular amino acid residues to the antigenic specificity. Thus, using the interaction with antibodies against the 'loop' determinant of lysozyme (Arnon and Sela, 1969), the reactivities of the lysozymes from turkey and quail were compared with that of hen egg white lysozyme. When the results are related to amino acid sequence data they reveal the strong influence of arginine at position 68, as compared to that of arginine at position 73, in conferring antigenic specificity (Fainaru *et al.*, 1974). Since most of the antigenic determinants in lysozyme are conformation dependent, it is clear that those 'permissible' amino acid substitutions that cause only minor alterations in the native three-

324

dimensional structure of the enzyme have relatively small effects on the antigenic properties of the molecule.

In connection with the evolution of lysozyme, it is of interest to note the relationship between hen egg white lysozyme and bovine α-lactalbumin. These two proteins show a striking similarity in their amino acid sequence; 49 out of 129 amino acid residues are identical, including an identity in the position of their disulphide bridges (Brew *et al.*, 1967; Canfield *et al.*, 1971; Jollés and Jollés, 1971). On this basis, it has been suggested that they might be related functionally (since α-lactalbumin participates in the lactose synthetase system) and that they may have similar molecular folding (Browne *et al.*, 1969; Tamaburro *et al.*, 1972).

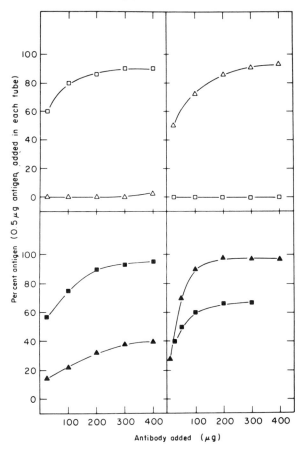

Figure 4 Antigen-binding capacity of native and open-chain egg white lysozyme obtained by reduction and carboxmethylation (RCM) of bovine α-lactalbumin, by isolated antibodies against native lysozyme (upper left), native lactalbumin (upper right), RCM lysoyme (lower left) and RCM lactalbumin (lower right). The antigens are: □, native lysozyme; △, native lactalbumin; ■, RCM lysozyme; ▲, RCM lactalbumin. From Arnon (1974)

According to physical calculation they also exhibit structural similarities (Lewis and Scheraga, 1971). It was postulated as a result that the two proteins are evolutionarily related, that is they may have been derived from a common ancestor gene by gene duplication (Brodbeck et al., 1967), and that this might explain the structural homology between them. Measurements of the physical properties of these two proteins does not lead, however, to a unified concept concerning the similarity in their structure.

In immunological studies carried out as a probe for the detection of a conformational relationship, antisera produced against either lysozyme or α-lactalbumin were tested for immunological interactions with the two antigens by several sensitive assays. The antisera towards each of the proteins revealed strong positive reactions with the homologous protein antigen, but showed no cross-reaction with the heterologous antigen (Arnon and Maron, 1970). On the other hand, when the unfolded peptide chains of lysozyme and lactalbumin (obtained by complete reduction and carboxymethylation) were used for immunization (Arnon and Maron, 1971), the resultant antisera showed an appreciable cross-reaction which could be measured by precipitin test and antigen binding capacities (Figure 4). These findings lead to the conclusion that (*i*) antibodies to the native conformation are apparently more specific than antibodies raised against the unfolded peptide chain and fail to recognize similarities in amino acid sequence *per se*; (*ii*) lysozyme and α-lactalbumin, which are obviously related, differ in their 'hydrophilic peripheries', that is those areas which may lead to the production of antibodies with similar specificities. They may still be similar in their three-dimensional overall conformation. The case of lysozyme thus can illustrate how information obtained from immunochemical investigations of immunogenicity and antigenicity can be utilized in studies on structure and evolution.

3.2.4 Staphylococcal Nuclease

Another globular protein which had been subjected to immunochemical analysis is staphylococcal nuclease. The biochemistry of this enzyme and its detailed structure have been characterized (Anfinsen et al., 1971). This nuclease, like myoglobin, is a protein free of disulphide bond, but its fragmentation results in the formation of a few, relatively large, polypeptide fragments which display antigenic specificity. Owing to the lack of disulphide bridges, these fragments can undergo alterations in their conformation resulting from the influence of the surrounding environment. Thus, this system has served for investigation of the affect of antibodies on the conformation of the antigen.

Antibodies specific towards the different antigenic regions of nuclease were obtained by immunoadsorption and elution on columns containing the isolated fragments (Sachs et al., 1972a, 1976). The peptides themselves retain, at least in part, the original, conformation-dependent antigenic specificity, but their immunogenicity is altered. This phenomenon was explained by Sachs et al. (1972b) as a consequence of conformational equilibria in the isolated peptides. In this explanation, antibodies can select the fraction of peptide in which the native conformation has been preserved, and can cause a further shift of the equilibrium towards formation of that particular conformational species. The antibodies to defined regions in the molecule (such as region 99–126) exhibit, as in the case of antibodies to the lysozyme loop, limited heterogeneity as indicated by binding curves (Sachs *et al.*, 1972*c*) and by isoelectric focusing (Eastlake *et al.*, 1974).

Antibodies against staphylococcal nuclease, as well as those fractions reactive with some of the defined antigenic determinants of nuclease, cause inhibition of enzymic activity. The convenient technique for determining antibody binding to the defined determinants by the inhibition of enzymic activity, has rendered this system amenable for studying several immunological phenomena such as the genetic control of immune response, and the characterization of anti-nuclease idiotypes and anti-idiotypes. This subject has been reviewed recently by Sachs and associates (1976) and will not be discussed here.

3.2.5 *Bovine Pancreatic Ribonuclease*

Immunological studies on this enzyme concern mainly the interrelationship between its globular structure and antigenicity. Early reports have indicated that the native ribonuclease carries only conformation-dependent determinants, since the native enzyme does not react with antiserum raised against the unfolded, performic acid-oxidized enzyme (Brown *et al.*, 1965, 1967; Brown, 1963) and the denatured enzyme reacts only very poorly with antibodies to the native enzyme. Subsequently, it was shown that the native conformation, which is essential for enzymic activity, can be conserved partially after the opening of only two disulphide bridges (Neuman *et al.*, 1967), and that in this derivative the antigenic integrity is retained as well. Ribonuclease exists in two forms, RNase A and RNase B, which differ in their degree of amidation (Tanford and Hanenstein, 1965), and consequently can be separated on ion-exchange columns. These two closely-related forms, which are similar in their structure, were shown by Brown *et al.* (1959) to be indistinguishable antigenically from each other.

Another point about ribonuclease, which is relevant to its antigenic properties, is the immunological interrelationship between the derivative known as RNase S and the native enzyme. RNase S is the product of cleavage of RNase A by subtilisin. The action of subtilisin results in the splitting of the peptide bond between alanine and serine at positions 20 and 21 respectively (Richards and Vithayathil, 1959) to yield a short, 20 residue peptide (referred to as the S peptide) and the remainder of the molecule (S protein), which are held together in an enzymically active species, but which can be separated. The two isolated fragments have no enzymic activity and lack antigenic capacity, since they show little or no antigenic cross-reactivity with RNase A (Singer and Richards, 1959; Merigan and Potts, 1966). Moreover, a novel enigmatic determinant can be detected, which is not present originally on RNase A. This may result either from the unmasking of an existing determinant when the S peptide is loosened from the remainder of the molecule, or from conformational changes occurring in the molecule upon cleavage (Kartha *et al.*, 1967; Wyckoff *et al.*, 1967). The loss of the original antigenic specificity of RNase A upon cleavage indicates either that the relevant determinants are located around the splitting point, or that they are composed of peptide segments present on both S peptide and S protein, which are situated in close proximity in the native enzyme. In this manner, the information from the antigenic analysis is correlated with the structural properties of the protein.

3.3 Antigens with Biological Activity

The interaction of antibodies with biologically active antigens and the resulting neutralization of their activity was one of the earliest observations in the history of modern immunology. In the previous sections, molecular parameters concerned with the antigenic properties of a variety of molecules have been discussed, including some biologically active antigens such as enzymes. The effect of antibody binding on the functional properties of these particular antigens will be considered now. Immunochemical studies on such biologically active molecules can not only help in the study of the mechanism of neutralization. Since the biological activity resides in a limited area of the molecule, and only antibodies specific towards this or related regions may have an effect on the catalytic activity. The contribution of different determinants to the immunological reactivity can be evaluated in the light of their relationship to the active site.

A very broad spectrum of molecules may be included in the category of biologically active antigens, including enzymes, hormones, antibodies and complement components, toxins, lectins and stimulants of cell activity such as mitogens, interferon, specific and non-specific factors that stimulate immunocytes. In this section, a few examples of enzymes and hormones will be examined, since these are the materials on which most immunological investigations have been carried out. Enzymes are particularly suited for such studies since they can be isolated and purified in relatively large amounts, they can be assayed accurately, and in many cases their structure and mode of action have been elucidated. Hence, the mechanism of their neutralization may be interpreted at a molecular level.

The interaction between enzymes and their respective antibodies leads generally to a reduction in the enzyme activity (reviewed by Arnon, 1971, 1973). In some cases, the enzyme is inhibited completely by the antibody, while in others only partially, and in a few cases no inhibition can be detected. Exceptions to this phenomenon also have been reported. It has been shown that sometimes an antibody can stimulate the activity of the enzyme. Several attempts have been made to elucidate the mechanism of the inhibition, however, it has not been found possible to arrive at a unified concept on the basis of results obtained with a large number of different enzymes (Cinader, 1957, 1967; Lee and Sehon, 1971). A number of factors is therefore used for evaluating the mechanism of inhibition for the enzyme to be investigated.

The extent of inhibition of an enzyme by an antibody is related frequently to the size of the substrate. This feature has been shown for several enzyme–anti-enzyme systems, such as ribonuclease (Brown *et al.*, 1959; Branster and Cinader, 1961), neuraminidase (Fazekas de St. Groth, 1963), trypsin (Arnon and Schechter, 1966), and papain (Shapira and Arnon, 1967). These results have led to the conclusion that the inhibition by antibody is attributable mainly to steric hindrance. The effect is not necessarily due to the formation of antigen–antibody aggregates, since it is observed also with soluble complexes obtained with monovalent fragments of antibodies.

An additional factor which has been found to participate in the inhibition involves conformational changes imposed on the enzyme by its interaction with the antibody. Direct evidence for the involvement of such conformational changes in enzyme–antibody interactions has been provided by enzyme systems, such as penicillinase, in which the interaction with the antibodies may bring about enhancement of the enzymic activity rather than inhibition (Citri and Zyk, 1965; Pollock *et al.*, 1967; Zyk and Citri, 1968). A similar phenomenon of stimulation of catalytic activity by specific antibodies has been observed with several other enzymes, including amylase (Okada *et al.*, 1963), takaamylase (Matsouka *et al.*, 1966), ribonuclease (Suzuki *et al.*, 1969; Pelichova *et al.*, 1970; Cinader *et al.*, 1971), β-lactamase (Gilboa-Garber *et al.*, 1971), and β-galactosidase (Rotman and Celada, 1968). In the last case, Messer and Melchers (1970), working with enzyme mutants, adduced direct evidence that the activation accompanying the interaction by the antibodies involves induced conformational changes.

One of the characteristic features of the inhibition of most enzymes by their respective antibodies is the residual catalytic activity which persists even in extreme antibody excess. This effect has been observed in many systems, especially when low molecular weight substrates were used for the activity assay (reviewed by Cinader, 1957, 1963, 1967). This phenomenon may be interpreted in two ways. One possible explanation is that the antibodies inhibit according to a uniform mechanism; each enzyme molecule is partially inhibited, while retaining a residual enzymic activity after combining with the antibody. Alternatively, the antibody population could be regarded as being inherently heterogeneous, consisting of species which differ in their inhibitory capacity. Undoubtedly, many antigenic determinants are present on the surface of each enzyme molecule, and these are apt to give rise to heterogeneous antibody populations. There is no reason to assume that all or any of these antigenic determinants should include the catalytic site or the substrate-binding site of the molecule. On the other hand, if antibodies should exist whose specificity were directed towards groupings associated with the active centre of the enzyme, their reaction with it would be expected to bring about inhibition of the enzymic activity, and the inhibitory capacity of such antibodies would be higher than that of the other antibody species. Indeed, it has been demonstrated that a fraction of stimulatory antibodies alongside 10 other fractions of neutralizing antibodies could be isolated from anti-ribonuclease by fractionation on ion-exchange columns (Cinader *et al.*, 1971).

Evidence that the inhibitory capacity of the antibodies is dependent on their narrow specificity, namely on the antigenic determinants of the enzyme with which they combine, was obtained using the papain–anti-papain system (Arnon and Shapira, 1967). In this case, antibodies with different inhibitory capacities were fractionated on the basis of their ability to cross-react with a related enzyme, chymopapain, which presumably contains similar antigenic determinants. Since the cross-reaction between the two enzymes is manifested also by cross-inhibition, it can be assumed that the regions which the two enzymes have in common include those antigenic determinants whose interaction with the antibodies is responsible for the decrease in catalytic activity of both enzymes. The fraction of the antibodies in anti-papain serum which cross-reacted with chymopapain was isolated as a consequence on a chymopapain immunoadsorbent, and was shown to possess high inhibitory capacity, much higher than that of the total antibody preparation. Thus it can be concluded that inhibition of enzymic activity is caused mainly by steric hindrance and conformational changes. The inhibitory properties of the antibodies are dependent on the determinants towards which they are specific.

Interaction of antibodies with hormones has attracted appreciable interest, mainly because of the broad clinical implications of these substances (Grodsky, 1965). The topic will be exemplified here by insulin (see reviews by Pope, 1966; Schwick, 1966; Wilson, 1967), and by chorionic gonadotrophin (Stevens, 1974).

The known primary structure of insulins from different species has allowed the elucidation of some structural–antigenic interrelationships. Human antibodies induced by repeated injections of beef insulin have been shown to be conformation dependent (Grodsky et al., 1959), since they do not react with the unfolded polypeptide chain of the hormone. Moreover, they have the capacity to react with the analogous human insulin, which probably has a similar gross structure to that of the beef hormone. However, the degree of cross-reaction between beef insulin and insulins of several other species was found to be proportional to the sequence homology between them (Berson and Yallow, 1959). Accordingly, the degree of neutralization of insulin by specific antibodies is related also to the structural differences between the insulin used for immunization and the tested hormone (Davidson and Haist, 1965; Davidson et al., 1969). Different antigenic determinants have been identified on the insulin molecule, and these have served not only for its immunochemical analysis but also for the elucidation of the genetic control of the immune response to this hormone, as will be discussed in more detail in Section 7.

An interesting application of the inhibition of a hormone activity by antibodies has been proposed as a means for fertility control (Stevens, 1974). It has been shown that the presence of antibodies to placental hormones such as human placental lactogen or human chorionic gonadotrophin (HCG) can neutralize the hormones in vivo, thus preventing, or even disrupting, gestation in baboons. Hence, attempts have been made to interfere deliberately with reproduction by active immunization with a hormone such as HCG. A hapten-conjugated HCG was used for immunization, to overcome the low immunogenicity due to the close similarity between the human and baboon hormones. The effect of the immunization is to reduce the level of gonadotrophin in the baboons; this results in the prevention of pregnancy. However, a concomitant effect is a lowering of levels of the structurally related luteinizing hormone, which is an essential hormonal component. A suggestion to overcome this problem was to use for immunization a fragment of the β-subunit of HCG which is completely absent from human luteinizing hormone (Stevens, 1974).

Although the results of clinical applications are not yet available, this technique is one of the best examples in which the molecular basis of antigenicity and immunogenicity of a material possessing biological activity might be utilized clinically, as well as for elucidating the mechanism of immunological interaction.

3.4 Synthetic Antigens

The obvious complexity of antigenic structure of native proteins has motivated immunochemists to look for simpler, synthetic molecules as models for protein antigens. As has been discussed in Section 1, the potential advantage of this approach is that through proper design of the antigens one may learn about many immunological phenomena and their molecular bases. Several review articles on this subject have appeared in recent years (see for example Sela, 1966, 1969; Gill, 1971), and therefore only a brief description of these antigens will be presented, with special emphasis on the relationships between molecular structure and their immunochemical properties.

It is necessary to distinguish between several types of synthetic antigens: (*i*) homopolymers of amino acids, (*ii*) random copolymers, either linear or branched; (*iii*) ordered linear copolymers with repeating sequences; and (*iv*) branched synthetic antigens containing ordered peptides with a desired sequence, as the antigenic determinants.

Homopolymers of amino acids are generally not immunogenic—with the exception of poly-L-proline in guinea-pigs (Jasin and Glynn, 1965a,b; Brown and Glynn, 1968). In contrast, copolymers of amino acids may be highly immunogenic, even when injected in low doses and thus can mimic, in many respects, protein antigens. This has been shown for linear copolymers (Gill and Doty, 1960) and for branched copolymers (Sela and Arnon, 1960b; Sela et al., 1962; Fuchs and Sela, 1963).

Attempts to pinpoint the requirements for immunogenicity have indicated that linear homopolymers behave like haptenic groups, and may be rendered immunogenic either by covalent attachment (Arnon et al., 1965; Schechter et al., 1966) or by electrostatic conjugation with a modified protein or peptide of opposite charge (Gill and Doty, 1962; Plescia et al., 1964; Maurer, 1965b; Goodman and Nitecki, 1967; Maurer and Pinchuck, 1968).

Homo-oligomers of amino acids not only become immunogenic by attachment to macromolecular carriers, but can also enhance the antigenicity of a poorly immunogenic protein, gelatin (Arnon and Sela, 1960; Sela and Arnon, 1960a,c). A detailed investigation of the immunochemical properties of many polypeptidyl gelatins, indicates that the best potentiator of the immune response in a specific manner is an oligopeptide containing either tyrosine only or tyrosine and glutamic acid (Sela and Arnon, 1960*a*; Arnon and Sela, 1960). This has led to the preparation of a completely synthetic antigen, which is a multichain, branched, synthetic polypeptide in which poly-DL-alanine side chains are attached to the ε-amino groups of a poly-L-lysine backbone, and the polyalanyl chains are in turn elongated with peptides containing L-tyrosine and L-glutamic acid (Sela and Arnon, 1960*b*; Sela *et al.*, 1962). This polymer is denoted (T,G)-A–L, and it has provoked the formation of antibodies specific for the peptides of tyrosine and glutamic acid, the (T, G) determinant.

Following the synthesis of this initial antigenic material, many analogues have been prepared and tested. From a knowledge of the chemistry of these compounds it seemed possible by studying copolymers which show only limited variations in their chemical formulae, to deduce the role of various structural features in their antigenic function. The problems considered over the years have included the role of shape, size, composition, and electrical charge of the macromolecule. Also, the importance of locus in the molecule of the area important for immunogenicity, as well as the optical configuration of its component amino acids and the steric conformation of the immunogenic macromolecule could be evaluated.

Homopolymers of amino acids are, as already mentioned, very poor immunogens, but the immunogenicity is improved by variations in composition. While macromolecular substances are more reliably immunogenic, low molecular weight peptide conjugates may still be effective provided that they have the right composition (de Weck, 1974). The presence of electrical charges on a macromolecule is not a minimal requirement for immunogenicity, but it affects the antigenic specificity (Fuchs and Sela, 1963). Moreover, when the antigen is charged, an inverse relationship exists between the net electrical charge of the immunogen and that of the antibodies it provokes (Sela and Mozes, 1966).

Peptides of opposite configuration are distinguished exquisitely by specific antibodies, which are usually stereospecific—totally unreative towards the other optical isomer—but polymers containing exclusively D-amino acids are poor immunogens and easily induce immunoglogical tolerance unless administered in very small doses. It seems that the inefficient formation of antibodies to polymers of D-amino acids in cases of tolerance is due to their slow and incomplete catabolism (Maurer, 1965*a*; Gill *et al.*, 1965, 1968).

One of the crucial factors affecting the antigenic properties of the molecule is the accessibility of the antigenic determinants (Sela *et al.*, 1962). The importance of the specific location of the determinant on the synthetic polymer was studied by comparing the response to the first synthetic antigen ((T,G)-A–L) with that elicited by an antigen of very similar composition, in which the (T,G)-peptides were attached directly to the ε-amino groups of the polylysyl backbone, and subsequently were elongated at their terminal positions with poly-DL-alaninyl chains (see Figure 1). As has been mentioned already in Section 2, it was found that the latter polymer, though of the same amino acid composition as

(T,G)-A–L, does not possess its immunogenicity, or the antigen specificity of the (T,G) group. Thus, by changing the locus of the functional antigenic group it is possible to render a macromolecule antigenic or non-antigenic, and the conclusion is that the antigenic determinant cannot be hidden in the interior of the molecule, but must be exposed or accessible in order to exert its effect.

One of the important conclusions drawn from the study of synthetic antigens concerns the crucial role that spatial conformation plays in the antigenic properties of protein molecules. As will be discussed in detail in Section 4, many studies with natural proteins where no immunological cross-reaction could be detected between the native protein and its denatured form indicate that the antibodies are directed mainly to conformation-dependent determinants. This phenomenon has been demonstrated clearly by the use of two systems of synthetic antigens. One such example involved the tripeptide Tyr-Ala-Glu, which was attached in one case to the branched poly-DL-alanine, and in the second case was polymerized to a high molecular weight periodic polymer, which exists under physiological conditions in an α-helical form (Ramachandran *et al.*, 1971). As will be discussed in Section 4, these two antigens (Figure 5) possess completely different specificities which reflect their three-dimensional conformations Schechter *et al.*, 1971*a*,*b*; Sela *et al.*, 1967).

Another interesting example is the synthetic ordered polypeptide (Pro-Gly-Pro)$_n$, which has been shown to have physical properties similar to those of collagen (Traub and Yonath, 1966). The detailed immunological properties of this polymer and its relation to collagen are described in detail in Section 4, but it should be mentioned here that the antigenic properties of this triple-helical polymer are completely different from those of a random polymer with the same amino acid composition, (Pro$_{66}$Gly$_{34}$)$_n$ (Maoz *et al.*, 1973*a*,*b*), emphasizing the role of conformation in antigenic specificity.

Another class of synthetic antigens is that containing peptides with ordered sequence. Such antigens make possible the detailed analysis of simple antigenic determinants. For example, in the synthetic antigen (T,G)-A–L, the determinant is a random oligopeptide containing tyrosine and glutamic acid. In a systematic study using a series of defined tetrapeptides, each composed of tyrosine and glutamic acid, attached to multichain poly-DL-alanine carrier, it is possible to demonstrate that the main antigenic determinant in the randomly polymerized (T,G)-A–L is the peptide with the sequence of Tyr-Tyr-Glu-Glu (T, T, G, G). The random and the ordered antigens exhibit similar antigenic specificities and have been found to be under the same genetic control. A similar determinant (T, G, T, G) attached to the polymeric carrier, yields a material which, although immunogenic by itself, shows almost no cross-reactivity with antibodies to the random polymer (Mozes *et al.*, 1974; Schwartz *et al.*, 1975). Thus, these two peptides—T, T, G, G and T, G, T, G—which differ from each other only in the exchange of position of two residues, confer completely different immunological properties on the macromolecular antigen of which they are a part.

The availability of methods for the synthesis of peptides with desired sequence (Merrifield, 1965; Fridkin and Patchornik, 1974) and the elucidation of the

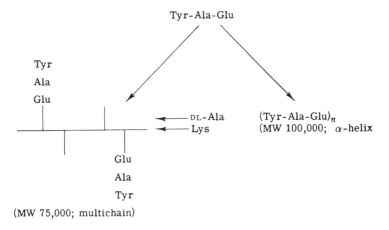

Figure 5 Synthetic branched polymer in which peptides of sequence Tyr-Ala-Glu are attached to the N-termini of polymeric side chains in poly-DL-alanyl-poly-L-lysine (left) and a periodic polymer of the tripeptide Tyr-Ala-Glu (right). From Schechter *et al.* (1971*a*)

amino acid sequences of many proteins, including those of defined antigenic regions within them, have permitted a synthetic approach to the study of antigenic determinants of native proteins. This approach has proved useful in the investigation of several proteins or polypeptide antigens such as bradykinin (Spragg *et al.*, 1967), lysozyme (Arnon *et al.*, 1971; Teicher *et al.*, 1973), and myoglobin (Atassi, 1975). The use of synthetic analogues of a given polypeptide antigenic determinant, in which either replacement or a change in size has been introduced, can define the role particular residues play in the antigenic specificity.

The use of synthetic ordered peptides has also made possible the preparation of antigens that elicit an antiviral antibody response. Thus, in an early study Anderer (1963*b*) showed that the C-terminal hexapeptide of tobacco mosaic virus, when conjugated to a protein carrier, elicits antibodies which reduce to some extent the infectivity of the virus. In a recent study (Langbeheim *et al.*, 1976), an effective antiviral action was provoked by a completely synthetic molecule containing an ordered peptide with the appropriate sequence. In this study, a synthetic peptide that corresponds to the amino acid sequence of a fragment (89–108) of the coat protein of MS-2 coliphage was conjugated to the synthetic carrier multichain polyalanine. This completely synthetic antigen induced in rabbits antisera able to effect almost total neutralization of MS-2 viability, nearly as efficiently as an antiserum prepared against the intact coat protein (Langbeheim *et al.*, 1976).

The use of ordered peptides of desired sequence in synthetic antigens might, therefore, not only contribute to the elucidation of the molecular basis of immunogenicity and antigenicity, but might also lead in the future to the development of appropriately designed materials with selected antigenic determinant(s) attached to an adequate polymeric carrier for production of a multivalent vaccine.

4 ROLE OF CONFORMATION IN ANTIGENICITY

The decisive role of conformation in determining the antigenic specificity of protein and polypeptide antigens is a widely recognized phenomenon and has been discussed in detail in a recent review by Crumpton (1974). Experimental evidence indicates that a drastic change in the antigenic properties occurs upon denaturation of native proteins (by heat or chemical modification) or upon unfolding of their polypeptide chains (Arnon, 1971; Benjamini et al., 1972). The denatured or unfolded proteins are usually still immunogenic, but their antigenic specificity is totally different from that of the corresponding native proteins. This was demonstrated convincingly for various proteins, such as ribonuclease (Brown et al., 1959; Neumann et al., 1967), papain (Shapira and Arnon, 1969), trypsin (Erickson and Neurath, 1943; Arnon and Neurath, 1970), lysozyme (Shinka et al., 1967; Gerwing and Thompson, 1968; Young and Leung, 1970), and albumin (Jacobsen et al., 1972). It is thus obvious that gross changes in the conformation of protein molecules are definitely accompanied by a major alteration of their antigenicity.

In many instances, more subtle conformational alterations in a protein also are accompanied by a change in antigenic reactivity. The best example of such systems concerns the change in the antigenicity associated with the removal of the haem group from sperm whale myoglobin (see Section 3.2.2). In this conversion of metmyoglobin to apomyoglobin the loss of haem is associated with only a small structural change, and in parallel, the antigenic properties of the two molecular species are not much different. However, the precipitate formed between metmyoglobin and anti-apomyoglobin was shown to be colourless and not to contain the ferrihaem group (Crumpton and Wilkinson, 1966), indicating that the antibodies specific towards the haem-free molecule induced a conformational change in the metmyoglobin and release the haem group from it during the antigen–antibody interaction.

It should be pointed out that not all conformational alterations have a measurable effect upon antigenicity and vice versa. There are, for example, several aberrant haemoglobins, with distorted, as indicated by X-ray crystallography, tertiary structures, and yet which cannot be distinguished antigenically from haemoglobin A (Reichlin, 1972), while the α and β chains of human haemoglobin do not show any antigenic resemblance in spite of the remarkable similarity in their conformation (Reichlin et al., 1966). However, these are probably exceptions to the general rule that there is an intimate relationship between conformation and antigenicity.

For a better assessment of the contribution of spatial conformation to the antigenic properties of a protein molecule, one should first analyse the various structural features affecting antigenic specificity. Antibodies produced in response to immunization with protein antigens are reactive with various antigenic determinants and may be directed against one or more of the structural aspects of the protein. These consist of the primary structure (the amino acid sequence of the polypeptide chain), the secondary structure (dictated by the backbone of the polypeptide, such as α helix and β-pleated sheet), the tertiary structure (conferred by interactions between various grouping in the chain and associated with its folding), and the quaternary structure (due specific association of several polypeptide chains to form a protein consisting of many subunits). The antigenic determinants are divided therefore, on a theoretical basis, into two broad categories, sequential and conformational (Sela *et al.*, 1967), depending on whether their specificity is due only to stretches of amino acid sequences in the protein or to the other structural features.

According to this classification a sequential determinant is defined as one due to a segment in the amino acid sequence in its unfolded or linear conformation, and antibodies to such a determinant would be expected to react with a peptide of identical or similar sequence. On the other hand, a conformational determinant is defined as one resulting from the steric conformation of the antigenic macromolecule, and leading to antibodies which would not necessarily react with peptides derived from that area of the molecule. Thus, conformational determinants would include those determinants composed of amino acid residues which are remote in the unfolded peptide chain but which occupy juxtapositions in the native folded structure.

Examination of the three-dimensional structures of a number of globular proteins reveals that they contain short sequences of adjacent amino acids whose side chains are partially or fully exposed on the surface of the protein, for example, residues 77–80 and 81–85 in sperm whale myglobin (Dickerson, 1964) and residues 53–63 of lamprey haemoglobin (Hendrickson and Love, 1971). Consequently, the existence of sequential determinants in globular proteins is feasible, at least theoretically. However, in practice, little convincing evidence in support of their occurrence has been reported. Indeed, the almost complete loss of antigenicity upon denaturation argues strongly that the vast majority of the determinants that elicit humoral antibody formation are conformational. In cases where short peptide fragments of a protein have been shown to interfere with the interaction of the native protein with its antibodies, this capacity is often due to the fact that the peptides are induced by the antibodies to refold into the structure that they assume in the native protein (Crumpton and Small, 1967). There are only a few, clear-cut cases where sequential determinants can be demonstrated, such as the terminal segments of collagen (Becker *et al.*, 1972) or silk fibroin (Cebra, 1961*a*,*b*), but as mentioned previously, antibodies to native proteins are directed mostly, and in several cases exclusively, against conformation-dependent determinants (Sela, 1969). A few examples will illustrate these points.

Native soluble collagen was shown to possess both sequential and conformational determinants. Thus as has been mentioned earlier (see Section 3.1.2), the majority of rabbit antibodies to native collagen is directed against the short, non-helical, N-terminal segments of the polypeptide chains of the native protein (Becker *et al.*, 1972). The sequential nature of these determinants was established by the observation that these antibodies also react with the terminal portions of the individual, randomly-coiled polypeptide chains of denatured soluble collagen.

On the other hand, rat antibodies recognize a portion of the triple-helical conformation of collagen. The conformational nature of these determinants was confirmed by failure of these antibodies to react with the uncoiled polypeptide chains, whereas restoration of the triple helix is associated with the recovery of reactivity (Beil et al., 1973). Silk fibroin is another protein in which the existence of a sequential antigenic determinant has been demonstrated unequivocally. The whole antigenic site of this protein comprises a sequence of approximately eight to twelve amino acid residues, mostly glycine and alanine, but containing one crucial tyrosine residue as well—Ala-(Gly-Ala)$_{3-4}$-Tyr. This determinant is probably a repeating unit in the protein, otherwise it could not account for the full antigenic specificity of the molecule.

In globular proteins, like haemoglobin, myoglobin, or lysozyme, the antigenicity is dependent almost exclusively on three-dimensional conformation. In sperm whale myoglobin, for example, even though the molecule lacks any disulphide bonds to stabilize its structure, the antigenic regions of the molecule have been shown to occupy 'corners' in the folded structure (Atassi and Saplin, 1968). A space-filling molecular model reveals that these corners coincide with the more exposed areas which, due to the folding of the polypeptide chain, are held in a fixed conformation. Moreover, the haem group, which is non-covalently bound to the protein moiety, and which can be removed to yield the haem-free apomyoglobin, also contributes to the antigenic properties. Thus, a difference in both conformation (Breslow et al., 1965) and antigenic specificity can be observed between myoglobin and apomyoglobin (Reichlin et al., 1963; Crumpton and Wilkinson, 1965; Atassi, 1967b). For lysozyme, at least two well-defined antigenic determinants have been characterized. One contains an intra-chain disulphide bridge (Arnon and Sela, 1969) and the other an inter-chain disulphide linking the N and C-terminal regions (Fujio et al., 1968a). While these determinants will be described in detail in Section 5, it should be mentioned here that both have been shown to be strictly conformation dependent.

In view of the role played by conformation in determining antigenicity, it is not surprising that antigenic cross-reactivity has been proposed as a sensitive probe for conformational differences and similarities between related proteins. However, whereas cross-reactivity could be taken as an indication for similarity, the lack of cross-reactivity does not necessarily imply gross differences in conformation. For example, native hen egg white lysozyme and bovine α-lactalbumin, which share 40 per cent of their amino acid sequences (Brew et al., 1969), do not cross-react (Arnon and Maron, 1970; Atassi et al., 1970; Habeeb and Atassi, 1971a) but, as shown in Figure 4, their unfolded polypeptide chains do display marked cross-reaction (Arnon and Maron, 1971). Although these results reveal obvious differences between the hydrophilic peripheries of the proteins, they are not unequivocally indicative of dissimilarity in their three-dimensional structure (Arnon and Maron, 1970). Similarly, the α and β chains of haemoglobin do not show any apparent antigenic resemblance since no cross-reaction between them has been detected using their respective antisera (Reichlin et al., 1966), in spite of the remarkable similarity in their conformation (Braunitzer et al., 1964).

The role of conformation in antigenic specificity was demonstrated most convincingly using two synthetic antigens containing the same tyrosyl-alanyl-glutamyl sequence mentioned earlier (see Figure 5). The first peptide is a high molecular weight, ordered copolymer composed of the repeated sequence of the tripeptide Tyr-Ala-Glu, previously shown to exist as a α helix (Ramachandran *et al.*, 1971). In the second antigen, the same tripeptide is attached to a branched polymer of alanine, and exists as a random coil. These two polymers bring about the formation of antibodies with distinct specificities, and no cross-reaction occurs between them (Schechter *et al.*, 1971*b*). Furthermore, the system of the branched polymer can be inhibited efficiently by the tripeptide, whereas the system of the helical peptide cannot. Inhibition of the latter system is achieved only with oligopeptides of the general formula (Tyr-Ala-Glu)$_n$, where n is from three to nine (Figure 6), the inhibitory capacity increasing with the value of n. Moreover, the oligopeptide (Tyr-Ala-Glu)$_{13}$ is able to cross-precipitate the antibodies to the helical polymer. Circular dichroism studies (Schechter *et al.*, 1971*c*) show that the above oligopeptides possess very little helical structure, but

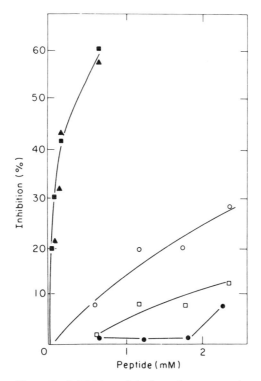

Figure 6 Inhibition of the homologous reaction in the (TAG)$_n$–anti-(TAG)$_n$ system, by ($\bullet$), Tyr-Ala-Glu; ($\square$), (Tyr-Ala-Glu)$_2$; ($\bigcirc$), (Tyr-Ala-Glu)$_3$; ($\blacktriangle$), (Tyr-Ala-Glu)$_7$; and ($\blacksquare$), (Tyr-Ala-Glu)$_9$. From Schechter *et al.* (1971*b*)

upon interaction with the Fab fragment of the antibody to the helical polymer their α-helical content increases. Thus it was concluded that the antigenicity of the α-helical copolymer is conformation dependent. In addition, the specific antibodies it elicits are capable of inducing a transconformation of the oligopeptides into a structure more like that of the high molecular weight helical polymer.

Therefore, structural conformation is an important factor affecting antigenicity. This will become even more obvious in Section 5, which describes in detail some defined antigenic determinants of proteins. It will emerge that most of these determinants depend on spatial conformation for integrity and specificity.

5 DEFINED ANTIGENIC DETERMINANTS IN PROTEINS

The approach used most commonly for the identification of antigenically reactive regions of proteins is fragmentation of the native protein either by chemical cleavage adjacent to specific residues or by controlled proteolysis. The resultant fragments are then fractionated and screened for immunologically active components, which either can bind to the antibodies, or can interfere with the interaction of the antibodies and the intact antigen. Since such fragments, by definition, embody antigenic determinants and can be analysed subsequently and defined, they have been utilized to characterize the antigenic structure of the parent molecule. Furthermore, by subjecting them to various chemical modifications, one can identify the particular residues which contribute to the antigenic reactivity and specificity. This technique, although very useful, is not without its shortcomings. (i) An isolated peptide will not necessarily maintain the conformation it had in the parent protein (Crumpton and Small, 1967; Taniuchi and Anfinsen, 1971). For this reason, a non-reactive fragment may still be a part of a reactive region in the intact protein. However, with some reactive region-carrying fragments, the antibody to the intact molecule may induce on the peptide the conformation necessary for binding with the antibody combining site (Schechter et al., 1971a). (ii) Cleavage of the protein may take place within a reactive region. Dissecting the reactive region into two (or more) peptides may result in the loss of most of the immunochemical reactivity of the site. This is a serious objection, since it may be difficult to locate all the antigenic determinants unless several cleavage techniques are used and overlapping fragments are analysed.

Notwithstanding these shortcomings, however, this technique is still one of the best approaches for studying antigenic determinants. When positive results are obtained with a given peptide, the data are useful, particularly if the same region is located as a part of several different overlapping peptides. This approach has led to the recognition of the antigenic make-up of several proteins.

The earliest attempts at antigenic analysis of proteins were made by Lapresle and Darieux (1957) using human serum albumin, and by Porter (1957) using bovine serum albumin. In both cases, the information gained was meagre, for two reasons. Firstly, the tested fragments were relatively large, since the methods for their preparation had not been developed fully, and secondly, the information then available on the structure or sequence of the proteins was very limited (Kaminski, 1965). Subsequent studies on several other proteins have yielded information on a number of antigenic determinants, culminating in the studies on myoglobin which have resulted in the complete antigenic mapping of the molecule. Several examples will be given to describe the defined antigenic determinants of several proteins, which have been elucidated.

5.1 Unfolded Globular Proteins

Studies with several unfolded proteins (prepared by reduction and alkylation, or by oxidation) have led to the location of some antigenic determinants, but those do not coincide necessarily with determinants in the native protein.

In the case of oxidized ribonuclease (Ribox), two peptides (comprising residues 38–61 and 105–124) have been isolated from a proteolytic digest of the protein. These peptides can inhibit the precipitation and complement fixation of the oxidized RNase with its antibody (Brown, 1962). These are, therefore, linear sequences which encompass antigenic determinants. In subsequent studies, it has been shown that the latter peptide can bind to antibodies against Ribox with an association constant of 3×10^6 M^{-1} and a homogeneity index of 0·98, indicating that the peptide is bound with relatively high affinity to a homogeneous fraction of the antibodies. It is calculated that the homogeneous fraction represents about 50 per cent of all the precipitating antibodies to this antigen (Isagholian and Brown, 1970), thus suggesting that the number of determinants on this unfolded polypeptide chain is small. By stepwise degradation it has been shown that the residues valine 116 and proline 117 make the principal contribution to the binding properties of this fragment (Brown and Liu, 1970) and are crucial for its antigenicity.

Similar behaviour was observed in the case of reduced and carboxymethylated lysozyme. Following cleavage with cyanogen bromide, Young and Leung (1970) obtained three peptides; two—the N and C-terminal fragments corresponding to residues 1–12 and 106–129, respectively—possessed marked inhibitory activity. In an independent study, Gerwing and Thompson (1968) reported that a single peptide (residues 74–96), isolated from a tryptic digest of the reduced and carboxymethylated lysozyme, gave a 60 per cent inhibition of the antigen–antibody precipitation. The reason for the variations in observations is not known and might be merely due to the different rabbits used for immunization. The results, however, do indicate that discrete portions of the unfolded polypeptide chain form defined antigenic determinants.

In the case of oxidized ferredoxin two fragments, the N-terminal heptapeptide and the C-terminal pentapeptide, are able to inhibit the interaction of oxidized ferredoxin with its antibody, to an extent of 40 and 55 per cent, respectively. Moreover, this inhibitory effect is cumulative–a mixture of the two peptides causes 90 per cent inhibition—demonstrating that these are two different, independent antigenic determinants (Mitchell and Levy, 1970; Kelly and Levy, 1971).

There are several similarities between the systems described above, which contain linear sequential determinants. (*i*) The antigenic determinant has to be of a certain minimal size—about eight to ten amino acid residues. When fragments of different size are available the efficiency of their inhibition increases with their size. (*ii*) The number of determinants is rather small—not more than two or three for a polypeptide chain of molecular weight 10 000. (*iii*) The contribution of the individual amino acid residues comprising the antigenically active site is not equal. In many cases, a particular residue, such as the tyrosine in silk fibroin or the valine and proline in Ribox, is crucial for the inhibitory effect on the respective antigen system, and may be considered as an immunodominant portion of the antigenic determinant, a phenomenon which has been observed in other antigens, especially carbohydrates (Luderitz *et al.*, 1966).

5.2 Tobacco Mosaic Virus and Its Coat Protein

Two antigenic systems of tobacco mosaic virus (TMV) were studied. These are the intact virus and the coat protein subunit (TMVP).

In the interaction of the intact virus and its antibodies, several peptides of the protein show inhibitory effect, but most of them are weak and are not efficient inhibitors. One of the more efficient inhibitory peptides is the C-terminal hexapeptide Thr-Ser-Gly-Pro-Ala-Thr (Anderer, 1963*a*). This peptide not only inhibits the precipitation of the virus by its antibodies, but also can elicit (when conjugated to a protein carrier) antibodies which can reduce the infectivity of the virus to some extent (Anderer, 1963*b*). Shorter peptides derived from this hexapeptide have lower activity (Anderer and Schlumberger, 1965). Although this and other linear peptides show inhibitory activity, there is considerable evidence that the tertiary structure of the protein is of great importance in the antigenicity of TMV (Anderer and Handschuh, 1962, 1963; von Sengbusch, 1965; Van Regenmortel, 1966). Evidence also suggests that these conformation-dependent determinants are created by the 'packing' of the protein subunits around the RNA core, resulting in the exclusive exposure of particular regions (Benjamini *et al.*, 1972).

Whereas these peptides, and in particular the C-terminal portion of the protein, constitue an antigenic determinant in the intact TMV, they are of minor importance, if any, in TMVP. In the latter case, an eicosapeptide, comprising the residues 93–112 of the protein, possesses the total inhibitory activity of a tryptic digest, and thus encompasses the single antigenic determinant (Benjamini *et al.*, 1964, 1965). Detailed studies have demonstrated that most of the activity of this peptide resides in its three terminal residues Ala-Thr-Arg (Young *et al.*, 1968; Benjamini *et al.*, 1969). Attempts to immunize experimental animals with the antigenic peptides of TMVP have been unsuccessful. Similarly, intact TMVP cannot inhibit the reaction between the peptides and their antibodies (Spitler *et al.*, 1970; Fearney *et al.*, 1971). This demonstrates and emphasizes the differences between antigenic specificity and immunogenicity, as a function of the structure of the material used for immunization.

5.3 Staphylococcal Nuclease

Staphylococcal nuclease is a single-chain protein lacking any disulphide bond to stabilize its three-dimensional structure, and yet its antigenic determinants that have been identified are conformation dependent. Several studies on its immunochemical characteristics have been carried out by Anfinsen and his coworkers. Fuchs *et al.* (1969) were interested mainly in the interaction of the enzyme with its antibodies and the resultant inhibition of the enzyme activity. Omenn *et al.* (1970*a,b*) investigated the antigenic determinants of nuclease by looking for immunologically active fragments. Fragmentation of the protein using either cyanogen bromide or tryptic digestion allows the antigenicity to be correlated with two regions. One of these, which includes residues 6–48, is restricted possibly to residues 18–47, whereas the second is located at the C-terminus, consisting of residues 99–149. The latter, as emerges from later studies (Sachs, 1972*a*), probably contains two determinants, one of which is localized in the linear sequence 127–149 and the second consists of residues 99–126. Examination of the three-dimensional structure of the molecule (Arnone *et al.*, 1971; Cotton and Hazen, 1971) reveals that each of these regions occupies corner(s) of the folded polypeptide chain, which are exposed on the surface of the native protein (Figure 7). Furthermore, comparison of the specificities of the antibodies formed against synthetic peptides corresponding to fragments of staphylococcal nuclease with those of the antibodies isolated from antisera to whole native nuclease, unequivocally demonstrates that the determinants possess

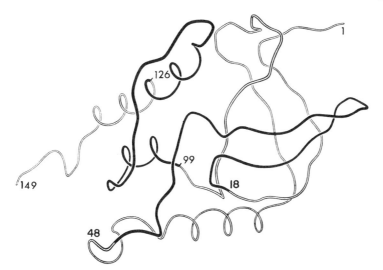

Figure 7 An artist's representation of the three-dimensional structure of staphylococcal nuclease. The drawing was made from a wire model based on the X-ray crystallographic structure (Cotton and Hasen, 1971). The sequences between amino acids 18 and 47 as well as 99 and 126, which contain the major antigenic determinants, have been shaded. From Sachs *et al.* (1972*c*)

conformation specificity (Sachs *et al.*, 1972*b*). Thus, although the nuclease has a low helical content and no disulphide bonds, its structural conformation influences its antigenic determinants. Antibodies to nuclease can serve consequently as sensitive indicators for the enzyme's conformation (Sachs *et al.*, 1972*c*).

5.4 Collagen and Synthetic Collagen-Like Polymer

The results of various studies have demonstrated clearly that native collagen possesses both sequential and conformational determinants. As mentioned earlier (see Section 3.1.2), vertebrate collagens are composed of three chains—two identical α_1 chains and one α_2 chain, which differ in their amino acid composition and sequence (Taub and Piez, 1971). Immunization with native collagens leads mainly to antibodies directed to the N and C-terminal non-helical regions of both types of chains (Piez *et al.*, 1968), which show considerable interspecies differences (Michaeli *et al.*, 1969; Pontz *et al.*, 1970; Timpl *et al.*, 1970; Furthmayr *et al.*, 1971; Becker *et al.*, 1972; Rautenberg *et al.*, 1972). Although some variations exist between the results of different studies, they still indicate that the specificities of the respective determinants depend almost entirely on their amino acid sequence. Thus, these are sequential determinants. In the case of human collagen, the relevant determinant has been identified as the sequence Glx-Leu-Ser-Tyr-Gly (Rautenberg *et al.*, 1972).

The helical region of collagen has been conserved during evolution to a greater extent than the other parts, yet some interspecies differences have been observed in this region as well, and they are expressed in conformational antigenic determinants. This was concluded from the finding that rat antisera against calf collagen, in contrast to rabbit and chicken antisera, interact primarily with the triple-helical conformation (Timpl *et al.*, 1971; Beil *et al.*, 1973).

Supporting evidence for the presence of conformational determinants in collagen was provided indirectly using a synthetic approach. As briefly mentioned in Section 3.1.2, a synthetic periodic polypeptide $(Pro-Gly-Pro)_n$, which was shown to have a collagen-like triple-helical structure (Engel *et al.*, 1966), was found to be immunogenic in guinea-pigs (Borek *et al.*, 1969). Immunization with this copolymer elicits antibodies that cross-react with collagens of several species (Maoz *et al.*, 1973*a,b*). Since a random copolymer of a similar composition, poly($Pro_{66}Gly_{34}$), does not cross-react with any collagen, it may be concluded that the polymer of ordered sequence reacts with the various collagens by virtue of the triple-helical conformation common to them and which serves as an important antigenic feature.

5.5 Myoglobin

Immunologically active fragments of myoglobin were first isolated from a chymotryptic digest (Crumpton, 1964; Crumpton and Wilkinson, 1965), and shown to comprise the residues 15–29, 56–69, 77–89, 139–146, and 147–153.

Fragments isolated later from tryptic digests (Atassi and Saplin, 1968) consist of the sequences 17–31, 79–96, 119–133, and 148–153. Although the similar distribution of the active peptides in these two studies may be fortuitous, this is not so likely since all antigenic fragments obtained by other methods of cleavage, such as near methionines (Crumpton, 1967; Atassi and Saplin, 1968), near prolines (Atassi and Singhal, 1970, 1972), and near arginines (Singhal and Atassi, 1971) also include the same regions of the molecule. That the C-terminal region of myoglobin constitutes a defined antigenic determinant was proven independently by Givas *et al.* (1968, 1972). These authors synthesized the C-terminal heptapeptide, Lys-Glu-Leu-Gly-Tyr-Glu-Gly, and used it for elution of a restricted antibody fraction from the total anti-myoglobin antibodies absorbed on a myoglobin immunoadsorbent, thus proving the presence of antibodies specific to this determinant.

These data indicate that a relatively large proportion of the total anti-myoglobin antibody population is directed towards a comparatively small portion of the total surface area of the antigen. Data also suggest that myoglobin has four to five independent determinants which are localized in the regions mentioned above, but do not necessarily include their whole length.

All of these regions include, or are adjacent to, corners in the folded polypeptide chain. Examination of a space-filling molecular model of myoglobin reveals that, although the overall shape of the molecule corresponds to a sphere, the surface comprises a series of hillocks and crevices, and that the corners of the folded polypeptide chain apparently coincide with some of the more exposed areas. While the significance of this relationship between location of the determinants and their degree of exposure on the surface is questionable, the results are consistent with the view that, assuming other requirements are satisfied, antibodies are formed preferentially against the most exposed portions of the surface structure (see Section 2) (Crumpton, 1974).

The role of individual amino acid residues in the antigenicity of myoglobin was studied by specific chemical modification of certain amino acids in the native protein or in its isolated peptides (Atassi, 1966, 1967*a,c*, 1969; Atassi and Caruzo, 1968; Atassi and Thomas, 1969; Andres and Atassi, 1973; Atassi *et al.*, 1975). According to these investigations no definite role can be assigned to any particular residue of the molecule.

A synthetic approach has been employed also in the study of individual determinants of myoglobin. Peptides with amino acid sequence corresponding to the antigenically active regions in the native molecule were synthesized. For each region, a series of peptides with increasing size has been prepared and tested (Koketsu and Atassi, 1974; Perlstein and Atassi, 1974; Atassi and Pai, 1975; Pai and Atassi, 1975). Results point to the role played by various residues in the antigenic properties of myoglobin.

Detailed investigation of the various immunologically active fragments, by stepwise degradation, by selective modification of particular amino acid residues in them, or by their chemical synthesis has led to accurate delineation of the antigenic determinants, and has culminated in a complete antigenic mapping of

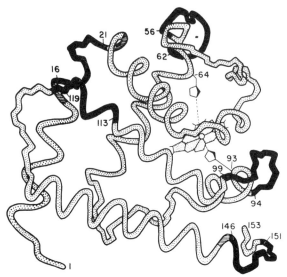

Figure 8 A schematic diagram showing the mode of folding of myoglobin and its antigenic structure. The solid black portions represent segments which have been shown accurately to comprise entire antigenic determinants. The striped parts, each corresponding to one amino acid residue only, can be part of an antigenic site with some antisera. The dotted portions represents areas which have been shown exhaustively to reside outside antigenically reactive regions. From Atassi (1975)

myoglobin. This has been described in detail in a recent review article by Atassi (1975), and is depicted in Figure 8. As shown, the defined antigenic determinants comprise the sequences 16–21 (between helices A and B), 56–62 (between helices D and E), 94–99 (between helices F and G), 113–119 (between helices G and H, and including part of helix G), and 146–151, (the random coil at the C-terminus of the molecule). All these regions are small, consisting of only six to seven amino acid residues each, and all the regions which separate them (which include essentially all the helical regions and the bends between B–C, C–D, and E–F helices) are non-immunogenic or antigenically silent.

5.6 Lysozyme

Studies on the antigenic determinants of hen egg white lysozyme utilized two approaches—either chemical modification and its influence on antigenicity and enzymic activity, or enzymic cleavage of the protein followed by analysis of the immunologically active fragments. Modification procedures for specific amino acids include modification of all or part of the tryptophans (Bonavida, 1968; Habeeb and Atassi, 1969; Strossberg and Kanarek, 1969), nitration of tyrosines (Bonavida, 1968; Atassi and Habeeb, 1969), or modification of ε-N amino group

Table 1 Effect of chemical modification on catalytic and antigenic
activity of lysozyme

Modified residues	Catalytic activity (per cent)	Antigenic reactivity* (per cent)
Tryptophans (all 6)	0	18
Tryptophans (5 out of 6)	0	85
Try 62 or Try 63	60	100
Try 62	0	100
Tyrosines (3 out of 6)	100	Limited decrease
Tyr20 and Tyr23	50	77–90
Lysines	0	60
Asp119 and Leu129	27	100
Arginines (all 10)	0	8–22
Arg61	83	100

* Extent of cross-reactivity with anti-lysozyme antibodies

of lysines by maleic anhydride, succinic anhydride, tetrefluorosuccinic anhydride, or citraconic anhydride, as well as by acetylation and carbamylation (Habeeb, 1967; Strossberg and Kanarek, 1968; Habeeb and Atassi, 1970, 1971*b*). Also, Atassi and coworkers have modified carboxyl groups in lysozyme (Atassi *et al.*, 1974; Atassi and Rosenblatt, 1974) or various arginines (Atassi *et al.*, 1972) and studied their effect. From these studies, summarized in Table 1, it can be concluded that in most cases changes in antigenic specificity reflect conformational changes conferred on the molecule upon modification, and antigenic specificity does not coincide always with a reduction in enzymic activity. However, this approach has only limited value in pinpointing the antigenically active regions of the molecule, mainly because most cases of modifications are not limited to a single amino acid residue but to several similar ones.

The approach of using degradative cleavage for studying antigenic determinants of lysozyme seems more fruitful. As in the case of other proteins, cleavage of hen egg white lysozyme yields several immunolocally active fragments (Arnon, 1976). The susceptiblility of this protein to trypsin is extremely low, like most other 'tight' proteins. Peptic digestion, however, leads to the isolation of two large fragments (Shinka *et al.*, 1962), the larger of which comprises the sequence 57–107, and contains two disulphide bridges and encompasses more than one antigenic determinant. The second large immunologically active fragment consists of the two terminal peptides—lysine 1–asparagine 27 and alanine 122–leucine 129—linked together by a single disulphide bond (cysteine 6–Cysteine 127) and was shown to contain an independent antigenic determinant (Fujio *et al.*, 1968*a,b*). This linked peptide does not give any precipitin reaction with anti-lysozyme antibodies, but as demonstrated by equilibrium dialysis studies, is capable of binding to these antibodies with an association constant of $1 \cdot 75 \times 10^5$ M^{-1}, and the percentage of antibodies directed towards it has been evaluated as 47 per cent (Fujio *et al.*,

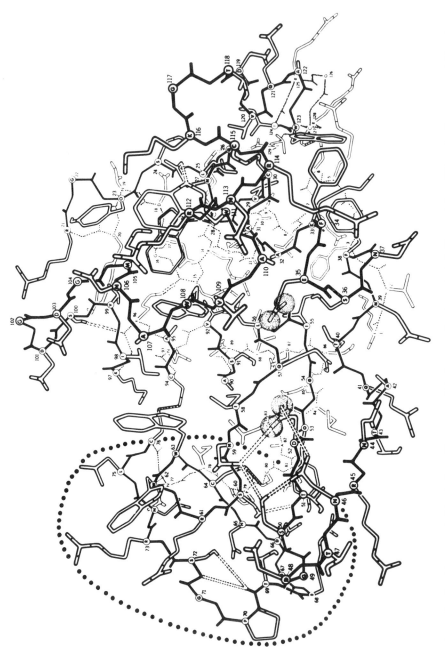

Figure 9 Backbone and side chains of lysozyme. The loop region is encircled. From *Atlas of Protein Sequence and Structure,* (Dayhoff, M. O., ed.)

1971). Its binding to anti-lysozyme antibodies is independent of and non-competitive with the binding of any other lysozyme fragment (Fujio *et al.*, 1968*b*).

The large fragment consisting of the region 57–107 can be split into smaller fragments which are immunologically active. Thus, by modifying the conditions of the peptic digestion, it is possible to obtain a relatively large fragment (Canfield and Liu, 1965), which after mild reduction yields a smaller peptide which still retains immunological activity (Arnon and Sela, 1969). This fragment, consisting of the amino acid sequence 60–83, and containing one intra-chain disulphide bond (Cysteine 64–Cysteine 80), was denoted 'loop'. Its location in the three-dimensional structure of lysozyme is shown in Figure 9, and as can be seen, it is exposed on the surface of the molecule. Antibodies specific to this region exclusively, prepared either by selective isolation from anti-lysozyme serum on loop-immunoadsorbent or by immunization with a conjugate containing the loop on a synthetic carrier, showed as predicted restricted heterogeneity (Maron *et al.*, 1971). The specificity of the loop–anti-loop reaction was studied by several techniques (Maron *et al.*, 1971), including a fluorometric method using a loop derivative in which a fluorescent chromophore was present (Pecht *et al.*, 1971). They all led to the conclusion that the loop is a conformation-dependent determinant. The anti-loop antibodies can distinguish between the loop and its open peptide chain and can recognize the loop structure in native lysozyme. Consequently, they are able to react with the intact enzyme (which is monovalent in terms of the loop), even though they can not precipitate it or inhibit its catalytic activity.

In later studies (Arnon *et al.*, 1971), it was shown that the loop peptide can be synthesized chemically. Attachment of this peptide to a synthetic carrier results in a completely synthetic conjugate which can elicit antibodies reactive with native lysozyme, and still recognizes the conformational determinant of the intact molecule (Arnon, 1974). Investigation of several synthetic analogues of the loop, each with one or two amino acid residues replaced by alanine (Teicher *et al.*, 1973), reveals the major role played by residues such as the prolines or the arginines in the antigenic specificity of this determinant. This information has been correlated with the calculated contribution of the various amino acid residues to the β bends that constitute the dominant structural feature in this region of lysozyme. A good agreement between the predicted values for β bend conservation and the antigenic reactivity of a particular analogue of the loop (Arnon *et al.*, 1974) provides further evidence for the crucial role of the spatial conformation in the specificity of this antigenic determinant.

As mentioned above, lysozyme displays very low susceptibility to tryptic digestion due to its 'tight' structure. Tryptic peptides can be obtained, however, if the molecule is treated appropriately beforehand by, for example, the reversible blocking of the amino groups of lysine with citraconic anhydride (Atassi *et al.*, 1973). The protein is then hydrolysed by trypsin at all the arginine residues. After deblocking it is possible to effect complete cleavage of all the lysine peptide bonds, thus yielding all the tryptic peptides of lysozyme, without rupturing the disulphide bonds. This mixture of peptides inhibits the reaction of lysozyme with its antibodies very strongly (85–89 per cent). The reactive fragments produced have been identified as consisting chiefly of the three disulphide-containing peptides, comprising the following sequences: 22–33 and 115–116, linked by Cystein 30–Cysteine 115, 62–68 and 74–96, linked by Cysteine 64–Cysteine 80 and Cysteine 76–Cysteine 94; and the sequences 6–13 and 126–129, linked by Cysteine 6–Cysteine 127. Most of these fragments are derived from the same regions as the N–C-terminal fragment reported by Fujio *et al.* (1968*a*), and the loop region (Arnon and Sela, 1969). This provides corroborating evidence to the premise that lysozyme, in common with other globular proteins such as myoglobin and nuclease, encompasses only a limited number, of antigenic determinants probably four to five, most of them being on the more exposed areas of the molecule surface.

6 MANIFESTATION OF ANTIGENICITY IN CELLULAR AND HUMORAL RESPONSES

Two types of cells are involved in the immune response, both arising from bone marrow stem cells. One set of cells are the T (thymus-derived) cells which are responsible for cell-mediated immunity, whereas the other type are B cells, which as mature cells are antigen-reactive and are responsible for antibody production, that is humoral immunity. T cells are often also necessary for the induction of antibody synthesis by a phenomenon termed cell co-operation. In this co-operation, it has been postulated that the B cells recognize the antigenic determinants, whereas the T cells recognize other portions of the antigen, termed the carrier determinants. Thus this phenomenon is dependent on the antigen structure, as will be discussed below. In several systems, it was observed that the formation of antibodies depends solely on B-cell activation. This phenomenon, termed thymus independency, is also a function of antigen structure and will be discussed at the end of this section.

The molecular structure of the antigen is thus expected to affect both cellular and humoral manifestations of antigenicity, and not necessarily in the same way or to the same extent. Indeed, the results of various studies suggest that the essential molecular requirements of size and conformation for cellular immune response are less stringent than those needed for humoral immunity. This concerns both immunogenicity and antigenic specificity.

In the case of immunogenicity there are several reports about protein fragments or small peptides that fail to stimulate detectable circulating antibody production, and yet elicit cellular immunity. For example, several fragments of the myelin basic protein (Lennon *et al.*, 1970; Eylar *et al.*, 1971) have been reported to induce cell-mediated delayed hypersensitivity to the intact protein, but which fail to react with antiserum against the whole protein. The encephalitogenic nonapeptide of this protein also is capable of eliciting cellular responses in guinea-pigs, but not humoral antibody production (Teitelbaum *et al.*, 1976). A low molecular weight peptic fragment of flagellin demonstrates similar behaviour (Ichiki and Parish, 1972). Fragmentation of flagellin with cyanogen bromide or its chemical modification also are associated with a reduction in the ability to initiate humoral immunity, but in contrast, cause a marked enhancement in the capacity to induce cellular immunity (Parish, 1971a,b; Parish and Liew, 1972). It seems likely that these effects arise from differences in presentation of the antigen to the cells involved in the immune response, and are the expression of the molecular requirements for T–B lymphocyte interaction.

The size of the molecule, as has been discussed previously, is also a decisive factor in immunogenicity. But again, this factor may be manifested in a different manner in cellular and humoral responses. Large polymeric structures are usually good immunogens, and in some cases aggregation of a poorly immunogenic protein may convert it into a much better immunogen for both humoral and cellular responses (Amkraut et al., 1969; Reichlin et al., 1970). However, with small molecules, differences between humoral and cellular manifestations of immunity are often observed, as has been demonstrated mainly by the use of synthetic peptides and their derivatives. For examples, whereas the p-azobenzenearsonate derivative of hexa-L-tyrosine, or even of tri-L-tyrosine, induce antibody production in rabbits as well as cellular immunity in guinea-pigs (Borek et al., 1965), the same derivative of N-acetyl tyrosine induces only delayed hypersensitivity in guinea-pigs, but no antibody production in rabbits (Borek et al., 1967).

The requirements for a minimal molecular size and for the presence of two different determinants for the endowment of a molecule with the capacity to induce antibodies, may be understood if the currently accepted concept and nature of T–B cell co-operation is correct. Hence, the two groups, such as the p-azobenzenearsonate and the tyrosine residue in the above-mentioned example, if adequately disposed and spaced, serve as 'determinant' and 'carrier'. This might not be an essential requirement for induction of an exclusive cell-mediated immune response.

Antigenic specificity is also manifested differently in humoral and cellular responses, and the molecular parameters involved in the two responses are not the same. Thus, as has been indicated before, most of the protein antigenic determinants which interact with humoral antibodies express conformation specificity. This relationship does not appear to hold for the determinants which mediate cellular immunity. For example, reduced and carboxymethylated lysozyme fails to cross-react with antiserum to the native enzyme and no cross-reactivity can be demonstrated between native lysozyme and antiserum to the unfolded chain. Yet, extensive cross-reactivity between native and unfolded lysozymes has been detected at the cellular level (Thompson et al., 1972). This reaction is manifested both in vivo by a marked delayed hypersensitivity reaction and in vitro by the inhibition of capillary macrophage migration (MIF technique).

A similar difference between the cellular and humoral responses has been observed in cross-reaction between related native proteins. Thus, collagen of Ascaris lumbricoides, which possesses a radically different structure from vertebrate collagens (McBride and Harrington, 1967a,b), appears to have completely distinct antigenic structure, and does not show any humoral cross-reactivity with the vertebrate collagens (Fuchs and Harrington, 1970). However, a cell-mediated cross-reaction has been observed between *Ascaris* and human collagens (Michaeli *et al.*, 1972).

Hen egg white lysozyme and bovine α-lactalbumin, which on the humoral level were observed to be completely non-cross-reactive (Arnon and Maron, 1970) (see Figure 4), have been reported to exhibit a definite cross-reaction at the cellular level. Hence, using both *in vivo* (delayed hypersensitivity) and *in vitro* (lymphocyte transformation) methods, a marked cross-reactivity has been observed between the two proteins (Maron *et al.*, 1972).

Another example is that of insulin. Whereas reduced and carboxymethylated B chain of insulin gives no detectable reaction with antisera to insulin, it elicits a delayed skin reaction in guinea-pigs previously sensitized with insulin (Clark and Munoz, 1970).

It appears that all these observations have a similar molecular basis, which leads to the conclusion that whereas the specificity of humoral antibodies is strict and, in many cases, these antibodies recognize and react mainly with conformational antigenic determinants; the determinants mediating cellular immunity are less conformation-dependent. In other words, the conformational integrity of a protein molecule, although not crucial for interaction with cell-bound receptors, is essential for eliciting humoral antibodies and reacting with them. Apart from emphasizing the different order of specificity recognized by humoral and cell-bound antibodies, the above results suggest that cell-mediated immunity represents a more informative parameter than humoral immunity for the study of amino acid sequence or phylogenetic relationships, especially between distantly related proteins (Michaeli *et al.*, 1972; Crumpton, 1974). On the other hand, humoral antibodies are more useful for the study of the structural relationships of proteins.

In some instances, it is possible to obtain information about the location and distribution of the determinants involved in cell-mediated immunity. In the case of myelin, which possesses an unfolded conformation (Oshiro and Eylar, 1970), several determinants that interact only with cell-bound antibodies were located in the molecule (Bergstrrand, 1972; Bergstrrand and Kallen, 1973). Another antigenic determinant of the same protein is the encephalitogenic nonapeptide residues 114–122 (Hashim and Eylar, 1969; Westall *et al.*, 1971), which can elicit the cell-mediated autoimmune phenomena associated with experimental allergic encephalomyelitis. It has been demonstrated recently that this nonapeptide can induce *in vivo* and *in vitro* cellular responses in guinea-pigs, (Teitelbaum *et al.*, 1976), although it does not stimulate antibody production. These data are in line with the previously mentioned observation that unfolded structures of proteins favour the production of cellular, rather than humoral immunity.

The structural requirements for the exclusive activation of B cells are completely different. The activation of B cells by antigens to form antibodies, in the case of most proteins, requires helper activity from T cells, (Mitchel and Miller, 1968; Feldman, 1972). It has been observed, however, that many antigens are able to activate B cells efficiently, *in vivo* and *in vitro*, in the absence of T cells, and this property is apparently dependent on the molecular structure of the antigen (Sela and Mozes, 1975). Such antigens are defined as thymus-independent antigens. The known T-independent antigens, most of which which are not proteins, include polymerized flagellin (Armstrong *et al.*, 1969; Feldmann and Basten, 1971), pneumococcal polysaccharide type SIII (Howard *et al.*, 1971), *Escherichia coli* lipopolysaccharide (Andersson and Blangren, 1971; Möller and Mitchell, 1971), polyvinyl pyrrolidone (Andersson and Blangren, 1971), levan (Del Guercio and Leuchars, 1972), dextran sulphate (Dorries *et al.*, 1974), some synthetic antigens (Sela *et al.*, 1972), and possibly collagen (Fuchs *et al.*, 1947*b*). The common feature of all these antigens is that they possess repeating antigenic determinants, and this has been considered to be the reason for their thymus independence (Sjöberg and Möller, 1970). However, while this may be a necessary requirement, it is not a sufficient one; many synthetic antigens with repeating determinants are known to require both T and B cells for eliciting a humoral immune response (Mozes and Shearer, 1971; Shearer *et al.*, 1972; Lichtenberg *et al.*, 1974). It appears that an additional requirement for thymus independence may be that the antigens are metabolized slowly (Sela *et al.*, 1972, Sela and Mozes, 1975).

It has been reported that collagen is thymus independent whereas gelatin, from which it is derived following denaturation, is thymus dependent (Fuchs *et al.*, 1974*a*; Mozes *et al.*, 1975). Thus, according to these data, two molecules with identical chemical structure, but differing only in the steric conformation, behave dramatically differently. It is interesting to note that the synthetic ordered polymer (Pro-Gly-Pro)$_n$ which possesses the collagen-like triple-helical structure is also thymus independent, whereas a random copolymer of the same composition is thymus dependent (Fuchs *et al.*, 1974*a,b*) thus indicating the role of spatial conformation in T-independent B-cell activation. It should be mentioned however, that other laboratories have reported that calf collagen is a T-dependent antigen (Timpl *et al.*, 1973*a*; Nowack *et al.*, 1976).

It has been reported recently that two synthetic polypeptides with defined repeating antigenic determinants, and differing only in the order of amino acids in their N-terminal side chains, vary in their capacity to activate B cells. Thus, the polymer (Tyr-Tyr-Glu-Glu)-Poly(DLAla)–Poly(L-Lys), which is similar in its pattern of immune response to the random polymer (T,G)-A–L, is T dependent, whereas the polymer (Tyr-Glu-Tyr-Glu)-poly(DL-Ala)–Poly(L-Lys) does not require T-cell help for efficient antibody production (Schwartz *et al.*, 1976). Since these two polypeptides, which are chemically similar, possess repeating antigenic determinants and would not be expected to differ in their rate of metabolism, one must look for other criteria or parameters which affect the triggering of B-cells, in order to understand the structural requirements for independent B-cell stimulation.

7 MOLECULAR BASIS FOR GENETIC CONTROL OF IMMUNE RESPONSES

The notion that the immune response may be controlled genetically, was proposed about 60 years ago for the phenomenon of hypersensitivity (Cook and Van Der Veer, 1916), but only in recent years have data become available for the molecular and cellular mechanisms of genetic control. This topic has been the subject of several recent reviews (Mozes and Shearer, 1972; Benaceraff and Katz, 1975; Mozes, 1975) and will be mentioned here only very briefly. The antigens employed in studies on this subject are mainly synthetic, but some information is available also on several proteins with defined antigenic structure and on alloantigens which have a very limited number of potentially immunogenic determinants.

The first immune response (Ir) gene described is the so-called PLL gene in guinea-pigs (Levine et al., 1963). This controls the carrier-specific response to hapten conjugates with various basic homopolymers or copolymers of amino acids, such as poly-L-lysine (PLL), poly-L-ornithine, poly-L-arginine and poly(L-lysine-L-glutamic acid), as well as the response to poly-L-lysyl side chains (Ben Ephraim et al., 1966). The PLL gene, which is present in strain 2 guinea-pigs but not in strain 13, is responsible for the differences between the immune responses of these two strains.

Ir genes have been identified more recently in inbred strains of mice mainly from the responses towards branched synthetic polypeptide antigens such as the series containing peptides of tyrosine, histidine, or phenylalanine and glutamic acid, attached to branched poly-DL-alanine ((T,G)-A–L, (H,G)-A–L and (Phe,G)-A–L) (McDevitt and Sela, 1965). Detailed genetic studies indicate that the response to these antigenes is controlled by a quantitative, unigenic dominant gene linked to the main histocompatibility complex, in a region defined as Ir-1 (McDevitt and Sela, 1967; McDevitt et al., 1972). For example, mice of CBA strain were found to be high responders to the histidine-containing polymer (H,G)-A–L whereas they responded poorly to (T,G)-A–L. C57BL Mice, on the other hand, demonstrated the reverse pattern. Moreover, the cell-mediated immune response (manifested as a delayed-type hypersensitivity reaction) to these antigens was shown recently to be under the same genetic control (Benacerraf and Katz, 1975).

The main conclusion, which could be drawn from these experiments, and from studies on other synthetic polypeptides (Benacerraf and Dorf, 1974; Dorf et al., 1975), is that the response to different antigens sharing antigenic specificities may be controlled by distinct Ir genes linked to the H-2 haplotype. Thus, the genetically determined capacity of an antigen to provoke a response is not dependent merely upon the ability to produce antibodies to the specific antigenic determinants, but is more complex and probably involves a recognition system with a much narrower specificity. The linkage to the H-2 locus was tested also for systems of polymers containing multichain polyproline (Pro–L) as a carrier, for example, (T,G)-Pro–L. In contrast to the A–L series, the responses were found not to be linked to the H-2 locus, indicating that the backbone peptide to which the determinants are attached may play an important role in the control of the response (Mozes *et al.*, 1969*a,b*).

Further analyses have demonstrated that the basis for the general phenomenon of this genetic control is inherent in the cellular make-up of the tested animal, and is due either to a defect or deficiency in one of the two cell types responsible for the immune response—T and B lymphocytes—or to interference in co-operation between them (Miller and Mitchell, 1969; Mozes, 1975).

As indicated above, most of the studies on the genetic control of the immune responses have been carried out using synthetic antigens. Similar studies with natural multiple-determinant antigens, such as proteins, are unapproachable, since the simultaneous production of antibodies of differing specificities complicates the study of the processes involved. A situation may be envisaged where the specificity of antibodies formed in various inbred strains against a particular protein may vary, due to different antigenic determinants, but this effect could escape notice, since the overall amount of antibodies against the whole protein molecule might still be similar. In effect, this phenomenon was observed even in the case of a simple synthetic antigen (multichain polyproline with peptides of phenylalanine and glutamic acid attached). Shearer *et al.* (1971) showed that two inbred strains immunized with this antigen responded equally well to the whole polypeptide, but one of them produced antibodies directed mainly towards the side-chain peptide portion of the molecule, whereas the antisera of the second strain react primarily with the backbone moiety of the immunogen, thus suggesting that two different genetic controls are operating for two determinants on the same molecule. With multideterminant proteins antigens the situation is expected to be much more complex. However, a limited number of investigations has been carried out on proteins, and on several defined antigenic determinants in them.

An interesting study has been carried out on the genetic control of the response to different insulin molecules (Keck, 1975). Bovine insulin differs from porcine in two amino acid residues (at residues 8 and 10) which are located in the intra-chain 'loop' of the A chain. The response to the two antigens, free or coupled to DNP, has been shown to be genetically controlled, H-2 linked. Thus $H\text{-}2^d$ mice show a high response to both insulins, $H\text{-}2^b$ mice respond only to the bovine insulin, whereas mice carrying $H\text{-}2^k$ are low responders to both.

Hen egg white lysozymes are under H-2-linked control also. The control gene for their response (denoted Ir-GEL gene), or its product, was shown to differentiate between highly related lysoymes that exhibit strain cross-reactivity. This emphasizes again the difference between the ability to bind to antibody and the capacity to stimulate the immune system (Hill and Sercaz, 1975). The response in mice to the isolated loop-peptide determinant of hen lysozyme, has also been shown to be under H-2-linked genetic control. In this case, advantage was taken of the feasibility of eliciting antibodies reactive specifically with this unique region of the protein by immunization with loop-A–L conjugate. Thus it was possible to analyse the immune response of various inbred mouse strains to the loop region, compared to their response to other portions of the lysozyme molecule (Mozes *et al.*, 1971; Maron *et al.*, 1973). The results demonstrate that most of the mouse strains tested respond well when immunized with lysozyme, but only some strains produce antibodies when injected with the loop-A-L conjugate or with a similar conjugate containing the loop attached to multichain polyproline (loop-Pro-L). The strains that do not respond to these conjugates are unable to produce antibodies specific towards the loop region even when they are injected with intact lysozyme, indicating that the immune response to different determinants of the protein is under separate genetic control.

Similar conclusions were arrived at in studies on staphylococcal nuclease. In this case, it was found that mice strains B10·A, A/J, and SJL respond to both peptide 1–126 and 99–149 of nuclease, whereas B10 mice respond to the first fragment only and DBA/1 does not respond to either (Berzofsky *et al.*, 1976; Sachs *et al.*, 1976).

Interesting studies on the genetic control of the immune response to different isozymes of lactic dehydrogenase have indicated that the response to these antigens is controlled also by an H-2-linked gene located between the Ir-1 and the Ss-Slp loci (Melchers *et al.*, 1975). It has been shown that mice that do not respond to LDH_B but that are high responders to the LDH_A isozyme may produce antibodies to LDH_B following immunization with the hetero-oligomeric form LDH_{AB}.

These experiments provide evidence that the genetic control of the immune response at the level of antigenic determinants holds not only for synthetic antigens on which most of the studies were performed, but for native proteins as well.

8 CONCLUDING REMARKS

This chapter has been concerned with the relationships between the molecular structure and the antigenic properties of proteins. The main emphasis has been placed on the involvement of the molecular parameters in immunogenicity—the capacity to induce an immune response—and in antigenic specificity—that is the ability to interact with antibodies. It has been demonstrated that structural features of the molecule affect both these properties, and thus play a major role in defining the distinct antigenic determinants. Moreover, many immunological phenomena are influenced by the molecular structure of the antigen.

The most crucial molecular parameters are size, accessibility of antigenic determinants, and the spatial conformation of the molecule, factors which dictate the immunological behaviour of the proteins. Size, in itself, is not a decisive requirement for immunogenicity since even low molecular weight molecules are capable of eliciting an immune response, particularly one of cell-mediated immunity, but it does affect the potency of the immune reaction—the higher the molecular weight of the antigen the stronger the response it elicits. Accessibility of the antigenic determinant is one of the most influential factors in determining the antigenic specificity, as most antigenic determinants of proteins are located at outer corners of the folded polypeptide chains. Similarly, the molecular conformation is a crucial parameter in defining the antigenic specificity, particularly for the induction of a humoral immune response.

An interesting conclusion from the investigation of the molecular basis of antigenicity of proteins is the existence of a relatively small number of distinct antigenic determinants (four to five per 10 000 molecular weight), in spite of the huge number of possible combinations in either folded or unfolded proteins. The elements which determine the selection of antigenic regions and their immunological potency are not yet defined. However, it is not only the antigenic determinants which affect the immune response, but also the remainder of the molecule plays a paramount role in both antigenicity and immunogenicity, as well as in other immunological phenomena exerted by the antigen.

What also emerges from work described in this chapter is that although remarkable progress in the elucidation of the many manifestations of immunity has been achieved during the last two decades, there are several points that still need elaboration for a complete understanding of this complicated biological function.

REFERENCES

Alving, C. R. (1976). In *The Antigens*, Vol. 4 (M. Sela, ed.), Academic Press, New York. 1976,

Amkraut, A. A., Malley, A., and Begley, D. (1969). *J. Immunol.*, **103**, 1301.

Anderer, F. A. (1963a). *Z. NaturForsch.*, **18b**, 1010.

Anderer, F. A. (1963b). *Biochim. Biophys. Acta*, **71**, 246.

Anderer, F. A., and Handschuh, D. (1962). *Z. NaturForsch.*, **17b**, 536.

Anderer, F. A., and Handschuh, D. (1963). *Z. NaturForsch.*, **18b**, 1015.

Anderer, F. A., and Schlumberger, H. D. (1965). *Biochim. Biophys. Acta*, **97**, 503.

Andersson, B., and Blangren, H. (1971). *Cell. Immunol.*, **2**, 411.

Andres, S. F., and Atassi, M. Z. (1973). *Biochemistry*, **12**, 942.

Anfinsen, C. B. (1973). *Science, N.Y.*, **181**, 223.

Anfinsen, C. B., Cuatrecasas, P., and Taniuichi, H. (1971). *The Enzymes*, Vol. IV (Boyer, P. D., ed.), Academic Press, New York and London, p. 177.

Armstrong, W. D., Diener, E., and Shellam, G. R. (1969). *J. Exp. Med.*, **129**, 393.

Arnheim, N., Prager, E. M., and Wilson, A. C. (1969). *J. Biol. Chem.*, **244**, 2085.

Arnheim, N., and Wilson, A. C., (1967). *J. Biol. Chem.*, **242**, 3951.

Arnon, R. (1968). *Eur. J. Biochem.*, **5**, 583.

Arnon, R. (1971). *Curr. Top. Microbiol. Immunol.*, **54**, 47.

Arnon, R. (1973). In *The Antigens*, Vol. I, (Sela, M., ed.), Academic Press, New York and London, p. 87.

Arnon, R. (1974). In *Peptides, Polypeptides, and Proteins*, (Lotan, N., Goodman, M., and Blout, E. R., eds.), John Wiley and Sons, New York and London, p. 538.

Arnon, R. (1976). In *Enzymes*, (Salton, R. J., ed.), John Wiley and Sons, New York and London, p. 1.

Arnon, R., and Maron, E., (1970). *J. Mol. Biol.*, **51**, 703.

Arnon, R. and Maron, E., (1971). *J. Mol. Biol.*, **61**, 225.

Arnon, R., Maron, E., Sela, M., and Anfinsen, C. B., (1971). *Proc. Nat. Acad. Sci. U.S.A.*, **68**, 1450.

Arnon, R. and Neurath, H. (1970). *Immunochemistry.* **7**, 241.

356

Arnon, R. and Schechter, I. (1966). *Immunochemistry*, **7**, 241.
Arnon, R. and Sela, M. (1960). *Biochem. J.*, **75**, 103.
Arnon, R. and Sela, M. (1969). *Proc. Nat. Acad. Sci., U.S.A.*, **62**, 163.
Arnon, R. Sela, M., Yaron, A. and Sober, H. A. (1965). *Biochemistry*, **4**, 948.
Arnon, R. and Shapira, E. (1967). *Biochemistry*, **6**, 3942.
Arnon, R., Teicher, E., and Scheraga, H. A. (1974). *J. Mol. Biol.* **90**, 403.
Arnone, A., Bier, C. J., Cotton, F. A., Day, V. W., Hazen, E. E., Richardson, J. S., and Yonath, A. (1971). *J. Biol. Chem.* **246**, 2302.
Atassi, M. Z. (1966). *Nature. (Lond.)*, **209**, 1209.
Atassi, M. Z. (1967*a*). *Archs Biochem. Biophys.*, **120**, 56.
Atassi, M. Z. (1967*b*). *Biochem. J.*, **103**, 29.
Atassi, M. Z. (1967*c*). *Biochem. J.*, **102**, 478.
Atassi, M. Z. (1969). *Immunochemistry*, **6**, 801.
Atassi, M. Z. (1975). *Immunochemistry*, **12**, 423.
Atassi, M. Z. and Caruzo, D. R. (1968). *Biochemistry*, **7**, 699.
Atassi, M. Z. and Habeeb, A. F. S. A. (1969). *Biochemistry*, **8**, 1385.
Atassi, M. Z., Habeeb, A. F. S. A., and Rydstedt, L. (1970). *Biochim. Biophys. Acta*, **200**, 184.
Atassi, N. Z., Habeeb, A. F. S. A., and Ando, K. (1973). *Biochim. Biophys. Acta*, **303**, 203.
Atassi, M. Z. and Pai, R. C. (1975). *Immunochemistry*, **12**, 735.
Atassi, M. Z. and Rosenblatt, M. C. (1974). *J. Biol. Chem.*, **249**, 4802.
Atassi, M. Z., Rosenblatt, M. C., and Habeeb, A. F. S. A. (1974). *Immunochemistry*, **11**, 495.
Atassi, M. Z. and Saplin, B. J. (1968). *Biochemistry*, **7**, 688.
Atassi, M. Z. and Singhal, R. P. (1970). *Biochemistry*, **9**, 3854.
Atassi, M. Z. and Singhal, R. P. (1972). *Immunochemistry*, **9**, 1057.
Atassi, M. Z., Suliman, A. M., and Habeeb, A. F. S. A. (1972). *Immunochemistry*, **9**, 907.
Atassi, M. Z. and Thomas, A. V. (1969). *Biochemistry*, **8**, 3385.
Atassi, M. Z., Litowich, M. T., and Andres, S. F. (1975). *Immunochemistry*, **12**, 727.

Becker, U., Timpl, R., and Kuhn, K. (1972). *Eur. J. Biochem.*, **28**, 221.
Beil, W., Timpl, R., and Furthmayr, H. (1973). *Immunology*, **24**, 13.
Benacerraf, B. and Dorf, M. E. (1974). In *Progress in Immunology II*, Vol. 2, (Brent, L. and Holborow, J. eds.), North Holland Publishing Co., Amsterdam, p. 181.
Benacerraf, B. and Katz, D. H. (1975). *Adv. Cancer Res.* **21**, 121.
Ben Ephraim, S., Arnon, R., and Sela, M. (1966). *Immunochemistry*, **3**, 491.
Benjamini, E., Michaeli, D., and Young, J. D. (1972). *Curr. Top. Microbiol. Immunol.*, **58**, 85.
Benjamini, E., Shimizu, M., Young, J. D., and Leung, C. Y. (1969). *Biochemistry*, **8**, 2242.
Benjamini, E., Young, J. D., Shimizu, M., and Leung, M. (1964). *Biochemistry*, **3**, 1115.
Benjamini, E., Young, J. D., Peterson, W. T., Leung, C. Y., and Shimizu, M. (1965). *Biochemistry*, **4**, 2081.
Bergstrrand, H. (1972). *Eur. J. Biochem.*, **27**, 126.
Bergstrrand, H., and Kallen, B. (1973). *Immunochemistry*, **10**, 229.
Berson, S. A., and Yallow, R. S. (1959). *J. Clin. Invest.*, **38**, 2019.
Berzofsky, J. A., Schechter, A. N., Shearer, G. M., and Sachs, D. H. (1976). *Fed. Proc.*, **35**, 627.
Blake, C. C. F., Koenig, D. F., Mair, G. A., North, A. C. T., Phillips, D. C., and Sarma, V. R. (1965). *Nature (Lond.)*, **206**, 757.
Bonavida, B. (1968). Dissertation, University microfilms.
Borek, F. (1968). *Curr. Top. Microbiol. Immunol.*, **43**, 126.
Borek, F., Kurtz, J., and Sela, M. (1969). *Biochim. Biophys. Acta*, **188**, 314.
Borek, F., Stupp, Y., and Sela, M., (1965). *Science, N.Y.*, **150**, 1178.
Borek, F., Stupp, Y., and Sela, M. (1967). *J. Immunol.*, **98**, 739.

Branster, M., and Cinader, B. (1961). *J. Immunol.*, **87**, 18.
Braunitzer, G., Hilse, K., Rudolp, V., and Hilschmann, N. (1964). *Adv. Protein. Chem.*, **19**, 1.
Breslow, E., Beychok, S., Hardman, K. D., and Gurd, F. R. N. (1965). *J. Biol. Chem.*, **240**, 304.
Brew, K., Castellino, F. J., Vanaman, T. C., Trayer, I. P. and Mattock, P. (1969). *Brookhaven Symp. Biology no. 21*, **1**, 139.
Brew, K., Vanaman, T. C., and Hill, R. L. (1967). *J. Biol. Chem.*, **242**, 3747.
Brodbeck, U., Denton, W. L., Tanahashi, N., and Ebner, K. A. (1967). *J. Biol. Chem.*, **242**, 1391.
Brown, P. C., and Glynn, L. E. (1968). *Immunology*, **15**, 589.
Brown, R. K. (1962). *J. Biol. Chem.*, **237**, 1162.
Brown, R. K. (1963). *Ann. N.Y. Acad. Sci.*, **103**, 754.
Brown, R. K., Delaney, R., Levine, L., and Van-Vunakis, H. (1959). *J. Biol. Chem.*, **234**, 2043.
Brown, R. K., and Liu, S. (1970). *Immunochemistry*, **7**, 852.
Brown, R. K., McEwan, M., Mikoryak, C. A., and Polkovsky, J. (1967). *J. Biol. Chem.*, **242**, 3007.
Browne, W. J., North, A. C. T., Philips, D. C., Brew, K., Vanaman, T. C., and Hill, R. L. (1969). *J. Mol. Biol.*, **42**, 65.

Canfield, R. E. (1963). *J. Biol. Chem.*, **238**, 2698.
Canfield, R. E. and Liu, A. K. (1965). *J. Biol. Chem.*, **240**, 1997.
Canfield, R. E., Morgan, F. J., Kammermann, S., Bell, J. J., and Agosto, G. M. (1971). *Rec. Prog. Hor. Res*, **27**, 121.
Cebra, J. J. (1961*a*). *J. Immunol.*, **86**, 190.
Cebra, J. J. (1961*b*). *J. Immunol.* **86**, 205.
Cinader, B. (1957). *Ann. Rev. Microbiol.*, **11**, 371.
Cinader, B. (1967). In *Antibodies to Biologically Active Molecules*, (Cinader, B., ed.), Pergamon Press New York and Oxford, p. 85.
Cinader, B. (1963). *Ann. N. Y. Acad. Sci.*, **103**, 495.
Cinader, B., Suzuki, T., and Pelichova, H. (1971). *J. Immunol.*, **106**, 1381.
Cinader, B., and Lafferty, K. J. (1964). *Immunology*, **7**, 372.
Citri, N., and Zyk, N. (1965). *Biochim. Biophys. Acta*, **99**, 427.
Clark, C. and Munoz, J. (1970). *J. Immunol.*, **105**, 574.
Cook, R. A., and and Van Der Veer, A. (1916). *J. Immunol.*, **1**, 201.
Cotton, F. A., and Hazen, E. E. (1971). *The Enzymes*, Vol. 4, Boyer, D. D., ed.), 3rd edn., Academic Press, New York and London, p. 153.
Cowan, P. M., McGavin, S., and North, A. C. T. (1955). *Nature (Lond.)*, **176**, 1062.
Crumpton, M. J. (1964). *Biochem. J.*, **91**, 4c.
Crumpton, M. J. (1967). *Nature (Lond.)*, **215**, 17.
Crumpton, M. J. (1974). In *The Antigens*, Vol. 2, (Sela, M., ed.), Academic Press, New York and London, p. 1.
Crumpton, M. J., and Small, P. S. (1967). *J. Mol. Biol.*, **26**, 143.
Crumpton, M. J., and Wilkinson, J. M. (1965). *Biochem. J.*, **94**, 545.
Crumpton, M. J., and Wilkinson, J. M. (1966). *Biochem. J.*, **100**, 223.

Davidson, J. K., and Haist, R. E. (1965). *Can. J. Physiol. Pharmacol.*, **43**, 373.
Davidson, J. K., Zeigler, M., and Haist, M. (1969). *Diabetes*, **18**, 212.
Davidson, R. F., Levine, L., Drake, M. P., Rubins, A., and Bump, S. (1967). *J. Exp. Med.*, **126**, 331.
Dayhoff, M. O., and Eck, R. V. (1969). In *Atlas of Protein Sequence and Structure*, National Biomedical Research Foundation. Silver Spring. 1969
Dehm, P., Olsen, B. R., and Prockop, D. J. (1974). *Euro. J. Biochem.*, **46**, 107.

358

Del Guercio, P., and Leuchars, E. (1972). *J. Immunol.*, **109**, 951.

de Weck, A. L. (1974). In *The Antigens*, Vol. II, (Sela, M., ed.), Academic Press, New York and London, p. 141.

Dickerson, R. E. (1964). In *The Proteins*, Vol. 2, (Neurath, H., ed.), 2nd edn. Academic Press, New York and London, p. 634.

Dickerson, R. E., Kopra, M. L., Borders, C. L., Varnum, J. C., Weinzierl, J. E., and Margoliash, E. (1968). In *Structure and Function of Cytochromes*, (Okuniki, Kamen, and Sekuzu, eds.), University of Tokyo Press, Tokyo, p. 225.

Dorf, M. E., Plate, J. M. D., Stimpfling, J. H., and Benacerraf, B. (1975). *J. Immunol.*, **114**, 602.

Dörries, R., Schimpl, A., and Wecker, E. (1974). *Eur. J. Immunol.*, **4**, 230.

Eastlake, A., Sachs, D. H., Schechter, A. N., and Anfinsen, C. B. (1974). *Biochemistry*, **13**, 1567.

Edmundson, A. B. (1965). *Nature (Lond.)*, **205**, 883.

Eisen, N. H. (1960). In *Cellular and Humoral Aspects of Hypersensitive State*, (Laurence, K. S., eds.), Harper (Hoeber), New York, p. 89.

Engel, J., Kurtz, J., Katchalski, E., and Berger, E. (1966). *J. Mol. Biol.*, **17**, 255.

Erickson, J. O., and Neurath, H. (1943). *J. Exp. Med.*, **78**, 1.

Eylar, E. H., Westall, F. C., and Brostoff, S. (1971). *J. Biol. Chem.*, **246**, 3418.

Fainaru, M., Wilson, A. C., and Arnon, R. (1974). *J. Mol. Biol.*, **84**, 635.

Fazekas de St. Groth, S. (1963). *Ann. N.Y. Acad. Sci.*, **103**, 674.

Fearney, F. J., Leung, C. Y., Young, J. R., and Benjamini, E. (1971). *Biochim. Biophys. Acta*, **243**, 509.

Feldmann, M. (1972). *J. Exp. Med.*, **135**, 1049.

Feldmann, M., and Basten, A. (1971). *J. Exp. Med.*, **134**, 103.

Fleischer, N., Givens, J. R., Abe, K., and Nicholson, W. E., (1965). *J. Clin. Invest.*, **44**, 1047.

Fleischer, N., Givens, J. R., Abe, K., Nicholson, W. E., and Liddle, G. W. (1966). *Endocrinology*, **78**, 1067.

Fridkin, M., and Patchornik, A. (1974). *Ann. Rev. Biochem.*, **43**, 419.

Fuchs, S., Cuatrecasas, P., Ontjes, D. A., and Anfinsen, C. B. (1969). *J. Biol. Chem.*, **244**, 943.

Fuchs, S., and Harrington, W. F. (1970). *Biochim. Biophys. Acta*, **221**, 119.

Fuchs, S., Maoz, A., and Sela, M. (1974*a*). *Israel. J. Chem.*, **12**, 681.

Fuchs, S., Mozes, E., Maoz, A., and Sela, M. (1974*b*). *J. Exp. Med.*, **139**, 148.

Fujio, H., Imanishi, M., Nishioka, K., and Amano, T. (1968*a*). *Bieken J.*, **11**, 207.

Fujio, H., Imanishi, M., Nishioka, K., and Amano, T. (1968*b*). *Bieken J.*, **11**, 219.

Fujio, H., Sakato, N., and Amano, T. (1971). *Bieken J.*, **14**, 395.

Furthmayr, H., and Timpl, R. (1972). *Biochem. Biophys. Res. Commun.*, **47**, 944.

Furthmayr, H., and Timpl, R. (1976). *Int. Rev. Conn. Tis. Res.*, 7,

Furthmayr, H., Beil, W., and Timpl, R. (1971). *FEBS Letters*, **12**, 341.

Geiger, B., and Arnon, R. (1974). *Eur. J. Immunol.*, **4**, 632.

Gelzer, J. (1968). *Immunochemistry*, **5**, 23.

Gerwing, J., and Thompson, K. (1968). *Biochemistry*, **7**, 3888.

Gilboa-Garber, N., Weisman, C., and Garber, N. (1971). *Abst. 41st Mtg Israel Chem. Soc.*, p. 47.

Gill, T. J. (1971). *Curr. Top. Microbiol. Immunol.*, **54**, 19.

Gill, T. J. and Doty, P. (1960). *J. Mol. Biol.*, **2**, 65.

Gill, T. J. and Doty, P. (1962). *Biochim. Biophys. Acta*, **60**, 450.

Gill, T. J., Kunz, H. W., and Papermaster, D. S. (1967). *J. Biol. Chem.*, **242**, 3308.

Gill, T. J., Papermaster, D. S., and Mawbray, J. F., (1965). *J. Immunol.*, **95**, 794.

Givas, J., Centeno, E. R., Manning, M., and Sehon, A. H. (1968). *Immunochemistry*, **5**, 314.

Givas, J., Sehon, A. H., and Manning, M. (1972). *Biochemistry*, **11**, 1351.

Goodman, J. W., and Nitecki, D. E. (1967). *Immunology*, **13**, 577.

Goodman, J. W., Nitecki, D. E., and Stoltenberg, J. M. (1968). *Biochemistry*, **7**, 706.

Grodsky, G. M. (1965). *Rep. Ross. Pediat. Res. Conf.*, **51**, 8.

Grodsky, G. M., Peng, C. T., and Forsham, P. H. (1959). *Archs Biochem.*, **81**, 264.

Gross, J. (1961). *Scient. Am.*, **204**, 120.

Habeeb, A. F. S. A. (1967). *Archs, Biochem. Biophys.*, **121**, 652.

Habeeb, A. F. S. A., and Atassi, M. Z. (1969). *Immunochemistry*, **6**, 555.

Habeeb, A. F. S. A., and Atassi, M. Z. (1970). *Immunochemistry*, **9**, 4939.

Habeeb, A. F. S. A., and Atassi, M. Z. (1971a). *Biochim. Biophys. Acta*, **236**, 131.

Habeeb, A. F. S. A., and Atassi, M. Z. (1971b). *Immunochemistry*, **8**, 1047.

Hakomori, S. J., and Kobata, A. (1974). In *The Antigens*, Vol. II, (Sela, M., ed.), Academic Press, New York and London, p. 79.

Harrison, S. C., and Blout, E. R. (1965). *J. Biol. Chem.*, **240**, 299.

Hashim, G. A., and Eylar, E. H. *Archs Biochem. Biophys.*, **129**, 645.

Haurowitz, F. (1950). *Chemistry and Biology of Proteins*, Academic Press, New York and London.

Hendrickson, W. A., and Love, W. E. (1971). *Nature, New Biol.*, **232**, 197.

Hill, S., and Sercarz, E. E. (1975). *Eur. J. Immunol.*, **5**, 317.

Howard, J. G., Christrie, G. H., Courtenay, B. H., Leuchars, E., and Davis, J. S. (1971). *Cell Immunol.*, **2**, 614.

Ichiki, A. T., and Parish, C. R. (1972). *Cell. Immunol.*, **4**, 264.

Isagholian, L. B., and Brown, R. K. (1970). *Immunochemistry*, **7**, 167.

Jacobsen, C., Fundling, L., Moller, N. P. H., and Steengaard, J. (1972). *Eur. J. Biochem.*, **30**, 392.

Janeway, C. A., and Humphrey, J. H. (1968). *Immunology*, **14**, 225.

Janeway, C. A., and Sela, M. (1967). *Immunology*, **13**, 29.

Jasin, H. E., and Glynn, L. E. (1965a). *Immunology*, **8**, 95.

Jasin, H. E., and Glynn, L. E. (1965b). *Immunology*, **8**, 260.

Jollés, J., and Jollés, P. (1971). *Helv. Chim. Acta*, **54**, 2668.

Jollés, J., Nieman, B., Herman, J., and Jollés, P. (1967). *Eur. J. Biochem.*, **1**, 344.

Jonsson, J., and Palens, S. (1966). *Int. Archs. Allergy. appl. Immunol.*, **29**, 272.

Kabat, E. A. (1960). *J. Immunol.*, **84**, 82.

Kabat, E. A. (1967). In *Structural Concepts in Immunology and Immunochemistry* Holt, Rinehard, and Winston Inc., New York, p. 82.

Kaminski, M. (1965). *Prog. Allergy*, **9**, 79.

Kartha, G., Bello, J., and Harker, D. (1967). *Nature (Lond.)*, **213**, 862.

Keck, K. (1975). *Nature, (Lond.)*, **254**, 78.

Kelly, B., and Levy, J. G. (1971). *Biochemistry*, **10**, 1763.

Kendrew, J. C., Watson, H. C., Standberg, B. E., Dickerson, R. E., Philips, D. C., and Shore, V. C. *Nature (Lond.)*, **190**, 666.

Kirrane, J. A., and Glynn, L. E. (1968). *Int. Rev. Conn. Tiss. Res.*, **4**, 1.

Kohn, L. D., Isursky, C., Zupnik, J., Pinars, A. L., Lee, G., and Lapiére, C. M. (1974). *Proc. Nat. Acad. Sci. U.S.A.*, **71**, 40.

Koketsu, J., and Atassi, M. Z. (1974). *Immunochemistry*, **11**, 1.

Landsteiner, K. (1942). *J. Exp. Med.*, **75**, 269.

360

Landsteiner, K. (1945). *The Specificity of Serological Reactions*, Harvard University Press, Cambridge, Mass.

Langbeheim, H., Arnon, R., and Sela, M. (1976). *Proc. Nat. Acad. Sci., U.S.A.*, **73**, 4636.

Lapresle, C., and Darieux, J. (1957). *Ann & Immunol. (Inst. Pasteur)*, **92**, 62.

Lee, W. Y., and Sehon, A. H. (1971). *Immunochemistry*, **8**, 743.

Lennon, V. A., Wilks, A. V., and Carnegie, P. R. (1970). *J. Immunol.*, **105**, 1223.

Levine, B. B., Ojeda, A., and Benacerraf, B. (1963). *J. Exp. Med.*, **118**, 953.

Lewis, P. N., and Scheraga, H. A. (1971). *Archs. Biochim. Biophys.*, **144**, 584.

Lichtenberg, L., Mozes, E., Shearer, G. M., and Sela, M. (1974). *J. Eur. Immunol.*, **4**, 430.

Luderitz, O., Staub, A. M., and Westphal, O. (1966). *Bacteriol. Rev.*, **30**, 192.

Maoz, A., Fuchs, S., and Michaeli, D. (1971). *Biochim. Biophys. Acta*, **243**, 106.

Maoz, A., Fuchs, S., and Sela, M. (1973a). *Biochemistry*, **12**, 4238.

Maoz, A., Fuchs, S., and Sela, M. (1973b). *Biochemistry*, **12**, 4246.

Margoliash, E., Nisonoff, A., and Reichlin, M. (1970). *J. Biol. Chem.*, **245**, 931.

Margoliash, E., and Schejter, A. (1966). *Adv. Protein Chem.*, **21**, 113.

Margoliash, E., Reichlin, M., and Nisonoff, A. (1967). In *Conformation of Biopolymers*, (Ramachandran, J., ed.) Academic Press, New York, and London p. 253.

Maron, E., Arnon, R., Sela, M., Perrin, J. -P., and Jolles, P. (1970). *Bìochim. Biophys. Acta*, **214**, 222.

Maron, E., Sher, H. I., Mozes, E., Arnon, R., and Sela, M. (1973). *J. Immunol.*, **111**, 101.

Maron, E., Shiozawa, C., Arnon, R., and Sela, M. (1971). *Biochemistry*, **10**, 763.

Maron, E., Webb, C., Teitelbaum, D., and Arnon, R. (1972). *Eur. J. Immunol.* **2**, 294.

Matsouka, Y., Hamaoka, T., and Yamamura, Y. (1966). *Jap. J. Biochem.*, **61**, 703.

Maurer, P. H. (1963). *J. Immunol.*, **90**, 493.

Maurer, P. H. (1964). *Prog. Allergy*, **81**, 1.

Maurer, P. H. (1965a). *J. Immunol.*, **95**, 1095.

Maurer, P. H. (1965b). *J. Exp. Med.*, **121**, 339.

Maurer, P. H., and Pinchuck, P. (1968). In *Nucleic Acids in Immunology*, (Plescia, O. J., and Braun, W., eds.), Springer Verlag, New York, p. 301.

McBride, O. W., and Harrington, W. F. (1967a). *Biochemistry*, **6**, 1484.

McBride, O. W., and Harrington, W. F. (1976b). *Biochemistry* **6**, 1499.

McDevitt, H. O., Deak, B. D., Shreffler, D. C., Klein, J., Stimpfling, J. H., and Snell, G. D. (1972). *J. Exp. Med.*, **135**, 2159.

McDevitt, H. O., and Sela, M. (1965). *J. Exp. Med.*, **122**, 517.

McDevitt, H. O., and Sela, M. (1967). *J. Exp. Med.*, **126**, 969.

Melchers, I., Rajewsky, K., and Shreffler, D. C. (1975). *Eur. J. Immunol.*, **3**, 754.

Merigan, T. C., and Potts, J. T. (1966). *Biochemistry*, **5**, 910.

Merrifield, B. B. (1965). *Science, N.Y.*, **150**, 178.

Messer, W., and Melchers, F. (1969). In *The Lactose Operon*, (Beckwith, J. R., and Zipser, D., eds.), Cold Spring Harbor, New York, p. 305.

Michaeli, D., Martin, G. R., Kettman, J., Benjamini, E., Leung, D. Y. K., and Blatt, B. A. (1969). *Science, N.Y.*, **166**, 1522.

Michaeli, D., Senyk, G., Maoz, A., and Fuchs, S. (1972). *J. Immunol.*, **109**, 103.

Miller, A., Bonavida, B., Stratton, S. A., and Secarz, E. (1971). *Biochim. Biophys. Acta*, **243**, 520.

Miller, J. F. A. P., and Mitchell, G. F. (1969). *Transplant. Rev.*, **1**, 3.

Mitchell, B., and Levy, J. G. (1970). *Biochemistry*, **9**, 2762.

Mitchell, G. F., and Miller, J. F. A. P. (1968). *J. Exp. Med.*, **128**, 821.

Möller, G., and Mitchell, G. (1971). *Cell. Immunol.*, **2**, 309.

Mozes, E. (1975). *Immunogenetics*, **2**, 397.

Mozes, E., Maron, E., Arnon, R., and Sela, M. (1971). *J. Immunol.*, **106**, 862.

Mozes, E., McDevitt, H. O., Jaton, J. -C., and Sela, M. (1969a). *J. Exp. Med.*, **130**, 1263.

Mozes, E., McDevitt, H. O., Jaton, J. -C., and Sela, M. (1969b). *J. Exp. Med.*, **130**, 493.

Mozes, E., Schmitt-Verhulst, A. -M., and Fuchs, S. (1975). *Eur. J. Immunol.*, **5**, 549.
Mozes, E., Schwartz, M., and Sela, M. (1974). *J. Exp. Med.*, **140**, 349.
Mozes, E., and Shearer, G. M. (1971). *J. Exp. Med.*, **134**, 141.
Mozes, E., and Shearer, G. M. (1972). *Curr. Top. Microbiol. Immunol.*, **59**, 167.

Neumann, H., Steinberg, I. Z., Brown, J. B., Goldberger, R. F., and Sela, M. (1976). *Eur. J. Biochem.*, **3**, 171.
Niedieck, B. (1975). *Prog. Allergy*, **18**, 353.
Nisonoff, A., Reichlin, M., and Margoliash, E. (1970). *J. Biol. Chem.*, **245**, 940.
Nolan, C., and Margoliash, E. (1968). *Ann. Rev. Biochem.*, **37**, 727.
Nossal, G. J. V., Ada, G. L., and Austin, C. M. (1964). *Aust. J. Exp. Biol. Med. Sci.*, **42**, 283.
Nossal, G. J. V., Austin, C. M., and Ada, G. L. (1965). *Immunology*, **9**, 333.
Nowack, H., Hahn, E., and Timpl, R. (1976). *Immunology*, **30**, 29.

O'Dell, D. S. (1968). In *Treatise on Collagen*, Vol. 2A, (Gould, B. S., ed.), Academic Press, London and New York, p. 311.
Okada, Y., Ikinaka, T., Yagura, T., and Yamamura, Y. (1963). *Jap. J. Biochem.*, **54**, 101.
Okada, Y., Watanoke, S., and Yamamura, Y. (1964). *J. Biochem.*, **55**, 342.
Omenn, G. S., Ontjes, D. A., and Anfinsen, C. B. (1970a). *Biochemistry*, **9**, 304.
Omenn, G. S., Ontjes, D. A., and Anfinsen, C. B. (1970b). *Biochemistry*, **9**, 313.
Oshiro, Y., and Eylar, E. H. (1970). *Archs Biochem. Biophys.*, **138**, 606.

Pai, R. C. and Atassi, M. Z. (1975). *Immunochemistry*, **12**, 285.
Parish, C. R. (1971a). *J. Exp. Med.*, **134**, 1.
Parish, C. R. (1971b). *J. Exp. Med.*, **134**, 21.
Parish, C. R., and Ada, G. L. (1969). *J. Biochem.*, **113**, 489.
Parish, C. R. and Liew, F. Y. (1972). *J. Exp. Med.*, **135**, 298.
Pecht, I., Maron, E., Arnon, R., and Sela, M. (1971). *Eur. J. Biochem.*, **19**, 368.
Pelichova, H., Suzuki, T., and Cinader, B. (1970). *J. Immunol.*, **104**, 195.
Perlstein, M. T., and Atassi, M. Z. (1974). *Immunochemistry*, **11**, 63.
Phillips, P. C. (1967). *Proc. Nat. Acad. Sci., U.S.A.*, **57**, 484.
Piez, K. A., Bladen, H. A., Land, J. M., Miller, E. J., Bornstein, P., Butler, W. T., and Kang, A. H. (1968). *Brookhaven Symp. Biology, No. 21*, **1**, 345.
Plescia, O. J., Braun, W., and Palczuk, N. C. (1964). *Proc. Nat. Acad. Sci., U.S.A.*, **52**, 279.
Pollock, M. R., Fleming, J., and Petrie, S. (1967). In *Antibodies to Biologically Active Molecules*, (Cinader, B., ed.), Pergamon Press, New York and Oxford, p. 139.
Pontz, B., Meigel, W., Rautenberg, J., and Kulin, K. (1970). *Eur. J. Biochem.*, **16**, 50.
Pope, C. G. (1966). *Adv. Immunol.*, **5**, 209.
Porter, R. R. (1957). *Biochem. J.*, **66**, 677.
Prager, E. M., Arnheim, M., Gross, G. A., and Wilson, A. L. (1972). *J. Biol. Chem.*, **247**, 2905.
Prager, E. M., and Wilson, A. C., (1971a). *J. Biol. Chem.*, **246**, 5978.
Prager, E. M. and Wilson, A. C. (1971b). *J. Biol. Chem.*, **246**, 7010.

Ramachandran, J., Berger, A., and Katchalski, E. (1971). *Biopolymers*, **10**, 1829.
Rautenberg, J., Timpl, R., and Furthmayr, H. (1972). *Eur. J. Biochem.*, **27**, 231.
Reichlin, M. (1972). *J. Mol. Biol.*, **64**, 485.
Reichlin, M., Bucci, E., Fronticelli, C., Wyman, J., Antonini, E., Loppolo, C., and Rossi-Fanelli, A. (1966). *J. Mol. Biol.*, **17**, 18.
Reichlin, M., Hay, M., and Levine, L. (1963). *Biochemistry*, **2**, 971.
Reichlin, M., Margoliash, E., and Nisonoff, A. (1968). *Fed. Proc.*, **27**, 276.
Reichlin, M., Nisonoff, A., and Margoliash, E. (1970). *J. Biol. Chem.*, **245**, 947.
Richards, F. M., and Vithayathil, P. J. (1959). *J. Biol. Chem.*, **234**, 1459.

362

Roelants, G. E., and Goodman, J. W. (1968). *Biochemistry*, 7, 1432.

Rotman, M. E. and Celada, F. (1968). *Proc. Nat. Acad. Sci., U.S.A.*, 60, 660.

Sachs, D. H., Berzofsky, J. A., Fathman, C. G., Piselsky, D. S., Schechter, A. N., and Schwartz, R. H. (1976). *Cold Spring Harbor Symp. Quant. Biol.*

Sachs, D. H., Schechter, A. N., Eastlake, A., and Anfinsen, C. B. (1972a). *J. Immunol.*, 109, 1300.

Sachs, D. H., Schechter, A. N., Eastlake, A., and Anfinsen, C. B. (1972b). *Proc. Nat. Acad. Sci., U.S.A.*, 69, 3790.

Sachs, D. H., Schechter, A. N., Eastlake, A., and Anfinsen, C. B. (1972c). Biochemistry, 11, 4268.

Schechter, B., Conway-Jacobs, A., and Sela, M. (1971a). *Eur. J. Biochem.*, 20, 321.

Schechter, B., Schechter, I., Ramachandran, J., Conway-Jacobs, A., Sela, M., Benjamini, E., and Shimizu, M. (1971b). *Eur. J. Biochem.*, 20, 309.

Schechter, B., Schechter, I., Ramachandran, J., Jacobs-Conway, A., and Sela, M. (1971c). *Eur. J. Biochem.*, 20, 301.

Schechter, I., Schechter, B., and Sela, M. (1966). *Biochim. Biophys. Acta*, 127, 438.

Schneider, D. R., Endahl, G. L., Dodd, M. C., Jesseph, J. E., Bigley, N. J., and Zollinger, R. M. (1967). *Science, N.Y.*, 156, 391.

Schwartz, M., Hooghe, R. J., Mozes, E., and Sela, M. (1976). *Proc. Nat. Acad. Sci, U.S.A.*, 73, 4184.

Schwartz, M., Mozes, E., and Sela, M. (1975). *Eur. J. Immunol.*, 5, 866.

Schwick, H. G. (1966). *Behringwerk Mitt.*, 46, 87.

Sela, M. (1966). *Adv. Immunol.*, 5, 29.

Sela, M. (1969). *Science, N.Y.*, 166, 1365.

Sela, M., and Arnon, R. (1960a). *Biochem. J.*, 75, 91.

Sela, M., and Arnon, R. (1960b). *Biochim. Biophys. Acta*, 40, 382.

Sela, M., and Arnon, R. (1960c). *Biochem. J.*, 77, 394.

Sela, M., Fuchs, S., and Arnon, R. (1962). *Biochem. J.*, 85, 223.

Sela, M., Katchalski, and Olitzki, A. L. (1956). *Science, N.Y.*, 123, 1129.

Sela, M., and Mozes, E. (1966). *Proc. Nat. Acad. Sci., U.S.A.*, 55, 445.

Sela, M., and Mozes, E. (1975). *Transplant. Rev.*, 23, 189.

Sela, M., Mozes, E., and Shearer, G. M. (1972). *Proc. Nat. Acad. Sci., U.S.A.*, 64, 2696.

Sela, M., Schechter, B., Schechter, I., and Borek, F. (1967). *Cold Spring Harbor Symp. Quant. Biol.*, 32, 537.

Shapira, E., and Arnon, R. (1967). *Biochemistry*, 6, 3951.

Shapira, E., and Arnon, R. (1969). *J. Biol. Chem.*, 244, 1026.

Shearer, G. M., Mozes, E., and Sela, M. (1971) *J. Exp. Med.*, 133, 216.

Shearer, G. M., Mozes, E., and Sela, M. (1972). *J. Exp. Med.*, 135, 1009.

Sherr, C. J., and Goldberg, B. (1973). *Science, N.Y.*, 180, 1190.

Shinka, S., Imanishi, M., Kuwahara, O., Fujio, H., and Amano, T. (1962). *Biken J.*, 5, 181.

Shinka, S., Imanishi, M., Miyagawa, N., Amano, T., Inouye, M., and Tsugita, A. (1967). *Biken J.*, 10, 89.

Singer, S. J., and Richards, F. M. (1959). *J. Biol. Chem.*, 234, 2911.

Singhal, R. P., and Atassi, M. Z. (1971). *Biochemistry*, 10, 1756.

Sjöberg, O., and Möller, E. (1970) *Nature (Lond.)*, 228, 780.

Spitler, L., Benjamini, E., Young, J. D., Kaplan, H., and Fudenberg, H. H., (1970). *J. Exp. Med.*, 131, 133.

Spragg, J., Schroder, F., Stewart, J. M., Austen, K. F., and Haber, E. (1967). *Biochemistry*, 6, 3933.

Stevens, V. D. (1974). In *Immunological Approaches to Fertility Control*, (Diczfalusy, E., ed.), Karolinska Institutet, Stockholm, p. 387.

Stollar, B. D. (1973). In *The Antigens*, Vol. 1, (Sela, M., ed.), Academic Press, New York and London, p. 1.

Storck, J., Rixier, T., and Uzan, A. (1964). *Nature (Lond.)*, **201**, 835.
Strossberg, A. D., and and Kanarek, L. (1968). *Archs. Int. Physiol. Biochim.*, **76**, 949.
Strossberg, A. D., and Kanarek, L. (1969). *FEBS Letters*, **5**, 324.
Stupp, Y., and Sela, M. (1967). *Biochim. Biophys. Acta*, **140**, 349.
Suzuki, T., Pelichova, H., and Cinader, B. (1969). *J. Immunol.*, **103**, 1366.

Tamaburro, A. M., Jori, G., Vidali, G., Scatturin, A., and Saccomani, G. (1972). *Biochim. Biophys. Acta*, **263**, 704.
Taniuchi, H., and Anfinsen, C. B. (1971). *J. Biol. Chem.*, **246**, 2291.
Tanford, C., and Hauenstein, J. D. (1965). *Biochim. Biophys. Acta*, **19**, 535.
Teicher, E., Maron, E., and Arnon, R. (1973). *Immunochemistry*, **10**, 265.
Teitelbaum, D., Webb, C., Arnon, R., and Sela, M., (1976). *Cell. Immunol*, in press.
Thompson, K., Harris, M., Benjamini, E., Mitchell, G., and Noble, M. (1972). *Nature, New Biol.*, **238**, 20.
Timpl, R. (1975). In *Biochemistry of Collagen*, (Ramachamdran, G. N., and Reddi, A. H., eds.), Plenum Press, New York.
Timpl, R., Fietzek, P. P., Furthmayr, H., Meigel, W., and Kuhn, K. (1970). *FEBS Letters*, **9**, 11.
Timpl, R., Beil, W., Furthmayr, H., Meigel, W., and Plotz, B. (1971). *Immunology*, **21**, 1017.
Timpl, R., Furthmayr, H., Hahn, E., Becker, U., and Stoltz, M. (1973a). *Behring Inst. Mitt.*, **53**, 66.
Timpl, R., Wick, G., Furthmayr, H., Lapiere, C. M., and Kuhn, K. (1973b). *Eur. J. Biochem.*, **32**, 584.
Traub, W., and Piez, K. A. (1971). *Adv. Protein Chem.*, **25**, 243.
Traub, W., and Yonath, A. (1966). *J. Mol. Biol.*, **16**, 406.

Unger, R. E., Eisentraut, A. M., McCall, M. S., Keller, S., Lanz, H. C., and Madison, L. L. (1959). *Proc. Soc. Exp. Biol. Med.*, **102**, 621.

Van der Mark, K., Click, E. M., and Bornstein, P. (1973). *Archs Biochem. Biophys.*, **156**, 356.
Van Regenmortel, M. H. V. (1966). *Adv. Virus Res.*, **12**, 207.
Van Vunakis, H., Kaplan, J., Lehrer, H., and Levine, L. (1966). *Immunochemistry*, **3**, 393.
Von Sengbusch, P. (1965). *Z. Verebungel.*, **96**, 364.

Westall, F. C., Robinson, A. B., Caccam, J., Jackson, J., and Eylar, E. H. (1971). *Nature, (Lond.)*, **229**, 22.
Wilson, A. C., and Prager, E. M. (1974). In *Lysozyme*, (Osserman, E. F., Canfield, R. E., and Beychok, S. eds.), Academic Press. New York and London, p. 127.
Wilson, S. (1967). In *Antibodies to Biologically Active Molecules*, (Cinader, B., ed.), Pergamon Press, New York and Oxford. p. 235.
Wyckoff, H. W., Hardman, K. D., Allewell, N. M., Inagami, T., Johnson, L. M., and Richards, F. M. (1967). *J. Biol. Chem.*, **242**, 3984.

Yagi, Y., Maier, P., and Pressman, D. (1965). *Science, N.Y.*, **147**, 617.
Young, J. D., and Leung, C. Y. (1970). *Biochemistry*, **9**, 2755.
Young, J. D., Benjamini, E., and Leung, C. Y. (1968). *Biochemistry*, **7**, 3113.

Zyk, N. and Citri, N. (1968). *Biochim. Biophys. Acta*, **159**, 327.

CHAPTER 10

Immunochemistry of the Classical and Alternative Pathways of Complement

D. T. Fearon and K. F. Austen

1 INTRODUCTION

The complement system consists of a group of plasma proteins whose sequential interaction may be initiated by immunoglobulins, microbial products, and tryptic enzymes. Activation is effected by generation and assembly of highly specific enzymes and is accompanied by limited proteolytic cleavage, resulting in the release of peptides and the formation of multimolecular complexes. Such complexes have diverse biological activities that are capable of recruiting essential ingredients of an inflammatory response. This review will describe the complement proteins, their chemistry, synthesis, and genetically controlled alterations, their molecular interactions, and the biologically active products generated by activation. Detailed discussions of the role of complement in human disease are available in several recent reviews (Ruddy *et al.*, 1972; Fearon and Austen, 1976a).

2 COMPLEMENT COMPONENTS AND ALTERNATIVE PATHWAY FACTORS

The complement system may be divided into four functional sections: two pathways for activation (the classical pathway and the alternative, or properdin pathway); an amplification mechanism for augmenting the activating pathways; and a final common effector pathway to which the activating sequences are directed and from which the biological activities are derived (Figure 1).

The constituent proteins of the classical complement system are signified by C and a number designating the component (C1, C4, C2, C3, C5–C9). The activated state of a component is indicated by a bar over the number (for example, C$\bar{1}$). Cleavage fragments are suffixed with letters (for example, C5a and C5b), while an inactive fragment is denoted with an i—as in C2i.

A provisional nomenclature for alternative pathway factors uses letters rather than numbers, maintaining the other conventions as for the classical components. The approximate molecular weights, electrophoretic mobilities, and serum concentrations of components and factors are given in Table 1.

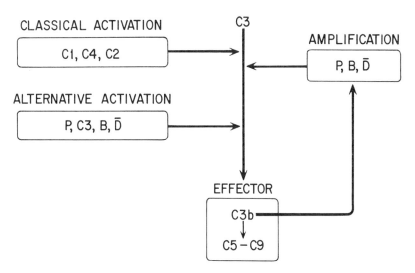

Figure 1 Four functional units of complement: two pathways for activation, the classical and alternative, which generate enzymes capable of cleaving C3; the amplification pathway, which utilizes C3b to form a C3-cleaving enzyme to augment activation of the effector sequence by either initiating pathway; and a terminal effector sequence, which is activated by the classical, alternative, and amplifying pathways, and from which are derived the biologically active products of complement

2.1 Classical Pathway of Complement Activation

The classical activating pathway is composed of three components—C1, C4, and C2. C1 is activated to $\overline{C1}$ following binding to certain antigen–antibody complexes. $\overline{C1}$ then cleaves its two complement substrates, C4 and C2, whose major cleavage products form a bimolecular complex (C4b2ab), the classical C3 convertase, which is capable of cleaving C3 to initiate activation of the effector complement sequence.

2.1.1 C1

The first component of complement consists of at least three subcomponents (C1q, C1r and C1s), which form a complex in the presence of Ca^{2+} (Lepow et al., 1956). The macromolecular complex of C1 contains one molecule of C1q, a dimer of C1r non-covalently held together, and a dimer of C1s linked by Ca^{2+} (Ziccardi and Cooper, 1977). The suggestion that an additional subcomponent, designated C1t, contributes to the C1 complex (Assimeh and Painter, 1975a,b) has not been confirmed by structural or functional studies of native C1 in serum or C1 reconstructed from purified C1q, C1r, and C1s (Ziccardi and Cooper, 1977).

Table 1 Physicochemical characteristics of proteins of the complement system

	Approximate molecular weight	Electrophoretic mobility	Serum concentration (μg/ml)	Cleavage fragments
Classical Pathway of Activation				
C1q	390 000	γ_2	190	
C1r	188 000	β	*	
C1s	110 000	α_2	120	
C4	209 000	β_1	430	C4a, C4b, C4c, C4d
C2	117 000	β_2	30	C2a, C2b
Alternative Pathway of Activation				
Properdin	223 000	γ_2	25	
Factor $\overline{\text{D}}$ (C3PAase, GBGase)	23 500	α	1–5	
Factor B (C3PA, GBG)	100 000	β_2	240	Bb(C3A, GGG), Ba(GAG)
C3 (β_1C)	210 000	β_1	1300	C3a, C3b, C3c(β_1A) C3d(α_2D)
Attack Sequence				
C3 (β_1C)				
C5	206 000	β_1	75	C5a, C5b
C6	95 000	β_2	60	
C7	120 000	β_2	*	
C8	163 000	γ_1	*	
C9	79 000	α	160	
Control Proteins				
C$\overline{\text{1}}$INH	105 000	α_2	180	
C3bINA (KAF)	100 000	β_2	25	
B1H	150 000	β_1	450	

* not known

Although the ratio of the subcomponents in the C1 complex is thought normally to be equimolar, disparate ratios of C1q, C1r, and C1s have been found in the sera of patients with classical X-linked agammaglobulinaemia (Stroud et al., 1970) and genetic deficiency of C1r (Day et al., 1972).

Ultrastructural studies of C1q by electron microscopy have shown six peripheral globular portions joined by strands to a central fibril-like region (Shelton et al., 1972). Since the valency of C1q for binding to immunoglobulin is six (Müller-Eberhard and Kunkel, 1961; Müller-Eberhard and Calcott, 1966), it is presumed that the globular portions correspond to these binding sites. C1q consists of six non-covalently linked subunits which have been found either to be identical in molecular weight (60 000) (Reid et al., 1972) or to be of two types with molecular weights of 60 000 and 42 000 (Yonemasu and Stroud, 1972). The subunits are composed of globular and collagen-like regions. The latter consists of three polypeptide chains covalently linked in a major triple helix, each chain having a $(X-Y-Gly)_n$ sequence and high levels of hydroxylated amino acids (Reid et al., 1972). A model for C1q proposes that the six subunits are joined at their collagen-like N-terminal ends to form a stem fibril from which branch the individual C-terminal globular regions carrying the immunoglobulin-binding sites. The IgG-binding site for C1q resides in the C_H2 domain of the Fc region (Ellerson et al., 1972), while in the case of IgM, it is found in C_H4 domain (Hurst et al., 1974).

Studies of the biosynthesis of C1q in tissue cultures have given variable results. The incorporation of $[^{14}C]$-amino acids into C1q, as assessed by radioimmunoelectrophoresis (Morse et al., 1967), has been reported for human peritoneal macrophages while guinea-pig peritoneal macrophages were not found to produce C1q as assayed by interaction of $C\overline{1}r$ with $C\overline{1}s$ to produce haemolytically active $C\overline{1}$ (Colten and Wyatt, 1972). Synthesis of a functionally intact C1 macromolecule, which presumably contains C1q, C1r, and C1s, was found in short-term cultures of guinea-pig columnar epithelial cells of the intestine, but intracellular assembly was not excluded (Colten et al., 1968).

Individuals with a genetic deficiency of C1q have not been observed, but depressed serum levels of C1q have been found in various immunodeficiency states. Patients with sex-linked aggammaglobulinaemia have subnormal serum levels of C1q (Müller-Eberhard and Kunkel, 1961), and in combined immunodeficiency diseases, C1q concentrations are diminished to 10–25 per cent of normal (O'Connell et al., 1967; Gewurz et al., 1968). Levels of C1r and C1s in these patients are normal or even elevated, indicating that different regulatory mechanisms exist for maintaining serum concentrations of the C1 subcomponents. That the C1q deficiency is not a primary defect is suggested by metabolic studies of radiolabelled C1q in hypogammaglobulinaemic patients. In this case synthetic rates are normal, fractional catabolic rates elevated, and volumes of distribution increased (Kohler and Müller-Eberhard, 1972). Since a direct correlation between serum IgG and C1q exists (Kohler and Müller-Eberhard, 1969), it has been postulated that C1q forms a reversible complex with IgG and thereby is maintained within the vascular compartment and protected from extravascular catabolism.

Activated C1r ($C\overline{1}r$), a γ-globulin with a molecular weight of 188 000, is the C1 subcomponent responsible for conversion of C1s to $C\overline{1}s$ (Naff and Ratnoff, 1968). The enzymic site on $C\overline{1}r$ has been characterized as an esterase, based on hydrolysis of certain synthetic amino acid esters and inhibition by phenylmethyl sulphonyl fluoride and the naturally occurring $C\overline{1}$ inhibitor ($C\overline{1}$ INH) (Naff and Ratnoff, 1968). The finding that ε-aminocaproic acid inhibits intrinsic activation of C1 may indicate an inhibitory effect on $C\overline{1}r$ generation (Soter et al., 1975). Although a trypsin-activatable precursor has been isolated by Valet and Cooper (1974a), the mechanisms responsible for proteolytic conversion of C1r to $C\overline{1}r$ in the intact macromolecule are not known. Reversible binding of $C\overline{1}r$ to C1q appears to be independent of cations, while the binding of C̄1r to C1s or C̄1s requires the presence of Ca^{2+}.

A well-documented family with genetic deficiency of C1r (Day *et al.*, 1972) and a patient without family studies (Pickering *et al.*, 1970) have been reported. Affected individuals had no total haemolytic activity or immunochemically detectable C1r, while some other family members, including both parents, had serum levels about one-half normal, indicating an autosomal recessive mode of inheritance. The cell responsible for synthesis of C1r has not been identified.

C1s, an α-globulin composed of a single polypeptide chain with a molecular weight of 80–110 000, is converted to C̄1s by C̄1r-induced cleavage of a peptide bond. C̄1s consists of a heavy and a light chain (molecular weights of 59 000 and 27 000, respectively) held together by a disulphide bridge (Sakai and Stroud, 1973). The esterase site of C̄1s resides in the light chain as indicated by binding of [^{32}P]diisopropylphosphofluoridate and an amino acid sequence near to the enzymic site similar to that of other serine esterases such as plasmin, thrombin, trypsin, and chymotrypsin (Barkas *et al.*, 1973). It appears that the single active site of C̄1s cleaves both complement protein substrates, C4 and C2. The site of synthesis of C1s is not known. A single patient with isolated C1s deficiency has been reported but genetic analysis was not performed (Pondman *et al.*, 1969).

A recently described additional subcomponent of C1 (C1t) is a 225 000 molecular weight $α_1$-glycoprotein composed of 10 non-covalently bound subunits of 22 600 molecular weight (Assimeh and Painter, 1975a, b). This subcomponent was reported to serve as a bridge between C1q and C1s, but its structural and functional contribution to C1 is now questioned.

2.1.2 C4

This component, a glycoprotein with a molecular weight of 209 000 and β electrophoretic mobility, is composed of three covalently linked polypeptide chains: an α chain of 93 000; a β chain of 78 000; and a smaller γ chain of 33 000 molecular weight (Schrieber and Müller-Eberhard, 1974). Cleavage of C4 by C̄1s releases a 7000–11 000 molecular weight fragment, designated C4a, from the N-terminus of the α chain; the residual major fragment is C4b. C4b is cleaved into additional fragments—C4c (molecular weight 157 000) and C4d (molecular weight 35 000)—by the action of partially purified C4b inactivator, which is a control protein probably identical to the C3b inactivator (Cooper, 1975). The former fragment appears to consist of unaltered β and γ chains and a portion of the α chain, while C4d is derived from the α chain.

Haemolytically active C4 has been harvested from tissue cultures of guinea-pig macrophages obtained from several organs (Burkholder *et al.*, 1970). Using the Jerne haemolytic plaque assay, individual peritoneal macrophages have been shown to synthesize both C4 and C2 (Wyatt *et al.*, 1972). In humans, a complex form of genetically determined polymorphism has been detected, and analysis of paired samples of maternal and foetal plasma has provided evidence for the foetal synthesis of C4 and absence of transplacental passage (Rosenfeld *et al.*, 1969a;

Bach *et al.*, 1971). Half-normal plasma levels of C4 were reported by Rosenfeld *et al.* (1969*b*) in four individuals from a family of 20, and two kindreds with homozygous C4 deficiency genetically linked to the major histocompatibility complex have been described (Hauptmann *et al.*, 1974; Rittner *et al.*, 1975; Ochs *et al.*, 1977).

2.1.3 C2

This component (C2) is a glycoprotein consisting of a single polypeptide chain (Nagasawa and Stroud, 1977) with a molecular weight of 117 000, which is cleaved by C$\overline{1}$s into two fragments—C2a (molecular weight 80 000) and C2b (molecular weight 37 000). The former carries the active site for cleavage and activation of C3 (Polley and Müller-Eberhard, 1968). Biosynthetic (Wyatt *et al.*, 1972; Colten, 1974) and genetic studies (Klemperer *et al.*, 1966; Ruddy and Austen, 1971*b*; Fu *et al.*, 1974; Lachmann, 1974) of C2 have been extensive. C2 is synthesized by guinea-pig peritoneal macrophages and human peripheral blood monocytes maintained in cultures for up to six weeks. Synthesis of C2 by macrophages is enhanced markedly following phagocytosis of heat-killed *Pneumococcus* species, demonstrating a potential regulatory mechanism for levels of complement at sites of inflammation. Monocytes from individuals with homozygous deficiency of C2 do not synthesize detectable C2 (Colten, 1974).

The first description of an inherited component deficiency was that of C2 by Klemperer *et al.* (1966), and has been followed by the analysis of 11 other kindreds (Ruddy and Austen, 1971*b*). C2 deficiency is inherited as an autosomal recessive trait and linkage to histocompatibility antigens has been described, especially with HLA-10 and W18 (Fu *et al.*, 1974). The occurrence of homozygous C2 deficiency in a normal blood donor population has been reported as one in 10 000 or less, implying heterozygosity in one in 100 individuals (Lachmann, 1974). The apparent increased frequency of 'collagen-vascular'-like diseases in individuals with homozygous deficiency in C2 (Ruddy and Austen, 1971*b*; Fu *et al.*, 1974) may be related either primarily to the complement abnormality (for example, impaired clearance of immune complexes) or to particular immune response genes with close linkages to C2 deficiency which predispose to these diseases or, most likely, to both.

2.2 Alternative Pathway of Complement Activation

The alternative (properdin) pathway of complement activation was described first more than twenty years ago as consisting of a group of serum factors interacting with zymosan, a yeast cell-wall polysaccharide at 37° to generate a zymosan–serum protein complex that is capable of activating C3 without the apparent utilization of C1, C4, and C2 (Pillemer *et al.*, 1954). Incubation of serum with zymosan at 17° renders the serum unable to generate C3-cleaving activity upon subsequent incubation with fresh zymosan at 37°. The eluate of zymosan which has been interacted with serum at 17° contains an active principle, termed properdin, which restores C3-cleaving activity of the adsorbed serum. Definitive evidence for the existence of an alternative route to complement activation awaited purification of some of the proteins involved. Properdin was purified to homogeneity less than 10 years ago and was shown to be distinct from immunoglobulin and known complement components (Pensky *et al.*, 1968). Since that time, other studies have demonstrated the importance of this pathway as an independent route for the activation of C3–C9 and as an amplifying system of both the classical and alternative pathways for the activation of C3–C9.

2.2.1 Properdin

Activated properdin ($\overline{P}$) is a γ-globulin of molecular weight 184 000–223 000, consisting of four apparently identical non-covalently linked subunits of 46 000 (Minta and Lepow, 1974). The precursor form (P) exhibits only weak binding to C3b (Götze *et al.*, 1977) and does not activate properdin-deficient serum in the absence of zymosan; and despite earlier reports (Minta, 1975), P does not differ in size or charge from $\overline{P}$. The site of P biosynthesis has not been identified.

2.2.2 Factor B

Factor B is a 100 000 molecular weight β-globulin, consisting of a single polypeptide chain (Götze, 1975), which is cleaved by $\overline{D}$ in the presence of C3b into (*i*) a minor fragment. Ba (molecular weight 20000), of α-electrophoretic mobility, and (*ii*) a major fragment, Bb (molecular weight 80 000), of γ-electrophoretic mobility (Müller-Eberhard and Götze, 1972). The enzymic site for C3 and C5 cleavage resides on Bb. Extensive electrophoretic polymorphism of B has been found and genetic analysis of the electrophoretic patterns is compatible with autosomal codominant inheritance (Alper *et al.*, 1972*a*). Family studies have demonstrated that the alleles controlling the polymorphism segregate with the major histocompatibility locus HL-A and the absence of recombinants in 44 informative analyses indicates close linkage (Allen, 1974). As mentioned above, C2 deficiency also is linked to histocompatibility antigens which, coupled with the findings of physicochemical and functional similarities between B and C2, suggests that one of these proteins arose by gene reduplication. Although the major site of B biosynthesis is not known, cultures of inflammatory rheumatoid synovial tissues have produced antigenically detectable B (Ruddy and Colten, 1974).

2.2.3 Factor D

The activated form of D ($\overline{D}$) is an α-globulin, with molecular weight of about 23 500, capable of cleaving B in the presence of C3b (Müller-Eberhard and Götze, 1972; Hunsicker *et al.*, 1973). The active site of $\overline{D}$ has been characterized as a serine esterase, based on its susceptibility to irreversible and competitive inhibition by diisopropylphosphofluoridate and *p*-tosyl-L-arginine methyl ester, respectively (Fearon *et al.*, 1974; Fearon and Austen, 1975*a*). $\overline{D}$ activity can be derived from a precursor, D, which is slightly larger and resistant to diisopropyl-phosphofluoridate inhibition, by brief treatment with trypsin (Fearon *et al.*, 1974). A plasma protein capable of converting D to $\bar{D}$ has not been identified, and a critical role for a precursor has not been established because of the invariable presence of $\bar{D}$ in plasma and serum.

2.2.4 C3

This component (C3), which was recognized first as the substrate for the classical C3 convertase, is now known to be identical to the factor A (Pillemer *et al.*, 1954) of the original description of the alternative pathway. The most abundant complement component in plasma (1·3 mg/ml), C3 is a β-globulin with a molecular weight of 210 000. Structural studies have demonstrated two polypeptide chains, α (molecular weight 140 000) and β (molecular weight 80 000), linked by disulphide bridges (Bokisch *et al.*, 1975; Nilsson *et al.*, 1975). Cleavage of C3 by C3 convertases, enzymes generated by the classical and alternative activating pathways, releases a 6000–8000 molecular weight fragment (C3a), from the N-terminus of the α chain, leaving a residual major fragment (C3b). Cell-bound C3b is rapidly inactivated by C3bINA (Ruddy and Austen, 1971a) and subsequently is cleaved into two additional fragments (C3c and C3d), possibly by the action of an additional protease. C3a consists of unaltered β chain and a portion of the α chain, while C3d is derived from the α chain (Bokisch *et al.*, 1975; Gitlin *et al.*, 1975).

More than 24 genetically controlled electrophoretic variants of C3 have been described and all variants are allelic (Alper and Propp, 1968; Rittner and Rittner, 1974). Inheritance of known allotypes is consistent with autosomal codominance and no linkage to histocompatibility antigens in the human has been observed. A 'blank' gene (C3⁻), which is allelic with other allotypes, codes for non-production of C3 and was observed in family members with half-normal serum levels of C3 (Alper *et al.*, 1969a). The presumption that these asymptomatic individuals are heterozygotes was confirmed subsequently when a subject with recurrent bacterial infections was found to have homozygous deficiency of C3 (Alper *et al.*, 1972b).

Biosynthesis of C3 appears to occur primarily in the liver as suggested by the demonstration of complete loss of recipient C3 allotype and the appearance of donor C3 allotype following a liver transplant (Alper *et al.*, 1969b). Although it has been suggested on the basis of immunofluorescent studies that the hepatocyte synthesizes C3, cultures of rheumatoid synovial tissues produce functionally and antigenically detectable C3 (Ruddy and Colten, 1974), raising the possibility of other sites of C3 synthesis.

2.2.5 C3 Nephritic Factor

An activity present in the sera of some patients with hypocomplementaemic membranoproliferative glomerulonephritis which is capable of inducing cleavage of C3 during incubation with normal serum was attributed to C3 nephritic factor (C3 NeF) (Spitzer *et al.*, 1969). This activity has been shown to reside in a γ-globulin of molecular weight 150 000 which effects cleavage of C3 by involvement of the alternative pathway. Although physical characteristics similar to IgG3 have suggested identity of C3 NeF with this immunoglobulin (Thompson, 1971), subsequent studies using purified C3 NeF failed to reveal reactivity with antisera to immunoglobulin light or heavy chains, or to IgG3 (Vallota *et al.*, 1974). Antiserum to C3 NeF reacts with a trace protein in normal serum, consistent with the existence of a precursor, non-active analogue to Ce NeF in normal individuals (Vallota *et al.*, 1974), termed initiating factor (Schreiber *et al.*, 1976). However, the subsequent findings that C3 NeF crosses the placenta (Davis *et al.*, 1977), exhibits antigenic determinants of immunoglobulins (Amos *et al.*, 1976), and when highly purified has the chain structure of an immunoglobulin (Daha *et al.*, 1978), indicate that it may be an autoantibody or immunoconglutinin to the amplification convertase, C3bBb.

2.3 Effector Complement Sequence

The effector sequence consists of C3 and five plasma proteins (C5, C6, C7, C8, and C9), forming a multimolecular complex which is the complement membrane attack unit. Convertases of both the classical and alternative pathways are capable of cleaving C3 and C5 to initiate formation of the C5–C9 complex.

2.3.1 C5

Like C3, C5 is a β-globulin of 206 000 molecular weight consisting of an α chain of 141 000 and a β chain of 83 000 molecular weight joined by disulphide bridges (Nilsson *et al.*, 1975). The structural changes that occur during the activation of C5 also are similar to those seen with C3; a peptide (C5a) of 11 000 molecular weight is cleaved from the α chain, yielding a residual major fragment (C5b). It has been suggested that C5b, like C3b and C4b, may be susceptible to further degradation by C3b INA (Kolb and Müller-Eberhard, 1975*a*), implying that C3, C4, and C5 may have several homologous peptide sequences.

One case of deficiency of C5 has been described in an individual with systemic lupus erythematosus and recurrent pyogenic infections (Rosenfeld *et al.*, 1974). The pedigree is consistent with autosomal recessive inheritance, heterozygotes having C5 haemolytic serum levels of 34–65 per cent of the normal mean.

2.3.2 C6

C6, a β-globulin (molecular weight 95 000), consists of a single polypeptide chain which does not appear to undergo cleavage during its participation in the complement sequence (Kolb and Müller-Eberhard, 1975*a*). Genetically determined microheterogeneity of C6 has been demonstrated by isoelectric focusing of plasma (Hobart *et al.*, 1975). A single instance of functional and immunochemical C6 deficiency has been described by Leddy and associates

(1974) in a woman with gonococcaemia and a previous history of good health. Five of six siblings and both parents had half-normal serum levels of haemolytically active C6. Coagulation studies of the homozygous deficient patient and her plasma were normal, in contrast to the prolonged clotting time observed in C6-deficient rabbits (Zimmerman and Müller-Eberhard, 1971; Heusinkveld et al., 1974). This disparity is probably due to the presence and absence of C3b receptors on rabbit and human platelets, respectively.

2.3.3 C7

C7 is a 120 000 molecular weight β-globulin which, like C6, has a single polypeptide chain which apparently remains intact during the complement reactions (Kolb and Müller-Eberhard, 1975a). Two families with C7 deficiency have been reported, with heterozygotes in both kindreds having approximately half-normal levels of haemolytically active C7 consistent with an autosomal recessive mode of inheritance (Nellek and Opferkuch, 1975; Boyer et al., 1976). The probands differed in that one persistently had no detectable C7 and the other had levels fluctuating between 0·4 and 3 per cent.

2.3.4 C8

This component (C8) is a γ-globulin (molecular weight 163 000) which has been found recently to consist of at least three chains: an α chain of 83 000; a β chain of 70 000; and a small γ chain of about 10 000 molecular weight (Müller-Eberhard, 1975). The α and β chains appear to be linked non-covalently while the γ chain is thought to be bound covalently to the α chain. No studies of genetic heterogeneity have been performed with C8, and one case of C8 deficiency has been described by Peterson et al. (1975) in an otherwise healthy individual with a prolonged episode of gonococcaemia.

2.3.5 C9

C9 is an α-globulin with a molecular weight of 79 000 comprising a single polypeptide chain (Kolb and Müller-Eberhard, 1975a). Examples of C9 deficiency have not been described and studies of biosynthesis or genetic variation are not available.

2.4 Control Proteins

Three plasma proteins, which have been well characterized, limit the extent of complement activation: the $C\overline{1}$ inhibitor ($C\overline{1}$ INH) (Pensky et al., 1961) which limits assembly of the classical C3 convertase by the inhibition of $C\overline{1}$; the C3b inactivator (C3b INA) (Tamura and Nelson, 1967) which limits function of classical and alternative C5 convertases and formation of the alternative C3 convertase; and β1H, which dissociates the alternative C3 convertase by displacing Bb from C3b. An additional type of control is represented by the anaphylatoxin inactivator (Bokisch and Müller-Eberhard, 1970) which inactivates the biologically active cleavage fragments, C3a and C5a, but which does not restrict activation of complement.

2.4.1 C$\bar{1}$ Inhibitor

This inhibitor (C$\bar{1}$ INH), which consists of a single polypeptide chain, is an α-globulin with a molecular weight of 105 000 and a high carbohydrate content (35 per cent) (Harpel et al., 1975). Inherited deficiency of C$\bar{1}$ INH is associated with hereditary angioedema (Donaldson and Evans, 1963), the most common disease resulting from a complement abnormality. Affected individuals in 42 kindreds had a mean serum concentration of 17·5 per cent (range 5–31 per cent) of that of normal (Rosen et al., 1971). Transmission of the deficiency occurs by autosomal dominant inheritance. Metabolic studies with radiolabelled purified C$\bar{1}$ INH indicate normal catabolic rates and impaired synthesis in deficient patients (Rosen et al., 1971; Brackertz et al., 1975). Immunofluorescent studies using antibody directed against C$\bar{1}$ INH show no fluorescent cells in liver biopsy specimens obtained from patients, as compared to specific fluorescence (Johnson et al., 1971) in 5–10 per cent of the hepatocytes of normal individuals, thereby confirming impaired synthesis.

The genetic variant form of hereditary angioedema, also inherited as an autosomal dominant trait, is associated with normal or elevated serum levels of a protein antigenically indistinguishable from normal C$\bar{1}$ INH, but which is incapable of inhibiting cleavage of C4 by C$\bar{1}$s (Johnson et al., 1971; Rosen et al., 1971). The variant inhibitor of a given kindred exhibits genetically determined variations in electrophoretic mobility, capacity to bind the C$\bar{1}$s, and ability to inhibit C$\bar{1}$s-induced esterolysis (Rosen et al., 1971). Chemical studies of a single variant C$\bar{1}$ INH protein indicate a molecular weight 3 per cent greater than that of normal C$\bar{1}$ INH and a small difference in the amino acid composition with respect to phenylalanine and acidic amino acids (Harpel et al., 1975). In none of the affected individuals in eight kindreds with the genetic variant form of hereditary angioedema was any normal C$\bar{1}$ INH functionally detected (Rosen et al., 1971). The capacity to synthesize normal C$\bar{1}$ INH exists in these patients, however, as demonstrated by their response to androgens (Gelfand et al., 1976; Rosse et al., 1976; Sheffer et al., 1977).

2.4.2 C3b Inactivator

The inactivator C3b INA, a β-globulin with a molecular weight of 100 000, inactivates C3b and leads to the fragments, C3c and C3d (Ruddy and Austen, 1971a), and probably C4b to C4c and C4d (Cooper, 1975). C3b INA is identical to the conglutinogen activating factor which renders cell-bound C3b reactive with bovine conglutinogen (Lachmann and Müller-Eberhard, 1968). Treatment of C3b INA with various inhibitors of proteases, such as diisopropylphosphofluoridate and soya bean trypsin inhibitor, does not alter its activity. However, function is abolished by treatment with metaperiodate, suggesting that carbohydrate residues may be required for the expression of its activity (Lachmann and Müller-Eberhard, 1968).

A patient with Klinefelter's syndrome, repeated pyogenic infections, and low serum levels of C3 and B has been shown by Alper *et al.* (1972*c*) to lack C3b INA. Family members had half-normal serum levels, consistent with an autosomal recessive mode of inheritance. Examination of the mechanisms responsible for hypercatabolism of C3 and B in this patient has permitted the identification of the C3b INA as a major control protein of the alternative complement pathway.

2.4.3 β1H

β1H is a β globulin with a molecular weight of 150 000; it consists of a single polypeptide chain (Whaley and Ruddy, 1976). β1H regulates the alternative pathway amplification reaction by increasing the rate of C3b inactivation by C3b INA (Whaley and Ruddy, 1976) and by dissociating Bb from the complex, C3b Bb, thereby abolishing activity of the amplification C3 convertase and exposing C3b to the irreversible action of C3b INA (Weiler *et al.*, 1976). The essential contribution of β1H-mediated decay-dissociation of C3b Bb to regulation of the alternative complement pathway is exemplified by the amplified C3 cleavage that occurs when this control function is circumvented by C3 NeF (Weiler *et al.*, 1976).

3 REACTION MECHANISMS

3.1 Classical Pathway of Complement Activation

The reactions leading to formation of the classical C3 convertase are summarized in Figure 2. Initiation of this pathway follows binding of the C1q subcomponent (Müller-Eberhard and Kunkel, 1961) to antigen–antibody complexes or non-specifically aggregated immunoglobulin containing IgM or IgG1–IgG3. Binding and activation of C1 has been described also with C-reactive protein complexed to type C polysaccharide of *Pneumococci* (Volanakis and Kaplan, 1974) and other polycation–polyanion complexes (Rent *et al.*, 1975). Activation of C1 requires the Ca^{2+}-dependent intact C1 complex and the interaction of at least two C1q-binding sites with immunoglobulin (Müller-Eberhard and Calcott, 1966); the reaction is time and temperature dependent. It has been suggested that bound C1q induces a steric change in the proenzyme (C1r) which permits autocatalytical self-activation. C̄1r converts to C1s to C̄1s by cleavage of a single peptide bond present within an intra-chain disulphide bond region, explaining why no cleavage fragment is released (Sakal and Stroud, 1973; Valet and Cooper, 1974*b*). Although the reaction is enzymic, the presence of Ca^{2+} results in a firm binding of C̄1r and C1s so that approximately equimolar amounts of C̄1r are required for complete activation of C1s (Valet and Cooper, 1974*b*). It has been suggested by Assimeh and Painter (1975*a*,*b*) that C1t serves as a bridge

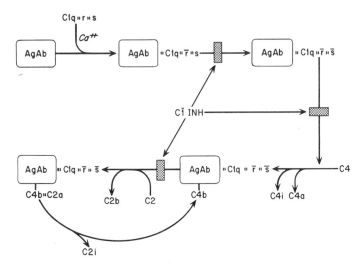

Figure 2 Classical pathway of complement activation and its initiation by an antigen–antibody complex (AgAb). Reactions subject to inhibition by C̄1 INH are shown

between C1q and C1s, and enhances activation of C1s by C̄1r. Once C̄1s is generated, an intact C̄1 complex is no longer required for assembly of the classical pathway C3 convertase since free C̄1s can cleave C4 and C2. However, the continued integrity of C1 directs the complement reaction to the initiating antigen–antibody complex to which the C1q subcomponent is bound.

C̄1s cleaves the low molecular weight C4a peptide from C4, thereby generating C4b which continues the complement reaction sequence (Patrick and Lepow, 1969; Schreiber and Müller-Eberhard, 1974). C4b serves five functions: (*i*) irreversible binding to immune complexes and cell membranes *via* a nascent site that otherwise undergoes rapid decay to fluid phase C4i, which is not capable of binding; (*ii*) binding to immune adherence receptors present on a variety of cells *via* a stable binding site on C4b (Cooper, 1969); (*iii*) interaction with C̄1 to allow more efficient cleavage of C2 (Gigli and Austen, 1969); (*iv*) binding to activated C2 to form C4b2a, the classical pathway C3 convertase (Müller-Eberhard *et al.*, 1967); and, (*v*) in the state of C4b2a, interaction with C3b to form C4b2a3b, which is the classical pathway C5 convertase. The hydrophobic binding site of C4b apparently resides in the α chain since the C4d fragment remains cell bound after C3b INA-induced cleavage of C4c from a cellular intermediate bearing C4b (Cooper, 1975). Fluid-phase C4i retains all the capacities of C4b except the binding to membranes by the nascent site, and these functions of C4i and C4b are lost after cleavage into C4c and C4d. Several proposals have been advanced for the effect of C4b/C4i on C2 cleavage by C̄1. These include an allosteric modification of the active site of C̄1, fully uncovering the specificity for C2 (Gigli and Austen, 1969), an allosteric modification of the substrate C2, exposing the site vulnerable to proteolytic attack by C̄1s, and the provision of a site for deposition of product (C2a) to allow interaction of C̄1s with additional substrate (C2) (Strunk and Colten, 1974).

Cleavage of C2 in the absence of C4b does not result in the appearance of C3-cleaving activity, presumably because the active site on C2a for C3 is not expressed without Mg^{2+}-dependent binding to C4b/C4i (Müller-Eberhard *et al.*, 1967; Polley and Müller-Eberhard, 1968). Thus, C2 has two interdependent sites uncovered by the action of $C\overline{1}s$: (*i*) an enzymic site on the C2a fragment for sequential cleavage of C3 and C5 and (*ii*), a binding site on the smaller C2b fragment (Nagasawa and Stroud, 1977) for C4b. C4b2ab undergoes temperature-dependent decay with a half life at 37° of five to 10 minutes due to release of the bound C2a fragment—designated C2i because it lacks the C2b binding site required for convertase function (Mayer, 1965). The residual C4b is capable of reforming new C4b2ab convertase upon cleavage of additional C2 by $C\overline{1}s$, indicating that decay of the convertase is secondary to loss of C2a and that native C2 displaces any residual C2b on the C4b site (Borsos *et al.*, 1961). Since C4b2ab may activate the effector sequence of complement, C3–C9, its formation completes the classical pathway of complement activation.

3.2 Alternative Pathway of Complement: Amplification Function and Activation

3.2.1 Cobra Venom Factor

Studies with cobra venom factor (CoVF), which forms a C3 convertase during incubation with serum (Nelson, 1966), have led to the initial recognition of $\overline{D}$ (Hunsicker *et al.*, 1973) and to the role of B (Götze and Müller-Eberhard, 1971) in forming alternative C3 convertases. CoVF and B form a Mg^{2+}-dependent

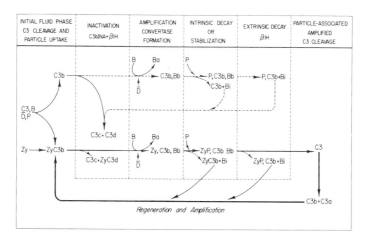

Figure 3 The alternative pathway of complement. Initial cleavage of C3 occurs slowly by the low grade interaction in the fluid phase of C3, B, $\overline{D}$, and P, which is normally prevented from advancing to C3b-dependent amplified C3 cleavage by the regulatory proteins, C3b INA and β1H. Binding of C3b to an activator, such as zymosan (Zy), results in amplified C3 cleavage with additional C3b deposition by surface-dependent circumvention of those regulatory proteins

reversible complex, CoVF–B, which has slight C3-cleaving activity (Cooper, 1973). The action of $\bar{D}$ on CoVF–B results in conversion of B into a minor fragment (Ba) and a major fragment (Bb). The latter remains firmly bound to CoVF forming CoVFBb, a Mg^{2+}-independent bimolecular complex with greatly increased C3-cleaving activity (Cooper, 1973; Hunsicker et al., 1973). CoVFBb undergoes decay with a half life of six hours at 37° by release of the Bb fragment, which is inactive and designated Bi. The residual CoVF is capable of reforming new CoVFBb complex upon incubation with additional B in the presence of $\bar{D}$ and Mg^{2+} (Fearon et al., 1973a). Thus, the active site on B for C3 cleavage is made partially available through reversible complexing with CoVF, while cleavage of B by $\bar{D}$ fully reveals this site. Like C2a, the integrity of the active site on Bb requires continued binding to an acceptor protein, C4b and CoVF, respectively, since dissociation results in irreversible loss of function. $\bar{D}$ and $C\bar{1}s$ are functionally analogous not only with respect to a serine esterase active site, but also in cleavage of B and C2, respectively, in the presence of their receptor proteins to reveal fully C3-cleaving potentials.

3.2.2 Alternative Pathway Amplification Convertases

The functional human counterpart of CoVF was shown to be C3b. The fluid-phase interaction of C3b, B, and $\bar{D}$ results in the cleavage of B to Bb and Ba and in the generation of C3 convertase (Figure 3) activity (Müller-Eberhard and Götze, 1972). This interaction may amplify cleavage of C3 that results initially from the action of any convertase, including classical C4b2ab that generates C3b. Thus this convertase (C3bBb), is termed the alternative pathway amplification convertase. The functional characteristics of this convertase were difficult to appreciate in the fluid phase and thus a suitable haemolytic intermediate was developed bearing C3b but lacking C2a. Interaction of EAC4b3b with B and $\bar{D}$ forms an intermediate, EAC4b3bBb, which is capable of activating C3–C9 so as to undergo lysis (Fearon et al., 1973b). These studies indicated for the first time that the composition of this alternative C3 convertase is probably C3bBb, a bimolecular complex analogous to CoVFBb and C4b2a. The number of convertase sites formed on the erythrocyte intermediate is related stoichiometrically to the input of B and to the cell-bound C3b. Decay of the labile convertase site is first order, with a half life of four minutes at 30°, and secondary to loss of Bb activity (Fearon et al., 1973b). Direct demonstration of the contribution of C3b and Bb to convertase function awaited a method for the stabilization of C3bBb in the fluid phase as described below.

3.2.3 Stabilization of Alternative Pathway Amplification Convertase by Properdin and C3 Nephritic Factor

$\bar{P}$ (Götze and Müller-Eberhard, 1974) and C3 NeF (Spitzer et al., 1969; Vallota et al., 1974), when added to serum, induce cleavage of C3 which is mediated by alternative pathway factors. The mechanisms by which this is accomplished were not known until these proteins were examined for their effects on amplification convertases and on the generation of initial convertases of the alternative pathway. $\overline{P}$ was found to bind on EAC4b3b in a temperature and cation-independent reaction, but not to EAC4b, indicating a specificity for C3b (Fearon and Austen, 1975*b*). Furthermore, binding of $\overline{P}$ to EAC4b3bBb results in a dose-related prolongation of the first-order decay of the convertase site, extending its half life of four minutes at 30° by as much as ten-fold. Although erythrocyte-bound $\overline{P}$ is resistant to washing, $\overline{P}$ is not irreversibly utilized at that site as demonstrated by transfer from EAC4b3b$\overline{P}$ to EAC4b3bBb with the consequent stabilization of the recipient convertase site (Fearon and Austen, 1975*b*). Thus, $\overline{P}$ enhances cleavage of C3 in the amplification portion of the alternative pathway by binding to C3b and stabilizing Bb whether $\overline{P}$ is present initially or taken up subsequently at that site by local generation or transfer. P has a similar functional effect but binds less firmly to C3b (Götze *et al.*, 1977).

Parallel experiments with C3 NeF have disclosed that it also retards decay of erythrocyte-bound C3bBb (Daha *et al.*, 1976*b*). Removal of fluid-phase C3 NeF after stabilization of the convertase site on EAC4b3bBb does not alter the previously retarded decay rate, so that C3 NeF either binds to the convertase site or alters a protein at that site. The capacity of C3 NeF to stabilize C3bBb in the fluid phase as well as on a cellular intermediate has led to the confirmation of the bimolecular state of the amplification convertase postulated initially to be present on EAC4b3bBb (Fearon *et al.*, 1973*b*; Daha *et al.*, 1976*b*). Interaction of C3 and B with $\overline{D}$ in the presence of C3 NeF followed by sucrose-density ultracentrifugation yields a complex with a sedimentation rate of 10 S which contains C3b and Bb and possesses C3-cleaving activity (Daha *et al.*, 1976*b*). In the absence of C3 NeF during the initial interaction, no convertase activity or complex has been found in sucrose-density fractions, despite the formation of a convertase in the initial reaction as indicated by inactivation of C3. It is noteworthy that the classical convertase C4b2ab, also was not isolated as a fluid-phase complex until a mechanism for stabilization of C2a was found by Polley and Müller-Eberhard (1967), namely the oxidation of C2. Studies with purified and radiolabelled C3 NeF have revealed that the stabilized convertase isolated as a complex on sucrose density gradients contains equimolar concentrations of C3b,Bb, C3 NeF (Daha *et al.*, 1977).

3.2.4 Formation of Amplification Convertases with Uncleaved B

Incubation of EAC4b3b with B in the absence of $\overline{D}$ results in the formation of an intermediate, EAC4b3bB, which is capable of activating C3–C9 with resultant haemolysis (Fearon and Austen, 1975). The C3-cleaving site is revealed without cleavage of B, presumably by a reversible conformation change in B induced by binding to C3b. This conformational change is of limited efficiency since addition of $\overline{D}$ to preformed and washed EAC4b3bB greatly increases convertase activity by cleaving B to reveal fully the enzymic site for C3 (Fearon and Austen, 1975). Binding of B to EAC4b3b is reversible so that functionally intact B can be recovered from EAC4b3bB by chelating Mg^{2+} with ethylene diamine tetra-acetate. Thus Mg^{2+} is essential for continued binding of B to C3b, whereas the cation is not required for binding of Bb after $\bar{D}$-dependent cleavage. Addition of either $\bar{P}$ or C3 NeF to EAC4b3bB decreases the rate at which B dissociates, resulting in stabilization of the convertase site. Indeed, the capacity of C3 NeF to stabilize fluid-phase C3bB has permitted the isolation by sucrose-density ultracentrifugation of a 10 S complex with C3-cleaving activity and containing C3b and uncleaved B, thereby directly demonstrating the composition of this convertase (Daha et al., 1976a).

3.2.5 Initial Cleavage of C3 by the Alternative Complement Pathway

As is depicted in Figure 3, formation of C3bBb or C3bB requires the presence of C3b, indicating that an additional C3 convertase must be formed during initial activation of the alternative pathway. Although the classical pathway may contribute to initial generation of C3b, an alternative mechanism independent of C4b2ab must exist since either zymosan or inulin is capable of inducing cleavage of C3 in serum of C2-deficient humans or C4-deficient guinea-pigs. Indeed, cleavage of C3 has been demonstrated to occur by interaction of C3 with B and $\bar{D}$ (Fearon and Austen, 1975d). Since the conclusion that C3 is capable of forming a convertase with B and $\bar{D}$ is contingent on excluding the presence of C3b during the initial reaction, the C3 used in these studies was shown to be devoid of C3b using immunoelectrophoresis, alkaline disc gel electrophoresis—with or without radiolabeled C3—and isoelectric focusing. In addition, preincubation of C3 with C3b INA does not diminish the former's subsequent capacity to permit the cleavage of B by $\bar{D}$, while C3b similarly treated loses 90 per cent of this activity. The composition of this initial convertase is not known but it may be a bimolecular complex between native C3 and B, which in the presence of $\bar{D}$ becomes C3Bb, analogous to, but less active than, the amplification convertase (C3bBb). Analysis of the dose-response characteristics and the kinetics of the interreaction of C3, B, and $\bar{D}$ indicate that the initial generation of C3b or exogenous addition of C3b markedly accelerates the reaction.

That $\bar{P}$ has a role in initiating the alternative pathway was suggested by the capacity of $\bar{P}$ to effect cleavage of C3 and B in the presence of $\bar{D}$ (Götze and Müller-Eberhard, 1974). However, these findings do not distinguish between a contribution by $\bar{P}$ to the generation of an initial convertase or to the stabilization of C3bBb generated after C3b is made available by interaction of C3, B, and $\bar{D}$. An initiating role for $\bar{P}$ was suggested by the finding of Fearon and Austen (1975c) that B and $\bar{D}$ may be so limited that detectable cleavage of C3 does not occur, except in the presence of $\bar{P}$. Furthermore, interaction of larger amounts of $\bar{P}$ and B with C3, in the absence of $\bar{D}$, leads to C3 cleavage without the breakdown of B, establishing a role for $\bar{P}$ in the formation of an initial convertase of the alternative pathway, presumably $\bar{P}C3B$ (Fearon and Austen, 1975c). Substitution of P or C3 NeF for $\bar{P}$ in the interaction of C3 and B, in the absence of $\bar{D}$ (Daha et al., 1976b) also results in C3 cleavage without cleavage or inactivation of

B. Even when the initiating C3 convertase containing native C3 and B progresses to the stage at which cleaved C3 is present, there is limited efficiency until $\overline{\text{D}}$ fully uncovers the convertase site on B. Initiation by $\overline{\text{D}}$, without P or C3 NeF, again yields a relatively inefficient convertase, which presumably contains native C3 and Bb, while progression to formation of a convertase with cleaved C3 yields an efficient, but highly labile, complex. The presence of $\overline{\text{D}}$ with either stabilizing factor greatly augments initial breakdown of C3 with $\overline{\text{D}}$ fully revealing the active site on B, and P or C3 NeF preventing decay of the complex.

3.2.6 Recognition Events in the Alternative Complement Pathway

A disparate group of substances is capable of activating the alternative complement pathway. These include complex microbial polysaccharides such as zymosan (Pillemer et al., 1954), endotoxin (Marcus et al., 1971), sulphated dextrans (Burger et al., 1975), rabbit erythrocytes (Platts-Mills and Ishizaka, 1974), and stroma of human erythrocytes (Poskitt et al., 1973). A characteristic common to three of these activating materials, zymosan, rabbit erythrocytes, and *E. coli*, is that their surfaces protect bound C3b from C3b INA and C3bBb from decay-dissociation by $\beta 1H$ (Fearon and Austen, 1977a, 1977b; Fearon, 1978). Thus, low grade fluid phase interaction of C3, B, $\overline{\text{D}}$, and P is held in check by C3b INA and $\beta 1H$ but provides C3b for initial deposition on activating surfaces, with subsequent amplification of C3b deposition because of circumvention of regulation of C3b and C3bBb on such surfaces.

Activation of the alternative pathway has been found also with certain immunoglobulin classes. Aggregates of $F(ab)_2$ fragments of guinea-pig IgG1 antibodies induce cleavage of C3 in guinea-pig serum without any apparent utilization of C1, C4, or C2 in a Mg^{2+}-dependent Ca^{2+}-independent reaction (Sandberg and Osler, 1971). Aggregated human IgA myeloma induces activations of the alternative pathway in human serum (Götze and Müller-Eberhard, 1971; Boackle et al., 1974), and a patient with an IgA-containing cryoglobulin was found to have depressed serum levels of C3, P, and B, but concentrations of C1, C4, and C2 were normals—results that are consistent with activation of the alternative complement pathway by the cryoglobulin (Soter et al., 1974). An additional antibody-dependent mechanism for activation of the alternative complement pathway has been described by May and Frank (1973a, b), which requires the intact C1 molecular complex.

3.3 Effector Complement Sequence

The classical and alternative C3 convertases cleave the C3a peptide from the N-terminus of the α-chain of C3 to generate C3b. C3b has four functions: (*i*) interaction with C4b2ab (Nilsson and Müller-Eberhard, 1967; Cooper and Müller-Eberhard, 1970), C3bBb (Fearon et al., 1973b), and C3bB to reveal their enzymic specificities for C5 (Daha et al., 1976c); (*ii*) initiation of the alternative pathway amplification reaction; (*iii*) binding to immune adherence receptors present on a variety of cells (Cooper, 1969); and (*iv*) irreversible binding to cell membranes *via* a nascent site which is extremely labile in an aqueous medium and only briefly available after cleavage of C3. As in C4, this nascent binding site resides in the C3d fragment since this portion of the α chain remains cell-bound after the C3b INA-induced cleavage of C3b (Ruddy and Austen, 1971*a*). The capacities to function in the alternative pathway, to reveal the C5 specificities of the C3 convertases, and to bind to immune adherence receptors are lost when C3b is broken down into C3c and C3d (Figure 4).

Cleavage of C5 by the C3b-modified C3 convertases releases the C5a fragment from the α chain and generates C5b. C5b may bind directly to membranes bearing the convertase, complex with C6 in the fluid phase to form C5b6, or remain in the fluid phase as C5i due to irreversible decay of the membrane binding site. Also membrane-bound C5b is labile, being subject to decay as C5i unless it complexes with C6 (Nilsson and Müller-Eberhard, 1967). The membrane binding site on fluid-phase C5b6 is not available until complexed with C7 to form C5b67 which is capable of transiently binding to unsensitized membranes, a mechanism known as reactive lysis, which extends the cytolytic effects of complement to 'innocent bystander' cells (Thompson and Lachmann, 1970; Goldman *et al.*, 1972). If C5b67 does not encounter an appropriate membrane, the binding site of C5b decays and the complex becomes C5i67, a cytolytically inactive, chemotactically active unit (Ward, 1972).

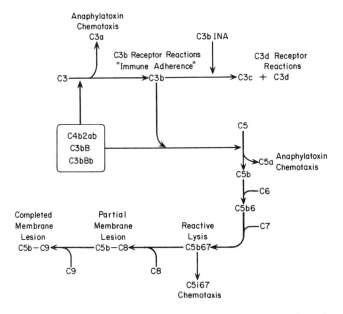

Figure 4 Effector pathway of complement which is activated by the classical or amplifying C3 convertases. Presumably, an initiating convertase of the alternative pathway may also activate C3–C9, but this has not been shown

Formation of membrane-bound C5b67 permits binding of C8 to the C5b fragment (Müller-Eberhard, 1975) to create a partial membrane lesion, resulting in slow lysis (Stolfi, 1968). Although C8 possesses as many as six binding sites for C9 (Kolb and Müller-Eberhard, 1973), formation of a complex using only one C9 accelerates the lytic reaction (Ruddy et al., 1971). These final steps in the complement sequence do not involve cleavage of C6–C9, but represent noncovalent assembly of the C5–C9 multimolecular complex, which reveals a neoantigen not present on the individual components (Kolb and Müller-Eberhard, 1975b). An additional serum protein, distinct from known complement components, has been found in C5–C9 complexes formed in the fluid phase. The function of this additional protein (Kolb and Müller-Eberhard, 1975a) is now believed to be regulatory (Kolb and Müller-Eberhard, 1977).

3.4 Control of the Complement Reaction

Two general mechanisms limit the extent of complement activation. The first is inherent and is represented by the rapid decay rates of C4b2ab, C3bBb, and C3bB, which restrict activation of C3–C9, and by the labile membrane binding sites of C4b, C3b, and C5b which limit cytolytic potential. The second type is extrinsic and exemplified by $C\bar{1}$ INH, C3b INA, and $\beta1H$.

$C\bar{1}$ INH controls assembly of C4b2ab by binding to the light chain of $C\bar{1}s$ which bears the serine esteric site, thereby irreversibly inhibiting its capacity to cleave C4 and C2 (Harpel and Cooper, 1975). Since complex formation between $C\bar{1}$ INH and $C\bar{1}s$ is firm, the inhibitor is removed by its reaction with the enzyme (Gigli et al., 1968). Although proteolytic degradation of some inhibitors occurs during interaction with their plasma enzymes, no breakdown of $C\bar{1}$ INH has been noted following inhibition of $C\bar{1}s$ (Harpel and Cooper, 1975). $C\bar{1}$ INH also blocks the esterolytic activity of $C\bar{1}r$ (Naff and Ratnoff, 1968). C3b INA serves as a major control protein of the alternative pathway amplification convertase by converting C3b into the inactive C3c and C3d fragments (Ruddy and Austen, 1971a). Haemolytic inactivation of C3b precedes fragmentation (Ruddy and Austen, 1972) and the latter may be facilitated by the presence of non-complement proteases (Gitlin et al., 1975). Genetic deficiency of C3b INA is associated with hypercatabolism of B and C3 (Alper et al., 1972c), presumably secondary to uncontrolled generation of C3bBb. Indeed, removal of C3b INA from serum facilitates Mg^{2+}-dependent breakdown of C3 and B without a requirement for the other usual activators of the alternative pathway (Nicol and Lachmann, 1973). Since intact C3b is necessary for immune adherence reactions and the modification of C3 convertases to C5 convertases, C3b INA also functions by controlling these reactions. As noted above (see Section 2.4.2), C4b is probably susceptible to cleavage by C3b INA, and the fragments C4c and C4d formed are incapable of participating in the formation of the classical convertase and in immune adherence reactions.

$\beta1H$ mediates extrinsic decay-dissociation of C3bBb even after stabilization by P (Weiler et al., 1976) and accelerates C3b inactivation by C3b INA (Whaley and

Ruddy, 1976). Thus, control of the amplification phase of the alternative pathway occurs at three levels: intrinsic decay of the labile C3bBb convertase, extrinsic decay by displacement of Bb from the convertase with β1H, and inactivation of C3b by C3b INA after removal of protective Bb by intrinsic or extrinsic decay.

4 BIOLOGICAL ACTIVITIES RESULTING FROM THE COMPLEMENT REACTION

The biological activities generated during activation of the complement pathways are derived primarily from C3 and the terminal sequence, C5–C9. Such activities may alter the target complex as occurs with cytolysis, may change the local microenvironment by increasing vascular permeability and attracting leucocytes, and also may have systemic effects. Although some activities are interdependent and derived at the same step, such as enhancement of phagocytosis and chemotactic stimulation of phagocytes, it is useful to classify the biological products of complement by their primary site of action.

4.1 Alteration of the Target Complex

4.1.1 Immune Adherence

The immune adherence reaction occurs between C3b-coated complexes and certain cells which bear specialized membrane-associated receptors (IA receptors) for C3b (Nelson, 1953). Human cells possessing the IA receptor comprise erythrocytes, polymorphonuclear leucocytes (neutrophilic and eosinophilic), macrophages and monocytes, and B lymphocytes. Although immune adherence to human erythrocytes by sheep erythrocytes heavily sensitized with C4b does occur (Cooper, 1969), adherence by C3b-coated particles is many times more sensitive. The presence or absence of other complement components does not influence adherence; C3b passively absorbed to tanned erythrocytes supports the reaction (Okada *et al.*, 1970). Immune adherence in man does not require divalent cations or energy metabolism but is temperature dependent, presumably because of aggregation of IA receptors is inhibited by the relative rigidity of the membrane at reduced temperatures. Treatment of cell-bound C3b with C3b INA abolishes the adherence to human erythrocytes (Tamura and Nelson, 1967), indicating the presence on this cell type only of receptors for intact C3b. However, human B lymphocytes (Ross *et al.*, 1973), peripheral blood monocytes (Ehlenberger and Nussenzweig, 1975), and lung macrophages (Reynolds *et al.*, 1975) bear additional receptors for C3d, the residual fragment of C3b remaining bound after cleavage by C3b INA. The IA receptor has not been characterized extensively. It has been shown, however, to be (Huber *et al.*, 1968) trypsin-sensitive and to contain sulphhydryl bonds which contribute to the integrity of the site (Dierich *et al.*, 1974). The biological consequences of immune adherence depend upon the cell type, and binding to the membrane IA receptor acts as a signal for which the cell response has been programmed. Translation of the membrane signals to cellular events such as phagocytosis, secretion, synthesis, or differentiation is appreciated already for polymorphonuclear leucocytes, platelets, and B lymphocytes, respectively.

Although complexes sensitized with IgG are subject to phagocytosis following binding to the membrane receptors for the Fc fragment of IgG, prior interaction of the immune complex with complement greatly increases the rate and extent of phagocytosis (Gigli and Nelson, 1968). The components required for enhanced phagocytosis are precisely those needed for immune adherence. Enhanced phagocytosis occurs only when C3b is present on the immune complex, and treatment of the bound C3b with C3b INA impairs phagocytosis. The two events can be dissociated, however, since only phagocytosis of immune complexes by polymorphonuclear leucocytes, monocytes, and macrophages is depressed by metabolic inhibitors, organophosphorus compounds, or chelation of divalent cations, while immune adherence is unaffected (Nelson, 1965; Pearlman et al., 1969). With regard to enhancement of phagocytosis, immune adherence may serve to effect a bond between the hydrophobic cell membrane and the hydrophilic immune complex, to act as a signal at the membrane to help to trigger the phagocytic process or, more likely, as a combination of the two. The importance of this activity of C3b in host defence is exemplified by patients with genetic or acquired deficiency of C3 who experience repeated bacterial infections. In the case of genetic deficiency, restoration of the C3 content with purified C3 results in correction of in vitro opsonic defects (Alper et al., 1972c).

Although such reactions generally benefit the host, immune adherence to phagocytes may be detrimental under certain circumstances. Neutrophils presented with particles not capable of being engulfed by phagocytosis and bearing C3b, such as C3b-coated millipore filters, release their lysosomal enzymes extracellularly, thus indicating that adherence may trigger secretion in addition to phagocytosis (Henson, 1972). A similar process may occur in diseases, typified by experimental nephrotoxic nephritis, in which neutrophils become adherent to basement membranes coated with antibody and complement components, including C3b, and contribute to inflammatory damage by enzyme secretion.

The adherence of C3b-coated particles to lymphocytes has been reviewed in detail by Nussenzweig (1974). Lymphocytes derived from the bone marrow (B lymphocytes) have membrane-associated receptors for C3 and its cleavage products, while lymphocytes processed by the thymus (T lymphocytes) do not. The receptors for C3–C3b and C3d are trypsin-sensitive as distinct from those for aggregated IgG. It appears that native C3 and C3b share a common receptor, whereas binding via C3d occurs through a separate receptor. Indeed, lymphocytes from some patients with chronic lymphatic leukaemia, a neoplasm of B lymphocytes, may bind immune complexes bearing C3d rather than C3b (Ross et al., 1973).

The functional implications of the interaction of the C3 receptors of B lymphocytes with immune complexes are being examined currently and several observations are available. The production of antibody to thymus-dependent antigens in mice is delayed by prior depletion of C3 using CoVF treatment (Pepys, 1974). Recent *in vivo* studies in the mouse indicate that complement, i.e., C3 is essential to the development of primary B memory cells but is not critical to the maintenance of established memory cells (Klaus and Humphrey, 1977). On the other hand, immune complexes bound to lymphocytes *via* their receptors for C3b are released by interaction with alternative pathway factors, suggesting that complement also may have a dampening effect on lymphocyte stimulation (Nussenzweig, 1974).

Although IA receptors on platelets occur only in non-primates and this review is concerned primarily with human complement reactions, studies using rabbit platelets have provided evidence of the ability of immune adherence to act as a membrane signal for secretion, and thus are of relevance to this discussion. Adherence of rabbit platelets to C3b-coated erythrocytes or zymosan particles results in non-cytolytic secretion of histamine, serotonin, and nucleotides (Henson and Cochrane, 1971). For secretion to occur, Ca^{2+}, energy metabolism, and activation of a platelet-associated serine esterase are essential. The multifaceted potential of the IA receptor thus is derived from the variety of cells bearing the receptor.

4.1.2 Cytolysis

Completion of the complement sequence with formation of the multimolecular complex C5–C9 on a membrane results in impairment of osmotic regulation which may cause cytolysis. Mathematical analysis and examination of the kinetics of complement-induced cytolysis suggest that a single membrane-bound C5–C9 complex is sufficient for lysis (Ruddy *et al.*, 1971). The early acting components of either the classical or alternative activating pathways are not required for the cytolytic lesion; fluid-phase C5b67 has the transient capacity to bind to cells lacking antibody or complement and to prepare them for lysis upon addition of C8 and C9. There appears to be no requirement for membrane-associated protein since liposomes, which are free of protein, are susceptible to the lytic action of the C5–C9 complex (Lachmann *et al.*, 1970).

Electron microscopy of erythrocytes that have been lysed by human complement has revealed characteristic 'doughnut-shaped' lesions on the outer leaflet which have a dark central portion with a diameter of 10–11° nm surrounded by a lighter ring (Humphrey and Dourmaskin, 1970). The dark central area may be a depression in the membrane or a hydrophilic region, while the outer ring may be a relatively raised or hydrophobic region. The lesions demonstrated by electron microscopy are removed by chloroform–methanol extraction but not by treatment with trypsin, suggesting that they are incorporated into the lipid layer of the membrane (Humphrey and Dourmaskin, 1970). However, it has been shown by freeze-etching technique that these ultrastructural changes are confined to the outer leaflet of the membrane with none being demonstrable on the inner leaflet (Iles *et al.*, 1973).

Several mechanisms have been proposed for complement-induced lysis and these fall into two general types: (*i*) production by the late-acting complement components of an enzyme that disrupts the membrane, or (*ii*) insertion of the C5–C9 complex, or a portion of it, into the membrane with the creation of a stable 'hole' through which salt and water can pass (Mayer, 1972). Support for the former hypothesis comes from the demonstration of an association between C7 and tributyrinase activity (Delage *et al.*, 1973). However, the action of complement on synthetic lipid bilayers is not accompanied by appearance of enzymatic degradation products of the lipids used (Inoue and Kinsky, 1970). The 'hole' model visualizes the insertion of a C5–C9 complex into the lipid bilayer with hydrophobic regions outside and an internal hydrophilic core which is not large enough to permit passage of the macromolecular content of cells, but which is sufficiently big to allow net uptake of salt and water by the cell. This would lead to gradual swelling of the cell, resulting in production of larger discontinuities in the membrane with resultant passage of macromolecules. A modified model proposes the insertion of the α and γ chains of C8 leading to the disruption of the membrane (Müller-Eberhard, 1975).

4.2 Alteration of the Microenvironment

Secondary mechanisms for affecting the microenvironment in which the complement reaction is occurring have been mentioned already such as IA-induced secretion of lysosomal enzymes from neutrophils. The complement reaction also generates products which may affect the microenvironment directly by increasing vascular permeability, contracting smooth muscle, and attracting phagocytic cells.

4.2.1 Permeability Factors and Smooth Muscle Contracting Principles

Patients with hereditary (Donaldson and Evans, 1963) or acquired (Caldwell *et al.*, 1972; Rosenfeld *et al.*, 1975; Schreiber *et al.*, 1975) deficiency of C$\bar{1}$ INH experience repeated attacks of localized non-inflammatory oedema of the subcutaneous tissue and mucous membranes. Such attacks may be fatal when they involve the larynx. Sera taken from patients during episodes of angioedema contain C$\bar{1}$ and profoundly depressed levels of its two substrates, C4 (Ruddy *et al.*, 1968) and C2 (Austen and Sheffer, 1965). *In vitro* incubation of sera taken between attacks results in generation of an activity capable of contracting the oestrous rat uterus, while prior treatment of the serum with antiserum to C4 and C2, but not C3, inhibits elaboration of this activity (Donaldson *et al.*, 1970). Characterization of this 'C-kinin' after partial purification from hereditary angioedemic serum showed that it is heat stable, susceptible to inactivation by trypsin, and has an estimated molecular weight of 5000 (O'Connell *et al.*, 1967). It has been suggested that this vasoactive principle is liberated from C2 by the action of C$\bar{1}$s in the presence of C4, and that it is distinct from other known permeability factors (Lepow, 1971). However, the report that intradermal injection of C$\overline{1}$s into an individual with homozygous deficiency of C3 does not result in an increase in vascular permeability (Alper and Rosen, 1974) indicates that the mechanisms for C$\overline{1}$s-induced increases in vascular permeability in normal subjects and the excessive response in patients with hereditary angioedema (Klemperer et al., 1968) awaits further definition.

Anaphylatoxin is the trivial name for the low molecular weight polypeptides C3a and C5a (Dias da Silva and Lepow, 1967; Jensen, 1967), and is derived from the term used by Friedberger (1909) to describe the active principle causing lethal bronchospasm in guinea-pigs following intravenous administration of antigen–antibody complexes. Human C3a and C5a contract isolated guinea-pig ileum at concentrations of 10^{-8} and 10^{-9} M, respectively, and cause degranulation of human skin mast cells with wheal and flare reactions at 10^{-12} and 10^{-15} M, respectively, which are blocked by antihistamines (Cochrane and Müller-Eberhard, 1968; Lepow et al., 1970). C3a and C5a do not exhibit cross-tachyphylaxis on the guinea-pig ileum, indicating that different spasmogenic receptors are involved. Furthermore, smooth muscle contractile activity that is independent of histamine release has been demonstrated. These activities of C3a and C5a are abolished rapidly by anaphylatoxin inactivator which removes the C-terminal arginine from both principles (Bokisch and Müller-Eberhard, 1970). Although unable to release histamine, the des-arginine derivative of C3a binds to mast cells and partially inhibits histamine release by active C3a (Johnson et al., 1975). This mode of receptor blockage may represent an additional control mechanism for limiting the biological activity of anaphylatoxins.

4.2.2 Chemotactic Factors

Three products generated during the complement reaction (C3 fragment, C5a and the haemolytically inactive fluid-phase complex, C5i67) have chemotactic activity for leucocytes in vitro (Ward, 1972). C3 fragment and C5a exhibit little chemotactic specificity, being capable of inducing directed migration of neutrophils, eosinophils, and monocytes, while C5i67 is chemotactic only for neutrophils and eosinophils (Ward, 1972; Goetzl and Austen, 1974). Generation of these chemotactic principles may occur not only by sequential activation of either the classical or alternative pathways, but also by the action of other proteolytic enzymes. Plasmin, trypsin, and a tissue protease found in most normal tissues produce fragments from C3 which possess chemotactic activity, while trypsin and a neutral protease present in lysosomal granules generate active fragments from C5 (Ward, 1972). Exposure of neutrophils to one chemotactic principle renders them unresponsive to the original as well as to others in a reaction termed 'deactivation' (Ward and Becker, 1968). Deactivation prevents further directed migration and may serve to hold the cell at an inflammatory focus so that other functions may be expressed.

In addition to these chemotactic factors representing haemolytically inactive products of complement reactions, CoVFBb has been shown to be chemotactic for neutrophils (Ruddy et al., 1975). The chemotactic activity of CoVFBb parallels its C3-cleaving activity. Furthermore, C3bBb deactivates neutrophils to subsequent chemotactic stimulation by C5a, indicating that this convertase is capable also of stimulating neutrophil chemotactic receptors (Ruddy *et al.*, 1975). Formation of such a convertase on cells fixing C3b by their IA receptors eventually may be shown to expand the functions mediated by that receptor.

Two serum proteins termed chemotactic factor inactivators which are capable of abolishing the chemotactic activities of C3 and C5-derived fragments, have been described by Till and Ward (1975). These inactivators which appear to exist in two chromatographically distinct forms, are not inhibited by metal ion chelators, distinguishing them from the metal-dependent anaphylatoxin inactivator.

4.2.3 Leucocyte Mobilizing Factor

A peptide released from C3 by C4b2a which is not chemotactic but which releases mature polymorphonuclear leucocytes from perfused, isolated bone has been described by Rother (1972). This fragment of C3 may influence accumulation of cells at sites of inflammation by inducing peripheral leucocytosis. Indeed, that this factor acts *in vivo* is suggested by the demonstration of leucocytosis in experimental animals after administration of CoVF which induces rapid cleavage of C3 (McCall *et al.*, 1974) and by the absence of leucocytosis during bacterial infections in a patient genetically lacking C3 (Alper *et al.*, 1972*b*).

5 SUMMARY

The complement system consists of at least 17 plasma proteins whose sequential interaction, which may be initiated by immunoglobulins, microbial products, and tryptic enzymes, results in generation of cleavage peptides and multimolecular complexes capable of recruiting the essential ingredients of an inflammatory response. All known constituent proteins have been isolated in highly purified states and some have been characterized partially with respect to their ultrastructure. Studies of genetically determined polymorphism and deficiencies of individual components have permitted analysis of their linkages to histocompatibility antigens and their homeostatic roles *in vivo*.

With respect to reaction mechanisms, complement consists of four functional portions—two pathways for initiation (the classical and alternative) an amplification pathway which augments activation of C3–C9 by the initiating sequences, and a final common effector pathway to which the initiating and amplifying pathways are directed and from which are derived most of the biological activities of complement. The classical pathway is usually initiated by certain antigen–antibody complexes which bind and activate C1. C$\overline{1}$ cleaves C4 and C2 whose major cleavage fragments form the classical C3 convertase, C4b2a. The alternative pathway is initiated by activating surfaces which protect C3b and C3bBb from the regulatory action of C3b INA and β1H. Such surfaces acquire

C3b by the continuous low grade turnover of fluid phase C3 and B in the presence of $\overline{D}$ and P. The fluid phase reaction does not amplify because it is regulated by C3b INA and β1H, whereas the surface reaction accelerates because the action of the regulatory proteins is impaired. It seems likely, but not proven, that the initial, evanescent fluid phase convertase has the form C3B, followed by C3Bb. In the amplification pathway, C3b, which is generated either by the classical or alternative initiating reactions, forms a reversible bimolecular complex with B, which is further activated when $\overline{D}$ degrades B to generate C3bBb, the amplification C3 convertase. This labile complex is stabilized by the binding of P to C3b, thereby greatly increasing its potential for activation of C3–C9.

C3b serves also to modify the substrate specificities of C4b2a and C3bBb to permit cleavage of C5. C5b, the major fragment, initiates the non-enzymic, non-covalent assembly of the multimolecular complex C5b6789, which is the membrane attack unit of complement. The biologically active products generated during activation of C3–C9 are: (*i*) the anaphylatoxins (C3a and C5a) which directly contract smooth muscle and release histamine from most cells; (*ii*) chemotactic principles (C3 fragment, C5a, and C5i67); (*iii*) C3b which binds to the initiating complex to promote its immune adherence to certain cells that bear the immune adherence receptor thereby initiating a response that is dependent on the cell type; and (*iv*) cell-bound C5b6789 which alters membranes to induce lysis.

ACKNOWLEDGEMENTS

Work from the author's laboratory is supported by grants AI-07722, AM-05577, and AI-10356 from the National Institutes of Health and a grant from the New England Peabody Home Foundation. D.T.F. is a Postdoctoral Fellow of the Helen Hay Whitney Foundation.

REFERENCES

Allen, F. H., Jr. (1974). *Vox Sang.*, **27**, 382.
Alper, C. A., and Propp, R. P. (1968). *J. Clin. Invest.*, **47**, 2181.
Alper, C. A., Boenisch, T., and Watson, L. (1972a). *J. Exp. Med.*, **135**, 68.
Alper, C. A., Colten, H. R., Rosen, F. S., Rabson, A. R., Macnab, G. M., and Gear, J. S. S. (1972b). *Lancet*, **ii**, 1179.
Alper, C. A., Johnson, A. M., Birtch, A. G., and Moore, F. D. (1969a). *Science, N.Y.*, **163**, 286.
Alper, C. A., Propp, R. P., Klemperer, M. R., and Rosen, F. S. (1969b). *J. Clin. Invest.*, **48**, 553.
Alper, C. A., and Rosen, F. S. (1974). In *Progress in Immunology II*, Vol. I, (Brent, L., and Holborow, I., eds.), North Holland Publishing Co., Amsterdam, p. 351.
Alper, C. A., Rosen, F. S., and Lachmann, P. J. (1972c). *Proc. Nat. Acad. Sci., U.S.A.*, **69**, 2910.
Amos, N., Sissons, J. G. P., and Peters, D. K. (1976). Third Eur. Complement Workshop, p. 2.

Assimeh, S. N., and Painter, R. H. (1975a). *J. Immunol.*, **115**, 482.
Assimeh, S. N., and Painter, R. H. (1975b). *J. Immunol.*, **115**, 488.
Austen, K. F., and Sheffer, A. L. (1965). *New Engl. J. Med.*, **272**, 649.

Bach, S., Ruddy, S., MacLaren, A. J., and Austen, K. F. (1971). *Immunology*, **21**, 869.
Barkas, T., Scott, G. K., and Fothergill, J. E. (1973). *Biochem. Soc. Trans.*, **1**, 1219.
Boackle, R. J., Pruitt, K. M., and Mestecky, J. (1974). *Immunochemistry*, **11**, 543.
Bokisch, V. A., Dierich, M. P., and Müller-Eberhard, H. J. (1975). *Proc. Nat. Acad. Sci.*, U.S.A., **72**, 1989.
Bokisch, V. A., and Müller-Eberhard, H. J. (1970). *J. Clin. Invest.*, **49**, 2427.
Borsos, T., Rapp, H. J., and Mayer, M. M. (1961). *J. Immunol.*, **87**, 326.
Boyer, J. T., Ball, E. P., Norman, M. E., Nilsson, U. R., and Zimmerman, T. S. (1975). *J. Clin. Invest.*, **56**, 905.
Brackertz, D., Isler, E., and Kueppers, F. (1975). *Clin. Allergy*, **5**, 89.
Burger, R., Hadding, U., and Bitter-Suermann, D. (1975). *Fed. Proc.*, **34**, 981a.
Burkholder, P. M., Kessler, D., and Littleton, C. (1970). *J. Immunol.*, **18**, 693.

Caldwell, J. R., Ruddy, S., Schur, P. H., and Austen, K. F. (1972). *Clin. Immunol. Patholog.*, **1**, 39.
Cochrane, C. G., and Müller-Eberhard, H. J. (1968). *J. Exp. Med.*, **127**, 371.
Colten, H. R. (1974). In *Progress in Immunology II*, Vol. 1, (Brent, L., and Holborow, J., eds.), North Holland Publishing Co., Amsterdam, p. 183.
Colten, H. R., Gordon, J. M., Rapp, H. J., and Borsos, T. (1968). *J. Immunol.*, **100**, 788.
Colten, H. R., and Wyatt, H. V. (1972). In *Biological Activities of Complement*, (Ingram, D. G., ed.), S. Karger, Basel, p. 244.
Cooper, N. R. (1969). *Science, N.Y.*, **165**, 396.
Cooper, N. R. (1973). *J. Exp. Med.*, **137**, 451.
Cooper, N. R. (1975). *J. Exp. Med.*, **141**, 890.
Cooper, N. R., and Müller-Eberhard, H. J. (1970). *J. Exp. Med.*, **132**, 775.

Daha, M. R., Austen, K. F., and Fearon, D. T. (1977). *J. Immunol.*, in press.
Daha, M. R., Austen, K. F., and Fearon, D. T. (1978). *J. Immunol.*, in press.
Daha, M. R., Fearon, D. T., and Austen, K. F. (1976a). *J. Immunol.*, **116**, 568.
Daha, M. R., Fearon, D. T., and Austen, K. F. (1976b). *J. Immunol.*, **116**, 1.
Daha, M. R., Fearon, D. T., and Austen, K. F. (1976c). *J. Immunol.*, **117**, 630.
Davis, A. E., III, Arnaout, M. A., Alper, C. A., and Rosen, F. S. (1977). *New Engl. J. Med.*, **197**, 144.
Day, N. K., Geiger, H., Stroud, R., de Bracco, M., Mancado, B., Windhorst, D., and Good, R. A. (1972). *J. Clin. Invest.*, **51**, 1102.
Delage, J. M., Lehner-Netsch, G., and Simard, S. C. (1973). *Immunology*, **24**, 671.
Dias da Silva, W., and Lepow, I. H. (1967). *J. Exp. Med.*, **125**, 921.
Dierich, M. P., Ferrone, S., Pelligrino, M. A., and Reisfeld, R. A. (1974). *J. Immunol.*, **113**, 940.
Donaldson, V. H., and Evans, R. R. (1963). *Am. J. Med.*, **35**, 37.
Donaldson, V. A., Merler, E., Rosen, F. S., Kretschmer, K. W., and Lepow, I. H. (1970). *J. Lab. Clin. Med.*, **76**, 986.

Ehlenberger, A. G., and Nussenzweig, V. (1975). *Fed. Proc.*, **34**, 854a.
Ellerson, J. R., Yasmean, D., Painter, R. H., and Dorington, K. J. (1972). *FEBS Letters*, **24**, 319.

Fearon, D. T. (1978). *J. Immunol.*, in press.
Fearon, D. T., and Austen, K. F. (1975a). *Ann. N.Y. Acad. Sci.*, **256**, 441.

394

Fearon, D. T., and Austen, K. F. (1975b). *J. Exp. Med.*, **142**, 856.
Fearon, D. T., and Austen, K. F. (1975c). *Proc. Nat. Acad. Sci., U.S.A.*, **72**, 3220.
Fearon, D. T., and Austen, K. F. (1975d). *J. Immunol.*, **115**, 1357.
Fearon, D. T., and Austen, K. F. (1976). *Essays Med. Biochem.*, **2**, 1.
Fearon, D. T., and Austen, K. F. (1977a). *Proc. Nat. Acad. Sci. U.S.A.*, **74**, 1683.
Fearon, D. T., and Austen, K. F. (1977b). *J. Exp. Med.*, **146**, 22.
Fearon, D. T., Austen, K. F., and Ruddy, S. (1973a). *J. Immunol.*, **111**, 1730.
Fearon, D. T., Austen, K. F., and Ruddy, S. (1973b). *J. Exp. Med.*, **138**, 1305.
Fearon, D. T., Austen. K. F., and Ruddy, S. (1974). *J. Exp. Med.*, **139**, 355.
Friedberger, E. (1909). *Z. Immun. Forsch.*, **2**, 208.
Fu, S. M., Kunkel, H. G., Brusman, H. F., Allen, F. H., Jr., and Fotino, M. (1974). *J. Exp. Med.*, **140**, 1108.

Gelfand, J. A., Sherins, R. J., Alling, D. W., and Frank, M. M. (1976). *New Eng. J. Med.*, **295**, 1444.
Gewurz, H., Pickering, R. J., Christian, C. L., Snyderman, R., Mergenhagen, S. E., and Good, R. A. (1968). *Clin. Exp. Immunol.*, **3**, 437.
Gigli, I., and Austen, K. F. (1969). *J. Exp. Med.*, **128**, 679.
Gigli, I., and Nelson, R. A. (1968). *Exp. Cell Res.*, **51**, 45.
Gigli, I., Ruddy, S., and Austen, K. F. (1968). *J. Immunol.*, **100**, 1154.
Gitlin, J. D., Rosen, F. S., and Lachmann, P. J. (1975). *J. Exp. Med.*, **141**, 1221.
Goetzl, E. J., and Austen, K. F. (1974). In *Chemotaxis: Its Biology and Biochemistry*, (Sorkin, E., and Davos-Platz, eds.), S. Karger, Basel, p. 218.
Goldman, J. N., Ruddy, S., and Austen, K. F. (1972). *J. Immunol.*, **109**, 353.
Götze, O. (1975). In *Cold Spring Harbor Symposium on Cell Proliferation*, (Reich, E. and Ritkin, D. B., eds.), Cold Spring Harbor, New York, p. 255.
Götze, O., Medicus, R. G., and Müller-Eberhard, H. J. (1977). *J. Immunol.*, **118**, 525.
Götze, O., and Müller-Eberhard, H. J. (1971). *J. Exp. Med.*, **134**, 905.
Götze, O., and Müller-Eberhard, H. J. (1974). *J. Exp. Med.*, **139**, 44.

Harpel, P. C., and Cooper, N. R. (1975). *J. Clin. Invest.*, **55**, 593.
Harpel, P. C., Hugli, T. E., and Cooper, N. R. (1975). *J. Clin. Invest.*, **55**, 605.
Hauptmann, G., Grosshans, E., and Heid, E. (1974). *Ann. Dermatol. Syph.*, **101**, 479.
Henson, P. M. (1972). In *Biological Activities of Complement*, (Ingram, D. G., ed.), S. Karger, Basel, p. 173.
Henson, P. M., and Cochrane, C. G. (1971). *J. Exp. Med.*, **133**, 554.
Heusinkveld, R. S., Leddy, J. P., Klemperer, M. R., and Breckenridge, R. T. (1974). *J. Clin. Invest.*, **53**, 554.
Hobart, M. J., Alper, C. A., and Lachman, P. J. (1975). In *Protides of the Biologic Fluids*, (Peeters, H., ed.), Pergamon Press, Oxford, p. 575.
Huber, H., Polley, M. J., Linscott, M. D., Fudenberg, H. H., and Müller-Eberhard, H. J. (1968). *Science, N.Y.*, **162**, 1281.
Humphrey, J. H., and Dourmaskin, R. R. (1970). *Adv. Immunol.*, **11**, 75.
Hunsicker, L. G., Ruddy, S., and Austen, K. F. (1973). *J. Immunol.*, **110**, 128.
Hurst, M. M., Volanakis, J. E., Hester, R. B., Stroud, R. M., and Bennett, J. C. (1974). *J. Exp. Med.*, **140**, 1117.

Iles, G. H., Seeman, P., Naylor, D., and Cinader, B. (1973). *J. Cell Biol.*, **56**, 528.
Inoue, K., and Kinsky, S. C. (1970). *Biochemistry*, **9**, 4767.

Jensen, J. A. (1967). *Science, N.Y.*, **155**, 1122.
Johnson, A. R., Hugli, T. E., and Müller-Eberhard, H. J. (1975). *Immunology*, **28**, 1067.
Johnson, A. M., Alper, C. A., Rosen, F. S., and Craig, J. M. (1971). *Science, N.Y.*, **173**, 553.

Klaus, G. G. B., and Humphrey, J. H. (1977). *Immunology*, **33**, 31.
Klemperer, M. R., Woodworth, H. C., Rosen, F. S., and Austen, K. F. (1966). *J. Clin. Invest.*, **45**, 880.
Klemperer, M. R., Donaldson, V. H., and Rosen, F. S. (1968). *J. Clin. Invest.*, **47**, 604.
Kohler, P. F., and Müller-Eberhard, H. J. (1969). *Science, N.Y.*, **163**, 474.
Kohler, P. F., and Müller-Eberhard, H. J. (1972). *J. Clin. Invest.*, **51**, 868.
Kolb, W. P., and Müller-Eberhard, H. J. (1973). *J. Exp. Med.*, **138**, 438.
Kolb, W. P., and Müller-Eberhard, H. J. (1975a). *J. Exp. Med.*, **141**, 724.
Kolb, W. P., and Müller-Eberhard, H. J. (1975b). *Proc. Nat. Acad. Sci., U.S.A.*, **72**, 1687.
Kolb, W. P., and Müller-Eberhard, H. J. (1977). *Fed. Proc.*, **36**, 1209.

Lachmann, P. J. (1974). *Boll. Ist. Sieroter, Milanese*, **53**, 195.
Lachmann, P. J., and Müller-Eberhard, H. J. (1968). *J. Immunol.*, **100**, 691.
Lachmann, P. J., Munn, E. A., and Weissman, G. (1970). *Immunology*, **19**, 973.
Leddy, J. P., Frank, M. M., Gaither, T., Baum, J., and Klemperer, M. R. (1974). *J. Clin. Invest.*, **53**, 544.
Lepow, I. H. (1971). In *Biochemistry of Acute Allergic Reactions*, (Austen, K. F., and Becker, E. L., eds.), Blackwell, Oxford, p. 205.
Lepow, I. H., Naff, G. B., Todd, E. W., Pensky, J., and Hinz, C. F., Jr. (1956). *J. Exp. Med.*, **117**, 983.
Lepow, I. H., Kretschmer, K. W., Patrick, R. A., and Rosen, F. S. (1970). *Am. J. Pathol.*, **61**, 13.

Marcus, R. L., Shin, H. S., and Mayer, M. M. (1971). *Proc. Nat. Acad. Sci., U.S.A.*, **68**, 1351.
May, J. E., and Frank, M. M. (1973a). *J. Immunol.*, **111**, 1661.
May, J. E., and Frank, M. M. (1973b). *J. Immunol.*, **111**, 1668.
Mayer, M. M. (1965). In *Ciba Foundation Symposium on Complement*, (Wolstenholme, G. E. W., and Knight, J., eds.), Little, Brown Co., New York, p. 4.
Mayer, M. M. (1972). *Proc. Nat. Acad. Sci., U.S.A.*, **69**, 2954.
McCall, C. E., DeChatelet, L. R., Brown, D., and Lachmann, P. J. (1974). *Nature, (Lond.)*, **249**, 841.
Minta, J. O. (1975). *Fed. Proc.*, **34**, 981.
Minta, J. O., and Lepow, I. H. (1974). *Immunochemistry*, **11**, 361.
Morse, J. H., Stecher, V. J., and Thorbecke, G. J. (1967). *Proc. Soc. Exp. Biol. Med.*, **124**, 433.
Müller-Eberhard, H. J. (1975). *Ann. Rev. Biochem.*, **44**, 697.
Müller-Eberhard, H. J., and Calcott, M. A. (1966). *Immunochemistry*, **3**, 500.
Müller-Eberhard, H. J., and Götze, O. (1972). *J. Exp. Med.*, **135**, 1003.
Müller-Eberhard, H. J., and Kunkel, H. G. (1961). *Proc. Soc. Exp. Biol. Med.*, **106**, 291.
Müller-Eberhard, H. J., Polley, M. J., and Calcott, M. A. (1967). *J. Exp. Med.*, **125**, 359.

Naff, G. B., and Ratnoff, O. D. (1968). *J. Exp. Med.*, **128**, 571.
Nagasawa, S., and Stroud, R. M. (1977). *Proc. Nat. Acad. Sci. U.S.A.*, **74**, 2998.
Nellek, B., and Opferkuch, W. (1975). *Clin. Exp. Immunol.*, **19**, 223.
Nelson, D. S. (1965). In *Ciba Symposium on Complement*, (Wolstenholme, G. E. W., and Knight, J., eds.), Little, Brown Co., New York, p. 222.
Nelson, R. A. (1953). *Science, N.Y.*, **118**, 733.
Nelson, R. A. (1966). *Surveys Ophthalmol.*, **11**, 497.
Nicol, P. A. E., and Lachmann, P. J. (1973). *Immunology*, **24**, 259.
Nilsson, A., and Müller-Eberhard, H. J. (1967). *Immunology*, **13**, 101.
Nilsson, U. R., Mandle, R. J., and McConnell-Mapes, J. A. (1975). *J. Immunol.*, **114**, 815.
Nussenzweig, V. (1974). *Adv. Immunol.*, **20**, 1.

396

Ochs, H. D., Rosenfeld, S. I., Thomas, E. D., Giblett, E. R., Alper, C. A., Dupont, B., Schaller, J. G., Gilliland, B. C., Hansen, J. A., and Wedgwood, R. J. (1977). *New Eng. J. Med.*, **296**, 470.

O'Connell, E. J., Enriguezi, P., Linman, J. W., Gleich, G. J., and McDuffie, F. C. (1967). *J. Lab. Clin. Med.*, **70**, 745.

Okada, H., Kawachi, S., and Nichioka, K. (1970). *Biochim. Biophys. Acta*, **288**, 541.

Patrick, R. A., and Lepow, I. H. (1969). *Fed. Proc.*, **28**, 817a.

Pearlman, D. S., Ward, P. A., and Becker, E. L. (1969). *J. Exp. Med.*, **130**, 745.

Pensky, J., Hinz, C. F., Jr., Todd, E. W., Wedgwood, R. J., Boyer, J. T., and Lepow, I. H. (1968). *J. Immunol.*, **100**, 142.

Pensky, J., Levy, L. R., and Lepow, I. H. (1961). *J. Biol. Chem.*, **236**, 1674.

Pepys, M. B. (1974). *J. Exp. Med.*, **140**, 126.

Peterson, B. H., Graham, J. A., and Brooks, G. F. (1975). *Clin. Res.*, **23**, 295a.

Pickering, R. J., Naff, G. B., Stroud, R. M., Good, R. A., and Gewurz, H. (1970). *J. Exp. Med.*, **131**, 803.

Pillemer, L., Blum, L., Lepow, I. H., Ross, O. A., Todd, E. W., and Wardlaw, A. C. (1954). *Science, N.Y.*, **120**, 279.

Platts-Mills, T. A. E., and Ishizaka, K. (1974). *J. Immunol.*, **113**, 348.

Polley, M. J., and Müller-Eberhard, H. J. (1967). *J. Exp. Med.*, **126**, 1013.

Polley, M. J., and Müller-Eberhard, H. J. (1968). *J. Exp. Med.*, **128**, 533.

Pondman, K. N., Hannema, A., Cormane, R., and Stoop, J. W. (1969). *Ned. T. Geneesk.*, **113**, 1462.

Poskitt, T. R., Fortwengler, H. P., Jr., and Lunskis, B. (1973). *J. Exp. Med.*, **138**, 715.

Reid, K. B. M., Lowe, D. M., and Porter, R. R. (1972). *Biochem. J.*, **130**, 749.

Rent, R., Ertel, N., Eisenstein, R., and Gewerz, H. (1975). *J. Immunol.*, **114**, 120.

Reynolds, H. Y., Atkinson, J. P., Newball, H. H., and Frank, M. M. (1975). *J. Immunol.*, **114**, 1813.

Rittner, C., Hauptmann, G., Grosse-Wilde, H., Grosshaus, E., Tongio, M. M., and Mayer, S. (1975). In *Histocompatibility Testing* (Kessmeyer-Nielson, F., ed.), Munksgaard, Copenhagen, p. 945.

Rittner, C., and Rittner, B. (1974). *Vox Sang.*, **27**, 464.

Rosen, F. S., Alper, C. A., Pensky, J., Klemperer, M. R., and Donaldson, V. H. (1971). *J. Clin. Invest.*, **50**, 2143.

Rosenfeld, S. I., Kelly, M. E., Baum, J., and Leddy, J. P. (1974). *J. Clin. Invest.*, **53**, 67a.

Rosenfeld, S. I., Ruddy, S., and Austen, K. F. (1969a). *J. Clin. Invest.*, **48**, 2283.

Rosenfeld, S. I., Ruddy, S., and Austen, K. F. (1969b). *Clin. Res.*, **17**, 358.

Rosenfeld, S. I., Staples, P. J., and Leddy, J. P. (1975). *J. Allergy Clin. Immunol.*, **55**, 104.

Ross, G. D., Polley, K. J., Rabelline, E. M., and Grey, H. M. (1973). *J. Exp. Med.*, **138**, 798.

Rosse, W. F., Logue, G. L., and Silberman, H. R. (1976). *Clin. Res.*, **24**, 482.

Rother, K. (1972). *Eur. J. Immunol.*, **2**, 550.

Ruddy, S., and Austen, K. F. (1971a). *J. Immunol.*, **107**, 742.

Ruddy, S., and Austen, K. F. (1971b). In *The Metabolic Basis of Inherited Disease*, (Stanbury, J. B., Wyngaarden, J. B., and Fredrickson, D. S., eds.), 3rd edn., McGraw-Hill Book Co., New York, p. 1655.

Ruddy, S., and Austen, K. F. (1972). In *Biological Activities of Complement*, (Ingram, D. G., ed.), S. Karger, Basel, p. 13.

Ruddy, S., Austen, K. F., and Goetzl, E. J. (1975). *J. Clin. Invest.*, **55**, 587.

Ruddy, S., Gigli, I., and Austen, K. F. (1972). *New Engl. J. Med.*, **287**, 489, 545, 592, 642.

Ruddy, S., and Colten, H. R. (1974). *New Engl. J. Med.*, **290**, 1284.

Ruddy, S., Everson, L. K., Schur, P. H., and Austen, K. F. (1971). *J. Exp. Med.*, **134**, 259s.

Ruddy, S., Gigli, I., Sheffer, A. L., and Austen, K. F. (1968). In *Allergology*, (Rose, B., Richter, M., Sehon, A., and Frankland, A. W., eds.), Excerpta Medica, Amsterdam, p. 351.

Sakai, K., and Stroud, R. M. (1973). *J. Immunol.*, **110**, 1010.
Sandberg, A. L., and Osler, A. G. (1971). *J. Immunol.*, **107**, 1268.
Schreiber, A. D., Abdon, N. I., Atkins, P., Goldwein, F., Layne, T., Cerbi, C., McDermott, P., and Zweiman, B. (1975) *Clin. Res.*, **23**, 296A.
Schreiber, R. D., Götze, O., and Müller-Eberhard, H. J. (1976). *J. Exp. Med.*, **144**, 1062.
Schreiber, R. D., and Müller-Eberhard, H. J. (1974). *J. Exp. Med.*, **140**, 1324.
Sheffer, A. L., Fearon, D. T., and Austen, K. F. (1977). *Ann. Int. Med.*, **86**, 306.
Shelton, E., Yonemasu, K., and Stroud, R. M. (1972). *Proc. Nat. Acad. Sci.*, *U.S.A.*, **69**, 65.
Soter, N. A., Austen, K. F., and Gigli, I. (1974). *J. Invest. Dermatol.*, **63**, 219.
Soter, N. A., Austen, K. F., and Gigli, I. (1975). *J. Immunol.*, **114**, 928.
Spitzer, R. E., Vallota, E. H., Forristal, J., Sudora, E., Stitzel, A., Davis, N. C., and West, C. D. (1969). *Science, N.Y.*, **164**, 436.
Stolfi, R. (1968). *J. Immunol.*, **100**, 46.
Stroud, R. M., Nagaki, K., Pickering, R. J., Gewurz, A., Good, R. A., and Cooper, M. D. (1970). *Clin. Exp. Immunol.*, **7**, 133.
Strunk, R., and Colten, H. R. (1974). *J. Immunol.*, **112**, 905.

Tamura, N., and Nelson, R. A. (1967). *J. Immunol.*, **99**, 582.
Thompson, R. A. (1971). Immunology, **22**, 147.
Thompson, R. A., and Lachmann, P. J. (1970). *J. Exp. Med.*, **131**, 629.
Till, G., and Ward, P. A. (1975). *J. Immunol.*, **114**, 843.

Valet, G., and Cooper, N. (1974*a*). *J. Immunol.*, **112**, 1667.
Valet, G., and Cooper, N. R. (1974*b*). *J. Immunol.*, **112**, 339.
Vallota, E. H., Götze, O., Spiegelberg, H. L., Forrestal, J., West, C. D., and Müller-Eberhard, H. J. (1974). *J. Exp. Med.*, **139**, 1249.
Volanakis, J. E., and Kaplan, M. H. (1974). *J. Immunol.*, **113**, 9.

Ward, P. A. (1972). In *Biological Activities of Complement*, (Ingram, D. G., ed.), S. Karger, Basel, p. 108.
Ward, P. A., and Becker, E. L. (1968). *J. Exp. Med.*, 127, 693.
Wyatt, H. V., Colten, H. R., and Borsos, T. (1972). *J. Immunol.*, **108**, 1609.

Yonemasu, K., and Stroud, R. M. (1972). *Immunochemistry*, **9**, 545.

Ziccardi, R. J., and Cooper, N. R. (1977). *J. Immunol.*, **118**, 2047.
Zimmerman, T. S., and Müller-Eberhard, H. J. (1971). *J. Exp. Med.* 134, 1601.

CHAPTER 11

Immunochemical Aspects of Polysaccharide Antigens

I. W. Sutherland

1 INTRODUCTION

The association of monosaccharide-containing structures with immunochemical specificity was an early contribution to the study of antigen–antibody interactions. Thus, the combination of a monosaccharide with a protein led to the formation of a new antigen distinct from the protein itself, and this antigen could react in the tests then available. At the same time, knowledge began to accumulate about the presence of polysaccharides and polysaccharide-containing structures at the surfaces of microbial and other cells. As more information about these cellular carbohydrates became available, possible explanations were provided for known serological cross-reactions between micro-organisms or between cells of prokaryotes and eukaryotes. Work was concentrated particularly on determining the structure of the polysaccharides from bacteria of medical significance and on blood group substances. Although studies on polysaccharide synthesis were slower to yield results, they too now provide much relevant information, which, taken together with the application of classical methods for determining carbohydrate structures, have done much to assist the immunochemist. A more recent development, which has been utilized quickly to provide more data on the antigenic determinants of polysaccharides and related molecules, has been the study of lectins (plant agglutinins) and their application. For these studies, many of the techniques originally developed for classical antigen–antibody reactions have been used. Some of the information provided has merely confirmed that obtained by other methods, but lectins have provided an additional specific and rapid source of information about the presence of specific monosaccharides in some configurations. Much of the more recent work on the immunochemistry of polysaccharides would have been impossible if improved micromethods for both serological and biochemical assays had not been developed, thus limiting the amount of pure antigen required. This has been even more important when features such as as the inhibition of antigen–antibody reactions by related compounds have been studied. Preparation of pure antigens of polysaccharide or glycoprotein in adequate amounts is not excessively difficult, but the provision of milligram, or greater quantities, of oligosaccharides for inhibition tests is still a laborious and expensive process, despite the development of mild hydrolytic agents (Painter, 1960) or of apparatus for the continuous removal of the oligosaccharides formed (Galanos *et al.*, 1969). The discovery of an increasing number of polysaccharide hydrolases (*endo*glycosidases), together with *exo*glycosidases, provides a simple and rapid method for obtaining relatively large amounts of oligosaccharides.

An account of the historical development of the immunochemistry of polysaccharide antigens with specific reference to blood group antigens is to be found in the review by Morgan (1970). The expansion of knowledge of the immunochemical specificities of microbial polysaccharides has been reviewed by Heidelberger (1973) who, with his colleagues, has been responsible for many of the developments in this field.

The aim of this chapter is not to examine the immunochemistry of polysaccharide antigens comprehensively; such a catalogue would require several volumes and, even then, be of doubtful value and completeness. Rather, emphasis has been placed on a more limited group of systems for which a general knowledge based on chemical, biochemical, genetic, and immunological studies is now available. Using these models, the importance of carbohydrate-containing immunological determinants can be placed in proper perspective, leading to the production of working models, and perhaps, the anticipation of some of the future developments in this field.

2 TYPES AND LOCATION OF MICROBIAL POLYSACCHARIDE ANTIGENS AND BLOOD GROUP ANTIGENS

In micro-organisms, whether eukaryotic or prokaryotic, the cell is enclosed frequently by a wall which confers strength and rigidity, in addition to containing and protecting the cytoplasmic (or plasma) membrane and its nucleus. The cell wall relies for its strength on polysaccharides, or similar polymers, and many of these compounds play important roles as antigens. Their location at or near the surface of the cell results in them being readily accessible to the immune mechanisms of the host. Furthermore, their resistance to non-specific enzymic degradation ensures their persistence even following phagocytosis or amoebic engulfment. Thus, polysaccharide antigens from the cell surface are important in many contexts, such as the invasiveness of the micro-organism in its host— exemplified by *Streptococcus pneumoniae* and *Cryptococcus* species—the epidemiology of food poisoning due to *Salmonella* species, and the routine use of serological typing of blood group antigens.

In addition to the polysaccharides which form a part of the cell wall structures, others are to be found outside the cell as extracellular polysaccharides (exopolysaccharides). These may be attached to the cell wall in the form of discrete capsules recognizable by the indian ink staining technique (Duguid, 1951) as in yeast such as *Cryptococcus* species or in the bacterial species *Klebsiella pneumoniae* and *Strept. pneumoniae*. Alternatively, the exopolysaccharide may be found in the form of loose slime unattached to the microbial cell surface. This is encountered frequently in *Escherichia coli*. Exopolysaccharides are usually haptenic, giving strong reactions with homologous antisera prepared using whole microbial cultures, but in the pure form are poor antigens.

In gram-negative bacteria, the major polysaccharide antigens are lipopolysaccharides. These exceedingly complex macromolecules, which are variously termed somatic antigens or O antigens, are a feature of the cell wall of gram-negative prokaryotes. In the bacterial wall, they form part of the outer membrane—composed of lipoprotein and lipopolysaccharide—found outside the rigid peptidoglycan layer (Figure 1). They are thus readily accessible to antibodies when mixed with whole cells, as well as playing important roles as

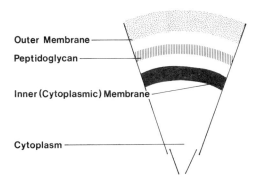

GRAM NEGATIVE CELL WALL

Figure 1 A diagrammatic representation of the cell wall of gram-negative bacteria

receptors for bacteriophages and bacteriocins. The importance of lipopolysaccharides as antigens has been reinforced by the development of serological methods in the epidemiology of enteric and other bacteria. Thus, the most intensively studied group of bacteria with respect to the immunochemistry of their lipopolysaccharides undoubtedly has been the family *Enterobacteriaceae*, which includes several human pathogenic genera such as *Salmonella*, *Shigella*, *Proteus*, *Escherichia*, and *Klebsiella*, as well as plant pathogens and harmless species. In quantitative terms, the lipopolysaccharides are also important, as in gram-negative bacteria, they represent 1–5 per cent of the microbial dry weight or 10–15 per cent of the dry cell walls. Lipopolysaccharide therefore can be obtained in relatively large quantities with comparative ease and, through the use of chemical and other techniques, free from contaminating macromolecules. Of particular value in this respect was the development of an extraction procedure utilizing hot aqueous phenol (Westphal *et al.*, 1952). In the hot single-phase mixture, all macromolecules from the cells are soluble, but on cooling the polysaccharides in the upper layer consisting of phenol-saturated water are separated from proteins in the lower layer consisting of water-saturated phenol. Purification of the lipopolysaccharide and separation from other water-soluble polysaccharides is achieved by ultracentrifugation. Separation of the antigenic portion of the molecule—the polysaccharide—from the complex lipid A, also is accomplished by mild acid hydrolysis relatively simply.

In gram-positive bacteria, two types of carbohydrate antigen are found in the cell walls (Figure 2). Some are apparently relatively simple polysaccharides of varying structure, but the second type are a group of unusual compounds termed *teichoic* acids. These are polymers of polyol phosphates (polyglycerol phosphate or polyribitol phosphate) or similar compounds such as polyhexosamine phosphates. Glycosyl substituents are also found on the linear macromolecules, increasing the number of possible antigenic determinants.

Yeasts contain a number of polysaccharides in their cell walls. Mannans—homopolymers of D-mannose—are linked covalently to protein in the cell wall

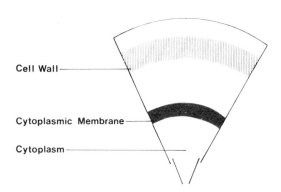

Cell Wall

Cytoplasmic Membrane

Cytoplasm

GRAM POSITIVE CELL WALL

Figure 2 The gram-positive bacterial wall

and are interspersed with the rigid glucan molecules which confer on the yeast cells their characteristic shape. Other yeast glycoprotein complexes are found as enzymes with varying activities. The yeast polysaccharides are much more difficult to extract and to isolate in a pure, undegraded form than are the bacterial cell wall polymers. Acetolysis provides one method which can be used to isolate the immunodominant mannans from yeast cell walls, as relatively pure haptens. The structure of the mannans found in yeast is more akin to that of the blood group substances than to those found in bacterial walls.

Some of the significance of the blood group substances lies in their presence on the surface of erythrocytes, but they, unlike microbial polysaccharide antigens located on the wall or extracellularly, are not confined to a single cellular location. Sources of blood group antigens include normal body fluids and secretions, such as saliva (containing 10–130 mg/l), meconium, and gastric juices. A particularly rich source from which the blood group antigens can be isolated relatively easily is ovarian cyst fluid. This source has the advantage that, unlike other tissues or mucosal linings, no peptic digestion is required and a purer product results.

The normal procedure for the preparation of blood group antigens is to extract the freeze-dried source material with cold 90–95 per cent phenol. The products are serologically active, but differ from the native form of the antigens. The desired degree of purification of the blood group active substances depends on the purpose for which the product is intended. Care has to be taken to avoid degradation of the glycoproteins by acid or alkali, but they are thermostable. Some specific purification procedures have been developed, such as precipitation with lectins, used by Kristiansen and Porath (1968) to isolate blood group A-active material from hog gastric mucin. The criteria for assessing the purity of the product may be chemical, physical, or immunological; problems are encountered with the first of these criteria, as the gross chemical composition of blood group antigens of all types (A, B, AB, H, and Le[a]) is very similar. Consequently, because of their chemical similarity, methods applicable to one type of blood group antigen are, in general, equally applicable to the other types.

3 EFFECTS OF CULTURAL CONDITIONS ON MICROBIAL POLYSACCHARIDE ANTIGENS

The architecture of the microbial cell surface is not, as was once thought, constant in composition, but instead is a dynamic structure. Changes occur both with the age of the microbial cell population and according to the conditions of culture, thus, the antigenic composition also is determined by these factors. Polysaccharide antigens on the microbial surface are particularly susceptible to alteration, with changes in the culture conditions leading to the virtual elimination of certain polysaccharide antigens together with the emergence of new antigenic determinants. Alternatively, the modifications may be merely quantitative. Many of these alterations have become appreciated only with the availability of improved methods of investigation.

Rapid growth leads to production of the largest quantity of total cell wall material, but may also cause undesirable characteristics in the polymers. Thus, the lipopolysaccharide of *Salmonella* species grown in continuous culture at high dilution rates of the order of 0.85 hr^{-1} contains relatively small amounts of the O-antigenic side chains (Collins, 1964), while bacteria with normal O-antigen content could be obtained by reducing the dilution (growth) rate. Such phenotypic changes are important therefore to the immunochemist wishing to produce material of uniform composition.

Much more marked changes have been observed in gram-positive bacteria exposed to alterations in the ionic composition of the growth medium. For example, bacteria such as *Bacillus* species grown with limiting nutrients including glucose, NH_4^+, K^+, or SO_4^{2-}, form cell walls containing 35–46 per cent teichoic acid (Ellwood and Tempest, 1972). Culture under conditions of Mg^{2+} limitation results in the teichoic acid content increasing to 62–74 per cent. This polymer disappears completely when the growth medium is phosphate limited, the polymer being replaced by teichuronic acids—compounds with completely different antigenic specificities. Teichuronic acids generally contain glucuronic acid and *N*-acetylgalactosamine. Besides these absolute changes in antigenic composition, alterations to substituents on the teichoic acid molecules have been noted. In *B. subtilis* var. *niger*, the teichoic acid is glucosylated normally but culture of the bacteria under conditions of glucose limitation leads to formation of a polymer with fewer glucose residues per teichoic acid molecule. Changes in nutrient limitation in continuous culture result in microbial population with different antigenic carbohydrate polymers in the cell walls (Ellwood and Tempest, 1969). This situation mimics certain aspects of batch culture which also may give rise to a mixed bacterial population containing both teichoic acids and teichuronic acids.

The immunochemist who wishes to prepare pure carbohydrate antigens from microbial cell walls, therefore, must choose the conditions of culture with care to ensure that they favour production of the desired antigen. He must also remember that continuous cultures, while useful in many ways, tend to produce fast-growing mutants which may differ greatly from the desired antigenic type.

4 ANTIGENIC DETERMINANTS IN POLYSACCHARIDES AND GLYCOPROTEINS

The polysaccharide macromolecule can possess one of several possible structures, for example it may be a homopolymer composed of a single type of monosaccharide, as in the case of dextrans and levans, polyglucoses and polyfructoses, respectively, formed by several groups of bacteria, and by the mannans found in many yeasts. Alternatively, the carbohydrate-containing structure of both homopolymers and heteropolymers can be subdivided further into uniform and non-uniform types. Typically, bacterial polysaccharides, including extracellular polysaccharides and *part* of the lipopolysaccharide molecule, are formed from repeating units. However, mammalian glycoproteins such as the blood group substances are formed from several monosaccharides giving structures which, while containing a strictly ordered sequence of monomers, normally lack repeating units. These variations in the polysaccharide structures are largely a reflection of different modes of synthesis by the micro-organisms and by eukaryotic cells, respectively.

Relatively few monosaccharides are used to form the components of most carbohydrate antigens. These include the three neutral hexoses, D-glucose, D-galactose and D-mannose; acetylamino sugars, especially N-acetyl-D-glucosamine and N-acetyl-D-galactosamine; the uronic acids of which D-glucuronic acid is the most commonly detected; and the methyl pentoses L-rhamnose and L-fucose (Figure 3). Other monosaccharides may be found,

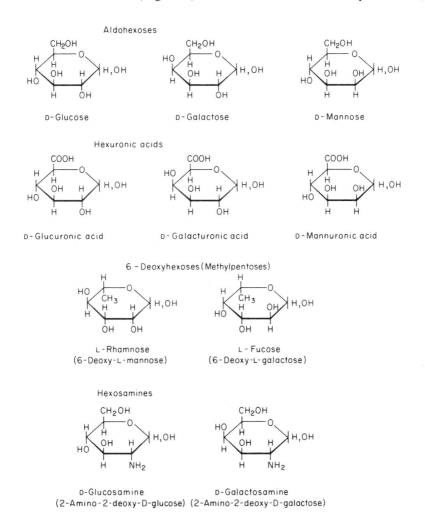

Figure 3 Common monosaccharides found in polysaccharides and glycoproteins

especially in microbial carbohydrate antigens, and contribute to the enormous number of potential antigenic determinants. This number is increased by the possibility of other substituents on the carbohydrate residues. Sulphated polysaccharides are confined mainly to eukaryotes but O-acetylated residues, ketals (divalent linkages between monosaccharides and compounds such as pyruvate), and phosphate groups all have been identified as components of polysaccharide antigens. Considerable care must be taken during polysaccharide isolation and purification as acyl groups are relatively labile, being lost under alkaline and acidic conditions.

4.1 Size of the Carbohydrate Antigenic Determinant

Polysaccharides are polymers with molecular weights of up to several millions. Despite the large size of the antigen (or hapten) molecule, the serological reaction with homologous antibody can often be inhibited by oligosaccharides as small as disaccharides, trisaccharides, or tetrasaccharides. This raises the question of the size of the combining site. Is it the same for all polysaccharide systems or is there considerable latitude even within a single system? An accurate measure of size can be obtained when a homopolysaccharide is studied and a series of oligosaccharides derived from it is readily available. Using such a system, optimal inhibition should be obtained with those oligosaccharides nearest in size to the combining site. If the oligosaccharides are smaller, and do not occupy the combining site completely, they should be less inhibitory than larger fragments. Very large fragments should be similar in potency on a molar basis to those of optimal size as they will approach the polysaccharide chain length found in the antigen itself.

In the case of the homoglycan dextran, the antigenic determinant is apparently isomaltohexaose. This oligosaccharide has a molecular weight of 990 and, in the fully extended form, has dimensions of approximately $3\cdot4 \times 1\cdot2 \times 0\cdot7$ nm. A determinant of similar size—a hexasaccharide—also has been postulated from inhibition studies, for the *Strept. pneumoniae* type III polysaccharide and its antisera (Mage and Kabat, 1963). In this system, the polymer is a heteropolysaccharide with alternating D-glucose and D-glucuronic acid residues. Not all systems need correspond to this optimal size; there have been suggestions that in some antigens the determinants may be as small as disaccharides, but never monosaccharides (see for example Kabat, 1968). The importance of small portions of polysaccharide molecules has been observed in numerous studies in which small oligosaccharides inhibit the antigen–antibody reaction even though they represent only a small portion of the total configuration present. The involvement of a small number of adjacent monosaccharides also accounts for the large number of cross-reactions detected by Heidelberger and his colleagues in their comprehensive studies with bacterial polysaccharides (1960, 1973).

The bacterial lipopolysaccharide (Figure 4) and the yeast mannan (Figure 5) are both complex structures despite the small number of monosaccharides forming the major components of the former, or mannose representing over 90

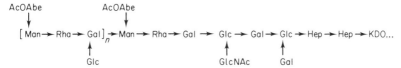

Figure 4 The structure of a bacterial lipopolysaccharide (based on *S. typhimurium*) Sugars: AcOAbe, *O*-acetylabequose; Man, mannose; Gal, galactose; Glc, glucose; Rha, rhamnose; GlcNAc, *N*-acetylglucosamine; Hep, heptose; KDO, ketodeoxyoctonic acid

per cent of the total carbohydrate of the latter. In theory, there is a large number of potential antigenic determinants in either type of molecule, but in practice, the number of antigenic regions is much more limited.

To take a specific example, the major antigenic portion of the lipopolysaccharide of *S. abortus-equi* is composed of a trisaccharide repeating unit, which forms a linear chain to which are attached glucose and abequose side chains

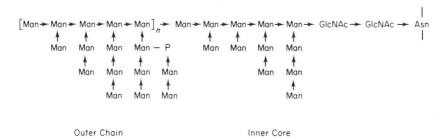

Figure 5 The structure of a yeast mannan (based on a *Saccharomyces cerevisiae* strain) Abbreviations as Figure 4, Asn; asparagine

(Figure 6). The antigenic formula for this structure according to the Kauffmann–White scheme is 4, 12, that is there are only two dominant antigens despite the many possible antigenic combinations. Studies have demonstrated that the antigen 12 is represented by a trisaccharide glucosyl-galactosyl-mannose, while antigen 4 is effectively the abequose substituent or the disaccharide abequosyl-glucose. The fifth sugar present, rhamnose, plays a relatively unimportant role. It is perhaps significant that in this example, as in most similar polymers, the side chains play the dominant role in the immunochemistry of these polysaccharides. The main-chain sugars are of less importance, almost certainly because they are

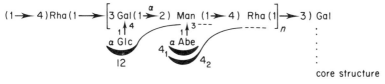

Figure 6 The structure of the antigens in *S. abortusequi* lipopolysaccharide. Abe, abequose; —, probable binding sites

unable to form such a close fit with antibody molecules as are the sugars forming the side chains.

Similar results have been found using glycoproteins such as yeast mannans or blood group substances. The monosaccharides at the outermost part of the polymer molecule are normally the immunodominant portion. The presumed antibody-binding sites for three different yeast glycoproteins studied by Raschke and Ballou (1972) conform to this pattern (see Figure 7).

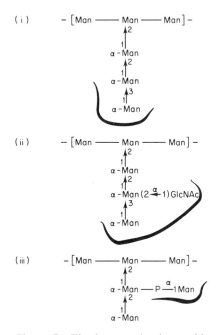

Figure 7 The immunodominant side chains of i) *Saccharomyces cerevisiae* (X2180), ii) *Kluyveromyces lactis*, and iii) *Kloeckera brevis*. —, probable binding sites are indicated

Even when a disaccharide is the immunodominant portion of the molecule there are numerous possible configurations. The terminal sugar may be either α or β-linked to any of four positions on the adjacent monosaccharide residue. There are, thus, eight possible disaccharides with the general configuration galactosyl-glucose, four of which are α and four are β-galactosyl-glucose compounds. When these disaccharides are attached to a third sugar as part of a polysaccharide, the number of potential trisaccharide determinants rises to 64 irrespective of whether the third sugar is glucose, galactose, or another monosaccharide. This accounts for the large number of serological 'species' in the genus *Salmonella*. Similarly, Nimmich (1968) detected only seven monosaccharides among the 72 capsular serotypes of the genus *Klebsiella*. As only a limited number of monosaccharides are found widely in micro-organisms, it is inevitable that, despite the number of possible linkages, there should be sufficient occurrence of common disaccharides or trisaccharides for serological cross-reactions to be observed. These are discussed later (see Section 4.2).

The size of the immunochemical determinant also may be relevant when the portion of the polymer molecule that is accessible to antibody is considered. Thus, in the lipopolysaccharides of gram-negative bacteria or the mannans of yeasts, there is a number of potential determinants but in the intact microbial cell not all determinants are realized. In the case of lipopolysaccharides, the side chains protrude slightly from the cell surface and are able to participate in immunological reactions. In wild-type bacteria, they are the only effective surface polysaccharide antigens. Loss of the side chains due to mutation leaves bacteria with R or rough surfaces still containing lipopolysaccharide with the 'core' portion of the molecule. This now becomes the dominant polysaccharide antigen on the surface (Figure 8). In yeast mannans, the dominant antigenic determinants

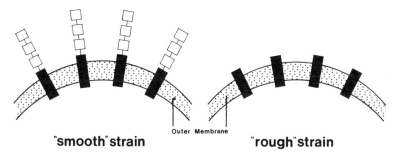

'smooth' strain   Outer Membrane   **'rough' strain**

Figure 8 Schematic representation of the dominant lipopolysaccharide antigens in wild type and mutant bacteria. The boxes represent the oligosaccharide repeating units and the shaded rectangles, the core structure, as designated in Figure 4

are again the outer portions of the molecule composed entirely of mannose (the outer chains in Figure 5), while the interior portions, including the N-acetylglucosamine residues, are of relatively minor importance.

4.2 Immunological Cross-Reactions

Serological cross-reactions are observed frequently when polysaccharides and glycoproteins are studied. A disadvantage when determining the reasons for such cross-reactions is the relatively small number of these polymers that have been characterized exhaustively. Cross-reactions have been noted between: (*i*) capsular antigens of the same bacterial species, for example, between *Kl. aerogenes* strains (Heidelberger and Dutton, 1973); (*ii*) capsular antigens of different species, for example, between *E. coli* and *Strept. pneumoniae* (Heidelberger *et al.*, 1968); (*iii*) lipopolysaccharides and capsular polysaccharides, as between

410

Shigella dysenteriae lipopolysaccharide and *Strept. pneumoniae* capsular polysaccharides (Heidelberger *et al.*, 1965); (*iv*) capsular polysaccharides and plant gums (Heidelberger, 1960); and (*v*) lipopolysaccharides and blood group substances—for example, group A substance and *Salmonella riogrande* lipopolysaccharide (Furukawa *et al.*, 1972).

In some of these examples, oligosaccharides of the same or closely related structure have been shown to be common to the cross-reacting systems, in others the reasons for the cross-reaction as yet can be postulated only from a partial knowledge of the polysaccharide components. One widely detected oligosaccharide is 3-*O*-β-D-glucuronosyl-D-galactose, which has been characterized positively in colanic acid (Figure 9) formed by *E. coli*, *Salmonella* species and

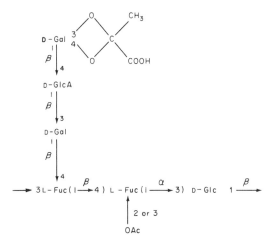

Figure 9 The structure of colanic acid from *E. coli* K 12. Results of Sutherland (1969) and Garegg *et al.* (1971*a* and *b*). Differences in acetylation and in the nature of the ketals attached to the galactose of the side chain are to be found in preparations from other strains.

Aerobacter cloacae (Roden and Markovitz, 1966; Lawson *et al.*, 1969). It is also known to form part of the linear trisaccharide repeating units identified in *E. coli* K30 capsular polysaccharide (see Table 3) (Hungerer *et al.*, 1967), and more recently, it has been identified as the side chain of the *K. aerogenes* K20 exopolysaccharide (see Table 2) (Choy and Dutton, 1972) attached to a main chain composed of mannose and glucose. It should, however, be remembered that this particular oligosaccharide also was characterized as a product of acid hydrolysis of chondroitin sulphate (Roden and Armand, 1966). It is thus found in prokaryotic and eukaryotic systems, and not unexpectedly, contributes to immunological cross-reactions between the different polysaccharides of which it is a component.

At the same time, it should be remembered that the presence of a common sequence of monosaccharides may not yield necessarily a cross-reaction which would be predicted from a knowledge of the carbohydrate structure. In the genus *Salmonella*, the serogroups B, D_1, D_2, E_1, E_2, E_3, and E_4 all contain the same trisaccharide sequence

$$\rightarrow 6)\,\text{mannosyl}(1 \xrightarrow{\alpha} 4)\text{rhamnosyl}(1 \rightarrow 3)\text{galactosyl}(1 \xrightarrow{\alpha}$$

Because other substituents are present, including O-acetyl groups and side chains of abequose, tyvelose, or glucose, not all these serogroups show serological cross-reactions. Common antigens also exist in a number of microbial groups. The effect of these is unconnected with serological cross-reactions, but represents the synthesis and presence of a polymer of the same chemical configuration in a number of (usually) closely related microbial strains. Two particular examples of polysaccharide common antigens are considered later—the C antigen of *Strept. pneumoniae* and the M antigen of the *Enterobacteriaceae*.

5 EXOPOLYSACCHARIDE ANTIGENS

As they are external to the cell wall and mask the antigenic components contained in it, extracellular polysaccharides are the dominant antigens in many micro-organisms. They are not confined to any one group of micro-organisms but have been detected in gram-positive and gram-negative bacteria, and in yeasts. Of added significance for these polymers is the absolute correlation between capsulation and virulence found in species such as *Strept. pneumoniae*. Non-capsulate mutants, obtained spontaneously on subculture or by muta-genesis, are devoid of virulence and fail to react with antisera to purified polysaccharides. The exopolysaccharide structure of several bacterial genera has been studied extensively because of the dominant role of these antigens. Most of the polymers for which complete carbohydrate structures have been determined are from *Strept. pneumoniae* and *K. aerogenes*, or *K. pneumoniae* strains. A feature of such polymers is the widespread occurrence of acid groups derived from uronic acids, ketals of pyruvate, or phosphate. The phosphorylated polymers, which are a feature of several *Strept. pneumoniae* strains, closely resemble the teichoic acids occurring commonly as cell-wall polymers in most gram-positive bacteria. Because of the presence of these acid groups, non-specific interaction with basic proteins is possible and must be distinguished from specific immunochemical reactions.

Eighty serotypes of capsular polysaccharides from *Strept. pneumoniae* have been recognized and the component monosaccharides of most of these have been determined. However, in only a small number of preparations has the exact chemical structure been elucidated. All these polymers are constructed from repeating units which range in size from the disaccharide aldobiouronic acid of type III to the much more complicated oligosaccharide of type XLI (Table 1).

Table 1 The structure of some representative *Strept. pneumoniae* exopolysaccharides

Type	Structure	Reference
I	. . . . D-GalA (1 → 3) GlcNAc (1 → 3) GalA. . . . . (part structure only)	Guy *et al.* (1967)
II	→ 3)α-L-Rha (1 → 3) α-L-Rha (1 → 3) β-L-Rha (1 → 4) α-D-Glc (1 — $\uparrow$ α-D-Glc $\uparrow$ α-D-Glc	Kenne *et al.* (1975)
III	→)3-β-D GlcA (1 → 4) β-D-Glc (1 —	Adams *et al.* (1941)
VI	→ 2)-Gal (1 $\xrightarrow{\alpha}$ 3) Glc (1 $\xrightarrow{\alpha}$ 3) Rha (1 $\xrightarrow{\alpha}$ 3) Rib-*O*-P	Rebers and Heidelberger (1961)
VIII	-Glc (1 $\xrightarrow{\beta}$ 4) Glc (1 $\xrightarrow{\alpha}$ 4) Gal (1 $\xrightarrow{\alpha}$ 4) GlcA 1 $\xrightarrow{\beta}$	Jones and Perry (1957)
XA	→ 2)D-Gal*f*(1 → 3) Gal*p* (1 → 4)-D-Gal*f*(1 → 6)-GalNAc (1 → 3) Gal*p* (1 Ribitol	Rao *et al.* (1966)
XIA	→ 3)-Gal (1 → 4) Glc (1 → 6) Glc (1 → 4) Gal (1 — | O-P-O-Glycerol	Kennedy *et al.* (1969)
XXIX	β-D-GalNAc (1 → 6) β-D-Gal*f*(1 → 3) β-D-Gal*p* (1 → 6) β-D-Gal*f*(1 → 1) Ribitol	Rao *et al.* (1969)
XXXIV	-D-Gal*f*(1 → 3) α-D-Glc*p* (1 → 2) D-Gal*f*(1 → 3) α-D-Gal*p* (1 → 2) Ribitol	Roberts *et al.* (1963)

Gal, galactose; GlcNAc, *N*-acetylglucosamine; Rha, rhamnose; Glc, glucose; Rib, ribose; GalNAc, *N*-acetylgalactosamine; GalA, galacturonic acid; GlcA, glucuronic acid; Gal*p*, galactopyranose; Gal*f*, galactofuranose

The close similarities in structure between type III and type VIII clearly indicate the reason for the cross-reaction between these two strains.

Also it has been possible, on the basis of immunochemical data, to eliminate some of the possible structures which have been proposed for particular polymers. Thus, Barker *et al.*, (1967) implied the involvement of cellobiouronic acid end groups for type II polysaccharide but a later study by Heidelberger *et al.* (1969) indicated that immune precipitation is strongly inhibited by α-D-glucuronosyl $(1 \rightarrow 6)$ D-glucose, less strongly by D-glucuronic acid, and less still by β-D-glucuronosyl $(1 \rightarrow 4)$ D-glucose (cellobiouronic acid). The effect of cellobiouronic acid and its higher analogues in inhibiting type III polysaccharide interaction with antibody indicates its role as the major antigenic determinant in this serotype (Heidelberger *et al.*, 1969). Cross-reaction with oxidised cellulose, a polymer rich in β-D-glucuronosyl $(1 \rightarrow 4)$ D-glucose segments, was noted also. A catalogue of the composition of pneumococcal exopolysaccharides and their serological interactions is to be found in the review by Heidelberger (1973).

Other *Streptococcus* species produce different polymers. These include dextrans of varying chain length and degrees of branching formed by *Strept. mutans* and related cariogenic strains (Baird *et al.*, 1973). Such polysaccharides are poorly antigenic and will not be considered further. Most other streptococcal strains are non-capsulated or produce a hyaluronic acid capsule for part of the growth cycle and degrade it by the subsequent production of hyaluronidase. Consequently, the dominant antigens are cell-wall polymers, which will be discussed later.

Other major bacterial groups for which the chemical structures of exopolysaccharide antigens have been elucidated are the genera *Klebsiella* and *Escherichia*. *K. pneumoniae* and *K.* (*Enterobacter*) *aerogenes* comprise a genus of capsulated gram-negative bacteria in which the dominant antigens are the exopolysaccharides. These are much more uniform in their carbohydrate structure than are the capsular polymers of other genera. Many are formed from tetrasaccharide repeating units, although *K. pneumoniae* serotype 1 (previously designated A) has been characterized recently as a trisaccharide (Erbing *et al.*, 1976). A few larger repeating units are known also and the structures presented in Table 2 represent the largest number known for a single bacterial genus. It should, however, be remembered that several investigations have used a single bacterial isolate. Thus, not all strains of the one serotype need possess identical carbohydrate structures and further work on this aspect is required. One study used three preparations from different type 2 strains and all had the same carbohydrate structure (Gahan *et al.*, 1967), but a re-examination of these and other polysaccharides of the same serotype (Sutherland, 1972a) indicates that the acyl groups present vary considerably. *O*-Acetyl, *O*-formyl groups, and pyruvyl ketals in various combinations are present but apparently do not play a significant role in the immunochemical reactions of this group. A number of cross-reactions occurs between *Klebsiella* exopolysaccharides. These reactions are not unexpected in view of the limited number of monosaccharides from which the different serotypes are formed (Nimmich, 1968). An example is that found between

Table 2 Repeating unit structures of *Klebsiella* exopolysaccharides

Type	Components	Structure	Reference
1	fucose, glucose, glucuronic acid, pyruvate	→ 3) Glc (1 $\xrightarrow{\beta}$ 4) GlcA (1 $\xrightarrow{\beta}$ 4) Fuc (1 $\xrightarrow{\alpha}$ 2‖3 Pyr	Erbing *et al.* (1976)
2	mannose, glucose, glucuronic acid (various acyl groups)	→ 4) Glc (1 $\xrightarrow{\alpha}$ 3) Glc (1 $\xrightarrow{\alpha}$ 4) Man (1 → 1↑3 α-GlcA	Gahan *et al.* (1967), Sutherland (1972*b*)
5	mannose, glucose, glucuronic acid, pyruvate, acetate	→ 4) GlcA (1 $\xrightarrow{\beta}$ 4) Glc (1 $\xrightarrow{\beta}$ 3) Man (1 — | 4‖6 Ac Pyr	Dutton and Yang (1973)
7	mannose, glucose, galactose, glucuronic acid, pyruvate	→ 3) GlcA (1 $\xrightarrow{\beta}$ 2) Man (1 → 3) Glc (1 — 1↑4 1↑3 4‖6 Gal Gal Pyr	Dutton *et al.* (1974)
8	glucose, galactose, glucuronic acid (acetate, pyruvate)	→ 3) Gal (1 $\xrightarrow{\beta}$ 3) Glc (1 $\xrightarrow{\alpha}$ 3) Glc (1 $\xrightarrow{\beta}$ ↑ GlcA	Sutherland (1970)
11	galactose, glucose, glucuronic acid, pyruvate	→ 3) Glc (1 $\xrightarrow{\beta}$ 3) GlcA (1 $\xrightarrow{\beta}$) Gal (1 $\xrightarrow{\alpha}$ 1↑4 Gal 4‖6 Pyr	Thurow *et al.* (1975)
20	mannose, glucose, galactose, glucuronic acid	→ 2) Man (1 $\xrightarrow{\alpha}$ 3) Gal (1 $\xrightarrow{\alpha}$ α1↑3 Gal β1↑3 GlcA	Bebault *et al.* (1973)

No.	Sugars	Structure	Reference

21	mannose, galactose, glucuronic acid, pyruvate	→ 3) GlcA (1 —α→ 3) Man (1 —α→ 2) Man (1 —α→ 3) Gal 1 —β
		  $\alpha,1\uparrow4$
		  Gal
		  4‖6
		  Pyr
			Choy and Dutton (1973)

24	mannose, glucose, glucuronic acid	→ 4) GlcA (1 —α→ 3) Man (1 —α→ 2) Man (1 —α→ 3) Glc (1 —β
		  $1\uparrow2$
		  β-Man
			Choy et al. (1973)

28	mannose, glucose, galactose, glucuronic acid	→ 2) Gal (1 —α→ 3) Man (1 —α→ 2) Man (1 —α→ 2) Glc (1 —β
		  $\beta,1\uparrow2$
		  GlcA
		  $1\uparrow3$
		  β-Glc
			Curvall et al. (1975a)

32	rhamnose, galactose, pyruvate	→ 4) Rha (1 → 4) Rha (1 → 3) Gal (1 → 3) Rha (1 → 4) Rha (1 → 3) Gal (1 —
		  2‖3
		  Pyr
			G. G. S. Dutton (unpublished results)

47	rhamnose, galactose, glucuronic acid	→ 3) Gal (1 —β→ 4) Rha (1 —α
		  $1\uparrow3$
		  GlcA
		  $1\uparrow4$
		  α-Rha
			Bjorndahl et al. (1973)

52	rhamnose, galactose, glucuronic acid	→ 4) Rha (1 → 2) Gal (1 —
		  $1\uparrow3$
		  GlcA
		  $1\uparrow4$
		  Rha
		  $1\uparrow2$
		  Gal
		  $1\uparrow3$
		  Gal
			Bjorndahl et al. (1973)

Table 2—*continued*

Type	Components	Structure	Reference
54	fucose, glucose, glucuronic acid (various acyl, no pyruvate)	→) Glc (1 →) GlcA (1 →) Fuc (1 — ↑4 1 β-Glc	Conrad *et al.* (1966), Sutherland (1967, 1970)
56	rhamnose, glucose, galactose, pyruvate	→ 3) Glc (1 —β→ 3) Gal (1 —β→ 3) Gal (1 → 3) Gal (1 —α— ‖ ↑2 Pyr α-Rha	Choy and Dutton (1973)
59	mannose, glucose, galactose, glucuronic acid, acetate	→ 3) Glc (1 —β→ 3) Gal (1 —β→ 2) Man (1 —α→ 3) Man (1 —β— ↑4 :6 :6 1 O.Ac O.Ac β-GlcA	Lindberg *et al.* (1975)
81	rhamnose, galactose, glucuronic acid	→ 2) Rha (1 —α→ 3) Rha (1 —α→ 4) GlcA (1 —β→ 2) Rha (1 —β→ 3) Gal (1 —β—	Curvall *et al.* (1975*b*)

Abbreviations as Table 1

serotypes 2, 30, and 69. All three polysaccharides contain D-mannose, D-glucose, and D-glucuronic acid, and D-galactose is found in types 30 and 69. Unpublished results from the author's laboratory have indicated the presence of several oligosaccharides common to all three polymers, but it is not yet certain whether any other components or portions of the molecule, so far unidentified, contribute to the serological cross-reactions.

The role of 2-*O*-linked, α-D-mannosyl residues in several *Klebsiella* exopolysaccharides also has been studied using lectins. Two chemotypes, K24 and K57, react with concanavalin A in precipitation tests, whereas K11 does not (Goldstein *et al.*, 1974). The reactions have been tested using the agar gel diffusion technique and by quantitative precipitation. The significance of this type of reaction, as opposed to a direct immunochemical one with homologous antisera, is the involvement of internal sugar residues rather than the terminal ones. This is in agreement with other reactions between concanavalin A and carbohydrate-containing structures with various terminal sugars but all containing at least one internal 2-*O*-αD-mannosyl residue.

The exopolysaccharide antigens of *E. coli* can be divided into three groups on the basis of their thermostability. The most stable are the A antigens which, in their gross morphology, resemble the capsular antigens of the genera *Streptococcus* or *Klebsiella*. The B and L antigens are less stable and also more difficult to detect, as they form a very thin layer surrounding the bacteria and cannot be visualized by the indian ink technique. Increased amounts of these antigens are formed at suboptimal growth temperatures (Ørskov, 1956), when the B or L antigens are apparent as capsules. The chemical composition of these antigens varies considerably according to the strain and frequently includes less common sugars such as fucosamine. Only a few of the chemotypes has been exhaustively studied, but several examples for which structures have been elucidated are given in Table 3. A more detailed account is to be found in the review by Luderitz and his associates (1968).

As well as the type-specific exopolysaccharide antigens found in *E. coli*, a further exopolysaccharide is found widely in the *Enterobacteriaceae*. This material has been called M antigen or colanic acid. Kauffmann (1936) noted the

Table 3 The structure of some *E. coli* exopolysaccharide antigens

Serotype (antigen type)	Structure	Reference
K27(A)	Gal → Glc → GlcA → Fuc	Jann *et al.* (1968)
K30(A)	Man → GlcA → Gal	Hungerer *et al.* (1967)
K42(A)	Gal → GalA → Fuc	Jann *et al.* (1965)
K85(B)	GlcA → Man → Man → GlcNAc ↑ Rha	Jann *et al.* (1966)

Abbreviations as Table 1

presence of material with the same serological specificity in various species of enteric bacteria; among the numerous subsequent reports were those of Goebel (1963) and of Linker and Evans (1968). These workers indicated the presence of an acid polysaccharide containing L-fucose, D-glucose, D-galactose, D-glucuronic acid, and acetate. The aldobiouronic acid portion of the molecule was identified by Roden and Markovitz (1966) as β-glucuronosyl $(1 \to 4)$ galactose. The repeating unit of the polymer was established later as a hexasaccharide to which a pyruvate group was attached (Figure 9) (Lawson *et al.*, 1969; Sutherland, 1969). This polysaccharide can be isolated from *E. coli* or *Salmonella* strains as well as from *Enterobacter cloacae*, and may be present as an extracellular slime or as a discrete capsule. Examination of polysaccharide preparations from different bacterial strains reveals that, although the carbohydrate structures are identical in all cases, considerable variations occur in the ketal derivative attached to the galactose side chain and in the presence, or absence, of the *O*-acetyl group (Garegg *et al.*, 1971a, b). The colanic acid may be the sole exopolysaccharide produced by the *E. coli* as occurs in *Salmonella* or *E. cloacae* strains, although it is not always formed under certain conditions of culture, or it may be present in addition to capsular antigens of the A, B, or L type. It also cross-reacts serologically with the *E. coli* K30 capsular antigen which contains the same aldobiouronic acid (Table 3).

The problem of masking of underlying cell-wall antigens can be overcome by removal of exopolysaccharide antigens. The ease with which this may be achieved varies with different bacteria. In some, stirring of the culture in a vortex mixer removes all the capsular material, but in others boiling or treatment with mild alkali is necessary. Although these methods are more drastic, little degradation of the cell wall occurs. The alkaline procedure does degrade the capsular polysaccharides by removal of *O*-acyl groups and this may be of immunochemical significance in some polymers. Pyruvate or other ketals are alkali resistant. It may be possible therefore to use the same preparation of bacteria to examine both exopolysaccharide and the underlying cell wall antigens.

6 LIPOPOLYSACCHARIDE ANTIGENS

The lipopolysaccharides or somatic antigens are found in the cell walls of virtually all gram-negative bacteria and are the subject of an enormous amount of literature because of their unique immunochemical and pharmacological properties. Many genera and species have been studied, but particular emphasis has been placed on pathogenic and closely related bacteria forming the family *Enterobacteriaceae*.

As can be seen in Figure 4, the structure of lipopolysaccharides is complex and, despite the presence of oligosaccharide repeating units in those polymers which have been examined rigorously, there are numerous structural permutations to account for the many known serological reactions. The genus *Salmonella* will be used to exemplify these polymers, as this group of bacteria probably has received most attention, but lipopolysaccharides are of equal importance in pathogenic

Pseudomonas aeruginosa (Chester *et al.*, 1973; Wilkinson and Galbraith, 1975), *E. coli* (Lüderitz *et al.*, 1968) and other strains.

The early serological work which produced the Kauffmann–White scheme for the serological differentiation of *Salmonella* isolates (summarized by Kauffmann, 1966) shows excellent correlation with the chemical studies of Lüderitz, Jann, and other workers (Lüderitz *et al.*, 1966; Lüderitz, 1970), although improved techniques in carbohydrate chemistry are revealing still further facets of lipopolysaccharide structure. The way in which the gross chemical composition is related to the serological group and to antigenic factors is shown in Table 4. The structures of some of the repeating units found in the polysaccharides or representative serotypes are shown in Table 5. The frequency with which the mannosyl-rhamnosyl-galactosyl sequence occurs can be noted easily, as can the numerous side chains attached to the repeating units. These side chains account for many of the major antigenic determinants. Other serogroups contain different oligosaccharide sequences, but also show the presence of immunodominant side chains never exceeding single monosaccharides attached to sugars in the oligosaccharide repeating units. The number of oligosaccharides forming the O antigens varies greatly, probably both as a result of the mechanism of their biosynthesis and as a consequence of slight degradation during extraction and purification. An unusual group of mutants (SR—Semi-rough) contains one oligosaccharide only attached to the core structure. In addition to the monosaccharides detailed in the O antigens, all *Salmonella* lipopolysaccharides possess a common core structure composed of D-glucose, D-galactose, *N*-acetyl-D-glucosamine, heptose, and ketodeoxyoctonic acid (Figure 10). Other genera of

Table 4 The serological and chemical relationships of *Salmonella* lipopolysaccharide antigens

Species	Group	Antigen factors [a]	O-specific sugars in the lipopolysaccharides
S. paratyphi A	A	1, 2, 12	mannose, rhamnose, paratose
S. paratyphi B	B	4, 5, 12	mannose, rhamnose, abequose
S. typhimurium		4, 5, 12	mannose, rhamnose, abequose
S. abortusequi		4, 12	mannose, rhamnose, abequose
S. paratyphi C	C	6, 7	mannose
S. cholera suis		6, 7	mannose
S. montevideo		6, 7	mannose
S. typhi	D	9, 12	mannose, rhamnose, tyvelose
S. enteritidis		1, 9, 12	mannose, rhamnose, tyvelose
S. sendai		1, 9, 12	mannose, rhamnose, tyvelose
S. anatum	E	3, 10	mannose, rhamnose
S. newington		3, 15	mannose, rhamnose
S. minneapolis		(3), (15), 34	mannose, rhamnose
S. senftenberg		1, 3, 19	mannose, rhamnose

Reproduced from Lüderitz (1970), with permission of Verlag Chemie

Table 5 The antigenic side-chains of some Salmonella serogroups

Group	Antigenic factors	Repeating units of side chains
B	1, 4, 12	α-Abe $\quad\quad\quad$ α-Glc $1\downarrow_3$ $\quad\quad\quad\quad$ $1\downarrow_6$ $\rightarrow$ [2) Man (1 $\rightarrow$ 4) Rha (1 $\rightarrow$ 3) Gal (1 $\xrightarrow{\alpha}$]
D_1	9, 12	α-Tyv $\quad\quad\quad$ α-Glc-O-Ac $1\downarrow_3$ $\quad\quad\quad\quad$ $1\downarrow_6$ $\rightarrow$ [2) Man (1 $\rightarrow$ 4) Rha (1 $\rightarrow$ 3) Gal (1 $\xrightarrow{\alpha}$]
D_2	(9), 46	α-Tyv $1\downarrow_3$ $\rightarrow$ [6) Man (1 $\xrightarrow{\alpha}$ 4) Rha (1 $\rightarrow$ 3) Gal (1 $\xrightarrow{\alpha}$]
E_1	3, 10	O.Ac | $\rightarrow$ [6) Man (1 $\xrightarrow{\alpha}$ 4) Rha (1 $\rightarrow$ 3) Gal (1 $\xrightarrow{\alpha}$]
C	6, 7	$\rightarrow$ [Man (1 $\rightarrow$ 2) Man (1 $\rightarrow$ 2) Man (1 $\rightarrow$ 2) Man (1 $\rightarrow$ 3) GlcNAc —] $1\uparrow^3$ Glc
L	21	$\rightarrow$ [Glc (1 $\xrightarrow{\beta}$ 3) GalNAc $\rightarrow$ GalNAc —] $\uparrow$ $\quad\quad\quad\quad\quad\quad$ $\uparrow$ Gal $\quad\quad\quad\quad\quad$ α-GalNAc
N	30	$\rightarrow$ [Glc (1 $\xrightarrow{\beta}$ 3) GalNAc (1 $\rightarrow$ 3) GalNAc $\rightarrow$ Fuc —] $1\uparrow^3$ Glc
U	43	$\rightarrow$ [Gal (1 $\xrightarrow{\beta}$ 3) GalNAc (1 $\rightarrow$ 3) GlcNAc (1 $\rightarrow$ 4) Fuc —] $1\uparrow^3$ α-Gal

Abbreviations as Table 1; Tyv, tyvelose

the *Enterobacteriaceae* possess similar structures in their lipopolysaccharides, that is side chains composed of oligosaccharides, together with a core structure, but have unique chemical structures and immunological specificities.

Other groups of gram-negative bacteria show greater divergence from the enterobacterial 'norm'. Some lack heptose or other sugars from the core structure, although all appear to contain ketodeoxyoctonic acid (Ellwood, 1970). Side chains are thought to be present in most lipopolysaccharides but vary greatly in their composition; many contain unusual amino sugars or monosaccharides such as *O*-methylxylose, while glucose, galactose, mannose, rhamnose, and fucose occur widely. It is not the author's intention to list all the possible structures, but the interested reader is referred to reviews by Luderitz (1970), Simmons (1971) and Wilkinson (1977).

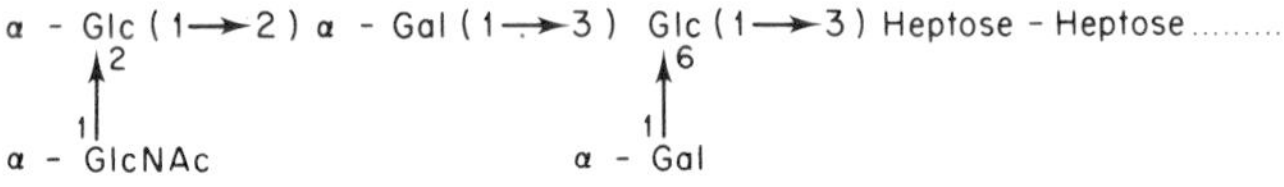

α - Glc (1 $\longrightarrow$ 2) α - Gal (1 $\longrightarrow$ 3) Glc (1 $\longrightarrow$ 3) Heptose - Heptose ....
$\quad\quad\uparrow^2$ $\quad\quad\quad\quad\quad\quad\quad\quad\quad\quad\quad\quad\quad\quad$ $\uparrow^6$
$\quad\quad\quad 1\mid$ $\quad\quad\quad\quad\quad\quad\quad\quad\quad\quad\quad\quad\quad\quad\quad\quad$ $1\mid$
α - GlcNAc $\quad\quad\quad\quad\quad\quad\quad\quad\quad\quad\quad\quad$ α - Gal

Figure 10 The structure of the core of *Salmonella* lipo-polysaccharides

There are numerous opportunities for cross-reactions with other antigens and these have been noted frequently. At the same time, it should be remembered that the different antigens ascribed to a given strain, for example, *S. paratyphi* has the antigenic formula 1, 2, 12, form part of a single polymer molecule. The actual determinant group comprising these factors is an oligosaccharide about the size of a hexasaccharide (Lüderitz *et al.*, 1968), that is the degree of polymerization ranges from four to seven or eight.

Numerous examples have been reported of immunochemical relationships between lipopolysaccharides and blood group substances. Several of these are listed in Table 6. The lipopolysaccharide of *E. coli* O86 has a carbohydrate

Table 6 Cross-reactions between bacterial lipopolysaccharides and blood group substances

Lipopolysaccharide	Bacterial		Reaction with blood group	Reference
	Group	Serotype		
Shigella dysenteriae		—	O(H)	Eisler (1930)
Salmonella paratyphi B		5	A	Yamamoto *et al.* (1963)
S. typhimurium				
S. poona	B	13	O(H)	Iseki (1952)
S. worthington				
S. bulawayo				
S. riogrande	R	40		
S. duval			A	Sakai *et al.* (1954)
E. coli	6			
S. milwaukee		43	B	Springer *et al.* (1961)
E. coli		086B7	B	Springer (1956)
Salmonella spp	U		B	Springer *et al.* (1961)

composition similar to that of blood group substances, containing D-galactose, *N*-acetyl-D-glucosamine, and L-fuctose, in addition to the core structure (Springer *et al.*, 1964). The partial structure was determined later and as can be seen in Figure 11 it is structurally very similar to the oligosaccharide structures found in blood group substances. Oligosaccharides derived from the *E. coli* also inhibit the blood group B system (Springer *et al.*, 1966). Furthermore, there is cross-reaction with lipopolysaccharides from *Salmonella* species belonging to serogroup U. All these polysaccharides, bacterial and eukaryotic, have a common disaccharide sequence of α-galactosyl(1 → 3)galactosyl, which is the probable cause of the cross-reaction. Lüderitz *et al.* (1965) characterized this

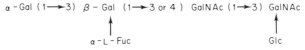

Figure 11 Lipopolysaccharide with blood group activity. The partial structure of *E. coli* O86 lipopolysaccharide conferring blood group B activity

disaccharide in *S. milwaukee* (serogroup U) as part of the pentasaccharide sequence α-D-galactosyl(1 → 3)β-D-galactosyl(1 → 3)*N*-acetylgalactosaminyl-(1 → 3)D-*N*-acetylglucosaminyl-(1 → 4)L-fucose.

A similar study with *S. riogrande* lipopolysaccharide led to isolation of the hexasaccharide α-*N*-acetylgalactosaminyl(1 → 3)mannosyl-glucosyl(1 → 3)*N*-acetylgalactosaminyl-glucosyl-(*N*-acetylglucosamine) (Furukawa *et al.*, 1972), which actively inhibits the blood group A system. The only portion of this oligosaccharide with a structure common to human blood group A substance is the terminal α-*N*-acetylgalactosaminyl residue. This is thus the most likely common antigenic determinant. The lipopolysaccharide (or whole cells) of *S. riogrande* fails to absorb anti-A agglutinin, although antiserum to the lipopolysaccharide reacts with group A erythrocytes and group A saliva. This is indicative of the failure of the anti-A agglutinin to form a close enough association with the bacterial cells due to the differences in the non-terminal portion of the oligosaccharide.

These particular interactions with blood group systems are absent in rough mutants of the bacteria, which lack the O-antigenic determinants. However, some strains, which have no blood group activity in the smooth (wild type) forms, reveal it in R mutants (Iseki and Onuki, 1960). Two *Citrobacter freundii* strains (B_{124} and B_{131}), which in the smooth form lack any blood group A activity, are strongly active in A systems after mutation to rough forms. Llpopolysaccharides from both rough mutants contained D-glucose, D-galactose, and *N*-acetyl-D-glucosamine. The core structure of *Citrobacter* and other enterobacterial species differs from that indicated in Figure 10 for *Salmonella*.

A further technique for demonstrating blood group activity and similar immunochemical relationships in lipopolysaccharides was reported recently by Hammarström *et al.* (1972). In this approach, use was made of A haemagglutinin from the snail *Helix pomatia*. This protein was purified extensively and was found to precipitate polymers containing a number of non-reducing terminal α-*N*-acetyl-D-galactosamine residues, including blood group A substance, streptococcal C polysaccharide, and certain teichoic acids. Polymers containing non-reducing β-*N*-acetyl-D-glucosamine residues do not react nor do lipopolysaccharides isolated from rough mutants reduced to the backbone or glucosylated backbone (Figure 10). Lipopolysaccharides from rough mutants containing terminal α-*N*-acetyl-D-glucosamine, α-D-glucose, or α-D-galactose were precipitated. The structure common to all the reactive rough lipopolysaccharides is α-D-galactosyl(1 → 6)D-glucose (melibiose) (see Figure 10) and this fragment was postulated as the dominant portion involved in recognition in a manner analogous to immunochemical reactions.

7 TEICHOIC ACIDS AND OTHER CARBOHYDRATE ANTIGENS OF GRAM-POSITIVE BACTERIAL WALLS

As well as polymers of glycerol phosphate and ribitol phosphate found in gram-positive bacteria and classically regarded as teichoic acids, several similar

Table 7   The immunodominant components of teichoic acids

Bacteria	Serogroup	Teichoic acid	Determinant
Lactobacillus spp.	A	glycerol	α-glucose . . . . . .
	D	ribitol	α-glucose . . . . .
	F	glycerol	α-glucose . . . . .
Streptococcus spp.	D	glycerol	α-glucosyl (1 → 2) glucose . . .
Strept. mutans	I	glycerol	β-galactose . . . .
	II	ribitol	β-galactose . . . .

polymers of sugar phosphates will be considered here. Antisera against these polymers are prepared readily, although the association of many glycerol teichoic acids with the bacterial membrane may necessitate prior cell breakage. As acid-extracted teichoic acids are haptenic but not immunogenic, Knox and Wicken (1973) suggested the use of lectins or the A haemagglutinin of *Helix pomatia* for their study. The polyol phosphates generally contain attached monosaccharides, particularly glucose and galactose, which are immunodominant portions of the molecules. Thus glycerol or ribitol-containing teichoic acids with common α-D-glucosyl residues cross-react with other polymers containing α-D-glucosyl residues (Knox and Wicken, 1972). Most of the group antigens of the genus *Lactobacillus* are teichoic acids, but the immunodominant component is neither glycerol nor ribitol (Table 7). Surprisingly, the D-alanyl substituent, which is widely found in teichoic acids (see Figure 12), relatively seldom is involved in immunochemical specificity (McCarty, 1964). Evidence was presented by Sanderson *et al* (1961) that in a teichoic acid preparation from *Staphylococcus aureus*, containing alanine, *N*-acetylglucosamine, and ribitol, the immunodominant components are α-*N*-acetylglucosaminyl residues. β-linked residues of the same amino sugar are also present in the preparation but are not immunologically important. An examination of two glycerol teichoic acids from streptococcal strains indicated that, although both contain glucosylated polyglycerol phosphates (Wicken and Baddiley, 1963), the determinant groups are not identical. In one strain, the disaccharide α-D-glucosyl(1 → 2)glucose (kojibiose) is attached to glycerol residues. The teichoic acid from the second strain contains the corresponding trisaccharide, namely α-D-glucosyl(1→2)α-D-glucosyl(1→2)-glucose. Considerable cross-reaction between polymers with such similar substituents would be expected and very careful analysis is required to distinguish the glycosyl substituents.

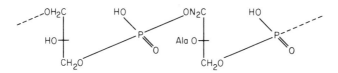

Figure 12   An alanine-containing teichoic acid structure

Knox *et al.* (1970) also indicated that misleading results might be obtained due to partial degradation of teichoic acids during their extraction from cell walls. In a study of an intracellular galactosylated polyglycerol phosphate representing the group F antigen in *Lactobacillus* species, they noted that partially degraded material of low molecular weight reacts poorly with antisera. A higher molecular weight product in the form of lipoteichoic acid—teichoic acid complexed with lipid—is a potent antigen.

Immunochemical specificity directed towards the polyol phosphate portion of teichoic acid molecules would account for several observed reactions between gram-positive bacteria. This was confirmed by McCarty (1959). An antiserum against group A *Streptococcus* species reacts with polyglycerol phosphate as well as with extracts from many gram-positive bacteria, and no such reaction has been noted using similar extracts prepared from gram-negative bacteria. The reaction can be ascribed to the presence of glycerol teichoic acids from gram-positive cocci. Other bacterial species have been reviewed by Knox and Wicken (1973).

The teichoic acids found as exopolysaccharide polymers in cultures of several serotypes of *S. pneumoniae* are generally more complex in their structure than those isolated from walls or membranes. Roberts *et al.* (1963) recognized that the exopolysaccharide of *S. pneumoniae* type XXXIV was formed from pentasaccharide repeating units

[*O*-D-galacto*furano*syl(1 ⟶ 3)*O*-α-D-gluco*pyrano*syl(1 ⟶ 2)*O*-D-galacto*furano*syl(1 ⟶ 3)*O*-α-D-galacto*pyrano*syl(1 ⟶ 2)ribitol]

The polymer is unusual in containing both furanosyl and pyranosyl, five and six-membered ring forms, respectively, of galactose. Galactofuranose has since been recognized as a component of various other polysaccharides. The exopolysaccharide from type XA is even more complex—a ribitol teichoic acid—which is composed of at least a hexasaccharide repeating unit in which galactose is present again in both furanose and pyranose forms, together with *N*-acetyl-D-galactosamine (Rao *et al.*, 1966).

Polymers of hexose phosphates, as opposed to polyol phosphates, occur widely in the cell walls of gram-positive bacteria and can be considered as being analogous to the phosphogalactans in yeasts (Slodki, 1966). In a *Micrococcus* species, Partridge *et al.* (1971) characterized a polymer of *N*-acetylgalactosamine 1-phosphate which comprises about 43 per cent by weight in the bacterial walls. It contains equimolar amounts of D-glucose, *N*-acetyl-D-galactosamine, and phosphate, and a repeating disaccharide unit has been postulated, having the structure 3-*O*-α-D-glucosyl-*N*-acetyl-D-galactosamine. The phosphate was linked to the C6 of the glucose and the C1 of the amino sugar.

Strept. pneumoniae cell walls contain a further type of polysaccharide, the so-called C substance, and also contains *N*-acetylgalactosamine phosphate, as well as *N*-acetylglucosamine, glucose, and choline. The chemical similarity of the C substance to depyruvylated type IV pneumococcal exopolysaccharide led to serological cross-reactions, and it was suggested that phosphorylcholine is an important antigenic determinant in the C substance (Heidelberger *et al.*, 1972).

By growing of the pneumococci in an ethanolamine-containing medium, the surface polymer can be altered from one containing choline to one containing ethanolamine (Tomasz, 1968). This causes changes in the surface properties of the bacteria which have been discussed extensively in a review by Tomasz (1973). Although 90 per cent of the choline in the walls of *Strept. pneumoniae* is accounted for by the presence of the C substance, a further choline-containing antigenic polymer has been reported (Briles and Tomasz, 1973). This material reacts with Forsmann antigens of mammalian cell surfaces and is similar in chemical composition to C substance, containing ribitol phosphate, glucose, and galactosamine.

From this account, it can be seen that even the walls of a single bacterial species may contain more than one polymer of antigenic importance in which the immunodominant portion is essentially carbohydrate.

8 POLYSACCHARIDE ANTIGENS OF YEAST CELL WALLS

The yeast cell wall contains two types of polysaccharides—glucan and mannan—polymers of D-glucose and D-mannose, respectively. The glucan is a structural polymer conferring rigidity on the microbial walls and plays only a minor role in the antigenicity of the walls. In intact cells, it is probably part of a complex to which are attached protein and mannan.

Although of less significance in the study of yeasts than of prokaryotes, the serology of yeast cell wall polysaccharides has become a subject of increasing

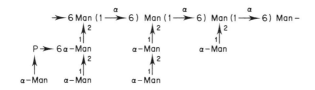

Kloeckera brevis

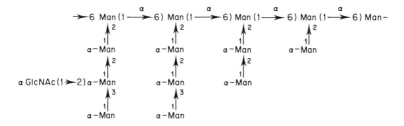

Kluyveromyces lactis

Figure 13   Two yeast mannan side chains containing the immunodominant part of the molecules

study (see, for example, Campbell, 1971). The mannan was recognized earlier as the major antigen on the yeast cell surface (Hasenclever and Mitchell, 1964). This polysaccharide could be prepared relatively easily and in reasonably high yield by acetolysis which involves the simultaneous hydrolysis and acetylation of the fragments produced.

The complexity of yeast mannans has been indicated in Figure 5. In the intact cell in which they exist as mannoproteins, protein may comprise between 5 and 50 per cent by weight of the complex. Gross differences in mannan preparations from different yeasts have been indicated by analysis of the acetolysis preparations (Ballou, 1974). Fragments identified from several yeast preparations include mannose, mannobiose, mannotriose, phosphorylated mannotriose, mannotetraose and pentaose, and a further pentasaccharide recognizable as a mannotetraose attached to N-acetylglucosamine. Several of these oligosaccharides inhibit agglutination of yeast cells by homologous antisera. As a result of such studies, Raschke and Ballou (1972) have identified the immunodominant side chains in several yeast species (Figure 13). Further details and examples are to be found in Ballou (1974).

9 BLOOD GROUP ANTIGENS

The gross chemical composition of preparations of highly purified blood group-active material is essentially similar even when this material displays the differing A, B, H, and Le^a immunological specificities. Each preparation contains L-fucose, D-galactose, N-acetylglucosamine, and N-acetylgalactosamine (Table 8). Sialic acid is found also in such preparations (Pusztai and Morgan, 1961). This component varies in amount from 1 to 18 per cent; high concentrations occur in preparations originating from cyst fluids (Morgan, 1963). Much wider variations in the composition of blood group substances are found if material from erythrocyte glycolipids is studied. Indeed, most of the information on the chemical nature of the carbohydrate determinants of blood group substances has derived from studies of material of non-erythrocytic origin. Thus, the analyses presented in Table 8 relate to blood group-active substances isolated from ovarian cyst fluids, but many of the oligosaccharides showing inhibition of the

Table 8 Carbohydrate composition of blood group substances

Specificity	Nitrogen (per cent)	Methyl-pentose (per cent)	Galactose (per cent)	Hexosamine (per cent)	Galactosamine (per cent)	Reducing sugar (per cent)
A	5·4	19	26	29	14	54
B	5·6	16	34	24	6	52
H	5·3	18	29	28	7	50
AB	5·6	17		26		54
Le^a	5·6	14		32		56

reaction between blood group substances and their homologous antisera have been obtained from human milk, urine, or meconium.

The similarity in chemical composition of the different blood group substances, extending even to the amino acid compositions of the peptide moieties, indicates that the serological differences must relate to the nature and configuration of glycosidic bonds that form part of the surface of the molecular structures. These differences are accentuated further by the non-uniformity of eukaryotic glycoproteins. Thus, attempts to obtain information about the polymer structure by the use of partial acid hydrolysis may lead to an extremely complex series of fragments. A further problem is seen in the results for A-active material. A number of oligosaccharides has been isolated and characterized from partial acid hydrolysates, but not all are active inhibitors of the A–anti-A serum system. The inactive fragments must be presumed to originate from underlying portions of the glycopeptide structure which are not involved directly in the immunochemical interactions. Of the eight oligosaccharides obtained by various workers (see Watkins, 1972), only three (a disaccharide with galactose as the terminal reducing sugar, and two trisaccharides containing equimolar amounts of N-acetylgalactosamine, N-acetylglucosamine, and galactose) are active inhibitors of anti-A serum.

A similar picture emerges from attempts to isolate fragments with activity in the blood group B–anti-B reactions. Fucose-containing oligosaccharides were obtained by Schiffman et al. (1960) from partial acid hydrolysates of group B material, but none of these reacted with the test system. Some oligosaccharides common to several blood group substances also have been isolated and are indicative of a basic underlying structure in the glycoprotein (Rege et al., 1963). However, Painter et al. (1962, 1963) have separated a disaccharide and two trisaccharides (Table 9) which are active inhibitors of anti-B serum. Although fucose is present in both A and B substances, it is clear from the results presented in Tables 9 and 10 that fucose-containing oligosaccharides are not responsible for either the A or B antigenic determinants. Fucose does not inhibit agglutination of Le^a erythrocytes by antisera, but the monosaccharide nevertheless does have an important role in determining the Le^a specificity. This was confirmed by the use of oligosaccharides isolated from human milk and characterized by Kun (1957). As with the oligosaccharides studied in the A system, not all are potential inhibitors even when the α-L-fucose residues are present.

Table 9 Active oligosaccharides isolated from blood group B material

Oligosaccharide	Reference
α-D-galactosyl (1 → 3) galactose	Painter et al. (1962)
α-D-galactosyl (1 → 3) β-D-galactose (1 → 3) N-acetyl-D-glucosamine	Painter et al. (1963)
α-D-galactosyl (1 → 3) β-D-galactose (1 → 4) N-acetyl-D-glucosamine	Painter et al. (1963)

Table 10   Oligosaccharides isolated from blood group A-active material

Oligosaccharide	Activity
β-D-Gal (1 → 3) GlcNAc	—
β-D-Gal (1 → 4) GlcNAc	—
β-D-GlcNAc (1 → 3) Gal	—
α-L-Fuc (1 → 6) GlcNAc	—
β-D-Gal (1 → 3) GalNAc	—
α-GalNAc (1 → 3) Gal	+
α-GalNAc (1 → 3) β-D-Gal (1 → 4) GlcNAc	+
α-GalNAc (1 → 3) β-D-Gal (1 → 3) GlcNAc	+

Use of the polystyrene sulphonic acid hydrolytic technique and of alkaline degradation methods has yielded other oligosaccharides from A and B substances, some of which contain α-fucosyl branches. These results indicate that fucosyl residues, although not required for the specific immunochemical activities are present on certain of the terminal oligosaccharide sequences of the blood group A and B substances. Examination of Le^a substances reveals the converse situation, namely a number of non-fucose-containing fragments devoid of activity and an immunologically active fucose-containing oligosaccharide, together with more complex fragments containing the same terminal structure (Figure 14). H and Le^b substances also have given rise to a number of

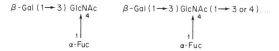

Figure 14   Oligosaccharides from Le^a material with Le^a activity

immunochemically active fucosylated fragments. Also present in the preparations are inactive oligosaccharides from which the fucose residues had been removed during the hydrolytic process (Figure 15). Many of the inactive compounds are similar in their chemical composition to those already isolated from A and B substances and known to be inactive in these systems. There is thus

H active β - Gal (1 → 4) GlcNAc β - Gal (1 → 3) GlcNAc
                    $_1\uparrow^2$ $_1\uparrow^2$
            α - Fuc α - Fuc

Le^b active β - Gal (1 → 3) GlcNAc β - Gal (1 → 3) GlcNAc (1 → 3) Gal
                    $_1\uparrow^2$ $_1\uparrow^4$ $_1\uparrow^2$ $_1\uparrow^4$
            α - Fuc α - Fuc α - Fuc α - Fuc

Figure 15   Oligosaccharides derived from H Le^b material

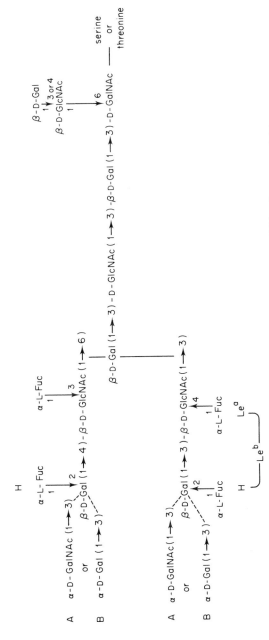

Figure 16 A composite picture of possible sources of blood group activities

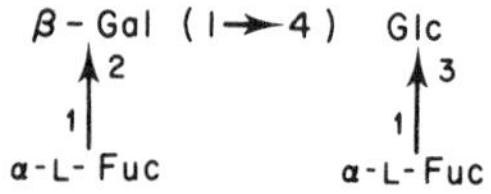

$$\beta - \text{Gal} \quad (1 \longrightarrow 4) \quad \text{Glc}$$

$$\begin{array}{ccc} \uparrow 2 & & \uparrow 3 \\ 1 & & 1 \\ \alpha - \text{L-Fuc} & & \alpha - \text{L-Fuc} \end{array}$$

From Bjorndal and Lindblad (1970)

Figure 17 Oligosaccharide isolated from the urine of O(H) secretors

considerable sharing of carbohydrate structure within the blood group substances. On the basis of the isolation of branched oligosaccharides by various workers and in particular of the branched pentasaccharide

β-galactosyl(1 $\longrightarrow$ 4)β-N-acetylglucosaminyl(1 $\longrightarrow$ 6)

galactose

β-galactosyl(1 $\longrightarrow$ 3)β-N-acetylglucosaminyl(1 $\longrightarrow$ 3)

Lloyd *et al.* (1968) suggested that the A, B, H, and Le activities derive from the structure shown in Figure 16.

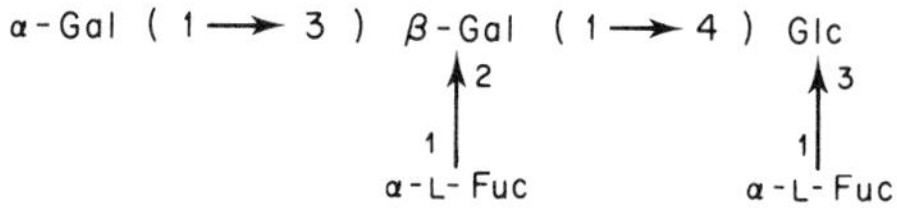

$$\alpha - \text{Gal} \quad (1 \longrightarrow 3) \quad \beta - \text{Gal} \quad (1 \longrightarrow 4) \quad \text{Glc}$$

$$\begin{array}{ccc} \uparrow 2 & & \uparrow 3 \\ 1 & & 1 \\ \alpha - \text{L-Fuc} & & \alpha - \text{L-Fuc} \end{array}$$

From Bjorndal and Lindblad (1970)

Figure 18 An oligosaccharide from urine of B secretors

As well as the oligosaccharides prepared by acidic or alkaline hydrolysis of polymeric blood group-active material, small molecular weight compounds with blood group activity have been isolated from other sources. Lundblad (1967, 1968) and Bjorndal and Lundblad (1970) used urine as a source of blood group-active oligosaccharides, which then were separated and purified by gel permeation chromatography and high voltage electrophoresis. In this way, two distinct pentasaccharides were isolated from A_1 and B secretors. Both contained glucose as the terminal reducing sugar, but one pentasaccharide (Figure 7) inhibited only the A_1–anti-A system, whereas the other (Figure 8) was active in the B–anti-B and O–anti-H systems. Another oligosaccharide from the urine of O(H) secretors (Lundblad, 1968) was identified tentatively as lactodifucotetraose (Figure 19). Bourillon and Goussauld (1968) obtained a polysaccharide with

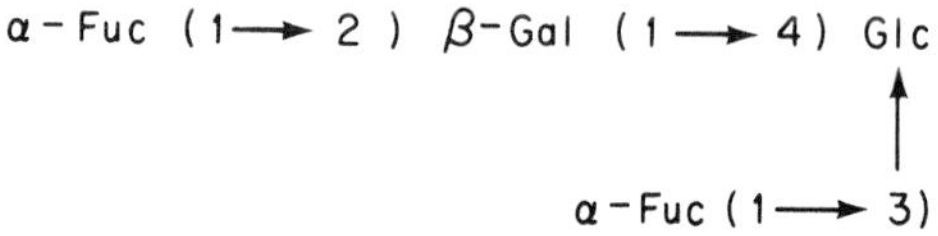

$$\alpha - \text{Fuc} \quad (1 \longrightarrow 2) \quad \beta - \text{Gal} \quad (1 \longrightarrow 4) \quad \text{Glc}$$

$$\begin{array}{c} \uparrow \\ \alpha - \text{Fuc} \quad (1 \longrightarrow 3) \end{array}$$

Figure 19 The structure of lactodifucotetraose

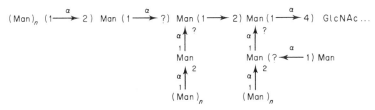

Figure 20 Thyroglobulin core structure as proposed by Arima and Spiro (1972)

O(H) activity from urine and the tetrasaccharide may be biosynthesized from this polymer. The polysaccharide contains 20 per cent fucose, with galactose and glucosamine as the other major components, as well as lesser amounts of other sugars, including mannose, glucose, and galactosamine. This polysaccharide inhibits both the eel antiserum and *Ulex* lectin systems.

The other major source of blood group-active oligosaccharides is human milk and a number of oligosaccharides from this source has been characterized. Originally, pooled milk samples were studied until it was realized that the compounds present varied with the blood group of the donor. Kobata *et al.*

$$..... Man\ (1\xrightarrow{\ \beta\ }4)\ GlcNAc\ (1\xrightarrow{\ \beta\ }4)\ GlcNAc\longrightarrow Asn..........$$

Figure 21 The possible structure of the glycoprotein core of ovalbumin. Results of Lee and Scocca (1972)

(1969), using single samples of milk, identified four oligosaccharides present in milk from Le[b] donors, but not from Le[a]. All contained the disaccharide sequence O-α-L-fucosyl($1 \rightarrow 2$)O-β-D-galactose. Huang (1971) has isolated several *N*-acetylneuaminic acid-containing oligosaccharides from human milk. The use of insolubilized lectins, already applied to the purification of polysaccharides by Lloyd (1970), will find wide application in the separation of oligosaccharides.

Eukaryotic cells contain numerous other glycoproteins, both at the surface and as intracellular or secreted products. Few of these have been studied as extensively as blood group substances; consequently much less is known about

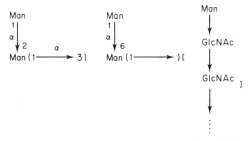

Figure 22 Core structure of γ-M-Immunoglobulin. From Hickman *et al.* (1972)

432

their immunochemistry. The close similarity in the carbohydrate structure of the core region of a number of glycoproteins is exemplified by thyroglobulin (Figure 20) (Arina and Spiro, 1972), ovalbumin (Figure 21) (Lee and Scocca, 1972), and other glycoproteins (Figure 22) (Hickman *et al.*, 1972). Similarities between these structures and the yeast mannans in their general mode of structure can be recognized. Hence, some of the results from studies on the immunochemistry of mannans from wild-type and mutant yeast mannans may be relevant to studies on other eukaryotic glycoproteins.

10 ALTERATIONS TO POLYSACCHARIDE ANTIGENS

10.1 Mutations

Changes in polysaccharide antigens due to mutation can occur in different ways, largely reflecting differences in their biosynthesis. Exopolysaccharides show an all-or-none effect, that is any mutation, other than in acyl groups, leads to loss of polymer production (Sutherland, 1972b). The only changes which have been recognized in exopolysaccharides derived from the same bacterial strain have been in the presence or absence of acetyl groups. These alterations do not seem to affect the synthesis of the polymer. In examining alterations to mannans in the yeast *Kluyveromyces lactis*, Smith *et al.* (1975) noted that whereas one side chain has the structure shown in Figure 13 and the mannotetraose, and its derivative containing *N*-acetylglucosamine, are immunodominant, mutants lack the amino sugar. Some mutants lack only *N*-acetylglucosamine, others contain neither the amino sugar nor the mannotetraose unit. Other portions of the mannon molecule are present still and apparently are unaltered.

Lipopolysaccharides resemble the mannans, as numerous mutations can occur, ranging from an almost complete loss of the monosaccharide residues, to a reduction in the O antigen from a chain of 10–20 repeating units to a single oligosaccharide attached to the core structure. Such alterations can occur due to, for example, the loss of a sugar transferase or a sugar synthetase. Reduction of the O antigen to a single repeat unit (SR or semi-rough mutation) leaves material capable of reacting with O antisera, wheras mutants lacking O material exhibit new R specificities (see p. 409 and Figure 8). The different types of mutations in lipopolysaccharide biosynthesis have been discussed in numerous reviews (see for example Nikaido, 1973) and are indicated in Figure 23. The other significant changes to the immunochemistry of lipopolysaccharide are those invoked by lysogenic conversion which will be discussed in Section 10.3.

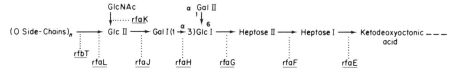

Figure 23 Rough mutations leading to loss of lipopolysaccharide

Studies also have been made on the probable changes in composition and immunochemistry of blood group substances due to mutation. These have been reviewed by Watkins (1974). The accumulation of knowledge on the structure and biosynthesis of blood group substances has enabled a projection of the likely results from mutational changes on several carbohydrate structures responsible for the activities in A, B, and other systems. The glycoproteins each possess several specificities, which can now be accounted for on a simple enzymic basis. Thus, galactosylation controlled by the B gene can result in the alteration of H structures, yielding B activity (Figure 24) (Watkins, 1974). Such studies need to be developed further before all the questions posed by blood specificities and carbohydrate structures can be answered.

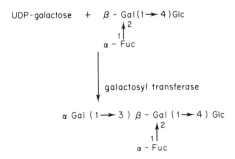

Figure 24   The mode of galactosylation of blood group substances

10.2 Enzymic Alterations

Two groups of enzymes are active on polysaccharide antigens—those that alter the nature of the monosaccharide residue at the point of chain breakage and those that cleave the glycosidic bond hydrolytically. A few of the enzymes of each type will be discussed here. Some of these enzymes are highly specific, acting only on a single polymer or a few structurally related polysaccharides, while others act on a specific component present in numerous polymers provided that the component is present in the correct configuration and linkage.

Exoglycosidases hydrolyse terminal monosaccharides. Some only act on relatively small oligosaccharides, while others act readily on terminal sugars of polysaccharides or glycoproteins. Typical of this latter type is an α-galactosidase studied by Springer *et al.* (1964). This enzyme removes terminal α-linked galactosyl residues from *E. coli* O86 lipopolysaccharide, an oligosaccharide also possessing group B activity, and B-active material in bovine erythrocytes. Simultaneously, blood group H(O) activity is unmasked in all three preparations (Table 11).

Although exoenzymes, in general, have provided more information about blood group substances or polymers of the yeast mannan type, some of the earlier results must be interpreted with caution as enzymes of unknown purity were

434

Table 11 Enzyme action on blood group substances

Enzyme source	Substrate	Products	Reference
Clostridium tertium	A substance	galactose, *N*-acetyl glucosamine Gal (1 → 3) GlcNAc	Schiffman *et al.* (1958)
	O(H) substance	galactose, amino sugar	
Trichomonas foetus	B substance	galactose, amino sugar (fucose)	Watkins (1959)
Clostridium sp.	B substance	galactose	Iseki *et al.* (1959)
Coffee beans (α-Galactosidase)	B substance	galactose	Zarnitz and Kabat (1960)
Bacillus cereus	O(H) substance	fucose (galactose)	Iseki *et al.* (1960)
B. cereus	Le^a substance	fucose, galactose	Furukawa and Iseki (1964)

Sugars in brackets indicate minor products of enzymic hydrolysis

used. Various exoglycosidases are frequently present in the source material and careful purification is required to ensure that the final product is a single enzyme, the specificity of which can be studied with confidence. The enzyme activity has been noted mainly using isolated blood group substances, but the corresponding glycolipids or erythrocytes also may provide suitable substrates.

As well as liberating monosaccharides, the exoglycosidases yield residual polymeric material which may (*i*) retain its original antigenic specificity (albeit at a reduced level), (*ii*) retain that specificity and exhibit new specificities, or (*iii*) lose the original specificity entirely and reveal completely new specificity. Examples of such actions have been reported during studies on enzymes acting on blood group substances and related polymers. When more than one enzyme is present, or when the polymer is treated sequentially with different enzymes, more than one specificity may be exposed then removed. The deliberate induction of a sequence of enzymes was used in the study of a glycoprotein carried out by Barker *et al.* (1963). Orosomucoid was used to induce an *N*-acetylneuraminidase and to release all terminal *N*-acetylneuraminic acid residues from the polymer. The residual polymeric material was subsequently used to induce an L-α-fucosidase. The non-diffusible product is reactive with antisera to *Strept. pneumoniae* type XIV polysaccharide, in which the immunodominant sugars are terminal β-D-galactosyl residues. Subsequent induction of a β-galactosidase removes terminal galactose residues and the immunochemical activity of the non-diffusible product with the pneumococcal antisera simultaneously. The identity of the bacteria in which this sequence of enzymes is capable of being induced was somewhat doubtfully reported as *Rhodopseudomonas palustris*, but the source and characteristics of this culture were not indicated.

Yeast cell-wall mannans are also substrates for an exoenzyme, exo-α-D-mannosidase prepared from an *Arthrobacter* species (Gorin *et al.*, 1969). Polymers containing mannose and galactose are resistant unless non-reducing terminal galactose residues are removed first using acid hydrolysis. The specificity of the enzyme is such that the sequence α-D-mannosyl(1 → 2)β-D-mannosyl(1 → 2)β-D-mannosyl(1 → ... is not a substrate. This has been interpreted as a requirement for two consecutive α-linked mannopyranose residues before a compound becomes a suitable substrate.

Endoenzymes have been reported usually from studies on polymers composed of regular repeating units such as microbial exopolysaccharides. The enzymes may be hydrolases which yield saturated products through addition of water

$$X-O-Y + H_2O \longrightarrow X-OH + Y-OH$$

or they may be lyases (eliminases), yielding both a saturated and an unsaturated fragment.

One eliminase, which is active against an exopolysaccharide from the yeast *Cryptococcus neoformans*, yields partially decapsulated cells which are more immunogenic than the original preparation (Gadebusch, 1960). Prolonged enzymic treatment removes all polysaccharide and antigenicity. A similar enzyme active on *Strept. pneumoniae* type VIII polysaccharide has been shown to produce a tetrasaccharide (Becker and Pappenheimer, 1966; Campbell and Pappenheimer, 1966a)

dehydroglucuronic acid(1 $\longrightarrow$ 4)glucosyl(1 $\xrightarrow{\beta}$ 4)glucosyl(1 $\xrightarrow{\beta}$ 4)galactose.

This oligosaccharide strongly inhibits precipitation of type VIII polysaccharide by homologous antisera, despite the introduction of the unsaturated uronic acid—a conformation not originally present in the polymer (Campbell and Pappenheimer, 1966b). The polysaccharide of *Strept. pneumoniae* type III also is depolymerized by an endoglycosidase, but this enzyme is a hydrolase, yielding a series of oligosaccharides of general structure

$$[\beta\text{-glucosyl}(1 \longrightarrow 3)\text{glucuronic acid}]_n$$

where n is from one to four, that is the oligosaccharides have a degree of polymerization (DP) of two to eight (Campbell and Pappenheimer, 1966b). These oligosaccharides inhibit the polysaccharide–antiserum reaction, the inhibition increasing with chain length.

Bacteriophage have been a much more fruitful source of endopolysaccharases for bacterial exopolysaccharides than have heterologous bacteria (Sutherland, 1972a). One such system was studied by Watson (1966). A phage-induced enzyme active against K. aerogenes type 2 polysaccharide effectively removes the polymer from coated erythrocytes, preventing agglutination with specific antisera. The enzyme has been identified as an endomannosidase, hydrolysing the type 2 polysaccharide to the component tetrasaccharide irrespective of the acyl groups also present

$$\text{glucose} \longrightarrow \text{glucose} \longrightarrow \text{mannose}$$
$$\uparrow$$
$$\text{glucuronic acid.}$$

Enzymes hydrolysing lipopolysaccharides, and teichoic acids are known also but, as their immunochemical significance has not been investigated, they will not be considered here.

10.3 Phage Conversion

The properties of many bacteria can be altered by the presence of a temperate (avirulent) virus (bacteriophage). The bacteriophage apparently carries genetic information acquired from a previous host and as long as the bacteriophage is maintained within the new host bacteria, new properties are expressed. Loss of the bacteriophage leads to a simultaneous loss of the new properties. Typical of such systems are the control of protein exotoxin production (toxigenicity) in Corynebacterium diphtheriae and the conversion of many lipopolysaccharides in gram-negative bacteria. The lipopolysaccharides of various genera and species have been shown now to be subject to phage conversion.

The process of phage conversion has been studied most thoroughly in Salmonella of serogroup E. Strains containing antigens 3 and 10, when infected with bacteriophage ε^{15}, show an almost immediate acquisition of a new antigen (15) and the loss of one of the original antigens (10). In the original bacteria, the lipopolysaccharide contains α-galactosyl residues which are also acetylated (Uchida et al., 1963). The new antigen lacks O-acetyl and contains β-linked galactose, thus three separate reactions affecting the immunochemistry of the lipopolysaccharide appear to occur: (i) O-acetyl groups are lost; (ii) α-galactose residues are lost; and (iii) β-galactose residues are formed. (Wright and Kanegasaki, 1971). These changes are due to the repression of the host enzymes involved in O-acetylation, the hydrolytic action of a phage-associated enzyme (Kanegasaki and Wright, 1973), and the induction of a new polymerase enzyme, respectively. The strains with antigenic specificity 3, 15 can be converted further by a second group-specific bacteriophage (ε^{34}) to antigen 34. The net result is the glucosylation of the O antigen (Figure 25). Although phage conversion affecting lipopolysaccharides occurs widely within the genus Salmonella, it has been

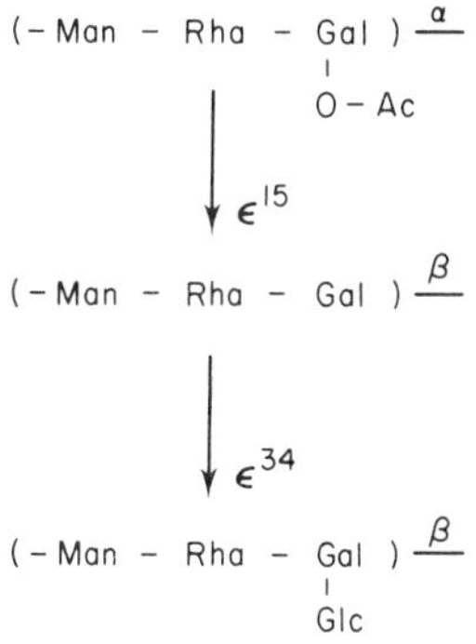

$$(- \text{Man} - \text{Rha} - \text{Gal}) \xrightarrow{\alpha}$$
$$| \\ O - Ac$$

$$\downarrow \epsilon^{15}$$

$$(- \text{Man} - \text{Rha} - \text{Gal}) \xrightarrow{\beta}$$

$$\downarrow \epsilon^{34}$$

$$(- \text{Man} - \text{Rha} - \text{Gal}) \xrightarrow{\beta}$$
$$| \\ Glc$$

Figure 25 Phage conversion in group E *Salmonella*

detected also in other genera of gram-negative bacteria such as *Shigella* (Itikawa, 1964). Because of the alterations which occur to the antigenic determinants, it is a process of considerable interest and importance to those studying the immunochemistry of lipopolysaccharides. Some of the known mechanisms involved in the alterations are listed in Table 12.

10.4 Chemical Alterations

Any chemical alteration of a carbohydrate-containing antigen is likely to change the immunochemical reactions of the polymer. When acidic (or alkaline)

Table 12 Examples of phage conversion

Phage	Alteration	Bacteria	Antigen structure	
			Before	After conversion
P22	glucosylation	*Salmonella* A, B, D	$\downarrow$ $\rightarrow$ Man $\rightarrow$ Rha $\rightarrow$ Gal —	α-Glc $\downarrow \qquad \downarrow$ $\rightarrow$ Man $\rightarrow$ Rha $\rightarrow$ Gal —
ε^{34}	glucosylation	*Salmonella* E	$\rightarrow$ Man $\rightarrow$ Rha $\rightarrow$ Gal —	α-Glc $\downarrow$ $\rightarrow$ Man $\rightarrow$ Rha $\rightarrow$ Gal —
ε^{15}	deacetylation	*Salmonella* E	O.Ac $|$ $\rightarrow$ Man $\rightarrow$ Rha $\rightarrow$ Gal —	$\rightarrow$ Man $\rightarrow$ Rha $\rightarrow$ Gal —
ε^{15}	polymer configuration	*Salmonella* E	O.Ac $|$ $\rightarrow$ Man $\rightarrow$ Rha $\xrightarrow{\alpha}$ Gal —	$\rightarrow$ Man $\rightarrow$ Rha $\xrightarrow{\beta}$ Gal —
ϕ 27	polymer configuration	*Salmonella* A, B, D	$\downarrow$ $\rightarrow$ 2 Man $\rightarrow$ Rha $\rightarrow$ Gal —	$\rightarrow$ 6 Man $\rightarrow$ Rha $\rightarrow$ Gal —

Further examples are to be found in the review by Nikaido (1973). The presence of a linkage on the mannose residues is indicative of a dideoxyhexose such as abequose or tyvelose

hydrolysis is used, the most frequent products are a series of oligosaccharides, some of which may be the same as those resulting from enzymic action. These fragments are, of course, extremely important in immunochemical studies as has been mentioned already with respect to all the major types of antigens discussed in this article. The oligosaccharides have been used widely as inhibitors of immune precipitation and, in a few examples, have been coupled to acceptors to form immunogens. The main drawback to the use of the products of partial acid hydrolysis is the need to isolate and purify relatively large amounts of oligosaccharides which are probably present as minor products of the hydrolysate. Fewer studies have been made on the macromolecular products remaining after partial acid hydrolysis. This could also yield significant information about polysaccharide antigens.

The *Strept. pneumoniae* type IV exopolysaccharide contains D-galactose, *N*-acetyl-D-galactosamine, *N*-acetyl-D-mannosamine, and a third amino sugar which is probably *N*-acetylfucosamine. There are also pyruvyl groups which are responsible for the type-specific reaction, resembling in this respect, certain polysaccharides from *Rhizobium* species in which pyruvylated sugars are also immunodominant groupings (Heidelberger *et al.*, 1970). Although stable in alkaline solutions, pyruvyl ketals are removed by mild acid hydrolysis using 0·01 N acid at 100°. Application of this procedure to *Strept. pneumoniae* type IV polysaccharide removes most of the pyruvate after 10–15 minutes, without causing any extensive degradation of the carbohydrate sequences (Higginbotham *et al.*, 1970). The depyruvylated polymer cross-reacts with antisera to other polymers that have shown no reaction with antisera to the intact polysaccharide. In particular, there is a new cross-reaction with *Strept. pneumoniae* C substance in which Gottschlich and Liu (1967) have shown that *N*-acetylgalactosamine 6-phosphate is the immunodominant sugar. Thus, the presence of pyruvate on the type IV polysaccharide is sufficient apparently to prevent interaction with the antiserum to C substance. Removal of the pyruvate residues, which are most likely to have been attached to D-galactose, exposes the *N*-acetylgalactosamine residues in a polymer which then shows some structural resemblance to C substance. As well as interaction with anti-C-serum, the depyruvylated polysaccharide reacts with the so-called 'C-reactive protein', whereas there is no precipitation of C-reactive protein by the original polysaccharide.

Pyruvate also plays a major role in the immunochemistry of exopolysaccharides prepared from *R. trifolii* and *R. meliloti* and was thought to be involved in the immune reaction of *Strept. pneumoniae* type 27 exopolysaccharide (Dudman and Heidelberger, 1969). Removal of pyruvate from the *R. trifolii* polysaccharide preparation produces a polymer incapable of interaction with antisera to the pyruvylated material or to type 27 polysaccharide. Instead, depyruvylated *R. trifolii* polysaccharide precipitates antisera to *Strept. pneumoniae* types VI, VII, VIII, IX, X, and XIV. In this case also, the removal of pyruvate from a polysaccharide exposes other monosaccharides as the new immunodominant components of the polymer.

Two other types of alteration can be applied to polysaccharides, namely reduction and oxidation. In those polymers which contain uronic acids, the process of carboxyl reduction converts the –COOH groups to —CH$_2$OH, thus glucuronic acid is converted to glucose, and mannose is formed from mannuronic acid. The stereochemistry of the monosaccharide and the anomeric nature of the linkages to adjacent sugars is conserved in each case. This technique can be applied to determine whether the uronic acid is important in the immunochemical reactions of the polymer. Oxidation is much less specific. The use of the mild oxidizing agent periodate oxidizes all monosaccharides which are neither branch points nor linked through the three position. The technique is used widely to characterize the linkages of sequences of monosaccharides, but Eriksen (1969) also has studied the immunochemistry of oxidized bacterial polysaccharides. She found that several oxidized polymers are immunologically active both in precipitation reactions and as antigens. *K. aerogenes* type 1 polysaccharide is essentially resistant to oxidation and retains the original antigenic specificity, whereas oxidized type 7 polysaccharide gains a new specificity. Antisera to oxidized type 7 polysaccharide do not react with unoxidized material. On the other hand, oxidized type 11 polysaccharide reacts with antisera to the original polymer, revealing both a line of identity with unoxidized polysaccharide and other precipitation lines. This was thought to indicate that antibodies to oxidized polysaccharide are induced in animals immunized with the natural polysaccharide, as was confirmed by quantitative precipitation tests. The antibodies against oxidized polysaccharide predominate early in the immunization period but decline later. The same phenomenon has been noted with *Klebsiella* type 21 polysaccharide. Oxidation and reduction can also be applied to oligosaccharides derived from the polymers, to determine the immunochemical significance of certain monosaccharides within the structures.

11 CONCLUSIONS

Polysaccharides and glycoproteins, whether from prokaryotic or eukaryotic sources, are an important group of antigens in which the immunodominant groupings vary considerably. The current knowledge of the chemistry, biosynthesis, and immunochemistry of these polymers makes it possible to present a clear picture of many of the structures involved. These may be subjected to alteration by chemical and biological means leading to changes in the antigenic determinant or, in some cases, to complete loss of the antigen. One polysaccharide or glycoprotein molecule can be the source of numerous antigenic determinants not all of which are exposed simultaneously. In several of the more complex polymers, mutation or enzymic treatment enables a previously masked determinant to become immunodominant. The examples provided in this chapter indicate the various types of polysaccharide and glycoprotein antigens which exist and some of the mechanisms by which they have been studied.

REFERENCES

Adams, M. H., Reeves, R. E., and Goebel, W. F. (1941). *J. Biol. Chem.*, **140**, 653.
Arima, T., and Spiro, R. G. (1972). *J. Biol. Chem.*, **247**, 1836.

Baird, J. K., Longyear, V. M. C., and Ellwood, D. C. (1973). *Microbios*, **8**, 143.
Ballou, C. E. (1974). *Adv. Enzymol.*, **40**, 239.
Barker, S. A., Pardoe, G. I., Stacey, M., and Hopton, J. W. (1963). *Nature, Lond.*, **197**, 231.
Barker, S. A., Somers, P. J., and Stacey, M. (1967). *Carb. Res.*, **3**, 261.
Bebault, G. M., Choy, Y. M., Dutton, G. G. S., Furnell, N., Stephen, A. M., and Yang, M. T. (1973). *J. Bacteriol.*, **113**, 1345.
Becker, G., and Pappenheimer, A. M. (1966). *Biochim. Biophys. Acta*, **121**, 343.
Björndal, H., Lindberg, B., Lönngren, J., Meszaros, M., Thompson, J. L., and Nimmich, W. (1973). *Carb. Res.*, **31**, 93.
Björndal, H., and Lundblad, A. (1970). *Biochim. Biophys. Acta*, **201**, 434.
Briles, E. B., and Tomasz, A. (1973). *J. Biol. Chem.*, **248**, 6394.
Bourillon, R., and Goussauld, Y. (1968). *Carb. Res.*, **8**, 175.

Campbell, I. (1971). *J. Appl. Bacteriol.*, **34**, 237.
Campbell, J. H., and Pappenheimer, A. M. (1966a). *Immunochemistry*, **3**, 195.
Campbell, J. H., and Pappenheimer, A. M. (1966b). *Immunochemistry*, **3**, 213.
Chester, I. R., Meadow, P. M., and Pitt, T. (1973). *J. Gen. Microbiol.*, **78**, 305.
Choy, Y. M., and Dutton, G. G. S. (1972). *J. Bacteriol.*, **112**, 635.
Choy, Y. M., and Dutton, G. G. S. (1973). *Can. J. Chem.*, **51**, 198.
Choy, Y. M., Dutton, G. G. S., and Zanlunga, M. (1973). *Can. J. Chem.*, **51**, 1819.
Collins, F. M. (1964). *Aust. J. Exp. Biol. Med. Sci.*, **42**, 255.
Conrad, H. E., Bamburg, J. R., Epley, J. D., and Kindt, T. J. (1966). *Biochemistry*, **5**, 2808.
Curvall, M., Lindberg, B., Lönngren, J., and Nimmich, W. (1975a) *Carb. Res.*, **42**, 73.
Curvall, M., Lindberg, B., Lönngren, J., and Nimmich, W. (1975b). *Carb. Res.*, **42**, 95.

Dudman, W. F., and Heidelberger, M. (1969). *Science, N.Y.*, **164**, 954.
Duguid. (1951). *J. Path. Bact.*, **63**, 673.
Dutton, G. G. S., Stephen, A. M., and Churms, S. C. (1974). *Carb. Res.*, **38**, 225.
Dutton, G. G. S., and Yang, M. T. (1973). *Can. J. Chem.*, **51**, 1826.

Eisler, M. Z. (1930). *ImmunForsch.*, **67**, 32.
Ellwood, D. C. (1970). *J. Gen. Microbiol.*, **60**, 373.
Ellwood, D. C., and Tempest, D. W. (1969). *Biochem. J.*, **111**, 1.
Ellwood, D. C., and Tempest, D. W. (1972). *Adv. Microbiol. Physiol.*, **7**, 83.
Erbing, C., Kenne, L., Lindberg, B., Lönngren, J., and Sutherland, I. W. (1976). *Carb. Res.*, **50**, 115.
Eriksen, J. (1969). *J. Immunol.*, **17**, 33.

Furukawa, K., and Iseki, S. (1964). *Proc. Japan. Acad.*, **40**, 588.
Furukawa, K., Kochibe, N., Takizawa, H., and Iseki, S. (1972). *Jap. J. Microbiol.*, **16**, 199.

Gadebusch, H. H. (1960). *J. Infect. Dis.*, **107**, 406.
Gahan, L. C., Sandford, P. A., and Conrad, H. E. (1967). *Biochemistry*, **6**, 2755.
Galanos, C., Lüderitz, O., and Himmelspach, K. (1969). *Eur. J. Biochem.*, **8**, 332.
Garegg, P. J., Lindberg, B., Onn, T., and Holme, T. (1971a). *Acta chem. scand.*, **25**, 1185.
Garegg, P. J., Lindberg, B., Onn, T., and Sutherland, I. W. (1971b). *A ta chem. scand.*, **25**, 2103.
Goebel, W. F. (1963). *Proc. Nat. Acad. Sci., U.S.A.*, **49**, 464.
Goldstein, I. J., Reichert, C. R., and Misaki, A. (1974). *Ann. N.Y. Acad. Sci.*, **236**, 283.

Gorin, P. A. J., Spencer, J. F. T., and Eveleigh, D. E. (1969). *Carb. Res.*, **11**, 387.
Gotschlich, E. C., and Liu, T. Y. (1967). *J. Biol. Chem.*, **242**, 463.
Guy, R. C. E., How, M. J., Stacey, M., and Heidelberger, M. (1967). *J. Biol. Chem.*, **242**, 5106.

Hammarström, S., Lindberg, A. A., and Robertson, E. S. (1972). *Eur. J. Biochem.*, **25**, 274.
Hasenclever, H. F., and Mitchell, W. O. (1964). *Sabouradia*, **3**, 288.
Heidelberger, M. (1960). *Prog. Chem. Org. Natur. Prod.*, **18**, 503.
Heidelberger, M. (1973). In *Research in Immunochemistry*, Vol. 3 (Kwapinski, J. B. G., ed.), University Park Press, Baltimore, p. 1.
Heidelberger, M., and Dutton, G. G. S. (1973). *J. Immunol.*, **111**, 857.
Heidelberger, M., Dudman, W. F., and Nimmich, W. (1970). *J. Immunol.*, **104**, 1321.
Heidelberger, M., Gotschlich, E. C. and Higginbotham, J. D. (1972). *Carb. Res.*, **22**, 1.
Heidelberger, M., Jann, K., Jann, B., Ørskov, F., Ørskov, I., and Westphal, O. (1968). *J. Bacteriol.*, **95**, 2415.
Heidelberger, M., Rao, C. V. N., and Davies, D. A. L. (1965). *Pathol. Microbiol.*, **28**, 691.
Heidelberger, M., Roy, N., and Glaudemanans, C. P. J. (1969). *Biochemistry*, **8**, 4822.
Hickman, S., Kornfeld, R., Osterland, C. K., and Kornfeld, S. (1972). *J. Biol. Chem.*, **247**, 2156.
Higginbotham, J. D., Heidelberger, M., and Gotschlich, E. C. (1970). *Proc. Nat. Acad. Sci., U.S.A.*, **67**, 138.
Hungerer, D., Jann, K., Jann, B., Ørskov, F., and Ørskov, I. (1967). *Eur. J. Biochem.*, **2**, 115.
Huang, R. T. C. (1971). *Hoppe Seylers Z. Physiol. Chem.*, **352**, 1645.

Iseki, S. (1952). *Gunma J. Med. Sci.*, **1**, 1.
Iseki, S., Furukawa, K., and Motegi, O. (1960). *Proc. Jap. Acad.*, **36**, 675.
Iseki, S., Furakawa, K., and Yamamoto, S. (1959). *Proc. Jap. Acad.*, **35**, 507.
Iseki, S., and Okunuki, E. (1960). *Jap. J. Microbiol.*, **4**, 123.
Itikawa, H. (1964). *Jap. J. Genet.*, **38**, 317.

Jann, K., Jann, B., Ørskov, I., and Ørskov, F. (1966). *Biochem. Z.*, **346**, 368.
Jann, K., Jann, B., Ørskov, I., Ørskov, F., and Westphal, O. (1965). *Biochem. Z.*, **342**, 1.
Jann, K., Jann, B., Schneider, K. F., Ørskov, F., and Ørskov, I. (1968). *Eur. J. Biochem.*, **6**, 456.
Jones, J. K., and Perry, M. B. (1957). *J. Am. Chem. Soc.*, **79**, 2787.

Kabat, E. A. (1968). *Immunology and Immunochemistry*, Holt, Rinehart and Winston, New York.
Kanegasaki, S., and Wright, A. (1973). *Virology*, **52**, 160.
Kauffmann, F. (1936). *Z. Hyg. InfektKrankh.*, **117**, 778.
Kauffmann, F. (1966). *The Bacteriology of the Enterobacteriaceae*, Munksgaard, Copenhagen.
Kenne, L., Lindberg, B., and Svensson, S. (1975). *Carb. Res.*, **40**, 69.
Kennedy, D. A., Buchanan, J. G., and Baddiley, J. (1969). *Biochem. J.*, **115**, 37.
Knox, K. W., Hewett, M. J., and Wicken, A. J. (1970). *J. Gen. Microbiol.*, **60**, 303.
Knox, K. W., and Wicken, A. J. (1972). *Archs Oral Biol.*, **17**, 1491.
Knox, K. W., and Wicken, A. J. (1973). *Bacteriol. Rev.*, **37**, 215.
Kobata, A., Ginsburg, V., and Tsuda, M. (1969). *Archs Biochem. Biophys.*, **130**, 509.
Kristiansen, T., and Porath, J. (1968). *Biochim. Biophys. Acta*, **158**, 351.
Kuhn, R. (1957). *Angew. Chemie*, **60**, 23.

Lawson, C. J., McLeary, C. W., Nakada, H. I., Rees, D. A., Sutherland, I. W., and Wilkinson, J. F. (1969). *Biochem. J.*, **115**, 947.

442

Lee, Y. C., and Scocca, J. R. (1972). *J. Biol. Chem.*, **247**, 5753.

Lindberg, B., Lönngren, J., Ruden, U., and Nimmich, W. (1975). *Carb. Res.*, **42**, 83.

Linker, A., and Evans, L. R. (1968). *Nature (Lond.)*, **218**, 774.

Lloyd, K. O. (1970). *Archs Biochem. Biophys.*, **137**, 460.

Lloyd, K. O., Kabat, E. A., and Licerio, E. (1968). *Biochemistry*, 7, 2966.

Lüderitz, O. (1970). *Angew. Chemie*, **9**, 649.

Lüderitz, O., Jann, K., and Wheat, R. (1968). In *Comprehensive Biochemistry*, Vol. 26a (Florkin, M., and Stotz, E. H., eds.), Elsevier, Amsterdam, p. 105.

Lüderitz, O., Simmons, D. A. R., and Westphal, O. (1965). *Biochem. J.*, **97**, 820.

Lüderitz, O., Staub, A. M., and Westphal, O. (1966). *Bacteriol. Rev.*, **30**, 192.

Lundblad, A. (1967). *Biochim. Biophys. Acta*, **148**, 151.

Lundblad, A. (1968). *Biochim. Biophys. Acta*, **165**, 202.

Mage, R. G., and Kabat, E. A. (1963). *Biochemistry*, **6**, 1278.

McCarty, M. (1959). *J. Exp. Med.*, **109**, 361.

McCarty, M. (1964). *Proc. Nat. Acad. Sci., U.S.A.*, **52**, 259.

Morgan, W. T. J. (1963). *Ann. N.Y. Acad. Sci.*, **106**, 177.

Morgan, W. T. J. (1970). In *British Biochemistry Past and Present* (Goodwin, T. W., ed.), Academic Press, New York and London, p. 99.

Nikaido, H. (1973). In *Bacterial Membranes and Walls* (Leive, L., ed.), Dekker, New York, p. 131.

Nimmich, W. (1968). *Z. Med. Mikrobiol. Immunol.*, **154**, 117.

Ørskov, F. (1956). *Acta path. microbiol. scand.*, **39**, 147.

Painter, T. J. (1960). *Chemy Ind.*, p. 1214.

Painter, T. J., Watkins, W. M., and Morgan, W. T. J. (1962). *Nature (Lond.)*, **193**, 1042.

Painter, T. J., Watkins, W. M., and Morgan, W. T. J. (1963). *Nature (Lond.)*, **199**, 282.

Partridge, M. D., Davison, A. L., and Baddiley, J. (1971). *Biochem. J.*, **121**, 695.

Pusztai, A., and Morgan, W. T. J. (1961). *Biochem. J.*, **78**, 135.

Rao, E. V., Buchanan, J. G., and Baddiley, J. (1966). *Biochem. J.*, **100**, 801.

Rao, E. V., Watson, M. J., Buchanan, J. G., and Baddiley, J. (1969). *Biochem. J.*, **111**, 547.

Raschke, W. C., and Ballou, C. E. (1972). *Biochemistry*, **11**, 3807.

Rebers, P. A., and Heidelberger, M. (1961). *J. Am. Chem. Soc.*, **83**, 3056.

Rege, V. P., Painter, T. J., Watkins, W. M., and Morgan, W. T. J. (1963). *Nature (Lond.)*, **200**, 532.

Roberts, W. K., Buchanan, J. G., and Baddiley, J. (1963). *Biochem. J.*, **88**, 1.

Roden, L., and Armand, G. (1966). *J. Biol. Chem.*, **241**, 65.

Roden, L., and Markovitz, A. (1966). *Biochim. Biophys. Acta*, **127**, 252.

Sakai, T., Serizawa, K., and Iseki, K. (1954). *Gunma J. Med. Sci.*, **3**, 239.

Sanderson, A. R., Juergens, W. G., and Strominger, J. L. (1961). *Biochem. Biophys. Res. Commun.*, **5**, 472.

Schiffman, G., Howe, C., and Kabat, E. A. (1958). *Fed. Proc.*, **17**, 534.

Schiffman, G., Howe, C., Kabat, E. A. (1969). *Fed. Proc.*, **17**, 534.

Simmons, D. A. R. (1971). *Bacteriol Rev.*, **35**, 117.

Slodki, M. E. (1966). *J. Biol. Chem.*, **241**, 2700.

Smith, W. L., Nakajima, T., and Ballou, C. E. (1975). *J. Biol. Chem.*, **250**, 3426.

Springer, G. F. (1956). *J. Immunol.*, **76**, 399.

Springer, G. F., Nichols, J. H., and Callahan, H. J. (1964). *Science, N.Y.*, **146**, 946.

Springer, G. F., Wang, E., Nichols, J., and Shear, J. (1966). *Ann. N.Y. Acad. Sci.*, **133**, 566.

Springer, G. F., Williamson, P., and Brandes, W. C. (1961). *J. Exp. Med.*, **113**, 1077.

Sutherland, I. W. (1967). *Biochem. J.*, **104**, 278.
Sutherland, I. W. (1969). *Biochem. J.*, **115**, 935.
Sutherland, I. W. (1970). *Biochemistry*, **9**, 2180.
Sutherland, I. W. (1972a). *J. Gen. Microbiol.*, **70**, 331.
Sutherland, I. W. (1972b). *Adv. Microbiol. Physiol.*, **8**, 143.

Thurow, H., Choy, Y. M., Frank, N., Niemann, H., and Stirm, S. (1975). *Carb. Res.*, **41**, 241.
Tomasz, A. (1968). *Proc. Natn. Acad. Sci., U.S.A.*, **59**, 86.
Tomasz, A. (1973). In *Bacterial Membranes and Walls* (Leive, L., ed.), Dekker, New York, p. 321.

Uchida, T., Robbins, P. W., and Luria, S. E. (1963). *Biochemistry*, **2**, 66.

Watkins, W. M. (1959). *Biochem. J.*, **71**, 261.
Watkins, W. M. (1972). In *Glycoproteins: Their Composition, Structure and Function* (Gottschalk, A., ed.), Elsevier, Amsterdam, p. 830.
Watkins, W. M. (1974). *Biochem. Soc. Symp.*, **40**, 125.
Watson, K. C. (1966). *Immunology*, **10**, 121.
Westphal, O., Lüderitz, O., and Bister, F. (1952). *Z. NaturForsch.*, **76**, 148.
Wicken, A. J., and Baddiley, J. (1963). *Biochem. J.*, **87**, 54.
Wilkinson, S. G. (1977). In *Surface Carbohydrates of Prokaryotes* (Sutherland, I. W., ed.), Academic Press, New York and London, p. 97.
Wilkinson, S. G., and Galbraith, L. (1975). *Eur. J. Biochem.*, **52**, 331.
Wright, A., and Kanegasaki, S. (1971). *Physiol. Rev.*, **51**, 748.

Yamamoto, S., Kogure, T., Ichikawa, H., and Iseki, S. (1963). *Gunma J. Med. Sci.*, **12**, 6.

Zarnitz, M. L., and Kabat, E. A. (1960). *J. Am. Chem. Soc.*, **82**, 3953.

CHAPTER 12

Interaction of Haptens with Proteins and their Immunogenicity

J. L. Turk and D. Parker

1 INTRODUCTION

The term 'hapten' was first described by Landsteiner in 1921 in a discussion of experiments on the immunogenicity of extracts of tissues containing the Forsmann antigen. A protein-free, alcohol extract of horse kidney was found to have a high affinity for Forsmann antibodies, but had no immunizing capacity. However, the immunizing capacity could be restored by addition of the alcohol precipitate which contained the protein. The term hapten was therefore first used to describe a substance with the capacity to react with antibody but not to immunize. The word is derived from the Greek, meaning to grab or fasten. In this original experiment, the hapten was a polysaccharide containing the antigen-determining site of a larger immunogenic molecule. The term hapten is now used to include artificial, as well as naturally occurring, chemical agents. These substances are mainly of low molecular weight and all are able to bind to antibody without inducing an immune response unless conjugated to a carrier protein.

The preparation of artificially conjugated antigens by Landsteiner and his colleagues bridged the gap that previously existed between immunology and chemistry. In the original experiments (Landsteiner and Lampl, 1918), a number of azo compounds were formed by diazotization of serum proteins. Rabbits injected with artifically prepared azo-proteins developed precipitating antibodies in their serum which were specific, within chemically defined limits, for the attached chemical grouping. The groupings, originally described by Landsteiner and Lampl (1918), were mainly azo dyes such as aniline and *o*-aminobenzoic acid which were bound to protein through a covalent linkage. Such dyes are not antigenic by themselves and only become so by means of their linkage to protein. It was therefore possible to extend the concept of haptens to these and similar compounds.

The use of artifically conjugated hapten–protein conjugates is essential in order to study the nature of antigenicity. By preparing proteins with chemically defined antigen-determining sites, it has been possible to investigate the antigen-recognition site of the immunoglobulin molecule and of the immunologically reactive lymphocyte. Artificially conjugated proteins also contribute to the present knowledge of the physical chemistry of the antibody combining site. Quantitative assessment of the binding strength of antibody for conjugated antigens provides further information on the stereochemical nature of the combination between the combining site on the antibody and the antigenic determinant.

Although much of the current data has been derived from artificial conjugates in which haptens have been linked covalently to the carrier protein, there is also evidence that, in some cases, the linkage may be of a weaker nature involving hydrogen bonding or even Van der Waal's forces.

2 ARTIFICIAL HAPTENS AND THEIR CONJUGATION THROUGH COVALENT LINKAGES

2.1 Hapten Specificity of Humoral Antibody

Much of the knowledge about the nature of the antigen determinant site stems from work using artificially conjugated antigens. The earliest synthetic antigens to be prepared were the azo-proteins formed by coupling proteins with diazonium compounds. These coloured products, which were developed by the aniline dye industry, depended on the preparation of *p*-hydroxyazobenzene from phenol and benzenediazonium chloride (Figure 1). It was found that when rabbits were injected with such dyes covalently linked to proteins, the antibody that developed had a greater specificity for the attached simple chemical grouping than for the carrier protein. Azo dyes bind to proteins covalently through the amino acids tyrosine and histidine. Although a molecule of serum albumin

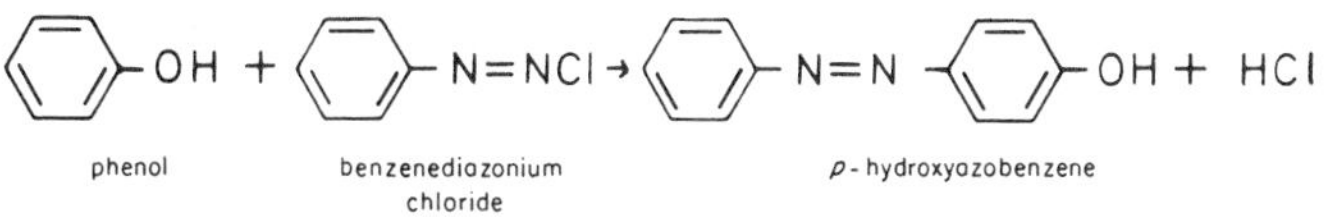

Figure 1 Preparation of *p*-hydroxyazobenzene

contains 30 such amino acids, only 10 residues need to be occupied to make the protein reactive, and over a certain concentration the protein will become unreactive (Haurowitz, 1936).

Experiments were performed in which the serum produced against an azo-protein from one species was as effective in precipitating a different protein linked to the same azo dye. Such experiments were decisive in establishing the specific reactivity of haptenic groups in artificial compound antigens. However, a crude antiserum prepared against an azo-protein not only contains antibodies specific to the hapten alone, but also possesses antibodies directed against the carrier protein itself, as well as antibodies which may be directed towards azo-proteins made from this or related proteins linked to the same or other azo dyes. These antibodies are of particular interest because of their carrier protein specificity and their direction to the linkage between the hapten and the protein.

Proof that the antibody can link directly to the hapten comes from hapten inhibition studies. The strength of the reaction between the hapten and the antibody can be quantified by the effect of increasing concentrations of hapten on the amount of precipitate formed in a solution in which the relative amounts of antigen and antibody remain constant. The antibody will react preferentially with the free hapten, and such complexes are unable to form a precipitate. As a result, there is a direct relationship between the extent of free hapten binding by the antibody and the inhibition of precipitation of the whole antigen (Pressman, 1964).

Another method of detecting antibody affinity for haptens is by fluorescence quenching (Eisen, 1964). The tyrosine and tryptophan residues of proteins absorb ultraviolet light and this absorbed radiant energy may be dissipated by fluorescence. Antibody fluorescence is excited maximally by light at about 280 nm (the absorption maximum for tryptophan and tyrosine) and the emitted light has a maximal intensity at 330–350 nm for tryptophan. When the antibody forms a soluble complex with certain haptens fluorescence is quenched as the energy absorbed from the irradiation of the tryptophan residues is transferred to the bound hapten and dissipated in other ways.

Hapten–antibody reactions obey the simple law of mass action. An affinity constant K can then be derived for the reversible reaction

$$\text{antibody site} + \text{hapten} \rightleftharpoons \text{antibody–hapten}.$$

Thus the affinity of an antibody for a univalent hapten may be determined simply by measuring the concentrations of free and bound hapten in an equilibrium mixture containing a known amount of antibody. This is achieved easily by equilibrium dialysis using radiolabelled haptens. Using this method, the average intrinsic association constant (K_0), defined as the reciprocal of the free hapten concentration at which half the total number of antibody sites are occupied by the hapten, may be calculated. The measurement of antibody affinity has been discussed in detail in Chapter 7 by Steward.

As mentioned above, much of the early work on hapten–protein conjugates was carried out using azo-proteins formed by coupling with diazonium compounds. Subsequently, a wide range of hapten–protein conjugates has been prepared by treating proteins with anhydrides, acyl chlorides, azides, isocyanates, aldehydes, halogenated compounds, oxazalones, and quinones. The most widely studied, artificially conjugated compounds are the halogen-substituted dinitrophenols, in which the link is mainly with lysine residues. In other systems, under biological conditions, more use may be made of the peptide linkage for hapten–protein conjugation. However to date, little evidence is available to support this assumption.

Antisera directed against hapten–protein complexes in which low molecular weight aliphatic or aromatic compounds are linked to proteins through a covalent linkage may contain antibodies which can discriminate exquisite differences in chemical structure. For example, sera against the lower molecular weight anilic acids (oxanilic and succanilic acids) can detect the lengthening or shortening of a chain by a single carbon atom. In other situations with haptens lacking a polar-carboxyl group specificity may be broader. Differences in molecular structure as well as in chemical constitution can also be discriminated. Thus d and l-*p*-aminobenzoyl phenylamino acetic acids conjugated through an azo-link can be distinguished as can the stereoisomers of tartaric acid after being converted into tartranilic acid, diazotized, and coupled to protein. This approach of determining differences in special configuration has been applied to the analysis of a range of mono and disaccharides derived from polysaccharides obtained, in particular, from *Pneumococcus* species, Friedlander's *Bacillus*, and plant gums.

More recently, the determination of the amino acid sequences in certain antibody areas has shown several chemical differences, which also may indicate variations in the three-dimensional structure of these antibodies. Using inbred guinea-pigs, Cebra and associates (1974) raised antibodies specific for three haptens. They analysed the first 83 amino acids of the N-terminal of the three IgG2 antibodies and compared these sequences with 'normal' IgG2. Each antibody was found to have a different and distinctive primary structure within each of the two hypervariable regions. The sequences of the hypervariable regions in the three antibodies were either unique or of restricted variability compared with those of normal IgG2. This aspect of antibody structure is discussed in detail in earlier chapters of this book (for example, see Richards *et al.*, Chapter 2).

Antigen formation by hapten–protein conjugation can occur *in vivo* as well as *in vitro*. Certain low molecular weight substances are able to bind to protein under normal biological conditions. These substances would then be able to bind to the animal's own proteins and convert these proteins into antigens. For example halogenated nitrobenzenes bind covalently to the ε-amino groups of lysine to form DNP–protein complexes. Other examples are *p*-phenylenediamine (which on oxidation combines covalently with proteins), neoarsphenamines, and the pentadecacatechols of poison ivy. Contact with such agents will induce both humoral antibody formation and delayed hypersensitivity.

2.2 Carrier Specificity in Delayed Hypersensitivity

A state of delayed hypersensitivity can be demonstrated by the intradermal injection of preformed hapten–protein complexes, by painting the agent onto the skin or by injecting the hapten intradermally so that it forms hapten–protein complexes *in vivo*. The role of the carrier in immunization was demonstrated first in experiments on the induction of delayed hypersensitivity to dinitrophenyl (DNP) and trinitrophenyl (TNP)–protein conjugates. In experiments of this type, the carrier protein is more than just a means of increasing the molecular weight of the complex to that which will induce an immune response, as it also contributes significantly to the overall antigenicity of the molecule (Benacerraf and Gell, 1959; Arnon and Geiger, Chapter 9).

Such carrier specificity is frequently more apparent in delayed hypersensitivity than with antibodies which tend to be more hapten specific. An example of this is found in guinea-pigs immunized with TNP–bovine γ-globulin. Antibody re-actions can be detected towards TNP conjugated with a wide range of carrier proteins. However, delayed hypersensitivity may be detected only to TNP coupled to the specific carrier used in immunization. Another example is when the hapten is coupled to one of the body's own proteins (Benacerraf and Levine, 1962). If guinea-pigs are sensitized with TNP–guinea-pig albumin, specificity in delayed hypersensitivity may be found directed to the immunizing antigen only. Antibody may, however, be detected reacting with a wide range of TNP conjugates, including TNP–rabbit albumin and TNP–ovalbumin. Similar carrier specificity may be demonstrated *in vitro* by the incorporation of [^{3}H]-thymidine into the DNA of lymph node cells from sensitized animals (Paul *et al.*, 1967) or by studying the inhibition of migration of peritoneal exudate cells from capillary tubes (David *et al.*, 1964). In these experiments, migratory cells from guinea-pigs sensitized to show delayed hypersensitivity to DNP–bovine γ-globulin were inhibited by DNP–bovine γ-globulin, but not by DNP–guinea-pig albumin, DNP–bovine serum albumin, or DNP–ovalbumin. The specificity of the carrier in cell-mediated immune reactions of this type is emphasized further by experiments in which guinea-pigs sensitized with DNP linked to a copolymer of L-glutamic acid and L-lysine react only to the immunizing antigen and will not react to the challenge with DNP conjugates of D-glutamic acid and D-lysine (Benacerraf *et al.*, 1970).

The optimum size of the carrier was demonstrated by Schlossman and coworkers (1966) in studies on the immunogenicity of oligo-L-lysines. In these studies, immunization was only possible with a molecule equal to or larger than the heptamer. Delayed hypersensitivity, however, could be elicited only with the octamer or nonamer. In contrast, antibody-induced Arthus reactions could be elicited with the hapten-substituted tetramer, pentamer, or hexamer. This would indicate that carrier specificity needs a chain length equivalent to that of the octamer, whereas hapten-specific reactions can be induced by the hapten-substituted tetramer.

2.3 Carrier Specificity in Humoral Antibody Production

Carrier specificity of the above type is however not limited to delayed hypersensitivity and may be found with antibodies elicited during the early phase of immunization. Thus, Borek and Silverstein (1965) found carrier and link specificity in antibodies between the 10th and 17th days after the immunization of guinea-pigs with p-aminobenzoate and p-nitroaniline coupled to guinea-pig albumin either by an azo link to tyrosine or histidine residues, or by a carbamido or thiocarbamido link to the ε-amino group of lysine. These antibodies, detected by passive cutaneous anaphylaxis, may be IgE or IgG1 homocytotropic antibodies. However, by four weeks after immunization all the antibody is hapten specific.

In other experiments, specifically purified hapten-specific anti-DNP antibodies have been shown to possess a significant, although limited, degree of carrier specificity, in systems in which the binding affinities were measured by fluorescence quenching or by equilibrium dialysis (Benacerraf *et al.*, 1970). It would appear, therefore, that there may always be some degree of carrier specificity in antibody prepared against artificially formed hapten–protein conjugates, although the extent of the contribution of the carrier to the antigenic specificity may vary according to the system. However, in many cell-mediated immune responses, the determinant encompasses both the hapten and a considerable part of the carrier. It has yet to be determined to what extent the binding energy provided by the carrier contributes to the binding affinity of the reaction as a whole.

The role of the linkage between the hapten and the carrier on the immunogenicity of the molecules must also be considered. Haptens coupled to carrier proteins by azo linkages may give only modest antibody levels, whereas those coupled through free amino groups induce considerably more hapten-specific antibody (Hoffman *et al.*, 1969). In other experiments, it has been found that guinea-pigs immunized with DNP coupled to free amino or carboxyl groups of bovine serum albumin respond with high levels of anti-DNP and low levels of anti-bovine serum albumin antibody, while those immunized with DNP coupled to the tyrosyl residues give the reverse response. It has been suggested therefore that DNP coupled to carboxyl or amino residues is on the outer surface of the protein molecule and is more likely to alter its surface configuration than when attached to a tyrosyl residue (Hanna *et al.*, 1972; see also Arnon and Geiger, Chapter 9). In other systems, there is no evidence for specificity related to the link between hapten and carrier. The introduction of a rigid polyproline spacer between the DNP hapten and the bovine serum albumin carrier does not alter the carrier effect in antibody production in the rabbit or in delayed hypersensitivity in the guinea-pig (Ungar-Waron *et al.*, 1973).

Carrier effects on antibody production have also been shown to occur in the induction of a secondary antibody response (Mitchison, 1971*a, b*). Such an effect can be demonstrated when a hapten–protein conjugate is injected into an animal, which has been primed previously with the same hapten conjugated to another serum protein. Under these conditions, the antihapten secondary response is less than that obtained when the animal is injected with a conjugate prepared with the carrier originally used for the priming. In addition, if animals are primed with a hapten–protein complex together with a second foreign protein, a normal secondary response can be induced when the hapten is injected conjugated to the second protein. As a result of these observations it has been postulated that a specific population of 'helper' cells that show marked carrier specificity are stimulated. These cells are independent of the hapten-specific antibody-forming cells and appear to be T cells similar to those involved in delayed hypersensitivity.

The relation between carrier specificity in delayed hypersensitivity to the carrier specificity of the helper cell in antibody production has been questioned (Liew and Parish, 1974). Delayed hypersensitivity to flagellin in the rat can be induced most effectively by acetoacetylated flagellin, not so well by flagellin itself and least well by polymerized flagellin. However, the specificity of the helper cells for the anti-DNP response to a range of DNP-flagellin conjugates is related inversely to that of cell-mediated immunity to the carrier, being in the order polymerized flagellin > flagillin > acetoacetylated flagellin. The mechanism by which carrier-specific T cells might co-operate with hapten-specific B cells has been the subject of a series of cell culture experiments (Feldmann *et al.*, 1974) involving both macrophages and an immunoglobulin-type molecule derived from specifically sensitized cells which cause the release of factors necessary for a normal IgG response.

2.4 Hapten Specificity in Delayed Hypersensitivity

As with humoral antibody, delayed hypersensitivity can discriminate under certain circumstances between variations in the molecular structure of the hapten. For example Silverstein and Gell (1962) found that delayed hyper-sensitivity could differentiate between *ortho*, *meta*, and *para*-substituted benz-oates conjugated to serum protein. However, the cross-sections observed are greater than those that occur using rabbit antibody *in vitro*.

Hapten specificity is particularly marked in delayed hypersensitivity in experiments using the azobenzenearsonate (ABA) group, which appears to behave differently to other haptens. Guinea-pigs sensitized to ABA–guinea-pig albumin react with guinea-pig albumin coupled to the azo-benzoate group (Benz–guinea-pig albumin). If desensitized with Benz–guinea-pig albumin, reactivity to this compound is diminished completely, but reactivity to ABA–guinea-pig serum albumin remains unaffected. Similar hapten specificity can be demonstrated in guinea-pigs immunized with ABA–polytyrosine, which reacts strongly to the ABA–hapten conjugated to a wide range of other carriers. Reactions to ABA–polytyrosine can be suppressed completely by systemic injection of the hapten ABA–N-acetyltyrosine, as also are reactions to other ABA conjugates (Leskowitz 1962, 1963).

Another feature of the ABA system is that guinea-pigs can be sensitized with ABA–hexa-L-tyrosine, ABA–tri-L-tyrosine, and ABA–N-acetyl-L-tyrosine amide. On incubating radiolabelled ABA–hexa-L-tyrosine with normal guinea-pig serum it was found that some of the conjugate is associated with serum protein, although ABA–hexa-L-tyrosine is not thought to form a covalent link with protein (Borek et al., 1965). A further feature of this sytem is that hapten specificity of delayed-type hypersensitivity reactions to ABA conjugates only occurs in systems in which the antigen is injected in Freund's incomplete adjuvant; the animal shows a milder, more transient form of reactivity known as Jones–Mote hypersensitivity. Animals sensitized with ABA–L-tyrosine in Freund's complete adjuvant show positive delayed reactions to ABA–bovine γ-globulin, whereas if sensitized with the former conjugate in Freund's incomplete adjuvant no such cross-reactivity occurs (Richerson et al., 1970). Thus, it has been suggested that the immunogenicity requirements for Jones–Mote hypersensitivity resemble those for antibody production rather than those for delayed hypersensitivity. This interpretation should be accepted with reservation as it depends mainly on the inability either to detect antibody after immunization with ABA–tyrosine in the complete adjuvant or to produce any delayed hypersensitivity after immunization with ABA–tyrosine in the incomplete adjuvant. The use of ABA–tyrosine as an immunogen would seem to present a rather special situation.

Both hapten and carrier specificity may exist together in delayed hypersensitivity. Guinea-pigs sensitized with DNP–guinea-pig albumin react with this antigen, but not with the DNP derivatives of ovalbumin, rabbit γ-globulin or keyhole limpet haemocyanin. In addition, guinea-pigs can discriminate between 2,4 and 2,6-dinitrophenyl and 2,4,6-trinitrophenyl derivatives of guinea-pig albumin (Fleischmann and Eisen, 1975).

2.5 Importance of the Density of the Hapten on the Carrier in the Induction of an Immune Response

Haurowitz (1936) intimated that only a few groups were needed for an antibody response to develop against the hapten; overloading would reduce the antigenic effect. In varying the number of DNP groups on albumin from five through 11 to 20 the ability to produce contact sensitivity to dinitrofluorobenzene is unaffected (Parker et al., 1970). Results of a more recent study, using polysaccharide carriers for the DNP group, showed that immunization occurs with a minimum number of DNP groups per molecule (in the region of one group per molecule) (Desaymard and Howard, 1975). However, tolerance could only be achieved with relatively highly substituted molecules (in the region of eight groups per molecule) when a high enough dose of antigen was used.

2.6 Polysaccharides as Haptens

Although antibodies can be produced regularly against polysaccharide antigens, it is frequently very difficult to demonstrate delayed hypersensitivity with these antigens. Whenever delayed hypersensitivity is demonstrated to polysaccharides there is usually the question of whether they contain a peptide moiety. It has been suggested that polysaccharides are unable to elicit delayed hypersensitivity because the binding affinities achieved by polysaccharide determinants seldom reach the high value that has been postulated to be necessary for delayed hypersensitivity (Karush and Eisen, 1962).

Polysaccharides, however, can be induced to stimulate delayed hypersensitivity if conjugated to a protein carrier so as to act as haptens. The mixed anhydride method has been used to prepare antigenic protein–polysaccharide conjugates containing glucuronic acid and galacturonic acid (Borek *et al.*, 1963). In addition, conjugates of monosaccharides and disaccharides through an azophenyl link with guinea-pig albumin and ovalbumin have been prepared. These compounds are able to sensitize guinea-pigs to exhibit delayed hypersensitivity. All these antigens display marked carrier specificity, and there are significant cross-reactions between haptens that would be recognized easily by conventional rabbit antibody. It has been suggested that the failure of purified polysaccharides to serve as elicitors of delayed hypersensitivity is due to the polysaccharide structure being unable to act as an antigenic carrier in this system (Borek *et al.*, 1963). It also appears that the linkage between the hapten group of the polysaccharide and the carrier protein plays an important part in delayed hypersensitivity reactions to saccharides, since certain polysaccharides, such as those of fungal or blood group origin, may be inactive even when associated with protein.

3 IMMUNOGENICITY OF HAPTEN–PROTEIN CONJUGATES FORMED *IN VIVO*

Natural conjugation between artificial haptens and body proteins occurs when a reactive compound, such as dinitrofluorobenzene, comes into contact with the skin or is injected into the body. The formation of such conjugates *in vivo* is the basis of chemical contact sensitivity, which is one of the major causes of industrial morbidity. Contact sensitivity involves mainly T-cell stimulation and delayed hypersensitivity. Drugs and other simple chemicals can also be introduced into the body by injection or by absorption through the gastrointestinal or respiratory tract, and induce the formation of humoral antibodies including IgE. A large number of allergic reactions to drugs falls into this group.

3.1 Chemical Contact Sensitivity to Organic Haptens

The earliest work on contact sensitivity to well-defined organic chemical sensitizers was that of Landsteiner and Jacobs (1935) who used chloro- and nitro-substituted benzenes. Sensitization with such simple chemicals was explained by assuming that these compounds link covalently with protein. The linkage was investigated by assessing the formation of substitution compounds with an organic base (aniline). A marked parallelism was found between the ability of these substituted benzenes to combine with aniline and their ability to sensitize guinea-pigs. Of the 20 compounds tested, 10 were found to react with aniline. These 10 compounds were found to produce contact sensitivity in guinea-pigs; those derivatives which did not sensitize guinea-pigs were not reactive with aniline. These findings were confirmed later by parallel studies in man (Sulzberger and Baer, 1938). Sensitization to agents of this type may be either by direct contact with the skin, in which case the conjugates are formed *in vivo* with skin proteins, or by injection of preformed stable conjugates of the chemical agents with serum proteins or erythrocyte stromata in Freund's complete adjuvant. A further method is by the intradermal injection of the sensitizer itself, with or without Freund's adjuvants.

A study of the actual compound formed *in vivo* in the skin was initiated by Eisen and colleagues (1952) who demonstrated that four DNP derivatives, which were able to sensitize humans, bound irreversibly through the formation of a covalent bond with bovine γ-globulin. However, four similar compounds that would not bind onto proteins were found not to be sensitizers. Most active sensitizers, such as dinitrochlorobenzene and dinitrofluorobenzene, when painted onto the skin may be recovered bound to lysine. However 2,4-dinitro-phenylsulphenylchloride and 2,4-dinitrophenylthiocyanate sensitize by binding to the disulphide bonds of the cystine residues in the proteins.

The nitro groups in the *ortho* and *para* positions of dinitrofluorobenzene and dinitrophenylthiocyanate ensure that the substitution at C-1 of the benzene ring is very active and readily replaced by any other negatively charged ion. Figure 2 shows how these haptens conjugate with proteins. As can be seen the fluoride atom of dinitrofluorobenzene is readily substituted for a hydrogen atom from the free ε-amino groups of lysines present in the proteins. In contrast, when the sulphur-containing dinitrophenyl derivatives are conjugated with protein, it is only the chloride or cyanide part of the substituent that is removed and the hapten is conjugated to the protein through a disulphide bond with one of the sulphur-containing amino acids in the protein chain. Reports of sensitization with amino acids such as DNP-S-glycine, DNP-S-cysteine, DNP-L-lysine, and DNP-S-glutathione (Frey *et al.*, 1969) should be viewed with caution as it may be that sensitization has occurred through a 'transconjugation' phenomenon in which the DNP group could be split from its amino acid carrier acid and conjugated with protein.

The afferent lymph draining from the site of application of a sensitizing dose of dinitrofluorobenzene in the pig has been found to contain many different DNP-conjugated proteins. None of these has been shown to induce contact sensivitiy if given as a single intralymphatic injection. However, repeated infusions of DNP–pig serum albumin administered at the same lymphatic site on three occasions, with an interval of 12 days between the infusions, induces strong contact sensitivity (Balfour *et al.*, 1974). There has been a number of reports of failure to

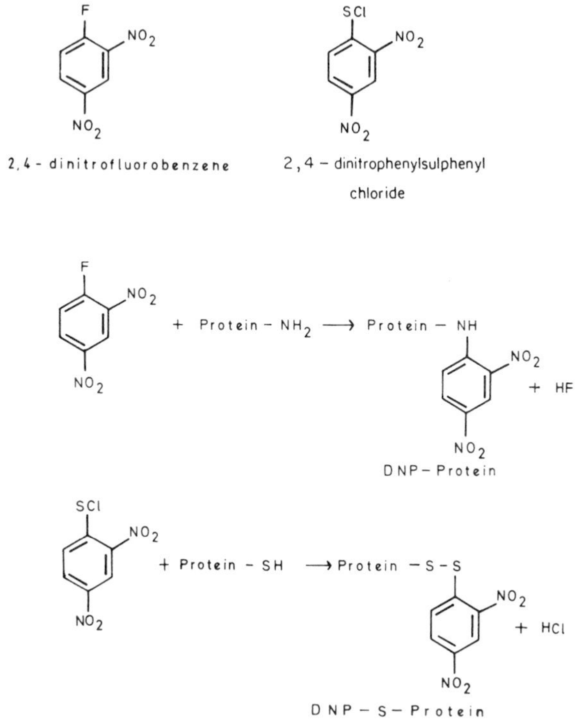

Figure 2 Chemical structure of dinitrofluorobenzene and dinitrophenylsulphenylchloride, and mechanism of conjugation with proteins

induce contact sensitivity in guinea-pigs with DNP-homologous serum proteins (Eisen *et al.*, 1959; Gell and Benacerraf, 1961; Salvin and Smith, 1961). However, in other studies (Parker *et al.*, 1970), contact sensitivity has been induced in guinea-pigs by conjugates of DNP with both homologous albumin and homologous γ-globulin as well as with soluble extracts of dinitrofluorobenzene-painted guinea-pig skin. Immunization was, in all cases, with the conjugates in Freund's complete adjuvant. Sensitization may be obtained also with subcellular particulate fractions of epidermis painted *in vivo* with dinitrofluorobenzene; microsomal fractions were found to be more active than mitochondrial fractions (Parker and Turk, 1970; Nishioka *et al.*, 1971).

Another potent contact sensitizer is 3-n-pentadecylcatechol, one of the active components of poison ivy. Guinea-pigs can be sensitized readily to this compound by its injection in Freund's complete adjuvant or by its percutaneous application (Bowser and Baer, 1963). Further work into the ability to induce contact sensitivity in guinea-pigs by pentadecylcatechol and related alkyl catechols has shown that neither the position of the alkyl group in the benzene ring nor the length of the side chain affects the ability to sensitize (Baer *et al.*, 1967). However, the introduction of carboxyl group into either the ring or the side chain abolishes completely the sensitizing capacity of the catechols. It has been shown that pentadecylcatechol itself does not combine with proteins *in vitro*, but first must be oxidized to the quinone (Mason and Lada, 1954). Quinones, prepared from the catechols, have been found to be better sensitizers than the corresponding catechols (Baer *et al.*, 1966).

3.2 Hapten–Protein Conjugates Formed by Non-Covalent Linkages

As described in Section 3.1 there are several classes of chemical compounds that are strong sensitizers in man and animals. The conjugation of these compounds with proteins by covalent linkages to form the immunogenic hapten–protein conjugate may be understood readily. However, in some instances in which sensitization is obtained, it would seem that linkage to protein may be by other, non-covalent forces. One example of a sensitizer that does not bind covalently to protein is the weak, contact sensitizer picric acid.

It was suggested originally by Landsteiner and Di Somma (1940) that picric acid was reduced *in vivo* to picramic acid which then could bind covalently to proteins. However, recent work has shown that it is only occasionally possible to sensitize using picramic acid (Chase and Maguire, 1974a). Studies on the reversible binding of picric acid to albumin (Fredericq 1954, 1955, 1956) have shown that the 2,4,6-trinitrophenoxide radical is attached to the albumin surface by hydrogen bonding, and not by Van der Waal's forces as previously suggested.

Good contact skin reactions to picric acid are induced in guinea-pigs by the split-adjuvant technique (Maguire and Chase, 1972). These reactions differ from the classical contact reactions in that the reactions reach a maximum three or more days after a skin test and histologically have an infiltrate consisting mainly of neutrophilic polymorphonuclear leucocytes. Animals sensitized to picrid acid cross-react readily, when skin tested by contact, with picryl chloride which rapidly binds covalently with proteins (Chase and Maguire, 1974b). However, animals showing good sensitivity to picric acid do not respond to intradermal tests using picric acid or picrylated proteins.

Using the split-adjuvant technique, no antibody could be detected to picrylated proteins, by passive cutaneous anaphylaxis, in these highly sensitive animals. When guinea-pigs are sensitized to picric acid by the technique of daily intradermal injections of picric acid and horse serum, good reactivity is obtained to intradermal injections of picric acid, although there is no contact reactivity. In these animals, passive cutaneous anaphylactic antibody can be detected using a two-step procedure with picrylated casein.

3.3 Immunological Unresponsiveness Induced by Organic Haptens

Some of the earliest chemicals to be investigated for their immunizing potential were the arsenical organic compounds arsphenamine and neoarsphenamine (Figure 3). Both humans and guinea-pigs can be sensitized with these compounds. Guinea-pigs given a single intradermal injection of neoarsphenamine

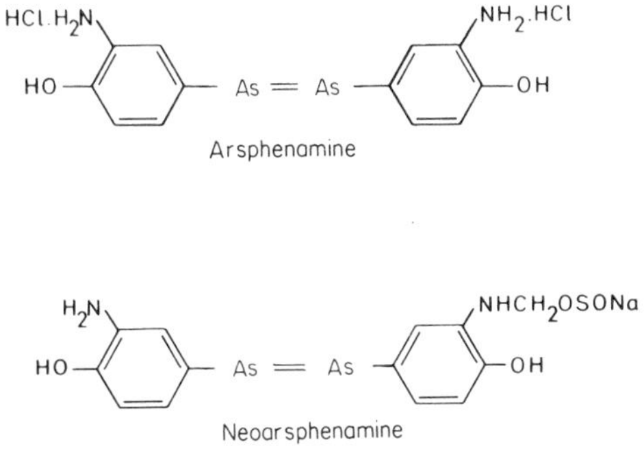

Figure 3 Chemical structure of arsphenamine and neoarsphenamine

(150 µg) showed delayed hypersensitivity if skin tested 28 days later with the same dose. However, if the animals are injected with an intravenous dose of neoarsphenamine before sensitization, a permanent state of unresponsiveness is induced (Sulzberger, 1929; Chase, 1963; Frey *et al.*, 1966). Similar tolerance to contact sensitivity with dinitrofluorobenzene can be induced by feeding this compound by mouth (Chase, 1946), or by intravenous injection of dinitrobenzenesulphonic acid (Asherson and Ptak, 1970). In the guinea-pig, it is possible to reverse this tolerance by pretreating the animal with cyclophosphamide three days before sensitization. Suppression of the immune response can be shown to be due to action of the specifically induced suppressor cells (Turk *et al.*, 1976). In the mouse, these suppressor cells have been shown to be T lymphocytes (Zembala and Asherson, 1973), although these cells have not been characterized fully in the guinea-pig. Similar suppressor cells, active in competing with effector cells in dinitrofluorobenzene sensitivity, can be induced by painting the skin with dinitrothiocyanate benzene (Sommer *et al.*, 1975). This compound can sensitize an animal only if injected in Freund's complete adjuvant. When painted on skin, it induces a state of specific immunological unresponsiveness. Another compound which induces unresponsiveness when applied to the skin is *p*-nitrosodimethylaniline, if applied in minute amounts (Lowney, 1970); larger doses will induce a state of hypersensitivity. It is likely that the smaller doses induce suppressor cell formation as in the dinitrothiocyanatebenzene system.

Intravenous injection of most sensitizers, after sensitization has developed, induces a state of temporary unresponsiveness usually referred to as desensitization. This state lasts 24 hours, and normal responsiveness can be detected again between three and seven days later. However, an intravenous injection of 60 mg neoarsphenamine followed by an intradermal injection of 150 µg of this compound can induce a state of permanent and complete unresponsiveness in an animal shown previously to be hypersensitive to this compound (Frey *et al.*, 1966). The only other sensitizer that so far has been shown to produce a state of permanent post-sensitization tolerance in the guinea-pig is potassium dichromate. As with neoarsphenamine, the intravenous injection of the dichromate (20 mg/kg) is associated with a skin contact test using 0·5 per cent of the dichromatic within 24 hours. Lack of skin contact, or positive skin contact after 24 hours, is due to a temporary state of unresponsiveness only (Polak and Turk, 1968).

3.4 Sensitivity to Inorganic Metal Compounds

In man, contact sensitivity can be induced with a number of inorganic metals, including beryllium, chromium, mercury, nickel, and zirconium. Sensitivity to potassium dichromate, beryllium fluoride, and mercuric chloride can be induced regularly in the guinea-pig.

Chromium is encountered usually as a sensitizer in its hexavalent form—as potassium dichromate—which penetrates the skin readily. In contrast, trivalent chromium penetrates the skin 10^4 times less effectively. A parallelism exists between the better sensitizing capacity of hexavalent chromium, compared with the trivalent compounds, and their ability to penetrate the skin when applied in corresponding doses onto undamaged skin surfaces. In numerous studies, it has been shown that it is the trivalent form of chromium, as opposed to the hexavalent form, which conjugates with protein both *in vitro* and *in vivo* (Polak *et al.*, 1973). The nature of the chromium–protein conjugate is unknown as attempts to sensitize animals with conjugates formed *in vitro* between chromium and serum, or skin proteins, have failed. Hexavalent chromium can be reduced both *in vivo* and *in vitro* to the trivalent form. The trivalent form possesses strong tanning properties and is also a sensitizer. This indicates that the hexavalent form, which is not a tanning agent, is transformed in the body to a complex tanning agent. It has been suggested, therefore, that chromium in the hexavalent form penetrates the skin, but is reduced there to trivalent chromium mainly by the sulphydryl groups of amino acids. The trivalent chromium then forms conjugates with skin proteins which are effective as full antigens. The fact that circulating antibodies to trivalent chromium conjugates are detected but not to conjugates with hexavalent chromium is consistent with this supposition. In addition, it has been possible to increase the number of animals sensitized to potassium dichromate by the addition of a carbostyril derivative which enhances the reduction of hexavalent chromium (Polak *et al.*, 1973).

Whereas guinea-pigs can be sensitized to beryllium fluoride and mercuric chloride by direct contact, sensitization is obtained only with any regularity with potassium dichromate if this last compound is injected in Freund's complete adjuvant. Other difficulties may be encountered as the ability to be sensitized and to react with these compounds is inherited as a single Mendelian dominant characteristic. Moreover, there are strain differences in reactivity. For example, 66 per cent of Hartley animals become sensitized to potassium dichromate, 79 per cent to beryllium fluoride and 46 per cent to mercuric chloride. Using inbred strain II guinea-pigs, 80 per cent become sensitized to potassium dichromate, and 72 per cent to beryllium fluoride, and none to mercuric chloride. On the other hand, 80 per cent of strain XIII become sensitized to mercury chloride but none to the other metals (Polak *et al.*, 1968). A similar clear-cut genetic difference has been found in studying the reactivity in guinea-pigs to linear copolymers and multichain polymers containing lysine or tyrosine and glutamic acid (Ben Efraim *et al.*, 1967). This suggests that variations in immune response may be related to the presence or absence of clusters of positive charges within the molecule.

Although *in vitro* tests of cell-mediated immunity are difficult to reproduce using the DNP–hapten or DNP–protein complexes, it may be possible to perform these tests with metal haptens in animals with metal sensitivity. This may be related to the solubility of the metal compounds in water, as most organic compounds are only soluble in organic solvents and are toxic at high concentration. Thus, inhibition of macrophage migration may be obtained using peritoneal macrophages from chromium-sensitive guinea-pigs. The best results have been obtained using potassium dichromate, which is effective at more than a hundred-fold lower concentration than chromium chloride. Inhibition also can be obtained with the whole antigen—chromium chloride conjugated to guinea-pig serum proteins. The increased effectiveness of hexavalent, as opposed to trivalent, chromium in this system is paradoxical. However, it is possible that because of the strong protein binding capacity of trivalent chromium, the majority of the chromium present may be bound to immunologically incompetent carriers, such as single amino acids, and so would be excluded from the reaction. Hexavalent chromium, on the other hand, could be bound after conversion directly to form immunocompetent conjugates. Another possibility is that it is necessary for the hapten to enter cells in order to conjugate with the relevant carrier. Hexavalent chromium is taken into cells very efficiently, whereas trivalent chromium will be bound to extraneous carriers and not be able to enter the cell (Polak *et al.*, 1973).

Activation of lymphocytes from specifically sensitized animals to produce macrophage migration inhibitory factor can also be induced in beryllium sensitivity. However, beryllium has to be complexed to sulphosalicylic acid to be effective; insoluble beryllium oxide and beryllium fluoride used to sensitize the animals are not effective. Sulphosalicylic acid is a chelating agent for beryllium and forms a complex with the metal ion if the latter is added in the form of beryllium hydroxides (Jones and Amos, 1974). Lymph node cells incubated with beryllium sulphosalicylic acid act as antigens in the induction of contact sensitivity to beryllium fluoride (Jones and Amos, 1975). Beryllium has been found to react selectively with certain proteins, for example, alkaline phosphatase and phosphoglucomutase, but does not appear to be able to bind very well to DNase, RNase, and chymotrypsin, although it binds well to nucleoproteins. When beryllium, complexed with a chelating agent such as sulphosalicylic acid, binds to nucleoprotein it is not known whether it binds as the complex or whether it first dissociates (Reiner, 1971).

4 MYELOMA PROTEINS WITH ANTI-HAPTEN ANTIBODY ACTIVITY

The demonstration of myeloma proteins with specificity for chemically defined haptens holds intriguing possibilities. These proteins bind haptens selectively and the binding site is on the Fab fragment as with a conventional antibody. In one series of experiments performed by Schubert *et al.* (1968), 240 mouse myelomas were screened against 21 hapten–protein conjugates. Of these conjugates, 28 were found to have antibody activity that reacted with purines, 5-acetyluracil, adenosine monophosphate, DNP, and TNP groups. At least one case of Waldenström macroglobulinaemia has been described in which the monoclonal protein has a low binding affinity for the DNP group. A number of the mouse myeloma proteins has antibody affinity for 5-acetyluracil and purines, as well as the DNP group. Moreover, purified anti-DNP antibody cross-reacts with 5-acetyluracil and purines, suggesting that the antibody activity is an autoimmune phenomenon.

One such mouse myeloma protein, from the IgA plasmacytoma MOPC 315 in BALB/c mice, has been studied extensively. This protein has a higher affinity for the DNP group than any of the other myeloma proteins studied. Thus, it precipitates with DNP–proteins and TNP–(picryl)-proteins but not with dansyl, tosyl, pipsyl, or 1,8-anilino-naphthalene sulphonyl-proteins. Moreover, the protein reacts with 2,4-DNP–aminocaproate better than with 2,6-DNP–aminocaproate in the same way as conventional rabbit and guinea-pig anti-DNP antibodies. An intriguing cross-reaction has been found with this protein as it is also bound specifically by the vitamin K-like molecule 2-(methyl)-1,4-naphthoquinone (menadione, Vitamin K_3) (Michaelides and Eisen, 1974).

Although there is a pronounced structural difference between DNP and menadione, the binding of both haptens by the same immunoglobulin cannot be taken as evidence in support of the idea that individual immunoglobulins are multispecific. It is suggested that menadione is bound specifically, and with considerable affinity, at a site that overlaps with the one binding DNP–haptens, as models of the two molecules have some structural similarities and can, to some degree, be superimposed. The results of experiments suggesting the presence of multiple combining sites within the antibody combining region of immunoglobulins have been discussed by Richards *et al.* in Chapter 2.

5 IMMUNOGENICITY OF HORMONES

Hormones, whether peptides or not, generally have relative low molecular weights and, as such, are non-antigenic. However, many non-antigenic hormones may be made antigenic by coupling covalently to a protein carrier. Also, some hormones, which are weakly antigenic, show increased antigenicity when coupled to proteins; sera prepared against such hapten–protein conjugates may then be used in radioimmunoassay. Among the compounds, which have been conjugated in this way to increase their antigenicity, are the peptide hormones, thyrotropin releasing hormone (tripeptide), vasopressin and bradykinin (9 amino acids), angiotensins (10), gastrin (17), secretin (27), glucagon (29), and ACTH (39).

To produce antibodies directed towards the peptide hormones, that is anti-hapten antibodies, most of these hormones are conjugated to homologous albumin. Techniques employing toluene diisocyanate or carbodiimide have been used frequently to couple these peptide hormones to the protein either by a direct peptide–peptide bond or with an organic compound between the two peptide molecules. In the toluene diisocyanate method, the diisocyanate is coupled first with one peptide molecule and the product, in the absence of any free diisocyanate, is coupled with another peptide (Figure 4). On the other hand, carbodiimides react first with the carboxyl groups of the peptide eventually forming an acid anhydride that can then react with the amino group of another peptide molecule forming a peptide–peptide bond between the peptide hormone and the protein (Figure 5) (Williams and Chase, 1967).

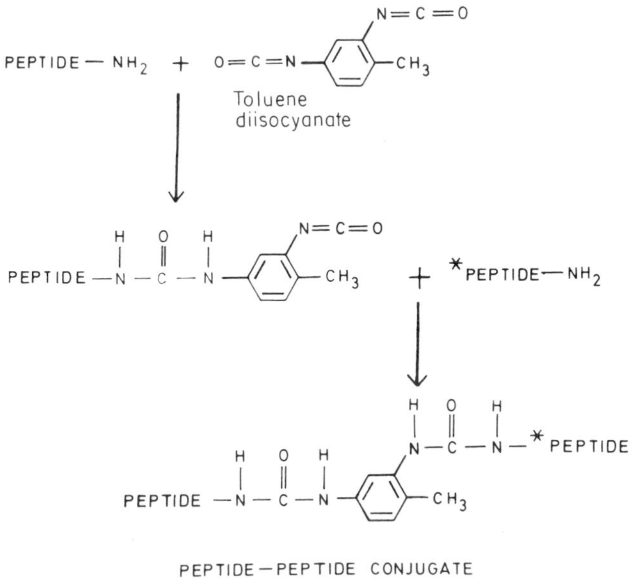

PEPTIDE—PEPTIDE CONJUGATE

Figure 4 Conjugation with toluene diisocyanate

Steroid hormones can be linked to the amino group of bovine serum albumin or other proteins either by the carbodiimide method or by the formation of a steroid–carboxymethyl oxime. In the latter method, the steroid is first conjugated to (*O*-carboxymethyl) hydroxylamine to produce a steroid molecule with a free carboxyl group. This complex is then conjugated directly to the protein carrier by a mixed anhydride technique. In some instances, hemisuccinate has been used instead of (*O*-carboxymethyl) hydroxylamine. This method has been applied to produce antibodies to testosterone, pregnenolone, progesterone, oestrone, cortisone, and desoxycorticosterone (Butler and Beiser, 1973).

6 IMMUNOGENICITY OF DRUGS

As originally suggested by Landsteiner and later by Eisen (1959), drugs produce allergic reactions by virtue of their ability to combine with proteins and,

462

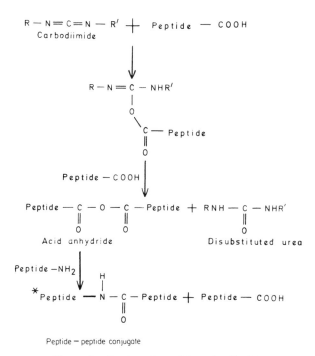

Figure 5 Conjugation with carbodiimide

in some cases, with polysaccharides (Schneider and De Weck, 1965). As a rule most drugs do not directly conjugate with endogenous macromolecules, but undergo metabolic degradation *in vivo*. The metabolites then conjugate covalently with proteins to become antigenic. Although this has been shown to be true in most cases of drug hypersensitivity, there are some instances, for example, hypersensitivity to Sedormid, where no evidence of metabolic degradation and binding with macromolecules has been produced (Ackroyd, 1975). It has been postulated that in these cases reactive metabolites are produced but they have not been detected so far. In other situations a contaminant, present in the preparation, has been shown to be responsible for the hypersensitive state. As there has been much investigation into penicillin allergy, this will be discussed in more detail to illustrate some of the mechanisms involved.

There are many metabolites of penicillin, some of which are depicted in Figure 6, and all of which could be responsible for an allergic reaction. Penicillenic acid, which is readily formed from penicillin in neutral, aqueous solution, is a highly reactive molecule at physiological pH. It can conjugate with protein either through the disulphide or sulphydryl groups to form penicillenate–protein or through the amino groups to yield penicilloyl–protein. Penicillin itself combines directly with protein to form a penicilloyl–protein conjugate (Batchelor *et al.*, 1965; Schneider and De Weck, 1965). In addition, the penicilloyl group is relatively unstable and yields successive degradation

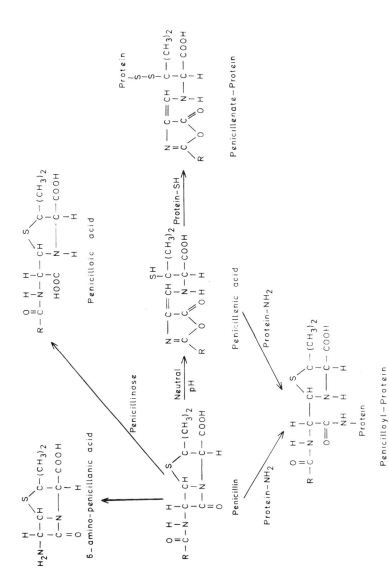

Figure 6 Some mechanisms of formation of antigen in penicillin allergy

products such as penicilloic acid. Penicilloic acid also is formed directly from penicillin when it is hydrolysed by the enzyme penicillinase (Parker, 1965).

It was thought originally that penicillenic acid was the main cause of penicillin allergy, but later work showed that the majority of antibodies detected in penicillin-sensitive patients was directed towards the penicilloyl conjugates, and it is now believed that this group is the major determinant (Parker *et al.*, 1962). Recent studies have demonstrated a close correlation between positive skin tests with penicilloyl–polylysine and penicilloyl-specific IgE antibodies, and it seems virtually certain that IgE and skin sensitizing antibodies are identical (Juhlin and Wide, 1972). Measurements of the agglutination of penicillin-coated erythrocytes have demonstrated IgG and IgM antibodies specific for the penicilloyl determinant in many cases of drug hypersensitivity. By skin testing with penicillin or other minor determinants it is possible to detect IgE antibodies with specificity not directed towards the penicilloyl determinant. However using haemagglutinating techniques, it has not been possible, as yet, to detect IgG and IgM antibodies other than those specific for the penicilloyl determinant. Intradermal injection of penicillin can give rise to delayed-type hypersensitivity reactions and it is believed that the incidence of this type of reaction is much higher than the incidence of an immediate-type reaction (Redmond and Levine, 1968; Ackroyd, 1975). The timing and the gross microscopic morphology of these delayed-type lesions are similar to those of classical delayed hypersensitivity reactions to intradermally injected tuberculin. A striking degree of carrier specificity has been observed in that giving delayed reactions to penicillin give no reaction to penicilloyl–polylysine or penicilloyl–human serum albumin, but good skin reactions to conjugates with human γ-globulin or with mixed human γ and β-globulins (Redmond and Levine, 1968).

Good delayed skin reactions can be induced in guinea-pigs using the spontaneously formed penicillin polymer and penicilloyl–polysaccharide conjugates such as penicilloyl–dextran (Schneider and De Weck, 1967). In these animals, no immediate reaction develops and no antibody can be detected by precipitation or haemagglutination and only in a few animals is anaphylactic antibody formed (Schneider *et al.*, 1971).

Stimulation of lymphocytes from penicillin-sensitive patients and guinea-pigs, measured by the incorporation of $[^3H]$-thymidine, has been investigated extensively. It was found that penicillin itself stimulates, whereas penicilloyl conjugated to several carriers, including human serum albumin and polylysine, has no effect. Furthermore, bivalent penicilloyl antigens, which are capable of 'firing' sensitized mast cells, have no effect (De Weck *et al.*, 1974). Further work showed that penicilloyl–protein conjugates stimulate lymphocytes but to a much lesser extent than penicillin itself. This is in contrast to results reported by Vickers and Assem (1974), who found that the penicilloyl conjugates are more effective lymphocyte stimulators than penicillin itself. However, the difference between these observations may be due to the different doses used. Further studies by De Weck (1975) have shown that penicilloyl–autologous lymphocytes are better stimulators of lymphocytes from penicillin-sensitive patients than is penicillin itself in the test system used. Additional work demonstrated that different classes of peripheral blood lymphocytes are stimulated by different forms of penicillin. Penicillin itself stimulates a class of lymphocytes that persists in the blood for a long time, whereas those stimulated by penicilloyl–polylysine disappear more rapidly. Stimulation of this latter class of lymphocyte is inhibited by anti-penicilloyl antibodies.

As mentioned previously, in some cases of drug allergy, a contaminant has been found to be responsible for the hypersensitivity. High molecular weight penicilloylated-proteins have been isolated from preparations of 6-amino-penicillanic acid (see Figure 6), from the penicillin nucleus, and from penicillin itself (Batchelor *et al.*, 1967; Stewart, 1967). It has been found that when this protein conjugate is removed, 6-amine penicillanic acid no longer stimulates an antibody response in rabbits. However, the situation with penicillin is not quite so simple, as when the purified penicillin (from which the penicilloylated-protein had been removed) is stored, a high molecular weight substance, probably a polymer, accumulates. This high molecular weight substance is a sensitizer. It would appear that the immunogenicity of these preparations of 6-amino penicillanic acid and penicillin may be due to both the penicillin product as well as to the impurity.

In comparison with penicillin hypersensitivity, very few investigations have been carried out into the mechanisms involved in aspirin intolerance—a relatively common occurrence. It is known that aspirin itself (acetylsalicylic acid) may conjugate with protein *via* one of two pathways (Figure 7). Acetylsalicylic acid can conjugate with the amino groups of proteins by direct acetylation. It has

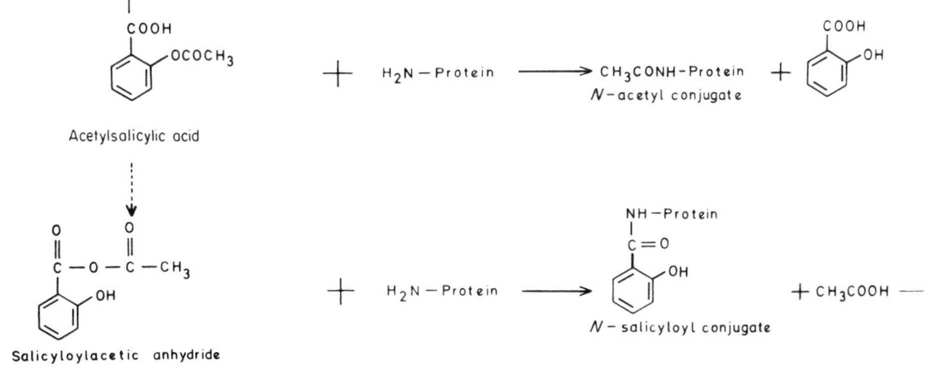

Figure 7 Some mechanisms of formation of antigen in aspirin allergy

been shown that, although aspirin acetylates most serum proteins *in vivo*, albumin is acetylated to the greatest extent (Farr, 1971). In the acidic environment of the stomach, aspirin is in the non-ionized form, however in the blood or duodenum, aspirin is hydrolysed rapidly forming salicylic acid and acetic acid. Whether it is salicylic acid or salicyloylacetic anhydride (an anhydride formed from salicylic acid and acetic acid) that conjugates with proteins is uncertain but salicyloyl–protein conjugates can be formed. Finally, it has been noticed that procedures used in the commercial synthesis of aspirin frequently promote the formation of aspirin anhydride, which under certain circumstances can also be formed spontaneously. The anhydride has been shown to be highly reactive with the amino groups in proteins, readily forming aspiryl–protein conjugates, which can be hydrolysed to salicyloyl conjugates (De Weck, 1971).

The presence of antibodies specific for the *N*-salicyloyl determinant has been reported in several instances, generally using passive haemagglutination with proteins conjugated with aspiryl chloride or aspiryl azide (Weiner *et al.*, 1963). More recently, reports of antibodies in possible aspirin-intolerant patients have been more controversial. Amos and coworkers (1971) have reported the presence of antibodies specific for the acetyl determinant in man but it has not been possible to correlate these antibodies with the clinical hypersensitive state. In a later study by Schlumberger *et al.* (1974), 27 aspirin-intolerant individuals were investigated for the presence of salicyloyl-specific homocytotropic antibodies. No such antibodies were detected either by skin testing or by passive transfer of serum into rhesus monkeys. Using several sensitive *in vitro* techniques, Lazary and associates (1972) failed to detect any antibodies specific to the aspiryl determinant but did produce positive skin test reactions with aspiryl-polylysine in these individuals.

The lack of reproducible results in investigations into antibodies in aspirin-intolerant humans may be due to the uncertainty of whether these individuals are truly sensitive to aspirin or its contaminants. However, it is relatively easy to produce hypersensitivity to aspirin in rabbits and guinea-pigs, and the antibodies produced are detected easily using the standard techniques. Although rabbits and guinea-pigs readily produce antibodies when immunized with a variety of aspirin derivatives and protein conjugates, it has not been possible to differentiate between anti-aspiryl and anti-salicyloyl antibodies (Hoffman and Campbell, 1969).

De Weck (1971) has shown that aspirin anhydride is a potent sensitizer in guinea-pigs. It is possible to induce hypersensitivity to this anhydride by either epicutaneous application or intradermal injection of the anhydride. Also, anti-aspiryl antibodies were detected regularly in these animals by passive cutaneous anaphylaxis. Using this contact hypersensitivity model in guinea-pigs, De Weck investigated the ability of commercial preparations of aspirin to induce contact skin reactions to the anhydride, with the subsequent development of anti-aspiryl antibodies. Although the number of animals used was small, the best contact reactions were elicited with the least pure commercial preparations of aspirin and the presence of antibodies paralleled this finding. The importance of aspirin anhydride in aspirin hypersensitivity was demonstrated further by Schlumberger (1975) who induced contact sensitivity in guinea-pigs with various salicylates. He showed that, whereas mild contact reactions could be elicited by several of the sensitizing agents, including salicylsalicylic acid and disalicylide, with aspirin anhydride a much stronger and more pronounced contact reaction was elicited, whatever the sensitizing agent. Therefore, it would seem that in aspirin intolerance, the contaminating anhydride could be the major antigenic determinant.

7 CONCLUSIONS

It is evident that Landsteiner's first use and definition of the term hapten is still essentially correct. It is a low molecular weight compound capable of binding to antibody, which is only capable of inducing an immune response when combined with a macromolecule. Haptens usually combine *in vivo* and *in vitro* with proteins and it is these hapten–protein conjugates which induce immune responses.

Hapten–protein conjugates prepared *in vitro* have been used successfully to study the specificity of many immune responses. Antibodies formed by immunization with hapten–protein conjugates show a large degree of hapten specificity but, at certain stages after immunization, carrier specificity of the antibody has been detected. Carrier specificity in antibody production has been found also in the induction of a secondary antibody response. The role of the carrier in delayed hypersensitivity appears to be more important than its role in antibody production. For example, animals immunized with a hapten–protein conjugate will develop delayed hypersensitivity reactions to the immunizing conjugate only, but antibodies towards the hapten can be detected with the hapten conjugated to a wide range of carrier proteins. However, a certain degree of hapten specificity has been detected in delayed hypersensitivity reactions, although this specificity is not as exacting as that encountered in antibody production. It would thus appear that in both types of immune reaction both hapten and carrier specificity can be found after immunization with hapten–protein conjugates.

There is a large range of different haptens encountered both *in vivo* and *in vitro*. From the evidence to date, it can be concluded that all immune reactions to low molecular weight compounds are as a result of these haptens conjugating to macromolecules. Although artificially prepared conjugates of hapten–polysaccharides have been used in investigations *in vivo*, it would seem that haptens conjugate preferentially with the body's own proteins. In most cases, haptens have been shown to conjugate covalently with proteins. However, the investigations into picric acid have demonstrated that the hapten does not necessarily have to conjugate with the macromolecule covalently. It may be that, in future, more examples of hapten–protein conjugation by non-covalent bonds will be found. Investigations into poison ivy and drug hypersensitivity have demonstrated that, in some instances, the hapten has to be metabolized by the body before it is conjugated with protein to form an antigen. In chromium sensitivity, evidence has been presented to show that the hexavalent form has to be transformed to the trivalent form in the body before it can sensitize.

It would appear therefore, that in all immune reactions to low molecular weight compounds investigated to date, these sensitizers, or their metabolites, first conjugate to proteins preferentially by covalent linkage, and it is these hapten–protein conjugates that are the true antigens. The use of artificially prepared hapten–protein conjugates has assisted in the investigation into the mechanisms and specificity of antibody production and delayed hypersensitivity.

REFERENCES

Ackroyd, J. F. (1975). In *Clinical Aspects of Immunology*, (Gell, P. G. H., Coombs R. R. A., and Lachmann, P. J., eds.), Blackwell, Oxford, p. 913.

Amos, H. E., Wilson, D. V., Taussig, M. J., and Carlton, S. J. (1971). *Clin. Exp. Immunol.*, **8**, 563.

Asherson, G. L., and Ptak, W. (1970). *Immunology*, **18**, 99.

Baer, H., Watkins, R. C., and Bowser, R. T. (1966). *Immunochemistry*, **3**, 479.

Baer, H., Watkins, R. C., Kurtz, A. P., Byck, J. S., and Dawson, R. C. (1967). *J. Immunol.*, **99**, 370.

Balfour, B. M., McFarlin, D. E., Sumerska, T., and Parker, D. (1974). In *Monograph on Allergy*, Vol. 8, (Parker, D. and Turk, J. L., eds.), Karger, Basel, p. 27.

Batchelor, F. R., Dewdney, J. M., and Gazzard, D. (1965). *Nature, (Lond.)*, **206**, 362.

Batchelor, F. R., Dewdney, J. M., Feinberg, J. G., and Weston, R. D. (1967). *Lancet*, **i**, 1175.

Benacerraf, B., and Gell, P. G. H. (1959). *Immunology*, **2**, 219.

Benacerraf, B., and Levine, B. B. (1962). *J. Exp. Med.*, **115**, 1023.

Benacerraf, B., Paul, W. E., and Green, I. (1970). *Ann. N.Y. Acad. Sci.*, **169**, 93.

Ben Efraim, S., Fuchs, S., and Sela, M. (1967). *Immunology*, **12**, 573.

Borek, F., and Silverstein, A. (1965). *Nature (Lond.)*, **205**, 299.

Borek, F., Silverstein, A. M., and Gell, P. G. H. (1963). *Proc. Soc. Exp. Biol. Med.*, **114**, 266.

Borek, F., Stupp, Y., and Sela, M. (1965). *Science, N.Y.*, **150**, 1177.

Bowser, R. T., and Baer, H. (1963). *J. Immunol.*, **91**, 791.

Butler, V. P., and Beiser, S. M. (1973). *Adv. Immunol.*, **17**, 255.

Cebra, J. J., Koo, P. H., and Ray, A. (1974). *Science, N.Y.*, **186**, 263.

Chase, M. W. (1946). *Proc. Soc. Exp. Biol. Med.*, **61**, 257.

Chase, M. W. (1963). In *La tolérance acquise et la tolérance naturelle a l'égard de substances antigeniques définies*, C.N.R.S., Paris, p. 139.

Chase, M. W., and Maguire, H. C. (1974*a*). In *Monograph on Allergy*, Vol. 8, (Parker, D., and Turk, J. L., eds.), Karger, Basel, p. 1.

Chase, M. W., and Maguire, H. C. (1974*b*). Int. Archs. Allergy, **45**, 513.

David, J. R., Lawrence, H. S., and Thomas, L. (1964). *J. Immunol.*, **93**, 279.

Desaymard, C., and Howard, J. G. (1975). *Eur. J. Immunol.*, **5**, 541.

De Weck, A. L. (1971). *Int. Archs Allergy*, **41**, 393.

De Weck, A. L. (1975). *Int. Archs Allergy*, **49**, 247.

De Weck, A. L., Spengler, H., and Geczy, A. F. (1974). In *Monograph on Allergy*, Vol. 8, (Parker, D., and Turk, J. L., eds.), Karger, Basel, p. 120.

Eisen, H. N. (1959). *Cellular and Humoral Aspects of the Hypersensitivity States*, Paul B. Hoeber, New York.

Eisen, H. N. (1964). *Meth. Med. Res.*, **10**, 115.

Eisen, H. N., Orris, L., and Belman, S. (1952). *J. Exp. Med.*, **95**, 473.

Eisen, H. N., Kern, M., Newton, W. T., and Helmreich, E. (1959). *J. Exp. Med.*, **110**, 187.

Farr, R. S. (1971). In *Mechanisms of Toxicity*, (Aldridge, W. N., ed.), Macmillan, London, p. 87.

Feldman, M., Basten, A., Boylston, A., Erb, P., Gorgyynski, R., Greaves, M., Hogg, N., Kilburn, D., Kontiainen, S., Parker, D., Pepys, M., and Schrader, J. (1974). In *Progress in Immunology II*, Vol. III, (Brent L., and Holborow, J., eds.), North Holland Publishing Co., Amsterdam, p. 65.

Fleischmann, J. B., and Eisen, H. N. (1975). *Cell. Immunol.*, **15**, 312.

Fredericq, E. (1954). *Bull. Soc. Chim. Belg.*, **63**, 158.

Fredericq, E. (1955). *Bull. Soc. Chim. Belg.*, **64**, 639.

Fredericq, E. (1956). *Bull. Soc. Chim. Belg.*, **65**, 631.

Frey, J. R., De Weck, A. L., and Geleick, H. (1966). *Int. Archs Allergy*, **30**, 385.

Frey, J. R., De Weck, A. L., Geleick, H., and Lergier, W. (1969). *J. Exp. Med.*, **130**, 1123.

Gell, P. G. H., and Benacerraf, B. (1961). *J. Exp. Med.*, **113**, 591.

Hanna, N., Jarosch, E., and Leskowitz, S. (1972). *Proc. Soc. Exp. Biol. Med.*, **140**, 89.

Haurowitz, G. (1936). *Z. Physiol. Chem.*, **245**, 23.

Hoffman, D. R., and Campbell, D. H. (1969). *J. Immunol.*, **103**, 655.

Hoffman, D. R., Aalseth, B. L., and Campbell, D. H. (1969). *Immunochemistry*, **6**, 632.

Jones, J. M., and Amos, H. E. (1974). *Int. Archs Allergy*, **46**, 161.

Jones, J. M., and Amos, H. E. (1975). *Nature*, **256**, 500.

Juhlin, L., and Wide, L. (1972). In *Mechanisms in Drug Allergy*, (Dash, C. H., and Jones, H. E. H., eds.), Churchill Livingstone, Edinburgh, p. 139.

Karush, F., and Eisen, H. N. (1962). *Science, N.Y.*, **136**, 1032.

Landsteiner, K. (1921). *Biochem. Z.*, **119**, 294.

Landsteiner, K., and Di Somma, A. A. (1940). *J. Exp. Med.*, **72**, 361.

Landsteiner, K., and Jacobs, J. L. (1935). *J. Exp. Med.*, **61**, 643.

Landsteiner, K., and Lampl, H. (1918). *Z. ImmunForsch.*, **26**, 293.

Lazary, S., Toffler, O., and De Weck, A. L. (1972). In *Mechanisms in Drug Allergy*, (Dash, C. H., and Jones, H. E. H., eds.), Churchill Livingstone, Edinburgh, p. 65.

Leskowitz, S. (1962). *J. Immunol.*, **89**, 434.

Leskowitz, S. (1963). *J. Exp. Med.*, **117**, 909.

Liew, F. Y., and Parish, C. R. (1974). *J. Exp. Med.*, **139**, 779.

Lowney, E. D. (1970). *J. Invest. Dermatol.*, **54**, 355.

Maguire, H. C., and Chase, M. W. (1972). *J. Exp. Med.*, **135**, 357.

Mason, H. S., and Lada, A. (1954). *J. Invest. Dermatol.*, **22**, 457.

Michaelides, M. C., and Eisen, H. N. (1974). *J. Exp. Med.*, **140**, 687.

Mitchison, N. A. (1971a). *Eur. J. Immunol.*, **1**, 10.

Mitchison, N. A. (1971b). *Eur. J. Immunol.*, **1**, 18.

Nishioka, K., Aoki, T., Nishioka, K., and Tashiro, M. (1971). *Dermatologica*, **142**, 232.

Parker, C. W. (1965). *Immunological Diseases*, (Samter, M., ed.), Little Brown and Co., Boston, p. 663.

470

Parker, C. W., Shapiro, J., Kern, H. M., and Eisen, H. N. (1962). *J. Exp. Med.*, **115**, 821.
Parker, D., Aoki, T., and Turk, J. L. (1970). *Int. Archs Allergy*, **38**, 42.
Parker, D., and Turk, J. L. (1970). *Int. Archs Allergy*, **37**, 440.
Paul, W. E., Siskind, G. W., Benacerraf, B., and Ovary, Z. (1967). *J. Immunol.*, **99**, 760.
Polak, L., Barnes, J. M., and Turk, J. L. (1968). *Immunology*, **14**, 707.
Polak, L., and Turk, J. L. (1968). *Clin. Exp. Immunol.*, **3**, 207.
Polak, L., Turk, J. L., and Frey, J. R. (1973). *Prog. Allergy*, **17**, 146.
Pressman, D. (1964). *Meth. Med. Res.*, **10**, 122.

Redmond, A. P., and Levine, B. B. (1968). *Int. Archs Allergy*, **33**, 193.
Reiner, E. (1971). In *Mechanisms of Toxicity*, (Aldridge, W. N., ed.), Macmillan, London, p. 111.
Richerson, H. B., Dvorak, H. F., and Leskowitz, S. (1970). *J. Exp. Med.*, **132**, 546.

Salvin, S. B., and Smith, R. F. (1961). *J. Exp. Med.*, **114**, 185.
Schlossman, S. F., Ben Efraim, S., Yaron, A., and Sober, H. A. (1966). *J. Exp. Med.*, **123**, 1083.
Schlumberger, H. D. (1975). *Int. Archs Allergy*, **48**, 467.
Schlumberger, H. D., Löbbecke, E. A., and Kallos, P. (1974). *Acta med. scand.*, **196**, 451.
Schneider, C. H., and De Weck, A. L. (1965). *Nature*, (*Lond.*), **208**, 57.
Schneider, C. H., and De Weck, A. L. (1967). *Immunochemistry*, **4**, 331.
Schneider, C. H., Michl, J., and De Weck, A. L. (1971). *Eur. J. Immunol.*, **1**, 98.
Schubert, D., Jober, A., and Cohn, M. (1968). *Nature*, (*Lond.*), **220**, 882.
Silverstein, A. M., and Gell, P. G. H. (1962). *J. Exp. Med.*, **115**, 1053.
Sommer, G., Parker, D., and Turk, J. L. (1975). *Immunology*, **29**, 517.
Stewart, G. T. (1967). *Lancet*, **i**, 1177.
Sulzberger, M. B. (1929). *Archs Dermatol. Syph.*, **20**, 669.
Sulzberger, M., and Baer, R. L. (1938). *J. Invest. Dermatol.*, **1**, 45.

Turk, J. L., Polak, L., and Parker, D. (1976). *Brit. Med. Bull.*, **32**, 165.

Ungar-Waron, H., Gurari, D., Hurwitz, E., and Sela, M. (1973). *Eur. J. Immunol.*, **3**, 201.

Vickers, M. R., and Assem, E. S. K. (1974). *Immunology*, **26**, 425.

Weiner, L. M., Rosenblatt, M., and Howess, H. A. (1963). *J. Immunol.*, **90**, 788.
Williams, C. A., and Chase, M. W. (1967). *Methods in Immunology and Immunochemistry*, Vol. 1, Academic Press, New York and London, p. 120.

Zembala, M., and Asherson, G. L. (1973). *Nature*, (*Lond.*), **244**, 227.

CHAPTER 13

Immunochemistry of Collagen

Helen K. Beard, W. Page-Faulk

L. E. Glynn, and L. B. Conachie

1 INTRODUCTION

Collagen is an important structural glycoprotein occurring in both vertebrates and invertebrates (except for protozoa) (Lowther, 1963). In mammals, it forms the major constituent of skeletal and connective tissues, and in skin, tendon, cornea, and demineralized bone, collagen accounts for more than 70 per cent of the tissue dry weight (Grant and Prockop, 1972a, b, c).

471

The fibrous nature of this protein is demonstrable readily by both electron microscopy and the use of histochemical techniques in association with light microscopy. The size, distribution, and alignment of collagen fibres varies enormously in tissues of differing functions (Causey, 1962; McCall, 1968; Forrester et al., 1969; Mohos and Wagner, 1969). The extent to which these variations are governed by factors, such as heterogeneity in primary structure (Miller and Matukas, 1974) or associations with other connective tissue components, including proteoglycans and glycosaminoglycans (Conochie et al., 1975; Lee-Owen and Anderson, 1975; Obrink et al., 1975), is still unknown.

Since the 1930s when the first X-ray diffraction studies of collagen fibres were published (Astbury, 1938), much information has been accumulated concerning the structure of collagen. The basic collagen molecule, tropocollagen, has been isolated, and its size, rod-like shape, and triple-stranded coiled-coil structure have been established firmly (Traub and Piez, 1971). Recently, great progress has been made towards the elucidation of the amino acid sequences, the nature of the carbohydrate linkages, and the identity of inter-chain cross-links. At present, four genetically distinct collagen types have been identified. Isolation of a biosynthetic collagen precursor, procollagen, has stimulated interest in the field of collagen metabolism.

The growth in the knowledge of the structure and biosynthesis of collagen has been accompanied by a complete reversal of the views concerning the immunogenicity of this molecule. Since Landsteiner (1936) declared collagen to be a classically non-immunogenic molecule, both antibodies and cell-mediated immunity to collagen have been demonstrated, and the nature of the antigenic determinants and the genetic control of the immune response have been studied in detail. In addition, antibodies to all four collagen types (I–IV), and to certain forms of procollagen have been produced successfully for use in the study of these molecules. The relevance of collagen immunochemistry in medicine is dealt with more fully elsewhere (see Beard et al., 1977a), but is touched upon in Section 5 of this chapter.

The structure and biosynthesis of collagen will be covered in this chapter only in sufficient depth to introduce immunochemical studies of collagen. Recent and detailed reviews on both aspects are available (Kuhn, 1969; Traub and Piez, 1971; Gallop et al., 1972; Grant and Prockop, 1972a, b, c; Bailey and Robins, 1973; Timpl et al., 1973a; Bornstein, 1974; Miller and Matukas, 1974; Martin et al., 1975).

2 COLLAGEN STRUCTURE

2.1 Chain Composition

The basic unit of collagen—tropocollagen—is a rigid rod-shaped molecule approximately 300 nm in length and 1·5 nm in diameter, with a molecular weight of 300 000. In all vertebrates so far identified, tropocollagen consists of three similar (but not always identical) polypeptide chains called α chains, each containing approximately 1000 amino acids. The three chains lie parallel to each other, being held together by hydrogen bonds and intra-molecular cross-links, and each α chain is twisted into a left-handed helix, while tropocollagen itself forms a right-handed superhelix. The so-called native triple-helical conformation of the tropocollagen molecule is maintained throughout its length with the exception of short regions at both ends of the molecule (Kang *et al.*, 1967; Stark *et al.*, 1971*b*; Fietzek and Kuhn, 1975), consisting of approximately 16 residues at the N-terminus and 25 residues at the C-terminus. Unlike the helical region, these residues are susceptible to attack by proteolytic enzymes such as trypsin, pronase, and pepsin (Kuhn *et al.*, 1966; Bornstein, 1969; Becker *et al.*, 1975*a*). The native conformation of tropocollagen in solution is lost readily on heating, the denaturation temperature varying according to the species from which the collagen is derived. Collagens from mammals such as rat, human, and cow begin to denature at $36°$, whereas the denaturation temperature of poikilotherms appears to correlate with the environmental temperature, that for antarctic ice-fish being $5·5°$ while cuticle collagen of earthworm denatures at $22°$ (Ramachandran, 1963; Rigby, 1968). On denaturation the α chains of tropocollagen assume a random conformation, and the resulting denatured collagen solution contains a varying mixture of randomly coiled monomers (α chains), dimers (β components), or trimers (γ components) depending on the degree of cross-linking (Piez *et al.*, 1963). Denatured collagen is often referred to as gelatin, but it differs considerably from the commercially available product which is derived usually from the insoluble collagen of cows' bones or hide by lime processing (Mees and James, 1966). Four different types of collagen have been identified, which differ in their subunit composition.

2.1.1 Type I Collagen

This was the first collagen type to be isolated and therefore the most thoroughly studied. It has the subunit composition $[\alpha_1(I)]_2\alpha_2$, having two identical α_1 (type I) chains and a third chain, α_2, with a different primary structure.

Type I collagen can be extracted from many tissues including skin, tendon and bone. Collagen becomes increasingly insoluble with age (Verzar, 1964; Sinex, 1968), but using tissues from young animals low yields of collagen may be obtained by extracting with neutral salt solutions, and usually up to 20 per cent of the collagen can be removed by $0·5$ M acetic acid. While acid-soluble collagen contains α, β, and γ components, monomeric α chains are the predominant component of the neutral salt extracts (Heikkinen and Kulonen, 1966), and the yield in these extracts may be increased markedly by the use of lathyrogen β-aminopropionitrile which, when fed to animals, reduces cross-linking by inhibiting the enzyme lysyl oxidase (see Section 2.4). Guanidine hydrochloride (5 M) or urea (8 M) also have been used to extract α chains for use in immunological studies and have been particularly useful because under these conditions the non-helical regions are protected from enzymic attack (Bornstein and Piez, 1964; Becker *et al.*, 1972).

The purification procedure for type I collagen involves the repeated precipitation of the molecule which can be achieved in a number of ways. Collagen can be precipitated from neutral solution by the addition of sodium chloride to 20 per cent (w/v) (Bornstein and Piez, 1964) by acidification to pH 3–4 (Piez *et al.*, 1963; Bornstein and Piez, 1964), and by the addition of ethanol to a final concentration of 14 per cent (by volume) (Gross, 1958). It is precipitated from an acidic solution by dialysis against 0·02 M disodium phosphate (pH 9·0) (Piez *et al.*, 1963; Michaeli *et al.*, 1971) or by the addition of sodium chloride to 5 per cent (w/v) (Piez *et al.*, 1963). Collagen also has been precipitated from neutral or acidic solution by dialysis against water (Gross *et al.*, 1955).

2.1.2 Type II Collagen

Type II collagen has so far been isolated from cartilage (Miller and Matukas, 1974), notochord (Linsenmeyer *et al.*, 1973) and intervertebral discs (Eyre and Muir, 1976). This has the composition $[\alpha_1(II)]_3$ having three identical α_1 (type II) chains which differ in primary structure from both the α_1 and α_2 chains of type I collagen. Soluble type II collagen has been obtained from the sternal cartilages of lathyritic chicks by extraction with neutral salt solutions (Miller, 1971; Trelstad *et al.*, 1972), but solubilization of type II collagen from non-lathyritic cartilage relies on the use of pepsin in an acid solution (Miller, 1972).

Removal of proteoglycan impurities from these preparations has been achieved by chromatography on DEAE–cellulose in 0·2 M sodium chloride (pH 7·5) (Miller, 1971) or by differential precipitation of the proteoglycans with cetyl pyridinium chloride (Miller and Matukas, 1969). Further purification can be achieved by dialysis against 0·02 M disodium hydrogen (pH 9·0) phosphate under conditions similar to those used for type I collagen.

Type II collagen, as well as type I, occurs in cartilage although in small amounts, and is mainly found in the perichondrium. The two collagen types may be separated by differential salt precipitation, type II remaining in solution at 2·2 M sodium chloride (pH 7·5) while type I is precipitated. The component α_1 chains, $\alpha_1(I)$ and $\alpha_1(II)$, may be separated from mixtures of these two by DEAE–cellulose chromatography using a stepwise pH gradient from 9·6 to 7·5 (Trelstad *et al.*, 1972).

2.1.3 Type III Collagen

This is the most recently characterized collagen and is described by the formula $[\alpha_1(III)]_3$, having three identical α_1 (type III) chains of unique primary structure. Type III collagen has been isolated from human placenta, infant skin and aorta, and uterine leiomyoma following limited pepsin digestion (Chung and Miller, 1974; Epstein, 1974; Chung *et al.*, 1976). Type III collagen is present also in neutral salt extracts of rat and bovine skin (Byers *et al.*, 1974; Lenears and

Lapiere, 1975; Timpl *et al.*, 1975) although it is detected in very small amounts—5–10 mg per 50 skins extracted in the case of rat tissue (Byers *et al.*, 1974) and 50–100 mg/kg. wet skin. This represents 5–10 per cent of the amount of Type I in the case of foetal bovine tissue (Timpl *et al.*, 1975).

Purification procedures for type III collagen are similar to those employed for type II, and acidic impurities can be removed by DEAE–cellulose chromatography using 0·2 M sodium chloride (pH 7·5) (Byers *et al.*, 1974; Timpl *et al.*, 1975). Again, types I and III collagens can be separated by differential salt precipitation, type III collagen precipitating out of 1·5 M sodium chloride solution (pH 7·5), while type I remains in solution (Chung and Miller, 1974; Epstein, 1974; Timpl *et al.*, 1975). An alternative method involves preferentially redissolving type I collagen in 1·5 M sodium chloride (pH 7·5) from a precipitate containing both type I and type III (Byers *et al.*, 1974).

2.1.4 Type IV Collagen

A feature of this collagen is that it is found exclusively in basement membranes from which it has been isolated, after limited pepsin digestion, and purified by repeated precipitation from acid solution using 15 per cent (w/v) potassium chloride (Kefalides, 1971). Although it was originally thought to have the chain composition $[\alpha_1(IV)]_3$, recent work suggests the presence of two distinct α chains in type IV collagen (Daniels and Hao Chu, 1975).

2.1.5 Structure–Function Relationships

The identification of these four types of collagen gives rise to some interesting speculations concerning their specialized functions in the body. While collagen types II and IV appear to be tissue-specific, types I and III co-exist in tissues such as skin and aorta, and any specialized function attributable to them may be non-structural. It has been suggested that type III collagen is a foetal type (Trelstad *et al.*, 1971; Epstein, 1971, 1974; Vinson and Seyer, 1974) but it also has been found that its capacity to aggregate platelets considerably exceeds that of types I and II (Balleison *et al.*, 1975). It seems likely that other types will be found, and indeed the collagen of cod-fish skin is known to have an entirely different subunit structure $(\alpha_1\alpha_2\alpha_3)$ (Traub and Piez, 1971).

2.2 Primary Structure

The amino acid compositions and carbohydrate contents of the component chains from all four collagen types are shown in Table 1. Certain features, namely the presence of at least one-third glycine and the high content of imino acids, are characteristic of all four types and are essential for the maintenance of the triple-helical structure (Traub and Piez, 1971; Jimenez *et al.*, 1973; Ramachandran *et al.*, 1973). The glycine contents of types III and IV are somewhat greater than

Table 1 Comparative amino acid and carbohydrate compositions of collagens types I–IV

Component	Concentration (residues/1000 total)				
	Type I (Skin)		Type II (Cartilage)	Type III (Skin)	Type IV (Glomerulus)
	α_2	α_1 (I)	α_1 (II)	α_1 (III)	α_1 (IV)
3-Hyp	1	1	2	NT	11
4-Hyp	89	99	99	121	130
Asp	43	41	42	48	51
Thr	18	17	20	15	23
Ser	35	38	27	41	37
Glu	66	74	90	71	84
Pro	113	131	120	102	61
Gly	335	329	333	355	310
Ala	109	115	100	92	33
Val	34	20	18	16	29
Met	5	7	9	7	10
Ile	14	7	9	13	30
Leu	32	20	26	21	54
Tyr	4	2	1	2	6
Phe	11	13	13	8	27
His	11	2	2	6	1Q
Hyl	9	5	14	5	45
Lys	22	30	22	30	10
Arg	51	50	51	46	33
$\frac{1}{2}$-Cys	0	0	0	2	8
units carbohydrate/ mole chain		1–2	10		36

Amino acid compositions refer to human collagens (Traub and Piez, 1971; Kefalides, 1971; Miller and Lunde, 1973; Epstein, 1974), carbohydrate compositions refer to animal species (Miller and Matukas, 1974). NT = not tested

one-third, and these two collagen types also have larger amounts of hydroxyproline than types I and II. Type II collagen is similar to type IV in having higher levels of glutamic acid, hydroxylysine, and hydroxylysine-linked carbohydrates than types I and III, but differs from all other types in its threonine : serine ratio. Particularly noteworthy is the presence of cysteine residues in types III and IV, while being absent from types I and II. Type IV also contains uniquely high levels of 3-hydroxyproline. The remaining amino acids, with the exception of alanine which is relatively high in type I, appear to be distributed similarly in all four types. Small variations in the numbers, as well as the distribution, of methionine residues are useful as cleavage at these sites by cyanogen bromide yields characteristic peptide mixtures for each collagen type.

The major carbohydrate components of collagen are glucose and galactose, which are linked to hydroxylysine either as glucosyl-galactosyl-hydroxylysine or as galactosyl-hydroxylysine units. As can be seen from Table 1, the carbohydrate content varies considerably. Digestion of α chains with cyanogen bromide and with enzymes, such as trypsin and collagenase, may facilitate the location of carbohydrate units. In type I, the carbohydrate appears to be restricted largely to the N-terminal regions of both chains, and has been located in the cyanogen bromide-cleaved peptides, α_1CB5 in rat and chick skin collagens (Butler, 1970; Aguilar et al., 1973; Kang et al., 1975), and α_2CB4 in rat and guinea-pig collagens (Aguilar et al., 1973; Clark et al., 1975). This portion, consisting of approximately 10 per cent of the total length from the N-terminus, coincides with the postulated hole region in the fibril (see Section 2.3), which could explain how this bulky side chain is accommodated within the collagen fibre (Morgan et al., 1970). The location of carbohydrate in types II–IV has not been investigated thoroughly, although it has been reported that the cyanogen bromide-generated peptides of the N-terminal half of the chick $\alpha_1(II)$ chain (CB 11 and 12) contain linked carbohydrate (Yonath et al., 1975).

Determination of the amino acid sequence of collagen is a formidable task because of the size of the chains; they contain approximately 1000 residues. However, the preparation of cyanogen bromide-cleaved fragments has provided a very useful method of obtaining more manageable sized peptides. The order of these peptides in the original chain can be deduced (i) by forming segment-long-spacing (SLS) precipitates of the peptides and the whole chain and comparing their band patterns, which are determined by the amino acid sequence, using electron microscopy; (ii) by characterization of uncleaved peptides; and (iii) by pulse-labelling experiments (Dintzis, 1961; Rauterberg and Kuhn, 1968; Piez et al., 1969; Igarashi et al., 1970; Vunst et al., 1970). Such peptides have been invaluable in immunochemical, as well as in sequence studies of collagen, and their order in types I and II collagens of several different species is shown in

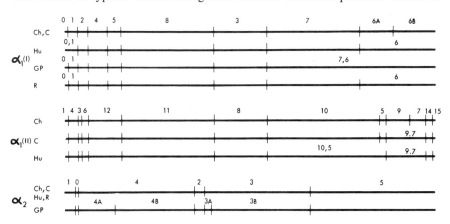

Figure 1 The order of the cyanogen bromide-produced peptides isolated from the α chains of collagen (Types I and II). The vertical lines show the positions of methionine residues, the distances between them are proportioned to the sizes of the peptides. Ch, chick; C, calf or adult bovine; Hu, human; GP, guinea-pig; R, rat. Data taken from Traub and Piez (1971), Volpin and Veis (1971), Miller and Lunde (1973), Miller et al. (1973), Clark et al. (1975).

Figure 1. In sequence studies many different enzymes, including trypsin, chymotrypsin, thermolysin, collagenase, and pepsin, have been used to produce further cleavage of the larger peptides (Balian *et al.*, 1972; Rexrodt *et al.*, 1973), and the complete sequence of the $\alpha_1(I)$ chain has been published using data obtained from rat and calf collagen (Fietzek and Kuhn, 1975*a*). The sequence of the α_2 chain also has been elucidated partially (Highberger *et al.*, 1971; Fietzek *et al.*, 1972). These data confirm previous evidence that the 1011 amino acids in the central helical region are distributed according to the formula Gly-X-Y. However, this sequence does not occur in the 16 residues at the N-terminus or the 25 residues at the C-terminus. In addition, the occurrence of individual amino acids in positions X and Y is not random, and it seems likely that this distribution is dictated by triple helical conformation, fibre formation, and cross-linking (Fietzek and Kuhn, 1975; Salem and Traub, 1975).

The sequence homology between collagens of different species and different types is an important consideration when studying the immune response to collagen. Early work showed similar amino acid compositions for collagens from many different sources (Eastoe, 1967). Comparison of type I collagens from human and rat indicates 97 per cent similarity in the helical region, but a greater variation in the non-helical portion (Bornstein, 1968). Correlation of the amino

Table 2   Sequence homology of type I collagen from several species

Region	Peptide	Number of amino acids sequenced	Species compared	Homology (per cent)
N-Terminal	α_1 CB0,1	20	chick/calf	80
		16	chick/rat	94
		20	man/rabbit	80
	α_1 CB2	36	chick/rat	97
			calf/rat	100
	α_1 CB4	47	chick/rat	96
			calf/rat	100
	α_1 CB5	37	chick/rat	97
			calf/rat	95
	α_1 CB8	26	calf/rat	88
	α_1 CB3	149	chick/calf	91
			chick/rat	89
	α_1 CB7	268	chick/calf	94
	α_1 CB6A	106	chick/calf	90
C-Terminal	α_1 CB6	25	calf/rabbit	68
N-Terminal	α_2 CB1	14	rabbit/rat	57
		12	rat/calf	83
	α_2 CB4	42	calf/rat	91
		39	calf/GP	92
	α_2 CB2	30	chick/rat	90
	α_2 CB3	21	calf/GP	86
			rat/GP	91

Data from Highberger *et al.* (1971), Traub and Piez (1971), Fietzek *et al.* (1972), Clark *et al.* (1975)
GP = Guinea-pig

acid sequences for type I collagens from several species is now possible, together with a comparison of sequences in the α_1 chain of bovine type I with corresponding sequences in Types II and III bovine collagen. Table 2 shows the percentage homology between short sequences occurring throughout the length of the α_1 and α_2 chains of type I collagens. As previously indicated by amino acid composition, the non-helical sequences are more variable than those in the central region, but it is interesting to note that the small peptides (CB2, CB4, and CB5) near the N-terminus of the α_1 chain appear, from these preliminary data, to be less variable than the rest. Comparison of sequences from α_1(I)CB3 of bovine type I and α_1(II)CB8 of bovine type II shows apparent clustering of variant and invariant regions (Butler et al., 1974), which may give rise readily to type-specific antigenic determinants in the central region. A similar effect is observed when bovine types I and III are compared by amino acid sequence data (Fietzek and Rauterberg, 1975) and human types I and III by the SLS band patterns seen using the electron microscope (Wiedemann et al., 1975).

2.3 Fibril Structure

Organized collagenous structures, such as the fibrous bundles in skin and tendon (Forrester et al., 1969), stacked sheets in cornea (Mohos and Wagner, 1969), and fine, mesh-like networks in interstitial tissue (Causey, 1962; Wick et al., 1975), are made up of fibrils comprising aggregated tropocollagen molecules. Current theories on the arrangement of the rod-like tropocollagen units within the fibril are represented diagrammatically in Figure 2. Electron microscopy of unstained (Spadaro, 1970) or negatively stained collagen fibres shows alternating light and dark bands with a periodicity of approximately 680 nm (Hodge et al., 1965). Different band patterns are obtained in SLS forms which are the short segments prepared by precipitating tropocollagen from solutions with ATP. The length of the SLS form (280 nm) corresponds closely to the length of the tropocollagen molecule, and careful analysis of SLS and native band patterns has provided convincing evidence for the 'quarter-stagger and overlap' alignment in the native fibril (see Figure 2) (Hodge and Schmitt, 1960; Kuhn et al., 1960). SLS is thought to consist of a single stack of tropocollagen molecules lying parallel to one another. The length of the tropocollagen molecule is $4.4 \times D$, where D is the native collagen period and the dark and light bands within the period correspond to the hole and overlap zones, respectively. The reason why the hole zone appears to be more electron dense than the overlap zone in unstained fibres is not understood (Spadaro, 1970; Traub and Piez, 1971). The way in which this quarter-stagger and overlap arrangement is maintained in three dimensions is still uncertain, but the pentameric microfibril theory (Smith, 1968) shown in Figure 2 fits well with recent X-ray diffraction data (Miller and Wray, 1971; Miller and Parry, 1973), which suggest that the tropocollagen molecules are twisted along the axis of the microfibril, thus becoming 'coiled, coiled coils' (Miller and Wray, 1971).

480

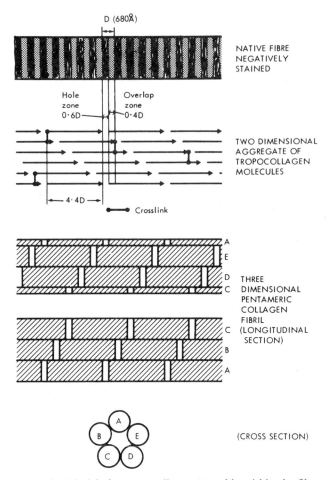

NATIVE FIBRE
NEGATIVELY
STAINED

Hole
zone
0·6D

Overlap
zone
0·4D

TWO DIMENSIONAL
AGGREGATE OF
TROPOCOLLAGEN
MOLECULES

4·4D

●— Crosslink

A
E

D THREE
C DIMENSIONAL
PENTAMERIC
COLLAGEN
FIBRIL
C (LONGITUDINAL
SECTION)
B
A

(CROSS SECTION)

Figure 2   Models for tropocollagen assembly within the fibre

2.4 Cross-Links

The supportive function of collagen requires both mechanical stability and tensile strength. These properties are maintained in the fibre by covalent cross-links between the aggregated molecules. The type of cross-links best studied are those formed from lysine and hydroxylysine-derived aldehydes, but these may be only intermediate in nature (Bailey and Robins, 1973). It is also possible that carbohydrate groups may have an indirect, if not a direct, role in collagen cross-linking (Bailey *et al.*, 1974). Also, in types III and IV collagen, the cysteine residues form disulphide bridges (Kefalides, 1971; Chung and Miller, 1974). The cysteine residues of type III collagen have been located in the C-terminal region (Chung *et al.*, 1974), and it has been postulated that the C-terminal extension of procollagen (see Section 3) also contains disulphide bridges (Murphy *et al.*,

1975), although in this precursor molecule their presence may be required for fibril formation rather than for stabilization (Martin *et al.*, 1975).

Both intra and inter-molecular cross-links are derived following the oxidation of lysine or hydroxylysine to its respective aldehyde by the enzyme lysyl oxidase. Intra-molecular bonds are formed by the reaction of two lysine-derived aldehydes to form the aldol, and inter-molecular cross-links arise from aldimine condensations of lysine and hydroxylysine with their aldehydes, in either combination (Traub and Piez, 1971). These cross-links differ in their stability and tissue distribution, and have been shown to decline with age, probably being replaced by other non-labile ones (Bailey and Shimokamaki, 1971; Bailey and Robins, 1973; Davis and Risen, 1974). This form of cross-linking may be inhibited by β-aminopropionitrile, which blocks the action of lysyl oxidase, or by D-penicillamine, which binds to aldehydes (Deshmukh and Nimni, 1969; Bailey and Robins, 1973).

Inter-molecular cross-links may form head-to-tail or side-to-side bonds between tropocollagen molecules in the fibre. Lysyl aldehydes have been located at the N-terminus of both $\alpha_1(I)$ and α_2, and at the C-terminus of $\alpha_1(I)$ (Stark *et al.*, 1971*b*; Furthmayr and Timpl, 1972; Rauterberg *et al.*, 1972), and the cross-linked peptides $\alpha_1(I)CB(1 \times 6)$, $\alpha_1(I)CB(6 \times 5)$, and $\alpha_1(II)CB(4 \times 9)$ have been isolated (Kang, 1972; Miller and Robertson, 1973; Becker *et al.*, 1975*b*), indicating the presence of head-to-tail cross-links originating from lysine aldehydes in both C and N-termini (see Figure 2).

3 COLLAGEN BIOSYNTHESIS

Collagen is produced by a wide variety of cell types including fibroblasts, chondrocytes, osteocytes, epithelial cells, and smooth muscle cells (Filton, Jackson and Smith, 1957; Green and Goldberg, 1964; Dehm and Prockop, 1973; May and Dodson, 1973; Trelstad *et al.*, 1973; Layman and Titus, 1975). The biosynthetic pathway, presented diagrammatically in Figure 3, involves the initial synthesis of the collagen precursor, procollagen, which undergoes several post-translational modifications, such as the hydroxylation of lysine and proline, and glycosylation, prior to the formation of the triple helix and secretion. Conversion of procollagen to collagen, fibril formation, and cross-linking are extracellular events controlled by factors not yet fully elucidated.

Synthesis of procollagen precursosrs whose component pro-α chains are longer than the α chains of collagen has been demonstrated repeatedly using tissue-culture techniques (Bellamy and Bornstein, 1971; Layman *et al.*, 1971; Smith *et al.*, 1972). Furthermore, procollagen has been isolated from the skin of dermatosporactic calves (Lenears *et al.*, 1971) as well as from normal rat and bovine skins (Clark and Veis, 1972; Veis *et al.*, 1973; Byers *et al.*, 1974; Lenears and Lapiere, 1975; Timpl *et al.*, 1975). Procollagen can be extracted from skin or fibroblast cultures using neutral salt solutions or 0·5 M acetic acid (Layman *et al.*, 1971; Clark and Veis, 1972; Sherr *et al.*, 1973), but its isolation from bone requires additional precautions such as rapid acidic extraction or the use of

482

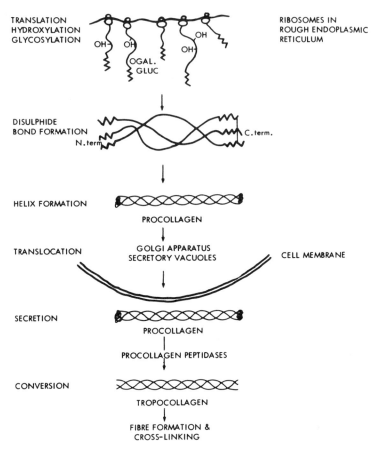

TRANSLATION
HYDROXYLATION
GLYCOSYLATION

RIBOSOMES IN
ROUGH ENDOPLASMIC
RETICULUM

OGAL.
GLUC

DISULPHIDE
BOND FORMATION

N.term

C.term.

HELIX FORMATION

PROCOLLAGEN

TRANSLOCATION

GOLGI APPARATUS
SECRETORY VACUOLES

CELL MEMBRANE

SECRETION

PROCOLLAGEN

PROCOLLAGEN PEPTIDASES

CONVERSION

TROPOCOLLAGEN

FIBRE FORMATION &
CROSS-LINKING

Figure 3 Diagrammatic representation of the biosynthetic pathway of
collagen

enzyme inhibitors to prevent breakdown of the molecule (Fessler *et al.*, 1973;
Monson and Bornstein, 1973). Purification has been achieved by precipitation
with ammonium sulphate, trichloracetic acid, ethanol, or sodium chloride (Byers
et al., 1974; Church *et al.*, 1974; Murphy *et al.*, 1975). Precursor molecules for all
four collagen types have now been identified (Grant *et al.*, 1972; Dehm and
Prockop, 1973; Anesey *et al.*, 1975). Recent evidence suggests that procollagens
contain three disulphide-linked pro-α chains which have polypeptide extension at
both the C and N-terminal ends (Tanzer *et al.*, 1974; Anesey *et al.*, 1975; Park *et
al.*, 1975), and it seems likely that isolated procollagen molecules which either
partially or totally lack disulphide bonds (Bellamy and Bornstein, 1971; Smith *et
al.*, 1972) or the C-terminal extension (Stark *et al.*, 1971) represent breakdown
products of the original precursor (Goldberg and Sherr, 1973; Monson and
Bornstein, 1973; Bornstein, 1974). The amino acid composition of the polypeptide extensions of procollagen differs markedly from that of tropocollagen,

having both cysteine and tryptophan, and containing higher levels of tyrosine, glutamic acid, aspartic acid and serine, while levels of proline and glycine are lower (Furthmayr *et al.*, 1972*a*; Schofield and Prockop, 1973). Preliminary results show that the C-terminal extension has higher levels of cysteine than that at the N-terminus, which agrees with the suggestion that the disulphide bonds are located in the former (Tanzer *et al.*, 1974; Murphy *et al.*, 1975).

Many functions have been postulated for procollagen, including (*i*) facilitation of transportation and/or secretion of the molecule, (*ii*) initiation of the triple-helical formation, (*iii*) inhibition of intracellular fibrillogenesis, and (*iv*) alignment of polypeptide chains in extracellular fibrillogenesis; none has been demonstrated experimentally. The presence of procollagen in adult tissues (Timpl *et al.*, 1973*b*; Veis *et al.*, 1973) prompts the speculation that this molecule may have post-biosynthetic functions.

Hydroxylation of proline and lysine in procollagen occurs under the control of the enzymes prolyl and lysyl hydroxylases, which have been shown by immunological and biochemical methods to be located in the rough endoplasmic reticulum (Diegelmann *et al.*, 1973; Olsen *et al.*, 1973; Al-Adnani *et al.*, 1974). Both enzymes require Fe^{2+}, molecular oxygen, α-ketoglutarate, and a reducing agent, which *in vivo* is probably ascorbate (Miller, 1971; Bornstein, 1974). The conversion of proline to 4-hydroxyproline by prolylhydroxylase is limited to proline residues in the position Y of the sequence Gly-X-Y, and lysyl hydroxylase only acts on lysine residues at this position. Hydroxyproline levels remain fairly constant, while hydroxylysine levels vary considerably in collagens from different tissues (Barnes *et al.*, 1971). However, hydroxylation of individual proline as well as lysine residues in the chain may be incomplete, leading to further microheterogeneity in collagen (Grant and Prockop, 1972*a*, *b*, *c*). Severe lysyl hydroxylase deficiency has been described in two siblings with a form of Ehlers–Danlos syndrome (Krane *et al.*, 1972).

Further modifications occur as hydroxylysine residues become oxidized by lysyl oxidase prior to cross-linking or become glycosylated by galactosyl and glucosyl transferases which are thought to act on nascent collagen chains (Brownwell and Veis, 1975). Defects in lysyl oxidase activity occur in diseased animals and humans (Rowe *et al.*, 1974; Danks *et al.*, 1972). Increased glycosylation of basement membrane collagen has been found in patients with diabetes mellitus (Beisswenger and Spiro, 1970). Basement membranes in this disease also have been shown by electron microscopy to be morphologically abnormal (Siperstein *et al.*, 1968).

The mode of cell transport and secretion of procollagen is uncertain. Formation of the triple helix and disulphide bonds occurs very soon after translation (Schofield and Prockop, 1973; Uitto and Prockop, 1974; Harwood *et al.*, 1975). Elegant ultrastructural studies using autoradiographic and immuno-histochemical techniques have indicated that procollagen molecules migrate from the rough endoplasmic reticulum to the golgi apparatus from where they are transported to the cell membrane in vesicles and released by exocytosis (Olsen and Prockop, 1974; Weinstock and Leblond, 1974). In addition, use of inhibitors such as colchicine, vinblastine, and cytochalasin B indicates that microtubules, but not microfilaments, are required for translocation of procollagen and its conversion to collagen (Ehrlich and Bornstein, 1972; Ehrlich et al., 1974). Collagen also has been reported to be membrane bound on fibroblasts, and the mobility of collagen within these membranes, as measured by the inhibition of antibody-generated cap-formation, is inhibited by colchicine. Thus, this further supports the suggestion of Faulk et al. (1975) that the process is mediated by microtubules.

Evidence for the extracellular conversion of procollagen to tropocollagen comes from the presence of both the precursor (Layman et al., 1971) and procollagen peptidase (Layman and Ross, 1973) in the medium of cultured fibroblasts. From pulse–chase experiments, it has been demonstrated that procollagen synthesized by chick tendons in organ culture is cleaved extracellularly (Jimenez et al., 1971). Procollagen peptidases, which convert acid-extracted bone procollagen—lacking in disulphide bonds—to collagen (Bornstein et al., 1972) or which remove N-terminal extensions from the procollagen found in the skin of dermatosparactic calves (Cohn et al., 1974), have been isolated. However, these enzymes do not remove necessarily inter-chain disulphide bridges from procollagen (Lenears and Lapiere, 1975; Murphy et al., 1975). Moreover, some evidence suggests that there may be many steps involved in the conversion of procollagen to collagen (Goldberg and Sherr, 1973; Davidson and Bornstein, 1975). Defects in this process have been detected in animals and man. For example, in dermatosparaxis of sheep and cattle, the peptide extensions are cleaved incompletely and the high levels of procollagen in the tissue prevent the formation of stable fibres (Bailey and Lapiere, 1973; Schofield and Prockop, 1973). Also, evidence has been found in humans for reduced procollagen peptidase activity in fibroblast cultures from patients with a form of Ehlers–Danlos syndrome (Lichtenstein et al., 1973).

4 IMMUNOLOGY OF COLLAGEN

Since the first definitive demonstrations of the immunogenicity of collagen by Watson et al. (1954) and Schmitt et al. (1964), there have been active studies in this field, with particular emphasis on structure in relation to antigenicity and, more recently, on the immunological characterization of the different collagens and procollagens. Investigations of biological controlling mechanisms in the immune response to collagen have been initiated also.

Several structural features of collagen make this study particularly rewarding. Firstly, approximately 95 per cent of the collagen molecule has a highly repetitive amino acid sequence with the formula Gly-X-Y (see Section 2.2), so that antigenic determinants within this region may require very precise methods of recognition. Information relevant to this question has been obtained from studies on the immune response to collagen-like synthetic polymers and from characterization of centrally located determinants in collagen (see Sections 4.5 and 4.1.3). Sequence analysis of the areas around antigenic sites in the non-helical region has contributed also to an understanding of the immunochemical basis of immuno-genicity, as will be discussed in Section 4.1.4. Secondly, collagen undergoes an unusually large number of post-translational modifications. Such variations in the degree of hydroxylation, glycosylation, and cross-linking give rise to a highly heterogeneous population of molecules. The degree to which these modifications are involved in the immune response to collagen is an important point, but one which so far has been only studied poorly, as will be seen in Section 4.1.4.

The ubiquitous, but structurally highly variable, nature of collagen raises the question of how the body recognizes and maintains tolerance to its own collagen, while being able to respond to collagens from other species which are structurally very similar. This problem is of more than academic interest in view of the reported presence of anti-collagen antibodies in both diseased and normal people (Maurer, 1954a; Steffen, 1969; Michaeli and Fudenberg, 1974). Studies on the genetic control of the immune response to 'foreign' collagen, which will be discussed in Section 4.6, may at least provide an approach to this problem.

4.1 Antibodies to Type I Collagen

4.1.1 Techniques

Insoluble (Steffen and Timpl, 1963), guanidine or urea-extracted (Becker et al., 1972; Rothbard and Watson, 1972), and salt and acid-extracted (Michaeli et al., 1968; Lindsley et al., 1971; Beil et al., 1972, 1973) collagens have been used in immunological studies. As well as being difficult to handle, insoluble collagen is characterized less readily than the soluble forms. The purity of the preparations is of great importance since the presence of minor contaminants, such as acidic (Leroy, 1969) or serum (Steffen et al., 1970a) proteins have been shown to give rise to antibodies. Although biochemical criteria, such as characteristic amino acid composition and electrophoretic mobility, low levels of hexose, and lack of hexosamines (Gross et al., 1958; Nagai et al., 1964; Eastoe, 1967), give an indication of purity, antisera to collagen should be characterized for specificity (Timpl et al., 1967). Salt and acid extracts of skin have been used frequently as a source of type I collagen, but there is evidence (Clark and Veis, 1972; Byers et al., 1974) to suggest that these extracts may also contain type III collagen, and types I and III procollagens. Immunological differences between salt and acid-soluble collagens have been reported (Paz et al., 1963) but incompletely characterized. Extraction of α chains from calf skin collagen using 8 M urea, however, preserves antigenic sites in the C-terminal region which are lost during acidic extraction (Becker et al., 1972).

Anti-collagen antibodies have been produced in rabbits, rats, mice, guinea-pigs, sheep, and chicken (Adelmann et al., 1973; Beil et al., 1972, 1973; Chidlow et al., 1974; Nowack et al., 1975b). The number of different immunization schedules employed almost equals the number of different investigations. Footpad, intradermal, intraperitoneal, intramuscular, and subcutaneous routes of in-jection have all been used, and although prolonged schedules were required in some cases (Michaeli *et al.*, 1968; Steffen *et al.*, 1968; Beil *et al.*, 1972; Timpl *et al.*, 1972), antibodies have been found after only a single injection (Schmitt *et al.*, 1964; Adelmann *et al.*, 1973). Freund's complete adjuvant has been employed usually, but extended immunization of rabbits with rat collagen in the absence of adjuvant gave rise to antibodies (Watson *et al.*, 1954) and Adelmann and coworkers (1973) found that guinea-pigs gave a better antibody response when collagen was emulsified in incomplete rather than in complete Freund's adjuvant. The nature of the immune response seems to vary greatly depending on the species of animal immunized, and on the origin of the collagen used (see Sections 4.1.2 and 4.1.3). In addition, marked differences in antibody specificity between early and late bleeds also have been found (Timpl *et al.*, 1972).

The methods used for the detection of anti-collagen antibodies include anaphylaxis (Rothbar and Watson, 1956), complement fixation (Schmitt *et al.*, 1964; Davidson *et al.*, 1967), cytotoxicity (Lustig, 1970; Duksin *et al.*, 1975), qualitative and quantitative immunofluorescence (Rothbard and Watson, 1961; Lustig *et al.*, 1969; Steffen *et al.*, 1971; Knapp *et al.*, 1974) and radioimmunoassay (Lindsley *et al.*, 1971; Adelmann *et al.*, 1973). Immunoprecipitation methods comprise quantitative precipitation in liquid media (Michaeli *et al.*, 1968), double diffusion in agar, and immunoelectrophoresis (Beil *et al.*, 1972; Furthmayer *et al.*, 1972*b*). Haemagglutination and haemagglutination inhibition studies have been considerably useful in the location of antigenic determinants using collagen fragments. These approaches have employed both glutaraldehyde or tannic acid-treated erythrocytes coated with native collagen, isolated α chains, or collagen fragments, and the reactions have been performed on glass plates or in micro-titre trays (Steffen *et al.*, 1967; Beil *et al.*, 1973).

4.1.2 Role of Conformation

Tropocollagen loses its native triple-helical conformation on heating to 45° for 15 minutes (Piez, 1967). The denatured collagen formed, gelatin, consists of randomly coiled chains. The immunogenicity of native and denatured molecules differs considerably, and direct comparison has been made in several cases (Michaeli *et al.*, 1971; Beil *et al.*, 1973).

Serum factors resembling antibodies, which react with gelatin or the gelatin derivative, oxypolygelatin, have been detected in healthy humans and in many animal species by quantitative precipitation (Maurer, 1954*a*, *b*). This is an important finding since oxypolygelatin has been considered for use as a blood plasma expander, but no significant increases in titre were obtained on immunization of human volunteers with this material (Maurer, 1954*a*), although rabbits were immunized weakly when adjuvants were used (Maurer, 1954*b*). Similar, so-called anti-gelatin factors (AGF) have been found in the sera of normal guinea-pigs and mice using radioimmunoassay (Adelmann *et al.*, 1973; Nowack *et al.*, 1975*b*), and in human, mouse, and guinea-pig sera by haemagglutination (Wolff *et al.*, 1967; Beard, 1974; Nowack *et al.*, 1975*b*). No reaction with native collagen has been detected in these systems. Binding of denatured collagen by mouse AGF in radioimmunoassay was shown to be unaltered following heating of the serum at 56° for 30 minutes, whereas haemagglutination of gelatin-coated erythrocytes by the same factor was abolished by this treatment (Nowack *et al.*, 1975*b*). Wolff and his colleagues (1967) obtained similar results using haemagglutination techniques and showed that this reaction is mediated by two components: (*i*) a heat-labile macroglobulin agglutinator; and (*ii*) a heat-stable macroglobulin activator which potentiates the agglutination. Although the AGF demonstrated by Maurer (1954*a*) reacts with antisera to human γ-globulin, the antibody nature of AGF has not been demonstrated unequivocally. Recently an IgM-like factor in normal guinea-pig sera with properties similar to AGF, was found to be cytophilic for normal macrophages (Hopper *et al.*, 1976), but the biological functions of AGF are unknown.

Immunization of animals with denatured collagen has produced varying results. Nowack and coworkers (1975*b*) found that denatured bovine type I collagen is non-immunogenic in mice, while the native molecule gives a good response. Similarly, guinea-pigs fail to respond to denatured collagens from several species when these antigens are injected in either complete or incomplete Freund's adjuvant (Geutner and Adelmann, 1976). Furthermore, $\alpha_1(I)$ chains of rat skin collagen fail to elicit an immune response in rabbits although antibodies are produced to the α_2 chain and to the native molecule (Lindsley *et al.*, 1971). In contrast, denatured rat type I collagen is able to elicit a good response in certain strains of mice (Fuchs *et al.*, 1974). Steffen and associates (1968) used both native and denatured bovine type I collagen in a large series of immunizations using rabbits and could not detect any differences between them. Native and denatured rat type I collagens have been shown to be equally good antigens in both chickens and rabbits (Beil *et al.*, 1973), although they produced antibodies of differing specificity. Antisera raised to denatured collagen reacts preferentially with this antigen, while antisera to native collagen recognizes both native and denatured molecules. Guinea-pig gelatin is also immunogenic in rabbits (Michaeli *et al.*, 1971) and once again the specificity of antisera differs from that raised to native collagen. Anti-gelatin antibodies and anti-collagen antibodies both recognized determinants in the N-terminus of the α_2 chain, but anti-gelatin antibodies recognize additional determinants in the α_1 chain. These apparently conflicting results on the immunogenicity of gelatin may result from species or strain differences in the animals used for immunization (Beil *et al.*, 1973).

The work discussed above suggests that rabbits and chickens are able to respond to immunization with gelatin, whereas guinea-pigs are not. Rats also may be unable to respond to gelatin because, although attempts to immunize them with gelatin have not been reported, animals immunized with native calf collagen fail to produce antibodies which recognize the denatured molecule (Beil *et al.*, 1973; Hahn and Timpl, 1973). The conflicting results concerning the antigenicity of gelatin in mice are difficult to compare since both the collagens and the strains of mice used are different. It is interesting to note that mice and guinea-pigs, which are unable to respond to immunization with gelatin, have been shown to possess the naturally occurring AGF in their sera (Maurer, 1954b; Adelmann *et al.*, 1973).

Immunization with native collagen gives rise to conformation-dependent and conformation-independent antibodies. The latter react equally well with native and denatured collagen. Once again, the species of animal used for immunization greatly influences the response obtained. For example, rabbits produce complement-fixing antibodies to calf collagen that are conformation-dependent (Schmitt *et al.*, 1964; Davidson *et al.*, 1967), but haemagglutinating rabbit antibodies, which recognize collagen and gelatin equally well, appear after immunization with native calf, guinea-pig, human and rat collagens (Michaeli *et al.*, 1968; Timpl *et al.*, 1968, 1972; Michaeli and Epstein, 1971; Chidlow *et al.*, 1974), although conformation-dependent antibodies also may appear in rare cases (Michaeli and Epstein, 1971; Stoltz *et al.*, 1973). Chickens produce a mixture of antibodies to rat collagen, some of which recognizes native and some of which recognizes denatured collagen preferentially (Beil *et al.*, 1973). As mentioned previously, only conformation-dependent antibodies have been produced in rats using bovine collagen (Beil *et al.*, 1973; Hahn and Timpl, 1973); similar results have been obtained in mice using bovine collagen (Nowack *et al.*, 1975b) and in guinea-pigs using chick, pig, calf, and rat collagens (Adelmann and Geutner, 1976).

4.1.3 Location of Determinants

Schmitt *et al.* (1964) postulated on theoretical grounds that the major antigenic sites in collagen are located at the terminal non-helical regions. They supported this theory experimentally by demonstrating that the antigenic determinants recognized by complement-fixing antibodies in rabbit antisera to bovine collagen are sensitive to limited pronase or pepsin digestion; enzymes known to remove the non-helical regions of the molecule. However, many different determinants exist in collagen as shown by Steffen and colleagues (1968) who using haemagglutination detected three discrete specificities to bovine collagen in rabbit antisera which they termed A, P, and S. Antibodies showing A, or general specificity, react with collagens from many different species, whereas antibodies displaying P or S specificity give more restricted reactions. P-specific determinants are located in the non-helical regions since they are pepsin labile, but both S and A-specific determinants are stable in the presence of pepsin. Further enzymic studies indicate that the A determinants, although insensitive to trypsin, chymotrypsin, pepsin, and pronase, are destroyed by collagenase, and amino acid analysis of active peptides suggests that these determinants are located in apolar regions (Steffen and Timpl, 1970; Steffen *et al.*, 1970b). S, as well as P, determinants are insensitive to collagenase, indicating that they do not lie in the central regions of the molecule (Steffen *et al.*, 1968).

The location of antigenic sites in collagen became considerably easier as techniques for cyanogen bromide cleavage of collagen, and the isolation and purification of the peptides were established (see Section 2.2). Location of the cyanogen bromide-cleaved peptides in the α_1 and α_2 chains of several species of type I collagen is shown in Figure 1. These isolated peptides have been used particularly in haemagglutination inhibition systems (Michaeli *et al.*, 1969; Timpl *et al.*, 1970*b*) but also in radioimmunoassays (Lindsley *et al.*, 1971) to map the position of antigenic determinants. Much of the work has so far been carried out using rabbit sera which, unlike the sera from other species, predominantly recognize sites in non-helical regions but determinants within the molecule also have been located. Beil *et al.* (1973) classified collagen determinants as non-helical, helical, or central according to their location in the molecule. Previous work, summarized in this way, is shown in Table 3. Central and non-helical determinants are almost invariably conformation-independent, whereas helical determinants are conformation-dependent. Rabbits recognize non-helical determinants at both ends of the α_1 and α_2 chains, but the determinants in $\alpha_1 CB6$

Table 3 Location of antigenic determinants in collagen

Region of molecule	Active peptides	Species immunized	Source collagen	Speci-ficity	Reference
Non-helical					
N-terminal	α_1 CB1	rabbit	man	S	Furthmayer *et al.* (1971)
	,,	,,	calf	S	Rauterberg *et al.* (1972)
	α_2 CB1	,,	rat	S	Timpl *et al.* (1972)
	,,	,,	guinea-pig	S	Michaeli *et al.* (1971)
C-terminal	α_1 CB6	rabbit	calf	P	Timpl *et al.* (1970*a*); Pontz *et al.* (1970)
	,,	,,	rat	S	Lindsley *et al.* (1971); Timpl *et al.* (1971*b*)
	,,	,,	man	S	Furthmayr *et al.* (1971)
	α_2 CB5	,,	calf	S	Pontz *et al.* (1970)
	,,	,,	rat	S	Lindsley *et al.* (1971); Timpl *et al.* (1970*b*)
Central	α_1 CB3; 8	rabbit	man	A	Furthmayer *et al.* (1971)
	,,	chicken	rat	A	Furthmayer *et al.* (1972*b*)
	α_1 CB7	rabbit	man	A	Furthmayr *et al.* (1971)
	,,	,,	calf	A	Timpl *et al.* (1971)
	,,	chicken	rat	A	Furthmayr *et al.* (1972*b*)
	α_1 CB6	rabbit	rat	A	Timpl *et al.* (1971)
	,,	chicken	rat	A	Furthmayr *et al.* (1972*b*)
	α_2 CB3; 5	rabbit	man	NT	Michaeli and Epstein (1971)
	,,	,,	calf	NT	Timpl *et al.* (1971)
	,,	,,	rat	NT	Timpl *et al.* (1971)
	,,	chicken	rat	NT	Furthmayr *et al.* (1972*b*)
	α_2 CB4	,,	rat	NT	Furthmayr *et al.* (1972*b*)
	,,	rabbit	man	NT	Michaeli and Epstein (1971)
Helical	α_1 CB6b	rabbit	rat	S	Stoltz *et al.* (1973)
	$(\alpha_1 I)_2 \alpha_2$ C78	mouse	calf	S	Nowack *et al.* (1975*b*)
	(helical)	rat	calf	NT	Hahn *et al.* (1974)

NT = not tested

(the C-terminus of α_1) are by far the most immunogenic in human and calf collagens (Timpl *et al.*, 1970*a*; Furthmayer *et al.*, 1971). Rabbits also produce antibodies more readily to the C-terminus than to the N-terminus of the α_2 chain of rat and calf collagens (Pontz *et al.*, 1970; Timpl *et al.*, 1972).

All determinants found in the non-helical regions are species specific, probably as a result of the inter-species variability of this region of the molecule (see Table 2). In contrast, antibodies to central sites show high levels of cross-reaction between species. Timpl *et al.* (1971) reported that 95 per cent of all rabbits immunized with mammalian collagens produce antibodies of this kind, but these antibodies usually form only a very minor component of the total response. Although such antibodies produced in rabbits after immunization with either rat or calf collagen show maximal activity with single peptides in the α_1 and α_2 chains (see Table 3) almost all the cyanogen bromide-produced peptides show some reaction. Extremely complex haemagglutination inhibition patterns have been obtained which are best interpreted as showing the presence of several different determinants in each peptide which cross-react with determinants in other peptides to varying degrees. In the case of calf collagen, evidence was given for at least nine discrete determinants in the central region. Species non-specific antibodies of much higher haemagglutination titres are obtained by immunizing of chickens with rat collagen (Beil *et al.*, 1972). While pronase digestion suggests that the non-helical regions are unimportant in this response, each of the large cyanogen bromide-produced peptides from the central regions of both α_1 and α_2 appears to possess unique antigenic sites (Furthmayer *et al.*, 1972*b*). The reasons for lack of species specificity for central determinants which are dependent on sequence and not conformation probably lie in the high inter-species homology in this region (see Table 2), but the heterogeneity observed suggests that the determinants involve structures more complex than the Gly-X-Y triplet.

Conformation-dependent determinants, which occur in native, but not in denatured collagen, are found almost entirely in the helical region. Antibodies to these determinants do not recognize denatured collagen, separated chains, or cyanogen bromide-cleaved peptides, but mouse and rat antibodies to calf collagen have been shown to react with a triple-helical fragment from the centre of the molecule obtained by limited collagenase digestion (Hahn *et al.*, 1974; Nowack *et al.*, 1975*b*). In one instance, a conformation-dependent determinant has been found which lies partly in the non-helical C-terminal end of rat collagen (Stoltz *et al.*, 1973).

4.1.4 *Nature of Determinants*

Elucidation of the structural requirements for conformation-dependent determinants is a difficult task since they may involve more than one polypeptide chain (Hahn and Timpl, 1973). Non-helical and central determinants are conformation-independent, and comprise particular regions of the amino acid sequence. Several studies have located non-helical determinants very precisely

(Becker *et al.*, 1972; Furthmayer and Timpl, 1972; Rauterberg *et al.*, 1972; Stoltz *et al.*, 1973) and attempts have been made to correlate these with the sequence homology between the particular species involved (Becker *et al.*, 1975*a*). Less detailed information is available in the case of central determinants, however, and many antigenic sites occur throughout this region in both chains, in spite of the apparent variation in species homology along the length of the α_1 chain (see Table 2).

The major non-helical determinants of calf collagen recognized in rabbits are located in the C-terminus of the α_1 chain and exhibit some degree of heterogeneity as a result of enzymic digestion of the antigen in this region (Timpl *et al.*, 1970*a*). However, Becker and coworkers (1972) detected two different determinants ('a' and 'b') which lie in a region of six amino acids and which are almost completely different in rabbit collagen. Rat skin collagen was shown to possess an antigenic determinant in this same position (Stoltz *et al.*, 1973). Several determinants in the N-terminus of the α_2 chain of rat collagen, again measured by immunization of rabbits, also have been located in regions that differed greatly between the two species (Furthmayer and Timpl, 1972; Becker *et al.*, 1975*a*). In contrast, N-terminal antigenic determinants in the α_1 chains of human and calf collagen showed only one or two amino acid variations from rabbit collagen (Rauterberg *et al.*, 1972; Becker *et al.*, 1975*a*). These determinants show few common features, with the exception of the presence of tyrosine in seven out of eight cases, although in two of these cases rabbit collagen also possesses tyrosine at identical positions. Thus the chemical requirements for antigenicity remain uncertain, and factors other than the variability of amino acid sequence seem likely to be involved in antigenic recognition. Almost complete sequence identity, however, can explain the lack of immunogenicity of rat α_1 CB1 and calf α_2 CB1 fragments in rabbits (Becker *et al.*, 1975*a*).

The role of cross-linking and carbohydrate linkages in collagen antigenicity has been ignored largely with the exception of a study by Furthmayr and Timpl (1972) who obtained variable results when they compared the reactivities of rat α_2 CB1 and its aldehyde derivative with rabbit antibodies which recognized this region of the rat α_2 chain.

4.2 Antibodies to Other Collagen Types

Type II collagen from bovine articular cartilage has been shown to be immunogenic in Wistar rats and in certain strains of mice (Hahn *et al.*, 1974; Nowack *et al.*, 1975*b*). Both species produce specific, conformation-dependent antibodies which do not react with either the denatured molecule or with bovine type I collagen. The response to bovine type II collagen in rabbits is different (Hahn *et al.*, 1975*b*). Rabbit antibodies can be separated into two fractions using collagen immunadsorbents, one of which reacts equally well with native and denatured bovine type II, while the specificity of the other is conformation-dependent; neither fraction shows any reaction with bovine type I collagen.

Rabbit antibodies reacting with denatured bovine type II collagen exhibit cross-reactions with chick type II collagen, and important determinants are located in $\alpha_1(II)$ CB11, which lies in the central region of the chain. Thus, rabbit, rat, and mouse antisera to type II collagen all appear to recognize either central and/or helical determinants. However, pepsin-digested molecules were used for immunization in all these studies, therefore the possibility of non-helical determinants cannot be ruled out.

The immunogenicity of type III collagen so far has been characterized incompletely, although recent evidence suggests that rabbit antibodies to soluble type III collagen from foetal calf skin recognize a cross-linked non-helical region in the N-terminus (Becker et al., 1976). Antibodies cross-reacting with human type III collagen (Nowack et al., 1976a) have been used to locate this collagen type in human aorta (Gay et al., 1975a) and in the livers of patients with hepatic cirrhosis (Gay et al., 1975b).

Antibodies which react with Type IV collagen from the basement membrane in sheep anterior lens capsule have been produced by immunizing rabbits with the purified collagen (Denduchis and Kefalides, 1970). These antibodies have been detected by precipitation reactions in gels and were shown to react with type IV collagen preparations from several different sources, but the nature of their specificity has not been defined so far. Antibodies raised to bovine type IV collagen from anterior lens capsule were shown to be type-specific by radioimmunoassay (Gunson and Kefalides, 1976), but their species specificity was not tested. The determinants appear to be in the central region in this case, since the antigenicity of type IV collagen are conformation-independent, and are unaffected by pepsin treatment.

4.3 Antibodies to Procollagen

Antibodies to procollagen have been obtained by immunizing rabbits with pro-$\alpha_1(I)$ from chick cranial bone (Von der Mark et al., 1973), and purified dermatosparactic procollagens have been extracted from skin (Timpl et al., 1973b) or produced in culture (Park et al., 1975), while type III procollagen was obtained from bovine amniotic fluid (Lee et al., 1975), and the culture medium of human diploid fibroblasts (Sherr and Goldberg, 1973). In each case, antibodies specific to the procollagen extensions were obtained which did not cross-react with the corresponding collagen chains. The antigenic determinants are dependent on the disulphide bridges in some cases, since the determinants are destroyed by reduction and alkylation (Timpl et al., 1973b; Park et al., 1975) but direct experiments to locate these determinants in the C or N-terminal extensions have not been performed. Procollagen synthesized by cloned dermatosparactic cells in tissue culture appears to have determinants in both C and N-terminal extensions, while dermatosparactic collagen (which lacks the C-terminal extension, see Section 3) has determinants in the N-terminal extension only (Park et al., 1975).

Antibodies to procollagen have been used in two interesting studies. In one case the intracellular transport of procollagen into fibroblasts was followed (Olsen and Prockop, 1974), and in the other the presence of procollagen in human serum was detected, with particularly high levels being found in human cord blood (Taubman *et al.*, 1974). Wick *et al.* (1975) have also used antibodies to procollagen from dermatosparactic calves to demonstrate the presence of this molecule in the subepithelial layers of normal calf skin and the interstitial tissue of normal calf kidney.

4.4 Cell-Mediated Immunity to Collagen

In comparison with the many studies of the humoral immune responses to collagen, cell-mediated responses have been largely neglected until recently. The first serious study of the cell-mediated responses was made by Adelmann and his coworkers (Adelmann *et al.*, 1968, 1972; Adelmann, 1972, 1973; Adelmann and Kirrane, 1973). They used highly purified preparations of human, calf, rat, and guinea-pig type I collagens extracted either using acidic or neutral salt solutions and employed the native or denatured form for immunization and subsequent testing. Immunization was induced with the aid of Freund's complete adjuvant incorporating 500 µg of antigen injected into the foot pads; the skin-test dose was 150 µg in saline (0·1 ml). For comparison, the reactions were expressed as an index based on the increase in skin thickness at 24 hours as well as on the diameter and degree of the associated erythema. It was clearly established that the complete adjuvant is essential in the immunizing schedule. Delayed-type skin sensitivity is maximal 20 days after immunization and persists for at least three months. Although the reactions are species specific, insofar as they are always greatest with the immunizing antigen, cross-reactions may be obtained readily using other mammalian collagens, except that of guinea-pig. Neither in guinea-pigs immunized with guinea-pig nor with heterologous collagen can any reaction be obtained indicative of cell-mediated immunity to guinea-pig collagen.

The ability of the individual α_1 and α_2 chains to induce cell-mediated reactions has also been reported (Adelmann, 1972). Both calf and rat skin collagens have been used and the free chains obtained by chromatography on carboxymethyl cellulose of neutral salt or urea-extracted collagen were employed both for immunization and subsequent skin testing. All eight specimens obtained by these procedures can induce cell-mediated reactions with considerable cross-reactivity, but the reactions are invariably strongest against the immunizing antigen, thus indicating a detectable degree of both species and chain specificity. Animals immunized with the salt-extracted materials cannot distinguish, however, between these and that extracted using urea. In the reverse situation, however, in which animals are immunized with urea-extracted chains, these always can be distinguished from the salt-extracted chains, thus indicating the recognition of some extra determinants in the urea extracts. In contrast to the antibody response to rat collagen α chains in rabbits, which is obtainable almost exclusively using the α_2 chains but not the α_1 chains (Lindsley *et al.*, 1971), the cell-mediated responses in the guinea-pig are induced readily with either chain. Moreover, the

N-terminal non-helical portion of the chain, which dominates the induction of the humoral response, plays no significant part in the cell-mediated reactions, since such reactions are as readily induced and elicited with samples from which the non-helical N-terminal portions have been removed by pepsin digestion. Furthermore, such treatment does not interfere with the species specificity of the reactions.

The effect of heat denaturation upon the capacity of collagen to induce cell-mediated immunity has proved particularly informative. It has been known for some years that denatured proteins are particularly effective in inducing this type of immunity (Gell and Benacerraf, 1959), and collagen is no exception. By using rat skin collagen, native and heat-denatured at either $40°$ or $50°$, Adelmann (1973) found that although in all cases cell-mediated reactions are induced, the maximal reaction in each instance is with the immunizing preparation, thus indicating the specific importance of the conformation itself despite the identity of amino acid sequence. Although there is a considerable degree of cross-reactivity indicated by these reactions, even between the native material and that denatured at $50°$, the serum from animals immunized with the denatured material is incapable of agglutinating sheep erythrocytes coated with the corresponding native collagen. It would appear, therefore, that conformation is of much greater significance for the specificity of humoral than of cell-mediated reactions.

Guinea-pigs immunized with native collagen can not only differentiate between the native and the denatured form of the homologous material, but can also distinguish the native from the denatured samples of heterologous material. Animals immunized with the denatured material, however, can not distinguish between the two varieties of collagen either homologous or heterologous.

Denatured collagen, even that denatured at $50°$, still retains species specificity, as revealed by delayed skin reactions. The loss of some of the native determinants resulting from denaturation suggests the possibility that in the native form some of these determinants embrace more than one of the chains of the triple helix, since the dissociation of the chains is one of the fundamental changes in collagen denaturation.

In view of the consistent failure of Adelmann and his colleagues (Adelamnn et al., 1972; Adelmann and Kirrane, 1973) to obtain any evidence of cell-mediated immunity to guinea-pig collagen in their guinea-pigs, whether immunized with heterologous or guinea-pig collagen, it is surprising that Senyk and Michaeli (1973) were able to demonstrate delayed hypersensitivity skin reactions to guinea-pig collagen in all eight guinea-pigs immunized with this collagen and in six out of eight immunized with human collagen. In most instances, the cell-mediated nature of these reactions was confirmed by migration inhibition tests on the peritoneal macrophages of the guinea-pigs in question, as well as by transformation tests on their lymph node cells. A comparison of the techniques employed by the two groups of investigators reveals a remarkable similarity that suggests, therefore, that the conflicting results must be attributable to the strain differences in experimental animals used—unspecified by Senyk and Michaeli and random-bred Pirbright by Adelmann et al.

To date virtually nothing is known of the distribution of the determinants responsible for the cell-mediated reactions along the individual chains in type I collagen. All that can be said at present is that some of the fragments present when collagen is digested with cyanogen bromide are still capable of inducing, as well as eliciting, delayed skin reactions in guinea-pigs when these have been immunized with the crude digest in Freund's complete adjuvant (Adelmann et al., 1972).

Cross-reactions between collagens and synthetic polypeptides related to collagen have been observed, especially reactions of delayed type. Such reactions are discussed in the section on synthetic polypeptides (see Section 5).

Cell-mediated immunity to type II chick collagen has been demonstrated in guinea-pigs (Beard et al., 1977b). Animals immunized with native or denatured chick collagen respond to both molecules and to the centrally located peptides CB8, 9, 10, 11, and 12, indicating the positions of conformation-independent determinants in cell-mediated immunity to this molecule. As found with type I collagens, the non-helical regions of type II chick collagen are unimportant in cell-mediated immunity since they could be removed by pepsin treatment without effect.

4.5 Antigenicity of Synthetic Polypeptides Related to Collagen

The repeating unit characteristic of the constituent peptide chains of collagen is a tripeptide with the sequence Gly-X-Y (see Section 2.2) where X is often proline, and Y is any α amino acid, including proline or hydroxyproline. By virtue of the invariable presence of glycine as the first residue and the frequent presence of proline as the second member of the sequence, the peptide chains adopt a characteristic helical configuration. X-ray diffraction and other studies have shown that, at least in the solid state, homopolymers of proline and hydroxyproline adopt a similar configuration to that of collagen. It is, therefore, of considerable interest to study the immunological properties of these polymers and their immunological cross-reactivity, if any, with collagen.

Although rabbits appear to be non-reactive to either the homopolymers or related random copolymers, guinea-pigs give both humoral and cell-mediated responses to several such polymers. These reactions, for example, are given by poly-L-proline of both form I and form II—with the peptide bonds in cis or trans arrangement, respectively—and by the random copolymers of L-proline and glycine, and of L-proline, glycine, and L-hydroxyproline. The two forms of poly-L-proline are distinct immunologically with no cross-reactivity other than that attributable to the spontaneous mutarotation of form I to form II. Cross-reactions between the various polymers indicate that the principal determinant in most of them consists of sequences of proline. This is true in animals immunized with the copolymer of $(Pro-Gly-Hyp)_n$ as shown by the positive reactions of skin testing with polyproline and the absence of reactions with polyhydroxyproline. Immunization with the acetylated derivative of $(Pro-Gly-Hyp)_n$ results in positive reactions at test sites with either polyproline or polyacetylhydroxyproline. Since guinea-pigs immunized with calf collagen give no reactions with either the polymer (Pro-Gly-Hyp)$_n$ or its acetyl derivative, but all animals immunized with acetylated collagen give a positive reaction to the acetylated polymer, it appears that the acetylated hydroxyproline behaves as a hapten in the system. This interpretation is supported by the positive skin reaction with acetylated polyhydroxyproline in animals immunized with acetylated calf collagen, and the occasional positive reaction to acetylated calf collagen in animals immunized with the acetylated copolymer.

Although the glycine residues play little part in the specificity of its copolymers with proline as shown by humoral responses, there is some evidence for their participation in reactions mediated by sensitized cells. Thus, although guinea-pigs immunized with poly(L-Pro-Gly) in Freund's adjuvant give delayed skin reactions to the immunizing antigen, as well as to polyproline with molecular weight of 17 000 or more. The converse does not occur and animals immunized with large molecular weight polyproline although displaying delayed skin reactions to itself do not give reactions with the copolymers. Even more convincing of the participation of glycine residues in the cell-mediated responses to poly(Pro-Gly) are the results obtained in animals made tolerant by previous injection of polyproline (molecular weight 14 000) in incomplete adjuvant (Brown and Glynn, 1968). In such animals, subsequent immunization with either polyproline or poly(Pro-Gly) fails to induce a humoral response and delayed skin reactions in the main are given only by the animals immunized with the copolymer. In contrast, when tolerance is induced by the copolymer itself, impairment of both humoral and cell-mediated responses results.

Despite the demonstrable immunogenicity of these various polymers as revealed by skin testing and passive agglutination, no evidence has been obtained of any cross-reactivity with collagen, either in the native or denatured form.

4.5.1 Sequential Polymers

The encouraging results obtained from studies with random copolymers related to collagen has led to the synthesis of several sequential polymers of the (Gly-Pro-X)$_n$ type, where X is usually alanine or proline, and the almost identical polymers (Pro-X-Gly)$_n$ where again X is usually alanine or proline. All these polymers have been shown to be antigenic, inducing both humoral and cell-mediated responses but, unlike the homo and random copolymers, also have been shown to be immunogenic in rabbits as well as in guinea-pigs. Furthermore, whereas the humoral antibodies to the non-sequential polymers are non-precipitating and non-complement fixing, the antibodies to the sequential polymers usually possess both these properties.

The structural similarity to collagen would be expected to be much closer for the sequential polymers than for the random copolymers or polyproline, since the former not only forms triple helices of the collagen type in the solid state (Engel *et al.*, 1966) but, by virtue of the available hydrogen bonds is able, at least in part, to resist the destabilizing effect of water when in aqueous solution (Brown *et al.*,

1972). Cross-reactivity with collagen is, therefore, more probable with sequential polymers than with either polyproline of the random copolymers. Such observations have been made.

Almost all the sequential polymers studied of the form $(Gly-Pro-X)_n$ or $(Pro-X-Gly)_n$ have been shown to be immunogenic, inducing both humoral and cell-mediated responses in both guinea-pigs and rabbits. Of particular interest is the observation that the response to these two varieties of polymer, where X is alanine, are indistinguishable, whereas the polymer $(Ala-Pro-Gly)_n$, although an equally good immunogen, shows no cross-reactivity with either of them. This implies that the determinants on this type of polymer are sited along the body of the peptide chain and not at either the free N or C-terminus. This is a striking contrast to the results obtained when polypeptides are used as haptens attached to another carrier protein (Schechter, 1970).

The probable explanation of this apparent difference in the behaviour of antibodies to immunogens and haptens is that the former are usually conformational and the latter sequential. Thus, in the case of the two polytripeptides, $(Gly-L-Pro-L-Ala)_n$ and $(L-Pro-L-Ala-Gly)_n$, it is evident that they only differ at their free ends. The antibodies raised against these two polymers are directed against conformational determinants as shown, for example, by their inability to react with the tripeptide or oligomers thereof and *vice versa*. The free ends of the polymers are unlikely however to be in the appropriate conformational arrangement since there are no residues beyond them to contribute to their stabilization, in the same way as the ends of a rope become frayed unless some external binding is applied. The terminal residues, therefore, in any helical chain will lack the conformation of the rest of the chain and consequently be exempt from immune reactions requiring a conformational determinant. On the other hand, these terminal sequences would be expected to react with antibodies directed against sequential determinants, provided the residues are in the correct sequence. The increasing cross-reactivity found by Maoz et al., (1973a) between antibodies to $(L-Pro-Gly-L-Pro)_1$ which is a sequential determinant and the corresponding polymer with decreasing size of the polymer is in complete agreement with this hypothesis since the smaller the polymer the greater is the ratio of terminal (sequential) to central (conformational) residues. If the hypothesis is correct this cross-reacting relationship between the antibodies to $(L-Pro-Gly-L-Pro)_1$ and the size of the polymer should not be shown with $(Gly-L-Pro-L-Pro)_n$ which lacks sequential identity at the ends although identical in its conformational part with $(L-Pro-Gly-L-Pro)_n$.

Of the many sequential polypeptides of the type $(Gly-Pro-X)_n$ studied the most immunogenic according to Brown and Glynn (1973) is $(Gly-Pro-Pro)_n$ or its equivalent $(Pro-Gly-Pro)_n$. In some guinea-pigs, it has proved so immunogenic that skin testing with a few micrograms of the polymer is sufficient to induce a humoral response, as shown by retesting two weeks later. There have been, however, some conflicting reports about the immunogenicitiy of $(Gly-Pro-Pro)_n$. Several authors have concluded that it is a weak antigen. This variation in observations is almost certainly attributable to some difference in composition resulting from differences in, for example, the technique of polymerization; cross-reactivity with native collagen was found in a small proportion of the animals immunized with these sequential polymers but was only of the cell-mediated variety. It was shown best in animals immunized with $(Gly-Pro-Pro)_n$ and this presumably is due to the strong immunogenicity of this polymer. No animal immunized with collagen gave any indication of cross-reaction with any of the polymers studied. This is not surprising since any one of these sequences is only sparsely represented on the collagen molecule and could therefore only play an extremely small part as determinant in competition with the many other determinants available. Nevertheless, in an animal already immunized with that determinant it might well be available on the collagen molecule in sufficient amounts to react with the sensitized cells. Maoz et al. (1973a, b) found a much higher incidence than Brown and Glynn (1973) of cross-reactivity to collagen in guinea-pigs immunized with their preparation of $(Pro-Gly-Pro)_n$. All eight animals tested gave positive delayed reactions to both rat tail tendon collagen and to guinea-pig skin collagen; several immediate cross-reactions were observed even with guinea-pig collagen.

It is of interest that no such cross-reactions, either humoral or cell-mediated, with collagen were found in guinea-pigs immunized with the random copolymer $L-Pro_{66}-Gly_{33}$. Despite the cross-reactions with collagen, no positive precipitin tests were obtained with sera from animals immunized with the sequential polymer and any of the collagens with the exception of Ascaris cuticle collagen. It is probably significant that of the various collagens used that from Ascaris, with about 26 per cent glycine residues and 30 per cent proline, is the closest in primary structure to the immunizing polymer (Maoz et al., 1973a, b).

An important observation which may explain partly the discrepancy between the results of different investigators concerning immediate skin reactions is the time difference between the induction of cell-mediated and immediate skin sensitivity. Since the cell-mediated form consistently antedates the humoral (immediate) form, early skin testing, that is between days 10 and 14, may miss the humoral response.

The immunogenicity of sequential polymers of the $(Gly-Pro-X)_n$ variety in which X is glutamic acid, ornithine, arginine, lysine, or tyrosine, has been studied recently (Brown and Glynn, unpublished results). All these polymers proved to be antigenic in guinea-pigs as shown by the appearance of precipitating antibodies and more consistent cell-mediated reactions. The polymer containing arginine is the most immunogenic for both humoral and cellular responses. Cross-reactions with native collagen are frequent, especially in the animals immunized with the tyrosine-containing polymer. This is surprising in view of the low incidence of this residue in the helical portion of the collagen molecule. Unfortunately the collagens used to test for cross-reactions did not include guinea-pig collagen.

The need for proline in a sequential polymer in order for it to induce a cross-reactivity to collagen in the immunized guinea-pig has been studied by using $(Ala-Gly-Pro)_n$-type polymers in which proline was replaced by either azetidine, pipecolic acid, or thiazolidine carboxylic acid. No cross-reactions with either native or denatured collagen developed in any of these immunized animals although all gave immediate reactions on homologous testing and the thiazolidine-containing polymer also induced delayed hypersensitivity.

The effect of substituting D for L amino acids also has been investigated. The polymer (D-Ala-Gly-D-Pro)$_n$ was found to be immunogenic, but only at the cellular level; no humoral response was detected by active cutaneous anaphylaxis. Despite the development of strong skin reactions of delayed hypersensitivity, no evidence of similar reactivity to native or denatured collagen was detected (Brown and Glynn, 1973).

4.6 Control of the Immune Response to Collagen

The requirement for cellular co-operation between thymus-dependent (T) cells and bone marrow-derived (B) cells in the antibody response to many antigens is well established (Claman et al., 1966; Miller and Mitchell, 1969). Some antigens such as *Escherichia coli* lipopolysaccharide (Sjoberg, 1971) pneumococcal polysaccharide type S III (Continho and Möller, 1973), and dextran sulphate (Dorries et al., 1974), are T cell-independent, and it has been suggested that this may result from their repetitive structure or their indigestibility (Sela et al., 1972; Feldmann et al., 1974). Conflicting results have been obtained in the case of collagen, and molecules of similar structure but differing species origin have been shown to vary in their T cell-dependence in mice. Thus, Fuchs and associates (1974) found that native (unlike denatured) rat collagen was T cell-independent in mice, whereas Nowack et al. (1976b) showed that native calf collagen was T cell-dependent in mice. These results are not readily comparable, however, since different strains of mice were used. In one case, mice were able to recognize native but not denatured calf collagen (Nowack et al., 1975b), while in the other case, mice gave a T cell-dependent response to rat gelatin but a T cell-independent response to rat collagen. The response to these two collagens would appear to be controlled by different genetic loci since the strain (SWR) that gave a good response to rat collagen (Fuchs et al., 1974) was almost totally unresponsive to calf collagen (Nowack et al., 1975a). Further studies using rat collagen showed that T cell-independent antigens, such as native collagen and (Pro-Gly-Pro)$_n$ are able to circumvent the T cell requirement of ovalbumin (normally a T cell-dependent antigen) when immunized simultaneously, but their effects on gelatin have not been tested (Mozes et al., 1975).

Studies on the genetic control of the antibody response to collagen indicate that several different genes may be involved. H2-Linked genes in mice, associated with alleles b and f confer high responsiveness to calf collagen type I, and the unresponsiveness of other strains may be overcome by use of a collagen carrier, such as procollagen, indicating that T cells may control the response (Nowack et al., 1975a; Hahn et al., 1975a). However, different genes control the antibody response of mice to calf type II collagen, and, as indicated above, to rat type I collagen (Nowack et al., 1975b).

5 FUTURE DIRECTIONS

Immunochemical studies of collagen over recent decades have provided sufficient information to make future research both exciting and potentially fruitful in several areas.

The usefulness of collagen as a model for the study of immunological questions, such as the nature of immunogenicity and the general control of the immune response, has been appreciated already, but work in these fields is only in infancy. One question of particular interest which has not been studied adequately is whether the body is tolerant to its own collagen. Although guinea-pigs have been induced to give a cell-mediated immune response to collagen from their own species (Steffen, 1965; Senyk and Michaeli, 1973), conflicting results have been obtained (Adelmann et al., 1972) and the effect of technical variations is not clear. Of relevance here is the presence of a naturally occurring anti-gelatin factor (AGF) (see Section 4.1.2) in normal sera, study of which may provide clues towards an understanding of the state of tolerance to collagen at least in its denatured form. However, further investigations of AGF are also warranted by the presence of these factors in animals unable to respond to immunization with gelatin (Nowack et al., 1975b). It has been postulated that naturally occurring antibodies to tissue antigens facilitate the clearance of tissue debris (Grabar, 1965). Normal guinea-pig macrophages have been shown to bind gelatin more efficiently than native collagen (Hopper et al., 1974, 1976). This property is abolished by treatment of the cells with trypsin, but can be restored by incubation with an IgM-like factor in normal guinea-pig serum which closely resembles AGF. Thus AGF, by interacting with macrophages may facilitate the clearance of denatured collagen, but this interaction may conceivably have an effect on the immune response to gelatin. In addition, the factors responsible for the activation of fibroblasts in a healing wound are unknown, but the involvement of AGF and macrophages in this process seems possible, especially in view of the presence of large numbers of macrophages and of denatured collagen at an inflammatory site.

Disorders of collagen are implicated in the pathology of many of the so-called connective tissue diseases. The proper functioning of collagen-containing tissues requires the development and maintenance of complex intercellular matrices which vary considerably according to the tissue. The biosynthetic process itself is very intricate in the case of collagen and several diseases are attributable to errors in this pathway (see Section 3). Recent evidence suggests that collagen may be active in the induction of tissue differentiation during embryogenesis (Shoshan and Gross, 1974), and it has also been suggested that the procollagen extensions released on conversion of procollagen to tropocollagen may have a regulatory role on collagen synthesis by fibroblasts (Murphy et al., 1975). It seems possible that native and denatured tropocollagen as well as the procollagen peptides, may modify fibroblast behaviour, and application of collagen to healing wounds has been shown to have profound effects on the inflammatory process (Shoshan and Finkelstein, 1970). A more obvious application of collagen immunochemistry in this field is the use of specific antisera to collagen and procollagen types and to the various enzymes involved in biosynthesis, in comparing normal and diseased conditions. A few studies have been carried out already which indicate the distributions of types I and III collagens (Rothbard and Watson, 1956; Gay *et al.*, 1975*a*, *b*) and type I procollagen (Wick *et al.*, 1975) in several tissues, and immunological means of detecting abnormal collagen structure in disease and of studying synthetic control mechanisms *in vitro* may prove to be very valuable.

Finally, immunological disorders are suggested in many diseases by the presence of antibodies to native and denatured collagen (Stefen, 1969; Wells *et al.*, 1973; Michaeli and Fudenberg, 1974). Immunochemical means are now available to detect the specificities of these antibodies and to investigate their reaction with procollagen and with collagen of types I–IV. Such an approach, as in the case of rheumatoid factors, may provide both basic and medically applicable information (Johnson and Faulk, 1976).

REFERENCES

Adelmann, B. C. (1972). *Immunology*, **23**, 739.
Adelmann, B. C. (1973). *Immunology*, **24**, 871.
Adelmann, B. C., Geutner, G. J., and Hopper, K. (1973). *J. Immunol. Meth.*, **3**, 319.
Adelmann, B. C., Glynn, L. E., and Kirrane, J. (1968). *Fed. Proc.*, **27**, 263.
Adelmann, B. C., and Kirrane, J. (1973). *Immunology*, **25**, 123.
Adelmann, B. C., Kirrane, J., and Glynn, L. E. (1972). *Immunology*, **23**, 723.
Aguilar, J. H., Jacobs, H. G., Butler, W. T., and Cunningham, L. W. (1973). *J. Biol. Chem.*, **248**, 5106.
Al-Adnani, M. S., Patrick, R. S., and McGee, J. O. D. (1974). *J. Cell. Sci.*, **16**, 639.
Anesey, J., Scott, P. G., Veis, A., and Chyatte, D. (1975). *Biochem. Biophys. Res. Commun.*, **62**, 946.
Astbury, W. T. (1938). *Trans. Faraday Soc.*, **34**, 378.

Bailey, A. J., and Lapiere, C. M. (1973). *Eur. J. Biochem.*, **34**, 91.
Bailey, A. J., and Robins, S. P. (1973). *Front. Matrix Biol.*, **1**, 130.
Bailey, A. J., Robins, S. P., and Balian, G. (1974). *Nature, (Lond.)*, **251**, 105.
Bailey, A. J., and Shimokamaki, M. S. (1971). *FEBS Letters*, **16**, 86.
Balian, G., Click, E. M., Hermodson, M. A., and Bornstein, P. (1972). *Biochemistry*, **11**, 3798.
Balleison, L., Gay, S., Marx, R., and Kuhn, K. (1975). *Klin. Wschr.*, **53**, 903.
Barnes, M. J., Constable, B. J., Morton, L. F., and Kodicek, E. (1971). *Biochem. J.*, **125**, 925.
Beard, H. K. (1974). Ph.D. Thesis, University of Bristol.
Beard, H. K., Faulk, W. P., Conachie, L. B., and Glynn, L. E. (1977). *Prog. Allergy*, **22**, 45.
Beard, H. K., Ueda, M., Faulk, W. P., and Glynn, L. E. (1977*b*). *Immunology*, in press.
Becker, U., Fietzek, P. P., Furthmayr, H., and Timpl, R. (1975*a*). *Eur. J. Biochem.*, **54**, 359.
Becker, U., Furthmayr, H., and Timpl, R. (1975*b*). *Hoppe-Seyler's Z. Physiol. Chem.*, **356**, 21.
Becker, U., Nowack, H., Gay, S., and Timpl, R. (1976). *Immunology*, **31**, 57.
Becker, U., Timpl, R., and Kuhn, K. (1972). *Eur. J. Biochem.*, **28**, 221.
Beil, W., Furthmayr, H., and Timpl, R. (1972). *Immunochemistry*, **9**, 779.
Beil, W., Timpl, R., and Furthmayr, H. (1973). *Immunology*, **24**, 13.

502

Beisswenger, P. J., and Spiro, R. G. (1970). *Science, N.Y.*, **168**, 596.
Bellamy, G., and Bornstein, P. (1971). *Proc. Nat. Acad. Sci., U.S.A.*, **68**, 1138.
Bornstein, P. (1968). *Science*, **162**, 592.
Bornstein, P. (1969). *Biochemistry*, **8**, 63.
Bornstein, P. (1974). *Ann. Rev. Biochem.*, **43**, 568.
Bornstein, P., Ehrlich, H. P., and Wyke, A. W. (1972). *Science, N.Y.*, **175**, 544.
Bornstein, P., and Piez, K. A. (1964). *J. Clin. Invest.*, **43**, 1813.
Brown, P. C., and Glynn, L. E. (1968). *Immunology*, **15**, 589.
Brown, P. C., and Glynn, L. E. (1973). *Immunology*, **25**, 251.
Brown, F. R., Hopfinger, A. J., and Blout, E. R. (1972). *J. Mol. Biol.*, **63**, 101.
Brownwell, A. G., and Veis, A. (1975). *Biochem. Biophys. Res. Commun.*, **63**, 371.
Butler, W. T. (1970). *Biochemistry*, **9**, 44.
Butler, W. T., Miller, E. J., Finch, J. E., and Inagami, T. (1974). *Biochem. Biophys. Res. Commun.*, **57**, 190.
Byers, P. H., McKenney, K. H., Lichtenstein, J. R., and Martin, G. R. (1974). *Biochemistry*, **13**, 5243.

Causey, G. (1962). *Electron Microscopy*, Livingstone, London.
Chidlow, J. W., Bourne, F. J., and Barley, A. J. (1974). *Immunology*, **27**, 665.
Chung, E., Keele, E. M., and Miller, E. J. (1974). *Biochemistry*, **13**, 3459.
Chung, E., and Miller, E. J. (1974). *Science, N.Y.*, **183**, 1200.
Chung, E., Rhodes, R. K., and Miller, E. J. (1976). *Biochem. Biophys. Res. Commun.*, **71**, 1167.
Church, R. L., Yaeger, J. A., and Tanzer, M. L. (1974). *J. Mol. Biol.*, **86**, 785.
Claman, H. N., Chaperon, E. A., and Triplett, R. F. (1966). *J. Immunol.*, **97**, 828.
Clark, C. C., and Veis, A. (1972). *Biochemistry*, **11**, 494.
Clark, C. C., Fietzek, P. P., and Bornstein, P. (1975). *Eur. J. Biochem.*, **56**, 327.
Cohn, L. D., Isersky, C., Zupnik, J., Lenears, A., Lee, G., and Lapiere, C. M. (1974). *Proc. Nat. Acad. Sci., U.S.A.*, **71**, 40.
Conochie, L. B., Scott, J. E., and Faulk, W. P. (1975). *J. Immunol. Meth.*, **7**, 393.
Continho, A., and Möller, G. (1973). *Eur. J. Immunol.*, **3**, 608.

Danks, D. M., Campbell, P. E., Walker Smith, J., Stevens, B. J., Gillespie, J. M., and Blomfield, J. (1972). *Lancet*, **i**, 110.
Davidson, J. M., and Bornstein, P. (1975). *Fed. Proc.*, **34**, 562.
Davidson, P. F., Levine, L., Drake, M. P., Rubin, A., and Bump, S. (1967). *J. Exp. Med.*, **126**, 331.
Davis, N. R., and Risen, O. M. (1974). *Biochem. Biophys. Res. Commun.*, **61**, 723.
Dehm, P., and Prockop, D. J. (1973). *Eur. J. Biochem.*, **35**, 159.
Denduchis, B., and Kefalides, N. A. (1970). *Biochim. Biophys. Acta*, **221**, 357.
Deshmukh, A. D., and Nimni, M. E. (1969). *Biochem. Biophys. Res. Commun.*, **35**, 845.
Diegelmann, R. F., Bernstein, L., and Peterkofsky, B. (1973). *J. Biol. Chem.*, **248**, 6514.
Dintzis, H. M. (1961). *Proc. Nat. Acad. Sci., U.S.A.*, **47**, 247.
Dixit, S. N., Kang, A. H., and Gross, J. (1975a). *Biochemistry*, **14**, 1929.
Dixit, S. N., Seyer, J. M., Oronsky, A. O., Corbett, C., Kang, A. H., and Gross, J. (1975b). *Biochemistry*, **14**, 1933.
Dorries, R., Schimpl, A., and Wecker, E. (1974). *Eur. J. Immunol.*, **4**, 230.
Duksin, D., Maoz, A., and Fuchs, S. (1975). *Cell*, **5**, 83.

Eastoe, J. (1967). In *Treatise on Collagen*, (Ramachandran, G. N., ed.), Academic Press, New York and London, p. 1.
Ehrlich, H. P., and Bornstein, P. (1972). *Nature, New Biol.*, **238**, 257.
Ehrlich, H. P., Ross, R., and Bornstein, P. (1974). *J. Cell Biol.*, **62**, 390.
Engel, J., Kurtz, J., Katchalski, E., and Berger, A. (1966). *J. Mol. Biol.*, **17**, 255.

Epstein, E. (1971). *Clin. Res.*, **19**, 359.
Epstein, E. H. (1974). *J. Biol. Chem.*, **249**, 3225.

Faulk, W. P., Conochie, L. B., Temple, A., and Papamichail, M. (1975). *Nature, (Lond.)*, **256**, 123.
Feldmann, M., Greaves, M. F., Parker, D. C., and Rittenberg, M. B. (1974). *Eur. J. Immunol.*, **4**, 591.
Fessler, L. I., Burgeson, R. E., Morris, N. P., and Fessler, J. H. (1973). *Proc. Nat. Acad. Sci.*, *U.S.A.*, **70**, 2993.
Fietzek, P. P., Kell, I., and Kuhn, K. (1972). *FEBS Letters*, **26**, 66.
Fietzek, P. P., and Kuhn, K. (1975a). *Mol. Cell. Biochem.*, **8**, 141.
Fietzek, P. P., and Kuhn, K. (1975b). *Eur. J. Biochem.*, **52**, 77.
Fietzek, P. P., and Rauterberg, J. (1975). FEBS Letters, **49**, 365.
Fitton Jackson, S., and Smith, R. H. (1957). *J. Biochem. Biophys. Cytol.*, **3**, 897.
Forrester, J. C., Hunt, T. K., Hayes, T. L., and Pease, R. F.W. (1969). *Nature, (Lond.)*, **221**, 373.
Fuchs, S., Mozes, E., Maoz, A., and Sela, M. (1974). *J. Exp. Med.*, **139**, 148.
Furthmayr, H., Beil, W., and Timpl, R. (1971). *FEBS Letters*, **12**, 341.
Furthmayr, H., Stolz, M., Becker, U., Beil, W., and Timpl, R. (1972). *Immunochemistry*, **9**, 789.
Furthmayr, H., and Timpl, R. (1972). *Biochem. Biophys. Res. Commun.*, **47**, 944.
Furthmayr, H., Timpl, R., Stark, M., Lapiere, C. M., and Kuhn, K. (1972a). *FEBS Letters*, **28**, 247.

Gallop, P. M., Blumenfeld, O. O., and Seifter, S. (1972). *Ann. Rev. Biochem.*, **41**, 617.
Gay, S., Balleison, L., Remberger, K., Fietzek, P. P., Adelmann, B. C., and Kuhn, K. (1975a). *Klin. Wschr.* **53**, 899.
Gay, S., Fietzek, P. P., Remberger, K., Eder, M., and Kuhn, K. (1975b). *Klin. Wschr.*, **53**, 205.
Gell, P. G. H., and Benacerraf, B. (1959). *Immunology*, **2**, 64.
Geutner, G. J., and Adelmann, B. C. (1976). *Immunology*, **31**, 87.
Goldberg, B., and Sherr, C. J. (1973). *Proc. Nat. Acad. Sci.*, *U.S.A.*, **70**, 361.
Grabar, P. (1965). In *Molecular and Cellular Basis of Antibody Formation*, (Sterzl, J., ed.), Academic Press, New York and London, p. 621.
Grant, M. E., Kefalides, N. A., and Prockop, D. J. (1972). *J. Biol. Chem.*, **247**, 3545.
Grant, M. E., and Prockop, D. J. (1972a). *New Engl. J. Med.*, **286**, 194.
Grant, M. E., and Prockop, D. J. (1972b). *New Engl. J. Med.*, **286**, 242.
Grant, M. E., and Prockop, D. J. (1972c). *New Engl. J. Med.*, **286**, 291.
Green, H., and Goldberg, B. (1964). *Nature (Lond.)*, **204**, 347.
Gross, J. (1958). *J. Exp. Med.*, **107**, 247.
Gross, J., Dumsha, B., and Glazer, N. (1958). *Biochim. Biophys. Acta*, **30**, 293.
Gross, J., Highberger, J. H., and Schmitt, F. O. (1955). *Proc. Nat. Acad. Sci.*, *U.S.A.*, **41**, 1.
Gunson, D. E., and Kefalides, N. A. (1976). *Immunology*, **31**, 563.

Hahn, E., Nowack, H., Gotze, D., and Timpl, R. (1975a). *Eur. J. Immunol.*, **5**, 288.
Hahn, E., and Timpl, R. (1973). *Eur. J. Immunol.*, **3**, 442.
Hahn, E., Timpl, R., and Miller, E. J. (1974). *J. Immunol.*, **113**, 421.
Hahn, E., Timpl, R., and Miller, E. J. (1975a, b). *Immunology*, **28**, 561.
Harwood, R., Bhalla, A. K., Grant, M. E., and Jackson, D. S. (1975). *Biochem. J.*, **148**, 129.
Hay, E. D., and Dodson, J. W. (1973). *J. Cell Biol.*, **57**, 190.
Heikkinen, E., and Kulonen, E. (1966). *Acta physiol. scand.*, **68**, 231.
Highberger, J. H., Corbett, C., Kang, A. H., and Gross, J. (1975). *Biochemistry*, **14**, 2872.
Highberger, J. H., Kang, A. H., and Gross, J. (1971). *Biochemistry*, **10**, 610.

504

Hodge, A. J., Petruska, J. A., and Bailey, A. J. (1965). In *Structure and Function of Connective and Skeletal Tissues*, (Fitton Jackson, S., Harkness, R. D., Partridge, S. M., and Tristam, G. R., eds.), Butterworths, London, p. 31.
Hodge, A. J., and Schmitt, F. O. (1960). *Proc. Nat. Acad. Sci., U.S.A.*, **46**, 186.
Hopper, K., Adelmann, B. C., Gentner, G., and Gay, S. (1974). *Z. Immunforsch.*, **147**, 316.
Hopper, K. E., Adelmann, B. C., Gentner, G., and Gay, S. (1976). *Immunology*, **30**, 249.

Igarashi, S., Kang, A. H., and Gross, J. (1970). *Biochem. Biophys. Res. Commun.*, **38**, 697.

Jimenz, S. A., Dehm, P., and Prockop, D. J. (1971). *FEBS Letters*, **17**, 245.
Jimenz, S., Harsch, M., and Rosenbloom, J. (1973). *Biochem. Biophys. Res. Commun.*, **52**, 106.
Johnson, P. M., and Faulk, W. P. (1976). *Clin. Immunol. Immunopath.*, **6**, 414.

Kang, A. H. (1972). *Biochemistry*, **11**, 1828.
Kang, A. H., Bornstein, P., and Piez, K. A. (1967). *Biochemistry*, **6**, 788.
Kang, A. H., Dixit, S. N., Corbett, C., and Gross, J. (1975). *J. Biol. Chem.*, **250**, 7428.
Kefalides, N. A. (1971). *Biochem. Biophys. Res. Commun.*, **45**, 226.
Knapp, W., Menzel, J., and Steffen, C. (1974). *Z. ImmunForsch.*, **148**, 132.
Krane, S. M., Pinnell, S. R., and Erbe, R. W. (1972). *Proc. Nat. Acad. Sci., U.S.A.*, **69**, 2899.
Kuhn, K. (1969). *Essays Biochem.*, **5**, 59.
Kuhn, K., Fietzek, P., and Kuhn, J. (1966). *Biochem. Z.*, **344**, 418.
Kuhn, K., Grassmann, W., and Hofmann, U. (1960). *Naturwissenschaften*, **47**, 258.

Landsteiner, K. (1936). *The Specificity of Serological Reactions*, Baillière Tindall, London, p. 28.
Layman, D. L., McGoodwin, E. B., and Martin, G. R. (1971). *Proc. Nat. Acad. Sci., U.S.A.*, **68**, 454.
Layman, D. L., and Ross, R. (1973). *Archs Biochem. Biophys.*, **157**, 451.
Layman, D. L., and Titus, J. L. (1975). *Lab. Invest.*, **33**, 103.
Lee, G., Tate, R., Martin, G., and Kohn, L. (1975). *Fed. Proc.*, **34**, 696.
Lee-Owen, V., and Anderson, J. C. (1975). *Biochem. J.*, **149**, 57.
Lenears, A., and Lapiere, C. M. (1975). *Biochim. Biophys. Acta*, **400**, 121.
Lenears, A., Ansay, M., Nusgens, B. V., and Lapiere, C. M. (1971). *Eur. J. Biochem.*, **23**, 533.
Leroy, E. C. (1969). *J. Immunol.*, **102**, 919.
Lichtenstein, J. R., Martin, G. R., Kohn, L. D., Byers, P. H., and McKusick, V. A. (1973). *Science, N.Y.*, **182**, 298.
Lindsley, H., Mannick, M., and Bornstein, P. (1971). *J. Exp. Med.*, **133**, 1309.
Lowther, D. A. (1963). *Int. Rev. Conn. Tiss. Res.*, **1**, 64.
Lustig, L. (1970). *Proc. Soc. Exp. Biol. Med.*, **133**, 207.
Lustig, L., Costantini, H., and Mancini, R. E. (1969). *Proc. Soc. Exp. Biol. Med.*, **130**, 283.

Maoz, A., Fuchs, S., and Sela, M. (1973*a*). *Biochemistry*, **12**, 4238.
Maoz, A., Fuchs, S., and Sela, M. (1973*b*). *Biochemistry*, **12**, 4246.
Martin, G. R., Byers, P. H., and Piez, K. A. (1975). *Adv. Enzymol.*, **42**, 167.
Maurer, P. H. (1954*a*). *J. Exp. Med.*, **100**, 497.
Maurer, P. H. (1954*b*). *J. Exp. Med.*, **100**, 515.
McCall, J. G. (1968). *Lancet*, **ii**, 1194.
Mees, C. E., and James, T. H. (1966). *The Theory of the Photographic Process*, Macmillan, London.

Michaeli, D., Benjamini, E., Leung, D. Y. K., and Martin, G. R. (1971). *Immunochemistry*, **8**, 1.

Michaeli, D., and Epstein, E. H. (1971). *Israel J. Med. Sci.*, **7**, 462.

Michaeli, D., and Fudenberg, H. H. (1974). *Clin. Immunol. Immunopath.*, **3**, 187.

Michaeli, D., Kamenecka, H., Benjamini, E., Kettman, J. R., Leung, D. Y. K., and Miner, R. C. (1968). *Immunochemistry*, **5**, 433.

Michaeli, D., Martin, G. R., Kettman, J., Benjamini, E., Leung, D. Y. K., and Blatt, B.A. (1969). *Science, N.Y.*, **166**, 1522.

Miller, A., and Parry, D. A. D. (1973). *J. Mol. Biol.*, **75**, 441.

Miller, A., and Wray, J. S. (1971). *Nature, (Lond.)*, **230**, 437.

Miller, E. J. (1971). *Biochemistry*, **10**, 1652.

Miller, E. J. (1972). *Biochemistry*, **11**, 4903.

Miller, E. J., and Lunde, L. G. (1973). *Biochemistry*, **12**, 3153.

Miller, E. J., and Matukas, U. J. (1969). *Biochemistry*, **64**, 1264.

Miller, E. J., and Matukas, V. J. (1974). *Fed. Proc.*, **33**, 1197.

Miller, E. J., and Robertson, P. B. (1973). *Biochem. Biophys. Res. Comm.*, **54**, 432.

Miller, E. J., Woodall, D. L., and Vail, M. S. (1973). *J. Biol. Chem.*, **248**, 1666.

Miller, J. F. A. P., & Mitchell, G. F. (1969). *Transplant. Rev.*, **1**, 3.

Miller, R. L. (1971). *Archs Biochem. Biophys.*, **47**, 339.

Mohos, S. C., and Wagner, B. M. (1969). *Archs Pathol.*, **88**, 3.

Monson, J. M., and Bornstein, P. (1973). *Proc. Nat. Acad. Sci., U.S.A.*, **70**, 3521.

Morgan, P. H., Jacobs, H. G., Segrest, J. P., and Cunningham, L. W. (1970). *J. Biol. Chem.*, **245**, 5042.

Mozes, E., Schmitt-Verhulst, A. M., and Fuchs, S. (1975). *Eur. J. Immunol.*, **5**, 549.

Murphy, W. H., Von der Mark, K., McEneany, L. S. G., and Bornstein, P. (1975). *Biochemistry*, **14**, 3243.

Nagai, Y., Gross, J., and Piez, K. A. (1964). *Ann. N.Y. Acad. Sci.*, **121**, 494.

Nowack, H., Hahn, E., David, C. S., Timpl, R., and Götze, D. (1975a). *Immunogenetics*, **2**, 331.

Nowack, H., Hahn, E., and Timpl, R. (1975b). *Immunology*, **29**, 621.

Nowack, H., Hahn, E., and Timpl, R. (1976b). *Immunology*, **30**, 29.

Obrink, B., Laurent, T. C., and Carlsson, B. (1975). *FEBS Letters*, **56**, 166.

Olsen, B. R., Berg, R. A., Kishida, Y., and Prockop, D. J. (1973). *Science, N.Y.*, **182**, 825.

Olsen, B. R., and Prockop, D. J. (1974). *Proc. Nat. Acad. Sci., U.S.A.*, **71**, 2033.

Park, E. D., Church, R. L., and Tanzer, M. L. (1975). *Immunology*, **28**, 481.

Paz, M. A., Davidson, O. W., Gomez, C. J., and Mancini, R. E. (1963). *Proc. Soc. Exp. Biol. Med.*, **113**, 98.

Piez, K. A. (1967). In *Treatise on Collagen*, (Ramachandran, G. N., ed.), Academic Press, New York and London, p. 207.

Piez, K. A., Eigner, E. A., and Lewis, M. S. (1963). *Biochemistry*, **2**, 58.

Piez, K. A., Miller, E. J., Lane, J. M., and Butler, W. T. (1969). *Biochem. Biophys. Res. Commun.*, **37**, 801.

Pontz, B., Meigel, W., Rauterberg, J., and Kuhn, K. (1970). *Eur. J. Biochem.*, **16**, 50.

Ramachandran, G. N. (1963). *Int. Rev. Conn. Tiss. Res.*, **1**, 127.

Ramachandran, G. N., Bansal, M., and Bhatnagar, R. S. (1973). *Biochim. Biophys. Acta*, **322**, 166.

Rauterberg, J., and Kuhn, K. (1968). *FEBS Letters*, **1**, 230.

Rauterberg, J., Timpl, R., and Furthmayr, H. (1972). *Eur. J. Biochem.*, **27**, 231.

Rexrodt, F. W., Hopper, K. E., Fietzek, P. P., and Kuhn, K. (1973). *Eur. J. Biochem.*, **38**, 384.

Rigby, B. J. (1968). *Nature*, *(Lond.)*, **219**, 166.
Rothbard, S., and Watson, R. F. (1956). *J. Exp. Med.*, **103**, 57.
Rothbard, S., and Watson, R. F. (1961). *J. Exp. Med.*, **113**, 1041.
Rothbard, S., and Watson, R. F. (1972). *Lab. Invest.*, **27**, 76.
Rowe, D. W., McGoodwin, E. B., Martin, G. R., Sussman, M. D., Grahn, D., Faris, B., and Franzblau, C. (1974). *J. Exp. Med.*, **139**, 180.

Salem, G., and Traub, W. (1975). *FEBS Letters*, **51**, 94.
Schechter, I. (1970). *Nature*, *(Lond.)*, **228**, 639.
Schmitt, F. O., Levine, L., and Drake, M. P. (1964). *Proc. Nat. Acad. Sci.*, *U.S.A.*, **51**, 493.
Schofield, J. D., and Prockop, D. J. (1973). *Clin. Orthop.*, **97**, 175.
Sela, M., Mozes, E., and Shearer, G. M. (1972). *Proc. Nat. Acad. Sci.*, *U.S.A.*, **69**, 2696.
Senyk, G., and Michaeli, D. (1973). *J. Immunol.*, **111**, 1381.
Sherr, C. J., and Goldberg, B. (1973). *Science*, *N.Y.*, **180**, 1190.
Sherr, C. J., Taubman, M. B., and Goldberg, B. (1973). *J. Biol. Chem.*, **248**, 7033.
Shoshan, S., and Finkelstein, S. (1970). *J. Surg. Res.*, **10**, 485.
Shoshan, S., and Gross, J. (1974). *Israel J. Med. Sci.*, **10**, 537.
Sinex, E. M. (1968). In *Treatise on Collagen*, Vol. 2B, (Ramachandran, G. N., ed.), Academic Press, New York and London, p. 410.
Siperstein, M. D., Ungar, R. H., and Madison, L. L. (1968). *J. Clin. Invest.*, **47**, 1973.
Sjoberg, O. (1971). *J. Exp. Med.*, **133**, 1015.
Smith, B. D., Byers, P. H., and Martin, G. R. (1972). *Proc. Nat. Acad. Sci.*, *U.S.A.*, **69**, 3260.
Smith, J. W. (1968). *Nature*, *(Lond.)*, **219**, 157.
Spadaro, J. A. (1970). *Nature*, *(Lond.)*, **228**, 78.
Stark, M., Lenears, A., Lapiere, C. M., and Kuhn, K. (1971*a*). *FEBS Letters*, **18**, 225.
Stark, M., Rauterberg, J., and Kuhn, K. (1971*b*). *FEBS Letters*, **13**, 101.
Steffen, C. (1965). *Ann. N.Y. Acad. Sci.*, **124**, 570.
Steffen, C. (1969). *Ann. Immunol.*, **1**, 47.
Steffen, C., Dichtl, M., and Brunner, H. (1970*a*). *Z. ImmunForsch.*, **140**, 408.
Steffen, C., Dichtl, M., Knapp, W., and Brunner, H. (1971). *Immunology*, **21**, 649.
Steffen, C., and Timpl, R. (1963). *Int. Arch. Allergy*, **22**, 333.
Steffen, C., and Timpl, R. (1970). *Z. ImmunForsch.*, **139**, 455.
Steffen, C., Timpl, R., and Wolff, I. (1967). *Z. ImmunForsch.*, **134**, 91.
Steffen, C., Timpl, R., and Wolff, I. (1968). *Immunology*, **15**, 135.
Steffen, C., Timpl, R., Wolff, I., and Furthmayr, H. (1970*b*). *Immunology*, **18**, 849.
Stoltz, M., Timpl, R., Furthmayr, H., and Kuhn, K. (1973). *Eur. J. Biochem.*, **37**, 287.

Tanzer, M. L., Church, R. L., Yaeger, J. A., Wampler, D. E., and Park, E. D. (1974). *Proc. Nat. Acad. Sci.*, *U.S.A.*, **71**, 3009.
Taubman, M. B., Goldberg, B., and Sherr, C. J. (1974). *Science*, *N.Y.*, **186**, 1115.
Timpl, R., Becker, U., Furthmayr, H., and Kuhn, K. (1970*a*). *Immunochemistry*, **7**, 876.
Timpl, R., Beil, W., Furthmayr, H., Meigel, W., amd Pontz, B. (1971). *Immunology*, **21**, 1017.
Timpl, R., Fietzek, P. P., Furthmayr, H., Meigel, W., and Kuhn, K. (1970*b*). *FEBS Letters*, **9**, 11.
Timpl, R., Furthmayr, H., and Beil, W. (1972). *J. Immunol.*, **108**, 119.
Timpl, R., Furthmayr, H., Hahn, E., Becker, U., and Stoltz, M. (1973*a*). *Behring Inst.Mitt.*, **53**, 66.
Timpl, R., Furthmayr, H., Steffen, C., and Doleschel, W. (1967). *Z. ImmunForsch.*, **134**, 391.
Timpl, R., Glanville, R. W., Nowack, H., Wiedemann, H., Fietzek, P. P., and Kuhn, K. (1975). *Hoppe Seyler's Z. Physiol. Chem.*, **356**, 1783.

Timpl, R., Wick, G., Furthmayr, H., Lapiere, C. M., and Kuhn, K. (1973*b*). *Eur. J. Biochem.*, **32**, 584.

Traub, W., and Piez, K. A. (1971). *Adv. Protein Chem.*, **25**, 243.

Trelstad, R. L., Kang, A. H., Cohen, A. M., and Hay, E. D. (1973). *Science, N. Y.*, **179**, 295.

Trelstad, R. L., Kang, A. H., and Gross, J. (1971). *Fed. Proc.*, **30**, 1196.

Trelstad, R. L., Kang, A. H., Toole, B. P., and Gross, J. (1972). *J. Biol. Chem.*, **247**, 6469.

Uitto, J., and Prockop, D. J. (1974). *Eur. J. Biochem.*, **43**, 221.

Veis, A., Anesey, J., Yuan, L., and Levy, S. J. (1973). *Proc. Nat. Acad. Sci., U.S.A.*, **70**, 1464.

Verzar, F. (1964). *Int. Rev. Conn. Tiss. Res.*, **2**, 243.

Vinson, W. C., and Seyer, J. M. (1974). *Biochem. Biophys. Res. Commun.*, **58**, 58.

Volpin, D., and Veis, A. (1971). *Biochemistry*, **10**, 1751.

Von der Mark, K., Click, E. M., and Bornstein, P. (1973). *Archs Biochem. Biophys.*, **156**, 356.

Vuust, J., Lane, J. M., Fietzek, P. P., Miller, E. J., and Piez, K. A. (1970). *Biochem. Biophys. Res. Commun.*, **38**, 703.

Watson, R. F., Rothbard, S., and Vanamee, P. (1954). *J. Exp. Med.*, **99**, 535.

Weinstock, M., and Leblond, C. P. (1974). *J. Cell Biol.*, **60**, 92.

Wells, J. V., Michaeli, D., and Fudenberg, H. H. (1973). *Clin. Exp. Immunol.*, **13**, 203.

Wick, G., Furthmayr, H., and Timpl, R. (1975). *Int. Archs Allergy*, **48**, 664.

Wiedemann, H., Chung, E., Fujii, T., Miller, E. J., and Kuhn, K. (1975). *Eur. J. Biochem.*, **51**, 363.

Wolff, I., Timpl, R., Pecker, I., and Steffen, C. (1967). *Vox Sang.*, **12**, 443.

Yonath, A., Traub, W., and Miller, E. J. (1975). *FEBS Letters*, **57**, 93.

CHAPTER 14

The Nature of Amyloid

M. Pras and J. Gafni

1 INTRODUCTION

Amyloidosis is the disease resulting from the systemic or localized extracellular accumulation of an abnormal fibrillar protein in the ground substance of the connective tissue. The systemic forms of the disease will form the bulk of this discussion. Since these forms are virtually always fatal, they have long aroused medical curiosity and have been thoroughly studied and debated.

Amyloid, the abnormal fibrillar protein, may be identified by its green birefringence on staining with Congo red and by a characteristic electron microscopic appearance. Until recently, its chemical characterization was hampered by peculiar physicochemical properties which made its extraction from tissues and its isolation in a pure form difficult. Eventually, exploitation of these properties has made possible its isolation, leading to rapid advances in the knowledge of its chemistry during the last five years. Their significance can be appreciated fully only against the background of controversy and confusion that has been rampant. To highlight these difficulties, the history of the disease will be reviewed briefly.

1.1 Historical Background

Systemic amyloidosis was discovered more than a century ago (Rokitansky, 1842) associated with chronic suppurative diseases such as tuberculosis, empyema, and osteomyelitis. Although now these diseases have been eradicated largely, amyloidosis has been found with increasing frequency associated with such non-suppurative inflammatory diseases as rheumatoid arthritis and Crohn's disease, and in two malignancies—hypernephroma and Hodgkin's disease. The clinical manifestations of the amyloidosis in these cases are dominated by nephropathy even though autopsy reveals, in addition to the underlying disease, severe renal involvement by amyloid and major deposits in the spleen, adrenal, and liver. On the assumption that the associated disease bears a causal relationship, this amyloidosis has been designated 'secondary' and the pattern of organ involvement as 'typical'.

Somewhat later, cases of amyloidosis were described in which there was no evidence during life, or at necropsy, of any associated disease (Wild, 1856). The clinical pictures in these cases are manifestations of the amyloidosis alone. One group of such patients presented with cardiomyopathy and/or macroglossia due to massive involvement of muscle in systemic amyloidosis. In another group, peripheral neuropathy due to neural involvement dominated the picture. In the absence of a predisposing disease, this amyloidosis has been designated as 'primary' and its pattern of organ involvement as 'atypical' (Lubarsch, 1929).

Expectations that these aetiological and pathological features would be paired always—primary amyloidosis with atypical distribution and secondary disease with typical distribution—were dispelled soon. The amyloidosis associated with multiple myeloma, undeniably secondary in nature, proved to be atypical in distribution, and was awarded a special classification (Reiman *et al.*, 1935; King, 1948). Furthermore, King (1948) predicted that when amyloidosis became understood the distribution of amyloid in the tissues would be more relevant than the presence or absence of predisposing disease. More difficult to establish was the converse situation with the possibility that amyloidosis of typical distribution could occur in the absence of any predisposing disease. Pathologists encountering this situation were prone to attribute pathogenic significance to irrelevant bronchiectatic and pyelonephritic lesions. In addition, a review of autopsy material has revealed that virtually all organs are involved in all cases of systemic amyloidosis, thus denying any relationship between the presence of predisposing disease, or its absence, and pattern of organ involvement (Symmers, 1956*a*,*b*).

The possibility of clinicopathological correlation was established by Missmahl

(1959). The distribution of amyloid in tissues was determined by its deposition initially along either reticulin or collagen fibres, producing a vascular lesion characteristic for each. It is the latter lesion which is present in virtually all organs of the body, regardless of whether the organ is one involved in typical or atypical amyloidosis or whether the amyloidosis is peri-reticulin or peri-collagen. At the level of parenchymal involvement, however, peri-reticulin amyloidosis roughly encompasses the organs of typical distribution and peri-collagen the atypical distribution (Heller *et al.*, 1964). This distinction has not been accepted universally (Cohen, 1972).

In the absence of chemical studies, there also has been considerable controversy on the nature of amyloid. Over the years, immunological mechanisms were often implicated in its pathogenesis. There were logical extrapolations of the frequent association of the disease with chronic inflammatory disorders, both suppurative and non-infectious, multiple myeloma (Magnus-Levi, 1956; Osserman *et al.*, 1964; Pick and Osserman, 1968), and states of hyperimmunity induced experimentally (Muckle, 1968; Teilum, 1968). Taking multiple myeloma and its amyloidosis as a prototype, Kyle and Bayrd (1961) found increased numbers of plasma cells in bone marrow and paraproteinemia in patients with primary amyloidosis. Many immunofluorescent studies demonstrated higher levels of globulin in deposits of primary, secondary, and experimental amyloidosis than in control tissues (Mellors and Ortega, 1956; Vasquez and Dixon, 1956; Schultz *et al.*, 1966, 1968). Complement also has been demonstrated in amyloid deposits (Vogt and Kochem, 1960; Lachmann *et al.*, 1962). Proponents of an immunoglobulin origin of amyloid suggested that amyloid could be called more appropriately 'gammaloid' and the disease 'gammaloidosis' (Osserman, 1961). On the other hand, Calkins *et al.* (1958) demonstrated only traces of γ-globulins in amyloid, and Benditt *et al.* (1962) failed to demonstrate a reaction between purified and anti-γ-globulin sera. In addition, Paul and Cohen (1963), using ferritin-conjugated antisera to γ-globulin, could not demonstrate ferritin granules on amyloid fibrils. Cathcart and Cohen (1966) demonstrated that amyloid fibrils failed to react with antisera to IgG, IgM and IgA and the κ and λ light chains. From these studies it was concluded that the amyloid was neither a simple antigen–antibody complex nor globulin an integral part of the fibril. It should be pointed out that the clinical source of these preparations often was not stated. However, it was not appreciated at that time that amyloid may be chemically heterogeneous and its source, therefore, of prime importance.

The emergence of several familial entities of amyloidosis during the last 25 years has introduced 'genetic thinking' into this subject (Gafni *et al.*, 1964). In all these cases, systemic amyloidosis was determined genetically and the only significant finding at necropsy was that the amyloidosis was primary. Its clinical expression was uniform in each entity. Entities manifested by nephropathy revealed peri-reticulin amyloidosis, clearly indicating that typical amyloidosis can be primary in nature. Entities manifested by cardiopathy or neuropathy had peri-collagen amyloidosis. The parallel histological segregation in the genetic

512

and non-genetic forms reflects fundamental differences in amyloid morphogenesis. The conception of the non-genetic forms of amyloidosis as phenocopies of the hereditary type suggests a classification designating amyloidosis as hereditary when there is genetic evidence, acquired, when a predisposing disease is found, and idiopathic, when neither of the above is established (Table 1). Thus the terms primary, secondary, typical, and atypical, which have been the source of confusion in the past, are avoided.

Table 1 Classification of the systemic amyloidoses

Classification	Peri-reticulin amyloidosis	Peri-collagen amyloidosis
Hereditary	FMF (Sohar *et al.*, 1967*a*)	Neuropathic—lower limbs (Andrade, 1952)
	Fever, urticaria and deafness (Muckle and Wells, 1962)	Neuropathic—upper limbs (Rukavina *et al.*, 1956) Cardiopathic (Frederiksen *et al.*, 1962)
Acquired	Associated with chronic infection (tuberculosis, leprosy, etc.)	Associated with multiple myeloma
	Associated with non-infectious inflammation (rheumatoid arthritis, Chron's disease, etc.) Associated with malignant tumors (hypernephroma, Hodgkin's disease)	Associated with macroglobulinaemia
Idiopathic	Primary with typical distribution (nephropathic)	Classical primary (cardiopathic and/or neuropathic)

FMF = familial Mediterranean fever

When mechanisms of genetic disorders are understood, they are found to be simple biochemical defects in a metabolic pathway. The constancy of the pathological pattern in each entity and the variation between them could reflect differences in their respective amyloids. Genetic concepts, therefore, have led to the suggestion that amyloid is a generic term for a family of different proteins (Heller *et al.*, 1965).

2 FIBRILLAR COMPONENT OF AMYLOID

Physico-chemical properties distinguish amyloid from other proteins in mammalian tissues. The physical properties of amyloid are unique and virtually identical regardless of its source. Chemical analysis has demonstrated variations in different preparations. These differences had been the source of debate as long as they could be attributed to lack of purity, but recent discoveries indicate the existence of at least two chemically distinct types of systemic amyloidosis.

2.1 Solubility Properties and Isolation

Only the classical protein solvents, concentrated urea and guanidine solutions, and sodium dodecyl sulphate can dissolve amyloid together with the other highly insoluble tissue proteins. Amyloid is highly insoluble in neutral aqueous media at ionic strengths commonly used (Hass and Schulz, 1940; Newcombe and Cohen, 1964), even after its extraction from the tissue. Surprisingly, amyloid fibrils are soluble in distilled water, but precipitate readily in saline solutions, even at concentrations as low as 0.01 M NaCl (Pras *et al.*, 1968). These unusual solubility properties are shown in Figure 1.

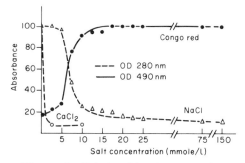

Figure 1 Relationship between the amount of amyloid left in solution and the concentration of added NaCl or CaCl$_2$. The amount of amyloid left in solution was determined by (a) the per cent of the initial absorbance at 280 nm left in the supernatant solution after adding salt and removing precipitated amyloid by centrifugation, and (b) measuring the per cent of Congo red in saline not precipitated when added to the same supernatant solution. The solid Congo red line was obtained with the supernatant solutions after the addition of NaCl

These features of amyloid fibrils have been exploited in their isolation and purification. To extract pure amyloid fibrils, it is necessary first to eliminate the normal tissue constituents by repeated extraction in saline and then to wash out the electrolytes from the suspension. The aqueous solution obtained after removal of all salts is straw-coloured and clear, and does not precipitate at 68 000 *g*. It abounds with fibrils when examined by electron microscopy. These stain with Congo red and show typical green birefringence. The distilled water extract is unstable and tends to precipitate on prolonged standing. It seems likely, therefore, that amyloid in distilled water represents either a suspension or a colloidal solution.

2.2 Morphological Forms

The fibrillar structure of amyloid was predicted on the basis of its dichroism and birefringent properties (Missmahl and Hartwig, 1953). Fibrils were shown in

514

electron micrographs published by Spiro (1959), but first recognized and described as such by Cohen and Calkins (1959) and Caesar (1960). Individual fibrils appear as straight, rigid structures, measuring about 10 nm in diameter. In many areas, the fibrils are organized parallel to collagen bundles or basement membranes (Heller *et al.*, 1964; Sohar *et al.*, 1967*b*). In others, particularly where parenchymal tissue is held in a loose fashion, such as in the spleen, renal interstitium, lymph nodes, and bone marrow, the fibrils criss-cross at random, no orientation being apparent (Zucker-Franklin and Franklin, 1970).

When isolated fibrils are examined by electron microscopy they appear identical to those seen in freshly fixed tissues (Figure 2). Many have a beaded substructure and may be twisted on one another. Often they appear as a pair of parallel filaments separated by a space of about 2 nm (Shirahama and Cohen, 1967). Such fibrils, measuring less than 10 nm and seeming to consist of paired filaments, also are seen when water-soluble amyloid is negatively stained without prior fixation (Pras *et al.*, 1968). High resolution studies have shown as many as

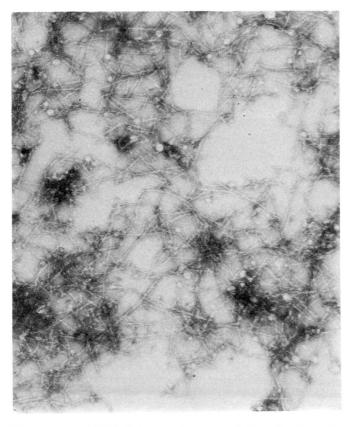

Figure 2 Amyloid fibrils isolated by water solubilization (magnification × 38 000)

five longitudinal protofibrils, each 2–3 nm wide and showing 3·5–5 nm beading (Shirahama and Cohen, 1967).

Bladen *et al.* (1966), and Benditt and Eriksen (1966) observed a second rod-like structure 10 nm wide with clear-cut 4 nm periodicity in amyloid isolated by sucrose-gradient centrifugation and sonicated. This rod could be disrupted to pentagonal structures consisting of five 2–2·5 nm units arranged around a hollow core. Originally described as the unit structure of amyloid, it is neither stained using Congo red nor displays green birefringence. Subsequently, it was shown by immunological and electron microscopic techniques to be identical to a newly discovered component of α_1-globulin (plasma P component) of normal individuals. The rod is not a part of the amyloid fibril and makes up only 5 per cent of amyloid deposits (Cathcart *et al.*, 1967; Shirahama and Cohen, 1967). The periodic rod structure, therefore, may represent another non-specific serum component contaminating amyloid fibrils extracted by certain techniques. In water-soluble amyloid preparations obtained from both peri-reticulin and peri-collagen sources, no such structure was found in a review of several hundred micrographs (Franklin and Zucker-Franklin, 1972).

2.3 Ultracentrifugation Studies

Most preparations of intact amyloid fibrils in distilled water sedimented as a single homogeneous component with a coefficient of about 45 S when examined immediately after isolation. In several preparations, however, and in those left standing, polymers with coefficients of 75 S and higher appear. After several weeks, such aggregates tend to precipitate from solution spontaneously but can be redispersed generally to the 45 S component by vigorous homogenization (Pras *et al.*, 1968, 1969). These properties are common to both peri-collagen and peri-reticulin preparations.

2.4 Chemical Characteristics

In view of the variety in the aetiological, clinical, and pathological features of amyloidosis, it was not a complete surprise when chemical analyses revealed marked differences in amyloid preparations. In retrospect, it can be said that even the sophisticated methods of isolation of whole amyloid fibrils yielded a product that was chemically impure, which was shown clearly in the amino acid analyses of amyloid fibrils isolated from various sources (Benditt *et al.*, 1962; Benditt and Eriksen, 1966; Cohen, 1966*a,b*; Pras *et al.*, 1968, 1969). Peptide mapping of primary, secondary, and myeloma amyloid preparations has demonstrated some common peptides and basic similarities (Pras *et al.*, 1969). Glenner and coworkers (1970*b*) showed, however, that amyloid preparations obtained from two organs of the same individual have identical peptide maps.

The carbohydrate moiety constitutes less than 2 per cent by dry weight of amyloid fibrils. Although its role is still uncertain, the sugar component does appear to be responsible for the metachromasia of amyloid (Pras and Schubert,

1969). However, various proteoglycans are responsible in different organs. Preparations derived from liver and spleen are metachromatic owing to heparitin sulphate, while chondroitin sulphate is responsible in kidney samples (Bitter and Muir, 1966; Dalferes, 1968; Muir and Cohen, 1968; Pras et al., 1971). It seems likely, therefore, that the carbohydrate moiety is entrapped or non-specifically adsorbed into the fibril mesh and is not an integral part of the amyloid molecule.

3 BASIC SUBUNITS OF AMYLOID FIBRILS

The realization that the 45 S component of water-soluble amyloid was a polymer prompted attempts to dissociate fibrils and to isolate a homogenous subunit. Early experiments were disappointing. Treatment with papain, pepsin, and trypsin not only failed to produce unique subunits but also left much of the fibrillar protein intact (Sorenson and Binington, 1964; Emerson et al., 1966; Ruinen et al., 1967; Kim et al., 1969; Pras et al., 1969). Miller et al. (1968) did obtain smaller fragments by cyanogen bromide cleavage, but they used an impure preparation unfortunately. Subsequently, Pras et al. (1969) degraded amyloid fibrils with 0·1 M sodium hydroxide to obtain a 1–2 S subunit (DAM) with a molecular weight of 30 000. Although not pure enough for chemical analysis, DAM was sufficiently antigenic to allow preparation of anti-amyloid fibril antibodies which proved useful in immunological studies (Franklin and Pras, 1969; Husby et al., 1972).

3.1 Methods of Preparation

Recent studies by several groups have used three different methods to obtain protein subunits from purified amyloid fibrils isolated by water extraction.

3.1.1 Urea Degradation

Although several investigators had treated amyloid fibrils with concentrated urea solutions, Benditt and his collaborators characterized the proteins resulting from the denaturation. Employing concentrated urea solutions at pH 3·5 and column chromatography, they demonstrated that amyloid fibrils derived from patients with tuberculosis and familial Mediterranean fever (FMF) are composed of several low molecular weight subunits (Benditt and Ericksen, 1966; Benditt et al., 1968, 1970). The major subunit constituted about 50 per cent of the fibrils and had a molecular weight of 6000–8000 (Benditt and Eriksen, 1971).

3.1.2 Guanidine Degradation

Glenner and his collaborators (1970a,b, 1971a,b,c; Harada et al., 1971) treated preparations of purified amyloid fibrils with 6 M guanidine hydrochloride and mercaptoethanol, and using column chromatography isolated subunits. These fractions constituted up to 70 per cent of fibril dry weight and ranged in molecular weight from 5000 to 30 000.

Zuckerberg *et al.* (1972) treated amyloid fibrils from patients with rheumatoid arthritis and FMF with 10 per cent sodium chloride and then 6 M guanidine hydrochloride, and using amicon PM-30 filtration isolated a protein with a molecular weight of 4000–5000 as estimated by SDS gel electrophoresis. After reconstitution the fibrils showed Congo red staining, green, birefringence, and electron microscopic dimensions of amyloid although appearing flexible.

Husby and his coworkers (1973) based their isolation procedure on treating the fibril preparations with 6 M guanidine and Sephadex G-100 gel filtration. They obtained a K_{av} 0·46 peak which contained 45–58 per cent of the original fibrils isolated from amyloidotic tissues of six patients suffering from non-suppurative inflammatory disease, FMF and hypernephroma, and one with Waldenström macroglobulinaemia. In six others, with primary amyloidosis and myelomatosis, and one with macroglobulinaemia, this fraction was detectable only after the fibrils were degraded with alkali; the yield was only 18–29 per cent.

3.1.3 Acid Solubilization

Pras and Reshef (1972) took advantage of the major protein component of amyloid fibrils derived from patients with FMF, tuberculosis, bronchiectasis,

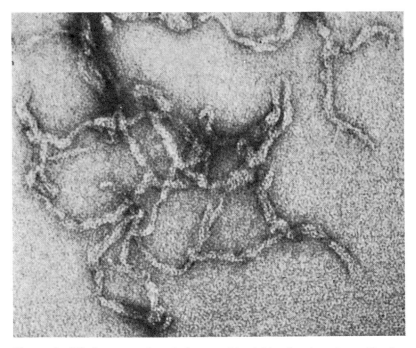

Figure 3 Fibrils reconstituted from acid-soluble fraction (magnification × 210 000)

rheumatoid arthritis, and Hodgkin's disease being soluble in 0·02 M hydrochloric acid. This acid-soluble fraction constitutes as much as 60 per cent dry weight of the purified amyloid fibrils and is a homogeneous protein with a molecular weight of about 8000. It reprecipitates when neutralized using dialysis or alkali as a fibrillar structure which is stained with Congo red and shows green birefringence. Instead of being straight, rigid and of uniform diameter, the reconstructed fibrils are undulating and flexible and vary in diameter from 3 to 20 nm along their lengths (Figure 3).

3.2 Amino Acid Analysis

The first clear-cut indications of chemical heterogeneity of amyloid were from the amino acid analyses of these subunits. In spite of differences in clinical background, organ source, and methods of isolation, their amino acid contents fall into one of two broad patterns:

(*i*) This is a very homogeneous pattern. It represents an unusual protein dominated by five amino acids—alanine, aspartic acid, arginine, glycine, and phenylalanine—accounting for 60 per cent of the residues. Cystine is absent, while threonine and proline are present at strikingly low levels. This amino acid pattern is present in preparations studied by Benditt *et al.* (1971), Pras and Reshef (1972), Zuckerberg *et al.* (1972), and Husby *et al.* (1973), and in one patient of Glenner *et al.* (1972).

(*ii*) Homogeneity in the amino acid composition of these proteins is much less striking. All amino acids are present, including cystine in proportions usually found in human proteins. The dominant amino acids are serine and glutamic acid, and the proline content is high. Such composition was found by Glenner and his associates (Glenner *et al.*, 1972; Terry *et al.*, 1973) in six patients, and in one each by Husby and coworkers (Husby *et al.*, 1974; Sletten *et al.*, 1974) and by Skinner *et al.* (1975).

By amino acid sequence studies it was established that the first pattern reflects a unique protein related to a previously unrecognized serum component, serum amyloid-A protein. The other is related to immunoglobulin light chain, usually being a fragment of its variable portion. The amino acid contents of respective amyloid preparations are shown in Tables 2 and 3.

4 AMYLOID RELATED TO SERUM AMYLOID-A PROTEIN

4.1 Sequence Studies on Amyloid Subunits—Amyloid-A Protein

The first amyloid subunit to be sequenced completely was the acid-soluble fraction derived from the spleen of a patient with FMF (Levin *et al.*, 1972). It proved to be a polypeptide comprising 76 amino acids, dominated by alanine, aspartic acid, arginine, and glycine. Together, these four amino acids accounted for 40 of the 76 residues. Arginine is the N-terminal amino acid and of five

Table 2 Amino acid analyses* of amyloid subunit preparations related to serum amyloid-A protein

	Benditt et al. (1971)	Zuckerberg et al. (1972)			Pras and Reshef (1972)		Glenner et al. (1972)	Husby et al. (1973)	
Method	Urea	Guanidine			Dilute Acid		Guanidine	Guanidine	
Disease	TB†	RA	FMF	FMF	FMF†	HD†	RA†	JRA†	MW
Organ	Liver	Liver	Liver‡	Spleen‡	Spleen	Liver	Spleen	Liver	Liver
Aspartic acid	13·4	12·6	11·1	11·4	12·6	10·5	15·5	3·0	13·5
Threonine	0·1	1·7	1·3	1·0	0·7	0	0	0·7	0·4
Serine	7·5	6·6	5·5	5·6	7·5	7·2	7·1	6·8	6·9
Glutamic acid	7·4	11·0	10·7	9·4	8·2	8·7	5·0	8·4	8·3
Proline	1·5	2·1	2·8	2·1	0·3	2·0	0	2·0	1·6
Glycine	12·2	11·5	10·9	11·0	10·8	9·6	10·3	11·1	11·6
Alanine	16·7	16·4	17·1	15·4	16·6	18·7	15·6	16·0	15·6
Cysteine	0·1	0	0	0	0	0	0	0·4	0·4
Valine	1·4	1·7	2·6	1·9	1·7	2·0	0	1·7	1·4
Methionine	2·8	1·7	2·0	2·4	2·8	2·8	4·4	3·0	2·7
Isoleucine	3·8	2·9	3·8	4·0	1·7	1·9	1·9	3·6	3·7
Leucine	1·5	4·1	4·5	3·8	2·7	1·8	2·5	2·5	2·0
Tyrosine	5·5	5·2	4·9	4·8	6·9	9·5	8·3	5·6	5·4
Phenylalanine	8·2	5·9	6·2	7·3	10·3	9·8	11·5	7·8	8·7
Lysine	2·8	2·8	3·3	4·6	3·0	2·4	2·5	2·0	2·5
Histidine	2·2	1·5	1·3	2·2	0	0	2·0	3·3	2·9
Arginine	10·8	9·6	8·5	10·2	11·6	10·9	11·1	10·0	10·7
Tryptophan	2·3	2·9	3·5	3·2	2·6	2·0	2·3	2·3	1·8

* Calculated as residues per 100 residues
† Specimens submitted to sequence study (see Table 5)
‡ Specimens from same patient
TB = tuberculosis, RA = rheumatoid arthritis, JRA = juvenile rheumatoid arthritis, FMF = familial Mediterranean fever, HD = Hodgkin's disease, MW = Waldenström's macroglobulinaemia

Table 3 Amino acid analyses of immunoglobulin light chain-related amyloid subunit preparations obtained from seven patients

Author	Glenner et al. (1972)*					Terry et al. (1973)†	Skinner et al. (1975)*
Method	Guanidine					Guanidine	Guanidine
Disease	Primary amyloidosis	Primary amyloidosis	Epidermolysis bullosa and TB‡	Primary amyloidosis‡	Primary amyloidosis	Plasma cell dyscrasia‡	Primary amyloidosis‡
Organ	Liver	Spleen	Spleen	Liver	Spleen	Intestine	Spleen
Aspartic acid	7·6	5·6	10·3	9·7	2·5	9·0	8·6
Threonine	8·0	6·4	7·6	8·5	6·6	6·7	8·0
Serine	11·2	12·3	10·3	10·9	11·8	11·5	14·8
Glutamic acid	10·6	9·8	11·2	10·7	9·7	13·0	10·3
Proline	7·8	6·3	5·6	7·7	7·9	6·1	7·1
Glycine	8·4	10·8	6·9	9·6	2·0	7·1	8·2
Alanine	9·2	8·3	6·3	6·0	8·9	6·6	8·1
Cysteine	2·3	2·3	2·0	2·1	1·8		1·4
Valine	7·5	5·8	5·9	4·4	6·7	7·5	6·8
Methionine	0·3	0	0·8	1·1	0	1·0	0·8
Isoleucine	3·0	4·1	4·6	4·8	5·1	3·3	3·6
Leucine	8·4	8·1	8·0	6·0	8·4	9·9	6·0
Tyrosine	3·2	4·4	3·9	5·2	4·0	3·6	4·6
Phenylalanine	2·2	2·4	4·6	4·5	3·5	4·5	2·8
Lysine	5·4	6·0	5·5	4·4	2·5	5·0	4·4
Histidine	1·2	1·7	1·3	0	1·3	1·4	1·6
Arginine	2·5	4·1	3·9	3·3	1·2	3·8	3·0
Tryptophan	1·4	1·3	1·1	1·4	1·1		

* Amino acids calculated as residues per 100 residues

† Amino acids calculated as moles per 100 moles; cystine and tryptophan not listed

‡ Specimens submitted to sequential study (see Tables 6 and 7)

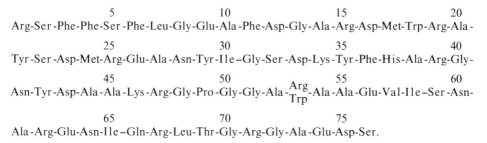

Arg-Ser -Phe-Phe-Ser -Phe-Leu-Gly-Glu-Ala -Phe-Asp-Gly-Ala -Arg-Asp-Met-Trp-Arg-Ala -

Tyr-Ser -Asp-Met-Arg-Glu-Ala -Asn-Tyr -Ile –Gly-Ser -Asp-Lys -Tyr -Phe-His-Ala -Arg-Gly-

Asn-Tyr-Asp-Ala -Ala -Lys -Arg-Gly-Pro -Gly-Gly-Ala -Arg/Trp -Ala -Ala -Glu-Val-Ile –Ser -Asn-

Ala -Arg-Glu-Asn-Ile –Gln-Arg-Leu-Thr-Gly-Arg-Gly-Ala -Glu-Asp-Ser.

Figure 4 Sequence of AA protein derived from patient with FMF. From Levin *et al.*
(1972)

phenylalanine residues, four are at positions 3, 4, 6, and 11, making a highly
characteristic N-terminal (see Figure 4). The chain contains no cysteine and only
one residue of threonine and proline (Table 4). Its molecular weight is 9100.

The uniqueness of the N-terminal portion was appreciated by Benditt *et al.*
(1971), who had highlighted this N-terminal region earlier in a urea-treated
preparation from a tuberculous patient. They had emphasized its remarkable
similarity in its first 24 amino acid residues to amyloid obtained from a monkey
with granulomatous (probably tuberculous) disease.

To date, complete amino acid sequencing has been carried out on only two
additional human amyloid preparations, both guanidine-treated fibrils. One,
derived from the liver of a juvenile rheumatoid arthritic, also consisted of 76
amino acid residues (Sletten and Husby, 1974), while the other, from the spleen of

Table 4 Complete amino acid content of
AA protein derived from a patient with FMF

Amino acid	Number of residues
Aspartic acid	10
Threonine	1
Serine	6
Glutamic acid	6
Proline	1
Glycine	9
Alanine	12
Cysteine	0
Valine	1
Methionine	2
Isoleucine	3
Leucine	2
Tyrosine	4
Phenylalanine	5
Lysine	2
Histidine	1
Arginine	9 (or 10)
Tryptophan	2 (or 1)

From Levin *et al.* (1972)

an adult with rheumatoid arthritis (Ein *et al.*, 1972), had only 45. Both specimens had the same phenylalanine-loaded N-terminal as the spleen preparation of Levin *et al.* (1972) and, if a single replacement of aspartic acid by asparagine is attributed to deamination during processing, were identical for the first 45 residues. Interestingly, the amyloid subunit derived from the tuberculous monkey also proved to be a 76-amino acid protein, very similar to the human (Hermodson *et al.*, 1972).

Such variation as is present in these completely sequenced subunits is in the C-terminal portion of the molecule. As a rule, this variance is expressed by the replacement of hydrophobic by hydrophobic residues and hydrophilic by hydrophilic residues, suggesting that hydrostatic polarity may be essential for the polymerization of subunits into fibrils (Franklin and Zucker-Franklin, 1972; Pras and Reshef, 1972; Zuckerberg *et al.*, 1972; Sletten and Husby, 1974). All sequence studies performed on this subunit of the amyloid fibril are shown in Figure 5. Sources of the AA protein subunit used together with the method of preparation are summarized in Table 5.

At the Helsinki conference on amyloidosis in 1974, this subunit was named

No.					5					10					15					20	
1	Arg-Ser	-Phe-Phe-Ser	-Phe-Leu-Gly-Glu-Ala	-Phe-Asp-Gly-Ala	-Arg-Asp-Met-Trp-Arg-Ala-
2	,,	,,	,,	,,	,,	,,	,,	,,	,,	,,	,,	,,	,,	,,	,,	,,	,,	,,	,,	,,	
3	,,	,,	,,	,,	,,	,,	,,	,,	,,	,,	,,	,,	,,	,,	,,	,,	,,	,,	,,	,,	
4	,,	,,	,,	,,	,,	,,	,,	,,	,,	,,	,,	,,	,,	,,	,,	,,	,,	,,	,,	,,	
5	,,	,,	,,	,,	,,	,,	,,	,,	,,	,,	,,	,,	,,	,,	,,	,,	,,	,,	,,	,,	
6	,,	,,	,,	,,	,,	,,	,,	,,	,,	,,	,,	,,	,,	,,	,,	,,	,,	,,	,,	,,	
7	,,	,,	,,	,,	,,	,,	,,	,,	,,	,,	_ _ _ _ _										
8	,,	,,	Trp	,,	,,	,,	,,	,,	,,	,,	Tyr	,,	,,	,,	,,	,,	,,	,,	,,		

No.					25					30					35					40	
1	Tyr-Ser	-Asp-Met-Arg-Glu-Ala	-Asn-Tyr-Ile	-Gly-Ser	-Asp-Lys	-Tyr-Phe-His-Ala-Arg-Gly-
2	,,	,,	Asn	,,	,,	,,	,,	,,	,,	,,	,,	,,	,,	,,	,,	,,	,,	,,	,,	,,	
3	,,	,,	Asp	,,	,,	,,	,,	,,	,,	,,	,,	,,	,,	,,	,,	,,	,,	,,	,,	,,	
4	,,	,,	,,	,,	,,	,,	,,	,,	,,	,,	,,	,,	,,	,,	,,	,,	,,	,,	,,	,,	
5	,,	,,	,,	,,	,,	,,	,,	,,	,,	,,	,,	,,	_ _ _ _ _								
6	,,	,,	,,	,,	_ _ _ _ _																
8	,,	,,	,,	,,	Lys	,,	,,	,,	,,	Lys-Asn	,,	,,	,,	,,	,,	,,	,,	,,	,,		

No.					45					50					55					60	
1	Asn-Tyr	-Asp-Ala-Ala	-Lys-Arg-Gly-Pro	-Gly-Gly-Ala	-Trp/Arg	-Ala-Ala	-Glu-Val-Ile	-Ser	-Asn-
2	,,	,,	,,	,,	,,	,,	,,	,,	,,	,,	,,	Val-Trp	,,	,,	,,	Ala	,,	,,	Asp-
3	,,	,,	,,	,,	,,	,,	,,	,,	,,	,,	,,	,,	,,	,,	_ _ _ _ _						
4	Asx	,,	Asx	,,	,,	.															
8	Asn	,,	Asp	,,	,,	Gln	,,	,,	,,	,,	,,	,,	,,	,,	,,	,,	Val	,,	,,	,,	

No.					65					70					75			
1	Ala-Arg-Glu-Asn-Ile	-Gln-Arg-Leu-Thr-Gly-Arg-Gly-Ala	-Glu-Asp-Ser.															
2	,,	,,	,,	,,	,,	,,	,,	Phe-Phe	,,	His	,,	,,	,,	Asn	,,	.		
8	,,	,,	,,	,,	,,	,,	Lys-Leu-Leu	,,	,,	,,	,,	,,	Asp-Thr.					

Figure 5 Sequence studies of AA protein subunits. Details of sources of protein and methods of isolation are listed in Table 5

Table 5 Sources and extraction methods used in preparing AA protein for sequence studies

Sequence number†	Species	Disease	Organ	Method	Reference
1	Human*	FMF	Spleen	Dilute acid	Levin *et al.* (1972)
2	,, *	Juvenile rheumatoid arthritis	Liver	Guanidine	Sletten and Husby (1974)
3	,,	Tuberculosis	Spleen	Dilute acid	Levin *et al.* (1972)
4	,, *	Rheumatoid arthritis	Spleen	Guanidine	Ein *et al.* (1972)
5	,, *	Hodgkin's disease	Liver	Dilute acid	Levin *et al.* (1972)
6	,, *	Tuberculosis	Liver	Urea	Benditt *et al.* (1971)
7	,,	Bronchiectasis	Liver	Dilute acid	Levin *et al.* (1972)
8	Monkey	Tuberculosis	Liver	Urea	Hermodson *et al.* (1972)

* Amino acid analysis presented in Table 2
† See Figure 5

amyloid-A protein (AA protein). It had been designated previously A (amyloid) by Benditt and Eriksen (1971), AUO (amyloid of unknown origin) by Glenner *et al.* (1972), AS (amyloid subunit) by Husby *et al.* (1973), F (fibril) by Zuckerberg *et al.* (1972), and ASF (acid soluble fraction) by Pras and Reshef (1972).

4.2 Identification and Characterization of Serum Amyloid-A Protein

Since the generation of protein comprising 76 amino acid requires many enzymes, it seemed more reasonable to assume that AA protein is derived from a naturally occurring protein than from a pathological one formed *de novo*. Indeed, antisera to chemically pure AA protein derived from a patient with FMF not only reacted in double diffusion with AA protein derived from patients with tuberculosis, bronchiectasis, and Hodgkin's disease but also recognized a hitherto unknown serum component, the serum amyloid-A (SAA) protein (Levin *et al.*, 1973).

When estimated by radioimmunoassay, this serum component was found in normal individuals. In many ways, the component acted as acute-phase reactants do—increasing in pregnancy, with ageing, and in a variety of acute inflammatory and chronic diseases with and without amyloidosis. SAA was isolated by gel chromatography of serum treated with 0·18 M hydrochloric acid. Using immunoelectrophoresis, it was identified in the α_1-globulin region (Levin *et al.*, 1973; Sletten and Husby, 1974; Benson *et al.*, 1975; Linke *et al.*, 1975), but was antigenically distinct from the plasma P component (Franklin *et al.*, 1975). Chromatographic studies suggest that SAA protein has a molecular weight of about 86 000 (Franklin *et al.*, 1975). The SAA protein isolated by Linke and associates (1975), using phosphate-buffered chromatography, from a non-amyloidotic patient with Hodgkin's disease had a molecular weight of 200 000, while that isolated by Benson *et al.* (1975), using gel and affinity chromatography from amyloidotic patients with FMF and granulomatous bowel disease had a molecular weight of 100 000–120 000.

4.3 The Subunit of Serum Amyloid-A Protein

Obviously, SAA protein is larger than the AA protein which has a molecular weight of 9100. A smaller subunit was isolated from SAA protein by column chromatography after degradation with 5 M guanidine (Linke *et al.*, 1975) and also after acid dissociation (Anders *et al.*, 1975; Rosenthal *et al.*, 1976). This subunit has a molecular weight of about 12 000. Its antigenic properties, amino acid analyses, and peptide maps relate it to AA protein. This relationship was established firmly when partial sequencing revealed an identical 11 amino acid N-terminal sequence (Anders *et al.*, 1975; Rosenthal *et al.*, 1976). There can be little doubt that AA protein represents the N-terminal fragment of the SAA subunit. The higher molecular weight of circulating SAA protein must be due to either polymerization or binding with serum α_1-globulin.

5 AMYLOID RELATED TO IMMUNOGLOBULIN LIGHT CHAIN

Glenner *et al.* (1971*c*) subjected subunits derived from amyloid fibrils obtained from two patients to analysis in an automatic sequencer. Partial sequences of 35 and 36 amino acid residues showed a striking homology to the first 30 residues of the N-terminal V region of κ light chain. Subsequently, they demonstrated homology of amyloid fibril subunits in a patient with plasma cell dyscrasia with his Bence–Jones protein—probably a complete κ light chain (Terry *et al.*, 1973). These comparisons are shown in Figure 6. However, in a case of amyloidosis studied by Pick *et al.* (1973) only five N-terminal residues were homologous to those described above. Glenner's group produced antisera against the subunits they had prepared and showed them to cross-react strongly with other amyloid subunits and with Bence–Jones proteins not only of the κ but also of the λ light-chain subclasses (Isersky *et al.*, 1972).

			5			10			15			20
$V_\kappa 1$*	Asp-Ile	–Gln-Met-Thr-Gln-Ser	-Pro	-Ser	-Ser	-Leu-Ser	-Ala	-Ser	-Val-Gly-Asp-Arg-Val-Thr-
Amyloid 1†	,,	,, ,, ,, ,, ,,	,,	,,	,,	,, ,,	,,	,,	,, ,, ,, ,, ,, ,,
,, 2‡	,,	,, ,, ,, ,, ,,	,,	Ala	,,	,, ,,	,,	,,	,, ,, ,, ,, ,, Ile
,, 3§	,,	,, Val ,, ,, ,,	,,	Pro-Leu	,,	,, Pro-Val-Thr-Pro	,,	Glu-Pro	-Ala-Ser
Bence–Jones‖ protein	,,	,, ,, ,, ,, ,,	,,	,,	,,	,, ,,	,,	,,	,, ,, ,, ,, ,, ,,

			25			30		35
$V_\kappa 1$*	Ile-Thr-Cys-Gln-Ala-Ser	-Gln-Asp-Ile-Lys	$-----$
Amyloid 1†	,, ,, ,, ,, ,, ,,	Asx ,, Gly-( )-Tyr-Leu-( )-Trp-	$------$
,, 2‡	,, (,,) ,, Glx ,, (,,)-Glx-	,, ,, (,,)-Pro- ,, ,, ,, (,,)-Tyr	$-----$
,, 3§	,, Ser ,, Arg-Ser-Ser ,,	$-------$	
Bence–Jones‖ protein	,, ,, ,, ,, ,, ,,	Gln $-------$	

* Milstein (1966, 1967)
† Obtained from spleen of patient with epidermolysis bullosa and TB using guanidine (Glenner *et al.*, 1971c)
‡ Obtained from liver of patient with primary amyloidosis using guanidine (Glenner *et al.*, 1971c)
§ Obtained from intestine of patient with plasma cell dyscrasia using guanidine (Terry *et al.*, 1973)
‖ Obtained from same patient as amyloid 3 (Terry *et al.*, 1973)

Figure 6 N-Terminal partial sequence studies of amyloid subunits compared with κ light-chain immunoglobulin

Clear homology with V_λ regions were established by Sletten *et al.* (1974) and confirmed by Skinner *et al.* (1975), each in a case of primary amyloidosis; the former was homologous for 45 N-terminal residues of an estimated 100 in the molecule and the latter for 16 (see Figure 7). In spite of the homology, this amyloid protein shows at least 50 per cent variance from known V_λ regions and does not react with them antigenically. Sletten *et al.* (1974) argued convincingly that it is the prototype of a new variable subgroup, termed $V_\lambda 5$, of λ light chains. In four other patients, including one with localized nodular pulmonary amyloidosis (Page *et al.*, 1972), there is evidence suggesting that the N-terminal tetrapeptide may be homologous to a fragment of λ light chain (Kimura *et al.*, 1972).

		5				10				15	
$V_\lambda 2$	His-Ser	-Ala	-Leu-Thr-Gln-Pro	-Ala	-Ser	-Val-Ser	-Gly-Ser	-Leu-Gly-			
Amyloid 1*	Asp-Phe-Met	,,	,,	,,	,,	His	,,	,,	,,	Glu	,,	(Pro) ,,
,, 2†	,,	,,	,,	,,	,,	Glu	,,	,,	,,	,,	,,	,, ,,

		20			25				30	
$V_\lambda 2$	Gln-Ser	-Ile-Thr-Ile	-Ser	-Cys-Thr-Gly-Thr-Ser	-Ser	-Asp-Val-Gly-				
Amyloid 1*	Lys-Thr-Val	,,	Phe	,,	(,,)	,,	Glu-Ser	-Asn-(,,)	-Ser	-Ile ‡
,, 2†	,,	− − − − − −								

		35			40			45	
$V_\lambda 2$	Gly-Tyr-Asn-Tyr	-Val-Ser	-Trp-Phe-Gln-Gln-His-Pro	-Gly-Thr-Ala	-Pro − − − − − −				
Amyloid 1*	Ala-Asp-Ser	-Phe	,,	Gln- (,,)	-Tyr-Glx-Glx- (,,)	,,	,,	Ser	,, ,, − − − − − −

* Case of primary amyloidosis, subunit isolated from spleen and liver using guanidine (Sletten *et al.*, 1974)

† Case of primary amyloidosis, subunit isolated from spleen using guanidine (Skinner *et al.*, 1975)

‡ Deletion to maximize homology

Figure 7 N-Terminal partial sequence studies of amyloid subunits compared with a λ light-chain immunoglobulin

Additional evidence, relating amyloid to light chains, was obtained by demonstrating that tryptic or peptic treatment of Bence–Jones proteins derived from patients with amyloidosis, or with multiple myeloma but no amyloidosis, produced fibrils which had the characteristic Congo red staining and X-ray diffraction of amyloid. (Glenner *et al.*, 1971*a*, 1974; Franklin and Zucker-Franklin, 1972). However their electron microscope appearance was undulating and more flexible. Shirahama *et al.* (1973) also succeeded in producing fibrils from variable light-chain fragments, but from only three of the 13 Bence–Jones proteins examined; two of these were κ light chains and the other λ.

The exciting conclusion from these studies is that, in some amyloid preparations, the major protein component is a fragment of immunoglobulin—usually the variable portion of light chain. This could account for the lack of homogeneity in the amino acid analyses of the various preparations.

6. CONCLUDING COMMENTS

6.1 Expectations

In general, new data seem to confirm the chemical heterogeneity of amyloid (Gafni *et al.*, 1964; Heller *et al.*, 1965), one form of which could be called gammaloid (Osserman, 1964). They also confirm the greater biochemical relevance of histological distribution compared with predisposing disease (King, 1948).

SAA protein-related amyloid has now been confirmed amply by independent groups using sequential studies of the genetic amyloidosis of FMF and the acquired amyloidosis associated with tuberculosis, bronchiectasis, juvenile and adult rheumatoid arthritis, and Hodgkin's disease. Striking homology also has been shown in non-human amyloids. For example, it has been observed in amyloidosis induced experimentally by endotoxin in mink (Nordstoga, 1972; Sletten and Husby, 1974, Natvig *et al.*, 1975) and by sodium caseinate in guinea-pig (Skinner *et al.*, 1974). Also, homology occurs in acquired amyloidosis associated probably with tuberculous granulomata in monkey (Hermodson *et al.*, 1972) and in the amyloidosis, possibly of a genetic nature, in duck (Eriksen *et al.*, 1974). Isolation of AA protein is dependent neither on organ source, for it is present in both hepatic and splenic amyloid, nor on whether the subunit is prepared by urea, guanidine, or dilute acid dissociation of the fibril.

The immunoglobulin light chain-related component has been found largely in guanidine-treated amyloid derived from cases of primary amyloidosis and amyloidosis associated with plasma cell dyscrasia (Glenner, 1971c; Kimura *et al.*, 1972, Pick and Osserman, 1973; Terry *et al.*, 1973; Sletten *et al.*, 1974; Skinner *et al.*, 1975).

In the main, therefore, SAA protein-related amyloid and immunoglobulin light chain-related amyloid would seem to account for the histological differentiation into peri-reticulin and peri-collagen distributions, respectively, and their clinical consequences.

6.2 Deviations

One of the two amyloid preparations in Glenner's initial study (1971c) was that from a patient with epidermolysis bullosa who had developed tuberculosis during steroid therapy (Harada *et al.*, 1971). The pathological description, although meagre, is compatible, in terms of the organs involved, with peri-reticulin amyloidosis as would be expected with tuberculosis. However, sequential analysis revealed the amyloid to be immunoglobulin-related (Figure 6, amyloid 1). These workers were able to establish SAA-related amyloid in association with rheumatoid arthritis (Figure 5, amyloid 4) (Ein *et al.*, 1972).

At the other extreme, Husby *et al.* (1973) found SAA-related amyloid, based on amino acid analysis (see Table 2) and immunochemical techniques, in the liver of a case of Waldenström IgM κ macroglobulinaemia, where peri-collagen amyloidosis would be expected normally. It should be noted that, in spite of peri-collagen amyloidosis in other organs, peri-reticulin involvement of the liver and kidney has been noted in macroglobulinaemia (Heller *et al.*, 1964). Furthermore, these investigators did not describe the isolation of immunoglobulin-related subunits from cases of primary amyloidosis and amyloidosis associated with multiple myeloma and macroglobulinaemia, although Husby *et al.* (1973), like Glenner's group had used guanidine dissociation of water-soluble amyloid. Indeed, the subunit they isolated chromatographically in seven out of eight such cases was AA protein, albeit in lesser quantity and usually after alkali degradation of the fibrils.

Employing acid solubilization on peri-collagen amyloids, Pras and Reshef (1973) failed to obtain any subunits at all. This, however, could be due to a limitation of acid solubilization when applied to a chemically different amyloid.

6.3 Provocations

In predicting the heterogeneity of amyloid, variation as great as that between immunoglobulin light chain-related and SAA protein-related amyloid was not anticipated. It had been visualized that, in the systemic amyloidoses, a family of closely related proteins exists, possibly differing in some specific amino acid residues or in the lengths of their polypeptide chains. However, it appears likely that even wider heterogeneity occurs. In localized amyloidosis, endocrine tissues are favoured sites of deposition. Considering the possibility that the amyloid may be an altered form of the respective polypeptide hormones, several investigators prepared 'amyloid' fibrils *in vitro* from purified insulin, glucagon, calcitonin, and parathormone (Glenner *et al.*, 1974; Westermark, 1974; Kedar *et al.*, 1976). Although Westermark (1974) showed that amyloid isolated from the islets of Langerhans cross-reacted with anti-insulin antibodies, chemical studies of comparable sophistication to those applied in the systemic amyloidoses have not yet been carried out on fibrils isolated from any of the localized forms.

However, in the systemic amyloidoses the discrepancies are disconcerting because they are at variance with clinical correlations. Of their possible explanations, one is that both components are present in all amyloid fibrils, but in different proportions. Interestingly, each of the major components isolated has constituted approximately 50 per cent of the fibril dry weight; therefore, about half the fibril weight is unaccounted for. It is possible that important protein constituents may have been discarded while isolating the major one. Such proteins certainly have not been studied as intensively as the major ones. Peptide mapping of lesser components of fibrils isolated from peri-reticulin amyloidoses, whose major component is AA protein, displays many similarities to those of light chains (Franklin *et al.*, 1975). The discovery by Husby *et al.* (1973) of SAA-related component in peri-collagen amyloids, whose major component was not described, may hint at a lesser component. However, Franklin and Zucker-Franklin (1972) earlier had been unable to demonstrate a reaction with antisera against the DAM subunit prepared from amyloid fibrils of both peri-reticulin and peri-collagen sources to each of the four major immunoglobulins and their light chains. It is disconcerting to think that one of the major constituents could prove to be a contaminant. Only a wider experience will explain the discrepancies and permit the replacement of histological criteria of classification by the much hoped for biochemical ones.

While a vast body of information has accumulated regarding the immunoglobulins, very little is known about the origins and functions of AA and SAA proteins. It is conceivable that the AA component of the amyloid fibril is derived by proteolysis or dissociation of serum AA protein, as has been suggested by Levin *et al.* (1973) and by Rosenthal *et al.* (1976). There is also the possibility that both are derived from an as yet unknown, common source. They could be related to an incompletely defined, normally occurring tissue protein as readily as to one in the serum. Indeed, it was postulated earlier that amyloid fibrils could be formed because of an error in the synthesis in normal fibrous proteins (Gafni *et al.*, 1964). Indeed, Zucker-Franklin and Franklin (1970) demonstrated, using immuno-flourescence, that antibodies to alkali-degraded amyloid (DAM) stain a component in the blood vessels of normal tissues.

Exploration of this possibility by the simple techniques that have proved fruitful in the studies of amyloid has yielded some exciting observations. By a modification of the method used for the preparation of amyloid fibrils, a component has been isolated by water extraction of the saline-insoluble residue of homogenates of normal spleen, liver, and kidney (Pras and Glynn, 1973). The water-soluble component has marked affinity for silver dyes, and antibodies to this component, produced in rabbits, show typical reticulin staining using immunofluorescence (Pras *et al.*, 1974). This component is distinguished from collagen by its failure to be stained by collagen-specific dyes, by the absence of hydroxyproline and by a glycine content of only 9 per cent. In saline and in acid, the behaviour of this reticulin component of normal tissues resembles that of amyloid. It is precipitated from the water-dispersed state by addition of sodium chloride (0·15 M). Acid solubilization yields a pure, low molecular weight protein

Table 6 Amino acid compositions* of SAA-protein and acid-soluble subunit of reticulin component of normal connective tissue

	SAA-protein (Rosenthal *et al.*, 1976)	Reticulin subunit	
		49-yr old subject	80-yr old subject
Aspartic acid	11·7	9	9
Threonine	3·7	5	5
Serine	6·2	6	6
Glutamic acid	10·5	12	13
Proline	3·5	5	4
Glycine	8·5	9	9
Alanine	13·2	8	8
Cysteine	1·8	2	2
Valine	3·4	5	4
Methionine	1·8	1	1
Isoleucine	1·6	3	4
Leucine	6·6	7	8
Tyrosine	2·7	3	3
Phenylalanine	5·6	3	3
Lysine	7·2	7	8
Histidine	4·0	4	4
Arginine	8·6	11	9

* Expressed as residues per 100 residues.

subunit which has a sedimentation coefficient of 1·4 S and a fibrillar structure when examined by electron microscopy (Sheinberg, 1976; Sheinberg and Pras, unpublished results). Its amino acid content bears closer resemblance to that of SAA than AA protein (Table 6). These similarities suggest that the AA protein and the acid-soluble fraction of the reticulin component of normal tissues may be related constitutionally. The more conclusive evidence that could be provided by immunochemical techniques is as yet incomplete and sequential studies have been thwarted by the unreactive N-terminal of the reticulin subunit.

ACKNOWLEDGEMENT

Research in the Author's laboratory cited here was supported by a grant from the United States–Israel Binational Science Foundation, Jerusalem, Israel.

ADDENDUM

The constancy of the N-terminal portion of the SAA-related amyloid subunit, in contrast to the C-terminus, is reinforced by Sletten *et al.* (1976*a*) who report another abbreviated AA protein constituting 45 per cent of fibrils obtained from a case of ankylosing spondylitis. It contained only 64 residues. Except for asparagine replacing aspartate at position 60, its N-terminal sequence was identical to the 76-residue AA protein they had sequenced earlier (Table 5, Number 2).

Westermark *et al.* (1976) demonstrated immunologically the coexistence of AA protein as the major component and a $V_\lambda 4$ region of light chain as a minor component in amyloid fibrils obtained from two cases of rheumatoid arthritis. In a case of primary amyloidosis, they found a mixture of homogenous λ 4 and λ 5 fragments.

The ubiquity of SAA-related amyloidosis in the animal kingdom has been augmented by sequence studies of amyloid fibrils, derived from mice (Eriksen *et al.*, 1976). Immunoglobulin-related amyloidosis has not yet been found other than in man.

In the localized amyloidosis of thyroid medullary carcinoma, Sletten *et al.* (1976*b*) established amino acid homology of amyloid fibril subunits with human calcitonin for 11 positions (9–19) sequenced. This additional evidence of chemical heterogeneity of amyloid strengthens the suggestion of Glenner that the staining and morphological features by which amyloid is identified reflect its β pleated sheet configuration and not its chemical composition.

REFERENCES

Anders, R. F., Natvig, J. B., Michaelsen, T. E., and Husby, G. (1975). *Scand. J. Immunol.*, **4**, 397.
Andrade, C. (1952). *Brain*, **75**, 408.

Benditt, E. P., and Eriksen, N. (1964). *Archs Pathol.*, **78**, 325.
Benditt, E. P., and Eriksen, N. (1966). *Proc. Nat. Acad. Sci., U.S.A.*, **55**, 308.

530

Benditt, E. P., and Eriksen, N. (1971). *Am. J. Pathol.*, **65**, 231.

Benditt, E. P., Eriksen, N., and Berglund, C. (1968). In *Amyloidosis* (Mandema, E., Ruinen, L., Scholten, J. H., and Cohen, A. S., eds.), Excerpta Medica, Amsterdam, p. 206.

Benditt, E. P., Eriksen, N., and Berglund, C. (1970). *Proc. Nat. Acad. Sci.*, *U.S.A.*, **66**, 1044.

Benditt, E. P., Eriksen, N., Hermodson, M. A., and Ericsson, L. H. (1971). *FEBS Letters*, **19**, 169.

Benditt, E. P., Lagunoff, D., Eriksen, E., and Iseri, O. A. (1962). *Archs Pathol.*, **74**, 323.

Benson, M. D., Skinner, M., Lian, J., and Cohen, A. S. (1975). *Arth. Rheumat.*, **18**, 315.

Bitter, T., and Muir, H. (1966). *J. Clin. Invest.*, **45**, 963.

Bladen, H. A., Nylen, M. U., and Glenner, G. G. (1966). *J. Ultrastruct. Res.*, **14**, 449.

Caesar, R. (1960). *Z. Zellforsch.*, **52**, 653.

Calkins, E., Cohen, A. S., and Gitlin, D. (1958). *Fed. Proc.*, **17**, 431.

Cathcart, E. S., and Cohen, A. S. (1966). *J. Immunol.*, **96**, 239.

Cathcart, E. S., Wollheim, F. A., and Cohen, A. S. (1967). *J. Immunol.*, **99**, 376.

Cohen, A. S. (1966a). *Lab. Invest.*, **15**, 66.

Cohen, A. S. (1966b). *Int. Rev. Exp. Pathol.*, **4**, 159.

Cohen, A. S. (1972). In *The Metabolic Basis of Inherited Disease* (Stanbury, J. B., Wyngaarden, J. B., and Fredrickson, D. S., eds.), 3rd edn., McGraw Hill Book Co., New York, p. 1273.

Cohen, A. S., and Calkins, E. (1959). *Nature (Lond.)*, **183**, 193.

Dalferes, E. R. (1968). *Proc. Soc. Exp. Biol. Med.*, **127**, 925.

Ein, D., Kimura, S., Terry, W. D., Magnotta, J., and Glenner, G. G. (1972). *J. Biol. Chem.*, **247**, 5653.

Emerson, E. E., Kikkawa, Y., and Gueft, B. (1966). *J. Cell Biol.*, **38**, 570.

Eriksen, N., Ericsson, L. H., Pearsall, L., Lagunoff, D., and Benditt, E. P. (1976). *Proc. Nat. Acad. Sci.*, *U.S.A.*, **73**, 964.

Eriksen, N., Fowler, H. S., and Ericsson, L. H. (1974). *Fed. Proc.*, **33**, 1563.

Franklin, E. C., and Pras, M. (1969). *J. Exp. Med.*, **130**, 797.

Franklin, E. C., Rosenthal, C. J., and Pras, M. (1975). In *Adv. Nephrol.*, **5**, 89.

Franklin, E. C., and Zucker-Franklin, D. (1972). *Adv. Immunol.*, **15**, 249.

Frederiksen, T., Gøtzshe, H., Harboe, N., Kiaer, A., and Mellemgaard, K. (1962). *Am. J. Med.*, **33**, 328.

Gafni, J., Sohar, E., and Heller, H. (1964). *Lancet*, *i*, 71.

Glenner, G. G., Eanes, E. D., Bladen, H. A., Linke, R. P., and Termine, J. D. (1974). *J. Histochem. Cytochem.*, **22**, 1141.

Glenner, G. G., Ein, D., Eanes, E. D., Bladen, H. A., Terry, W., and Page, D. (1971a). *Science, N.Y.*, **174**, 712.

Glenner, G. G., Ein, D., and Terry, W. D. (1972). *Am. J. Med.*, **52**, 141.

Glenner, G. G., Harada, M., Isersky, C., Cuatrecasas, P., Page, D., and Keiser, H. (1970a). *Biochem. Biophys. Res. Commun.*, **41**, 1013.

Glenner, G. G., Harbaugh, J., Ohms, J. I., Harada, M., and Cautrecasas, P. (1970b). *Biochim. Biophys. Res. Commun.*, **41**, 1287.

Glenner, G. G., Page, D., Isersky, C., Harada, M., Cuatrecasas, P., Eanes, E. D., DeLellis, R. A., Bladen, H. A., and Keiser, H. R. (1971b). *J. Histochem. Cytochem.*, **19**, 16.

Glenner, G. G., Terry, W., Harada, M., Isersky, C. and Page, D. (1971c). *Science, N. Y.*, **172**, 1150.

Harada, M., Isersky, C., Cuatrecasas, P., Page, D., Bladen, H. A., Eanes, E. D., Keiser, H. R., and Glenner, G. G. (1971). *J. Histochem. Cytochem.*, **19**, 1.

Hass, G., and Schulz, R. Z. (1940). *Archs Pathol.* **30**, 240.

Heller, H., Gafni, J., and Sohar, E. (1965). In *The Metabolic Basis of Inherited Diseases* (Stanbury, J. B., Wyngaarden, J. B., and Fredricksen, D. S., eds.), 2nd edn. McGraw-Hill Book Co., New York, p. 995.

Heller, H., Missmahl, H. P., Sohar, E., and Gafni, J. (1964). *J. Pathol. Bacteriol.*, **88**, 15.

Hermondson, M. A., Kuhn, R. W., Walsh, H., Neurath, H., Eriksen, N., and Benditt, E. P. (1972). *Biochemistry*, **11**, 2934.

Husby, G., Natvig, J. B., and Sletten, K. (1974) *J. Exp. Med.*, **139**, 773.

Husby, G., Sletten, K., Michaelsen, T., and Natvig, J. B. (1972). *Scand. J. Immunol.*, **1**, 393.

Husby, G., Sletten, K., Michaelsen, T. E., and Natvig, J. B. (1973). *Scand. J. Immunol.*, **2**, 395.

Isersky, C., Ein, D., Page, D. L., Harada, M., and Glenner, G. G. (1972). *J. Immunol.*, **108**, 486.

Kedar, I., Ravid, M., and Sohar, E. (1976). *Israel J. Med. Sci.*, **12**, 1137.

Kim, I. C., Franzblau, C., Shirahama, T., and Cohen, A. S. (1969). *Biochim. Biophys. Acta*, **181**, 465.

Kimura, S., Guyer, R., Terry, W. D., and Glenner, G. G. (1972). *J. Immunol.*, **109**, 891.

King, L. S. (1948). *Am. J. Pathol.*, **24**, 1095.

Kyle, R. A., and Bayrd, E. D. (1961). *Archs Int. Med.*, **107**, 344.

Lachmann, P. J., Müller-Eberhard, H. J., Kunkel, H. G., and Paronetto, F. (1962). *J. Exp. Med.*, **115**, 63.

Levin, M., Franklin, E. C., Frangione, B., and Pras, M. (1972). *J. Clin. Invest.*, **51**, 2773.

Levin, M., Pras, M., and Franklin, E. C. (1973). *J. Exp. Med.*, **138**, 373.

Linke, R. P., Sipe, J. D., Pollock, P. S., Ignaczak, T. F., and Glenner, G. G. (1975). *Proc. Nat. Acad. Sci., U.S.A.*, **72**, 1473.

Lubarsch, O. (1929). *Virchows Archs Pathol. Anat.*, **271**, 367.

Magnus-Levi, A. (1956). *J. M Sinai Hosp.*, *N.Y.*, **19**, 8.

Mellors, R. C., and Ortega, L. G. (1956). *Am. J. Pathol.*, **32**, 455.

Miller, H. I., Rotman, Y., Ben-Shaul, Y., and Ashkenazi, Y. (1968). *Israel J. Med. Sci.*, **4**, 982.

Milstein, C. (1966). *Biochem. J.*, **101**, 352.

Milstein, C. (1967). *Nature*, (*Lond.*), **216**, 330.

Missmahl, H. P. (1959). *Verh. dt. Ges. inn. Med.*, **65**, 439.

Missmahl, H. P., and Hartwig, M. (1953). *Virchows Arch. Pathol. Anat.*, **324**, 480.

Muckle, T. J. (1968). *Israel J. Med. Sci.*, **4**, 1020.

Muckle, T. J., and Wells, M. (1962). *Quart. J. Med.*, **31**, 235.

Muir, H., and Cohen, A. S. (1968). In *Amyloidosis* (Mandema, E., Ruinen, L., Scholten, J. H., and Cohen, A. S., eds.), Excerpta Medica, Amsterdam, p. 280.

Natvig, J. B., Husby, G., Sletten, K., Nordstog, K., Michaelsen, T. E., and Anders, R. F. (1975). *J. Immunol.*, **4**, 760.

Newcombe, D. S., and Cohen, A. S. (1964). *Biochim. Biophys. Acta*, **104**, 480.

Nordstoga, K. (1972). *Acta Path. microbiol. scand.*, **80**, 159.

Osserman, E. F. (1961). *Ann. Int. Med.*, **55**, 1033.

Osserman, E. F., Takatsuky, K., and Talal, N. (1964). *Semin. Hematol.*, **1**, 3.

Page, D. L., Isersky, C., Harada, M., and Glenner, G. G. (1972). *Res. Exp. Med.*, **159**, 75.

Paul, W. E., and Cohen, A. S. (1963). *Am. J. Pathol.*, **43**, 721.

Pick, A. I., and Osserman, E. F. (1968). In *Amyloidosis* (Mandema, E., Ruinen, L., Scholten, J. H., and Cohen, A. S., eds.), Excerpta Medica, Amsterdam, p. 100.

Pick, A. I., Schreibman, S., Lavie, G., and Fröhlichman, R. (1973). In *Protides of the Biological Fluids* (Peeters, H., ed.), Pergamon Press, New York and Oxford, p. 63.

Pras, M., and Glynn, E. L. (1973). *Brit. J. Exp. Pathol.* **54**, 449.

Pras, M., Johnson, G. D., Holborow, J., and Glynn, E. L. (1974). *Immunology*, **27**, 469.

Pras, M., Nevo, Z., Schubert, M., Rotman, J., and Matalon, R. (1971). *J. Histochem. Cytochem.*, **19**, 443.

Pras, M., and Reshef, T. (1972). *Biochim. Biophys. Acta*, **271**, 193.

Pras, M., and Reshef, T. (1973). In *Protides of the Biological Fluids* (Peeters, H., ed.), Pergamon Press, New York and Oxford, p. 103.

Pras, M., and Schubert, M. (1969). *J. Histochem. Cytochem.*, **17**, 258.

Pras, M., Schubert, M., Zucker-Franklin, D., Rimon, A., and Franklin, E. C. (1968). *J. Clin. Invest.*, **47**, 924.

Pras, M., Zucker-Franklin, D., Rimon, A., and Franklin, E. C. (1969). *J. Exp. Med.*, **130**, 777.

Reiman, H. A., Koucky, R. F., and Eklund, C. M. (1935). *Am. J. Pathol.*, **11**, 977.

Rokitansky, C. (1842). In *Handbuch der Pathologischen Anatomie*, Vol. 3, Braumuller and Seidel, Vienna, p. 311.

Rosenthal, C. J., Franklin, E. C., Frangione, B., and Greenspan, J. (1976). *J. Immunol.*, **116**, 1415.

Ruinen, L., Scholten, J. H., and Mandema, E. (1967). *Genetics Elements; Properties and Functions*, Symposium, 1966, p. 325.

Rukavina, J. G., Block, W. D., Jackson, C. E., Falls, H. F., Carey, J. H., and Curtis, A. C. (1956). *Medicine*, **35**, 239.

Schultz, R. F., Calkins, E., Milgrom, F., and Witebsky, E. (1966). *Am. J. Path.* **48**, 1.

Schultz, R. F., Kasukawa, R., Calkins, E., and Milgrom, F. (1968). In *Amyloidosis* (Mandema, E., *et al.*, eds.), Excerpta Medica, Amsterdam, p. 400.

Sheinberg, A. (1976). M. D. Thesis, Tel-Aviv. University, Israel.

Shirahama, T., Benson, M. D., Cohen, A. S., and Tanaka, A. (1973). *J. Immunol.*, **110**, 21.

Shirahama, T., and Cohen, A. S. (1967). *J. Cell Biol.*, **33**, 679.

Skinner, M., Benson, M. D., and Cohen, A. S. (1975). *J. Immunol.*, **114**, 1433.

Skinner, M., Benson, M. D., Cohen, A. S., Cathcart, E. J., and Lion, J. B. (1974). *Fed. Proc.*, **33**, 618.

Sletten, K., and Husby, G. (1974). *Eur. J. Biochem.*, **41**, 117.

Sletten, K., Husby, G., and Natvig, J. B. (1974). *Scand J. Immunol.*, **3**, 833.

Sletten, K., Husby, G., and Natvig, J. B. (1976a). *Biochem. Biophys. Res Commun.*, **69**, 19.

Sletten, K., Westermark, P., and Natvig, J. B. (1976b). *J. Exp. Med.*, **143**, 993.

Sohar, E., Gafni, J., Pras, M., and Heller, H. (1967a). *Am. J. Med.*, **43**, 227.

Sohar, E., Merker, H. J., Missmahl, H. P., Gafni, J. and Heller, H. (1967b). *J. Pathol. Bacteriol.*, **94**, 89.

Sorenson, G. D., Binington, H. B. (1964). *Fed. Proc.*, **23**, 550.

Spiro, D., (1959). *Am. J. Pathol.*, **35**, 47.

Symmers, W. C. (1956a). *J. Clin. Pathol.*, **9**, 187.

Symmers, W. C. (1956b). *J. Clin. Pathol.*, **9**, 212.

Teilum, G. (1968). In *Amyloidosis* (Mandema, E., Ruinen, L., Scholten, J. H. and Cohen, A. S. eds.), Excerpta Medica, Amsterdam, p. 37.

Terry, W. D., Page, D. L., Kimura, S., Takashi, I., Osserman, E. F., and Glenner, G. G. (1973). *J. Clin. Invest.*, **52**, 1276.

Vasquez, J. J., and Dixon, F. J. (1956). *J. Exp. Med.*, **104**, 727.

Vogt, A., and Kochem, H. G. (1960). *Z. ZellForsch. mikrosk. Anat.*, **52**, 640.

Westermark, P. (1974). *Histochemistry*, **38**, 27.
Westermark, P., Natvig, J. B., Anders, R. F., Sletten, K., and Husby, G. (1976). *Scand. J. Immunol.*, **5**, 31.
Wild, C. (1856). *Beitr. Pathol. Anat.*, **1**, 175.

Zucker-Franklin, D., and Franklin, E. C. (1970). *Am. J. Pathol.*, **59**, 23.
Zuckerberg, A., Gazith, J., Rimon, A., Reshef, T., and Gafni, J. (1972). *Eur. J. Biochem.*, **28**, 161.

CHAPTER 15

Immunological Aspects of Cell-Surface Chemistry

N. A. Staines

1 INTRODUCTION

A conspicuous feature of mammalian cells is the range of polymorphic histocompatibility antigens on their surface. While the normal physiological role of these antigens remains partly obscure—polymorphism may not be related to function directly—it is obvious that they both elicit transplantation reactions and are involved in the expression of immune responsiveness and all that this entails.

Chemical analysis of surface antigens might reveal structural and immunogenetic information, and identify methods of preparing antigens which could be used to manipulate the graft-rejection machinery. Neither hope has been realized yet to any great extent. In view of the recent explosion of interest in histocompatibility systems and their relationship to transplantation, the failure to identify a suitable soluble antigenic preparation for the generation of effective donor-specific immunosuppression (DSI) is disappointing. All attempts to induce permanent DSI in adults, without the intervention of non-specific suppressive agents, have failed.

It is known that the immunogenic properties of antigens are altered drastically when they are removed from the cell. What was not suspected widely until recently is that at least two categories of antigens are involved in transplant rejection and that those most readily detected serologically may be less important in the generation of DSI.

2 GENETICS OF HISTOCOMPATIBILITY SYSTEMS

In every mammalian species so far studied, the rapid rejection of transplants depends very heavily upon incompatibility coded by a highly polymorphic major histocompatibility complex (MHC). The genetic and functional homology between, for example, H-2 in mouse, HLA in man*, and Ag-B in rat, is a strong cohesive force in studies on transplantation immunology. It should be stressed, however, that turning the homology into a generality could obscure real phylogenetic and tissue-specific differences. Many minor histocompatibility (H) systems exist, but individually they have little effect upon rejection in the face of an MHC difference although, in the absence of MHC differences, minor systems can cumulatively generate vigorous graft rejection.

The H-2 system is the main source of information on the genetics of MHC systems. The way this knowledge has evolved in recent years is well documented

---

* HLA nomenclature as proposed by WHO Nomenclature Committee HLA-A = LA, SD1; HLA-B = 4, SD2; HLA-C = AJ, SD3; HLA-D = LD1.

in reviews by Snell and Stimpfling (1966), Klein snd Shreffler (1971), Demant (1973), Snell *et al.* (1973), Klein (1974, 1975), and Shreffler and David (1975). The important features of MHC genetics are outlined below, concentrating mainly upon H-2, as most chemical and biological studies have been carried out in mice.

Much information about the MHC has been derived from serological techniques. As the definition of antibody specificity, antigen specificity, and gene identity is a closed process, genetic information is only as precise as the last serological test. It seems inevitable in serology that almost any monospecific reagent becomes polyspecific with enough testing and therefore, what is seen now must be a very incomplete picture.

2.1 K and D Regions of the H-2 Complex

Classical H-2 antigens are products of two independently segregating regions, K and D, mapping about 0·5 cM apart on chromosome 17 (Klein and Shreffler, 1971). In man, the HLA-A and HLA-B series antigens are products of segregating regions of the HLA system separated by a similar map distance (Bodmer, 1972). The K,D antigens are highly polymorphic and each homozygous inbred strain will express several of the more than 40 specificities so far identified. Private specificities are rare in the sense that they are found in only one strain (and its derivatives). Other specificities are found in several unrelated strains and these are the public antigens. The private antigens are exclusive to either K or D region and within a region may be allelic. They are expressed in a codominant fashion in heterozygous (hybrid) cells (Cullen *et al.*, 1972), thus each heterozygote expresses two K and two D-region specificities which is analogous to the expression of two HLA-A and two HLA-B series antigens in man. (For review of HLA genetics and functions see Thorsby, 1974.)

It is presumed that public antigens are also expressed codominantly, although this has not been tested exhaustively. Some public H-2 specificities are not exclusively products of either the K or D region. That public H-2 specificities (1, 3, and 5, for example) may be coded by either or both regions led Shreffler *et al.* (1971) to propose that the two regions arose by gene duplication. Functional and chemical studies support this proposal. This is an important proposition because it may indicate why the MHC has such a profound effect upon transplant survival; it is an accumulation of loci which individually elicit weak histocompatibility reactions but which together combine or act synergistically.

2.2 I Immune Response Region of the H-2 Complex

An association between H-2 haplotype and immune responsiveness (Ir) was reported by McDevitt *et al.* (1972) to be a function of Ir genes mapping between the K and D regions. This led ultimately to the definition of an I region. In the hope of raising antibodies against Ir gene products, cross-immunizations between K,D-identical and Ir-different strains were performed. Antisera were raised between Ir-congenic strain combinations by a number of workers (David *et al.*, 1973, 1974; Hauptfeld *et al.*, 1973; David and Shreffler, 1974; Hämmerling *et al.*, 1974*a*). Most sera produced in this way are preferential B-cell reactors, although T-cell reactions are observed occasionally in cytotoxicity testing (Frelinger *et al.*, 1974). All serologically detectable products of the I region are referred to as Ir-associated (Ia) antigens. The I region has been subdivided so far into three regions which map from K in the sequence I-A, I-B, I-C. Most of the Ia specificities so far mapped are products of the I-A region (David and Shreffler, 1974; Shreffler *et al.*, 1974; Shreffler and David, 1975; Sachs *et al.*, 1975).

It is convenient when constructing models of the MHC to refer to separate regions. However, genetic information derived from the study of recombinant halotypes defines only relative gene positions (or mutational sites) on the chromosome, and the region boundaries are imposed artificially by the observer. Hence one should not be surprised to find either subdivision of regions—segregation of previously unseparated genes—or antigens mapping in a region where they appear anomalous in terms of structure or function.

2.3 G and S Regions of the H-2 Complex

The S region maps between I-C and D and controls the Ss (serum serological variant) and Slp (sex-linked protein) traits of a serum β-globulin. The Ss trait involves quantitative differences in serum levels of the β-globulin between strains and sexes, and Slp is an allotypic marker on the same molecule (see reviews by Shreffler and Passmore, 1971, and Shreffler and David, 1975). In addition, the S region controls serum complement levels (Démant *et al.*, 1973). There is no evidence that the region codes for cell-surface antigens or takes part in histocompatibility reactions, its function is therefore rather distinct from those of other H-2 regions.

The G region, which maps between S and D, was described recently by David *et al.* (1975). This region codes for an erythrocyte antigen absent from lymphoid cells. This is specificity H-2.7 defined by haemagglutination reactions. The typing reactions of haemagglutinating and lymphocytotoxic H-2.7 sera are anomalous but it appears that the erythrocyte antigen is a product of the G region, while the lymphocyte antigen is produced by the I region. No alternative alleles have been identified for H-2G.7, but one may draw an analogy between this locus and the HLA-C (SD3) locus in man which defines a third segregant series of serologically detected antigens (Svejgaard *et al.*, 1972; Pierres *et al.*, 1975).

Apart from the relocation of H-2.7 to another region (G), there are other H-2 specificities, which have been known for some time, that are not K or D products. Several H-2 specificities, defined by cytotoxic rather than haemagglutination techniques (for example 34 and 46), are really products of the I regions (Staines *et al.*, 1975*a*).

2.4 Mixed Lymphocyte Culture and Graft-*versus*-Host Reactions

The antigens that stimulate both in mixed lymphocyte culture reactions (MLR) and in graft-*versus*-host reactions also map in the MHC. Rychlikova *et al.*

(1970) first demonstrated that K end antigens are generally stronger stimulators in MLR than D end antigens. Subsequently, Widmer *et al.* (1973) and Meo *et al.* (1973) showed that the K-end activity is attributable to MLR-stimulating antigens which map in the I regions. Shreffler and David (1975) concluded that the I-A and I-B regions are predominantly responsible but that other regions also may code for MLR stimulating antigens active under the appropriate conditions. I-C region MLR-stimulating antigens are expressed on T cells, while those of other I regions appear to be represented on both T and B cells (Lonai and McDevitt, 1974).

A sequel to cell stimulation in MLR is the production of killer cells which are detectable by techniques for cell-mediated lympholysis. The important feature of this reaction is that the cell-mediated lympholysis-target antigens are not the same as the MLR-stimulating antigens in either mouse (Bach *et al.*, 1973) or man (Eijsvoogel *et al.*, 1972). The antigens of cell-mediated lympholysis are largely, although probably not exclusively, products of the K and D regions in mouse. Anti-K,D sera block the lympholysis (Nabholz *et al.*, 1974), whereas anti-Ia sera block MLR (Meo *et al.*, 1975; Fish *et al.*, 1976). Production of killer cells occurs only in combinations with both I and K,D-region differences (Schendel and Bach, 1974), indicating that killer-cell production involves stimulation by two types of antigen and co-operation between cells.

This account is much simplified and the article by Shreffler and David (1975), in addition to those cited above, gives a more detailed analysis. The mixed lymphocyte–lympholysis system is important in order to understand experiments on the biological activity of soluble antigens, although it is an *in vitro* system and similar functional differences between antigens may not occur *in vivo*. Recent evidence shows that private, not public, antigens are the targets in cell-mediated lympholysis (Forman and Möller, 1975), but public antigens can immunize for second set rejection *in vivo* (Klein and Murphy, 1973).

Antigens that stimulate strong graft-*versus*-host reactions are associated with the I regions of the MHC and, as in MLR, weak stimulatory activity is associated with K and D regions (Klein and Park, 1973; Livnat *et al.*, 1973). The analysis of graft-*versus*-host reactions at the cellular level has never been pursued extensively, but the large host proliferative component in some systems (Fox, 1962) and the reaction of F_1 to inactivated parental cells in mixed lymphocyte reaction (Gebhardt *et al.*, 1974) indicate that the situation is highly complex and involves unidentified genetic factors.

The I regions of the H-2 complex code for several different activities; whether or not these are functions of single gene products is uncertain. In man (Van Rood *et al.*, 1975a) and the rhesus monkey (Balner, personal communication), there are MHC antigens expressed by B rather than T cells. These are Ia analogues, but unlike the mouse, they are products of several loci which appear to be distinct from MLR-stimulating and Ir loci. The fact that murine Ia sera inhibit some I region functions may indicate only that the sera contain cryptic components. Alternatively, the homology between rodents and primates may break down at this point.

The compartmentalization of different activities into particular gene regions may be aesthetically satisfying but it can be misleading. The functional differences between antigens of different regions are not absolute. It is likely that individual antigens are multifunctional, in the sense that on their own they may elicit one type of reaction, but in the presence of other incompatibilities may elicit another. There are alternative pathways of sensitization, and the net result of the interaction between different antigens is the measured immune response.

2.5 Minor Histocompatibility Loci

In the mouse, there is a large number of H loci outside the MHC (identified H-1, H-3, and so on), and certainly enough for at least one to be present on each chromosome including X and Y (Klein, 1975). Alleles of these H loci are identified by grafting rather than by serological methods—many do not appear to induce antibodies. Individually some induce an insidious rejection often only after suitable preimmunization. One of their features is that there is frequently a disequilibrium of rejection between congenic partners. Thus, in one direction, rejection is achieved rapidly but in the reverse case rejection either does not occur at all or takes place slowly over several months (Graff et al., 1966), accompanied by reversible rejection crises. Generally, Ea antigenic differences do not lead to graft rejection, but there is, for example, an H locus (H-Ea-2) closely linked to, but distinct from, the Ea-2 locus (Flaherty and Bennett, 1973a).

Of the numerous erythrocyte antigen systems in man only the ABO system clearly has any effects upon skin (Dausset and Rapaport, 1966) and kidney-graft survival (Joysey et al., 1973). The presence of other minor H loci in man is inferred from the rejection of transplants by ABO-matched HLA-identical siblings but none are defined clearly.

2.6 Tissue-Specific Histocompatibility Antigen Systems

The products of minor H loci (non-H-2) have a wide distribution in different tissues. Tissue-specific differentiation antigens are, by definition, not distributed widely, but may play a little appreciated role in transplantation. Skin-specific antigens (Sk-1) have been described in the mouse by Scheid and coworkers (1972), but there is no clear evidence for the existence of tissue-specific transplantation antigens, although, for example, in the case of the kidney, heart or liver, such antigens could be invoked to account for the variation in acceptance of different tissue transplants. Thy-1 antigens can be detected upon epidermal cells but TL and Ly antigens cannot (Scheid et al., 1972). Mice congenic for these antigen systems reject skin grafts (Flaherty and Bennett, 1973a,b), but second-set grafts exchanged between them are not always rejected (John et al., 1972; Flaherty and Bennett, 1973a,b; Staines and O'Neill, 1975), probably due to the production of enhancing antibody.

Skin-graft rejection due to TL and Ly differences is a function not of the serologically recognized markers but of closely linked H loci (H(Tla) and H(Ly), respectively) (Flaherty and Bennett, 1973a). There may be an inverse relationship between graft rejection and antibody production in these cases. Whether or not the serological and transplantation antigens act in concert to effect rejection is not known.

Thy-1 differences also provoke skin-graft rejection but in this case genes controlling serological markers and transplantation antigens have not been separated, although it is possible that they could be because antibody production and graft rejection are not always associated (John et al., 1972; Staines and O'Neill, 1975). The author has observed that whereas A strain mice readily reject grafts from their Thy-1 congenic partner (A/Thy1.1) the reverse is not true. Thus, it has been postulated that the inability of A/Thy-1.1 mice to reject Thy-1.2-carrying tissues is due to a deletion of an Ir gene (in the germ line of the A strain mouse) following its long association with the Thy-1.2 antigen (Staines and O'Neill, 1975). The generality of such a model is not proved, but it is supported by the disequilibrium of rejection in other minor H loci systems and by the observations that MHC recombinant I-region congenic strains will not produce antibody against I-A products if the I-C region of the recipient has the same haplotype of origin as the I-A region of the donor (David, personal communication).

3 MEASUREMENT OF ANTIGENIC ACTIVITY

Many serological assays are available to measure alloantigenic activity (for review see Klein, 1975). Unfortunately, alloantibodies and soluble antigenic preparations do not precipitate directly; as a result, the most widely used assay systems employ a target cell of some type.

The original definition of H-2 by Gorer (1936) depended upon haemagglutination reactions but because human erythrocytes do not carry HLA antigens their detection involved platelet (Dausset et al., 1960) and leucocyte agglutination (Van Rood and Van Leeuwen, 1963). The evolution of mouse and human histocompatibility testing has followed different paths but it is obvious that some serological techniques are appropriate for all species. It has been assumed that antigens (H-2, HLA) detected by conventional serology are involved in transplant rejection. This assumption has obscured the fact that there are other important antigenic systems (such as Ia), which are not so easily detectable by conventional serology.

Purification of soluble antigens starts from highly heterogeneous materials and as MHC antigens have no marked characteristics their isolation depends upon serological methods. Alloantisera are active in a number of test systems and most, if not all, can be inhibited by soluble antigens. Most inhibition tests involve either a two-stage procedure or a competitive inhibition system, usually under antibody-limiting conditions.

3.1 Haemagglutination Assays

For the mouse, dextran and normal human serum (Gorer and Mikulska, 1954) or some other high molecular weight 'developer' must be added (Stimpfling, 1961) before alloantibodies can agglutinate erythrocytes. Tests are performed in tubes or trays. Another technique described by Severson (Severson and Thompson, 1968; Severson *et al.*, 1974) measures the rate of break up of an agglutinated cell pellet in an inverted microcapillary tube. This approach is claimed to be highly sensitive but, surprisingly, has not been used to assay soluble antigens.

3.2 Lymphocytotoxicity Assays

Complement-dependent assays employ the uptake of supravital (Gorer and O'Gorman, 1956) or fluorochromatic (Bodmer *et al.*, 1967) dyes or the release of ^{51}Cr from radiolabelled cells (Sanderson, 1965; Wigzell, 1965) as criteria for cell death. The general technique is suitable for lymphoid cells of any species—although cell numbers and complement source will vary—and for epidermal cells (Cooper and Lance, 1971), macrophages (Archer and Davies, 1974), and some tumour cells. The release of ^{51}Cr has been adapted for HLA typing as a microcytotoxicity test (Welsh and Cresswell, 1971), which normally depends upon supravital staining. Current practice in human tissue typing is reviewed by Ray *et al.* (1974).

Whereas haemagglutination reactions detect only antigens that are products of the K,G,D regions of the H-2 complex, and certain other non-MHC antigens (Ea) in the mouse and their homologues in other species, cytotoxicity testing can detect, as far as can be seen, any antigen present on the cell surface. With the ^{51}Cr-test system, cytotoxic negative absorption positive phenomena (CYNAP) frequently arise and therefore the distribution of antigens is best defined by absorption rather than by direct testing. The amount of radiolabel released is proportional to the number of cells killed in the target population. Therefore, a depressed release of radiolabel argues for the representation of the antigen on a subset of the cells in the target population. Activity of antigen preparations is measured by reacting doubling dilutions of the test material with limiting amounts of antibody.

3.3 Direct Precipitation

Alloantisera do not precipitate soluble MHC antigens, perhaps because the molecules are monovalent. On the other hand, xenoantisera will precipitate soluble antigens and can be used in this way (and by cytotoxicity inhibition) to monitor chromatographic purification, presumably because the sera recognize allotype and xenotype determinants on the same molecule (see Section 5.2).

3.4 Indirect Precipitation and Radioimmunoassay

Indirect precipitation of alloantibody–antigen complexes is possible using anti-immunoglobulin reagents. Such approaches are very sensitive and are able to detect small amounts of soluble antigenic material and have been used to precipitate antigens either labelled in culture with radioactive sugars or amino acids (Nathenson *et al.*, 1972; Creswell *et al.*, 1973), or radioiodinated *in vitro* (Tanigaki *et al.*, 1973). In these cases, it is necessary to remove all normal serum components from the antigen preparations before adding alloantiserum and the developing anti-immunoglobulin reagent. A disadvantage of such techniques is that biologically active material cannot be recovered from the precipitates. Other radioimmunoassay techniques have been described by Lucas (1970) and by Foschi and Manson (1970).

4 CHEMICAL AND PHYSICAL PROPERTIES OF HISTOCOMPATIBILITY ANTIGENS

4.1 Distribution

H-2 and HLA antigens appear in all adult tissues. I-region antigens appear to have a more restricted distribution (Hämmerling *et al.*, 1974*b*) than K,D specificities, being absent from erythrocytes, platelets, and liver parenchyma. They are easily detectable by direct cytotoxic reaction on B cells and by other techniques on T cells. Little is known about the quantitative differences in expression of MHC antigens on different tissues and cells. When antigens are reported absent from a particular cell the sensitivity of the assay system used must be considered; very low levels may not be detected easily as in the case of HLA on erythrocytes. Non-MHC H antigens have a wide distribution while differentiation antigens are by definition more restricted.

H antigens are located on the cell-surface membrane. Whether they exist in large amounts in the free state or on the endoplasmic reticulum within the cell is doubtful (Haughton, 1966; Wilson and Amos, 1972; Wilson and Boyle, 1972). However, Albert and Davies (1973) reported the association of these antigens with the outer leaflet of the nuclear membrane.

H antigens are not structural proteins, rather they are inserted in and are free to move about the lipid membrane matrix as proposed by Singer and Nicholson (1972). That they are neither buried nor immobile in the membrane is indicated by the ease with which they are solubilized (see Section 4.2) and by antibody-induced redistribution, respectively. Capping experiments have shown that: (*i*) K and D antigens in the mouse, and A, B, and C antigens in man are on separate molecules (Bernoco *et al.*, 1972; Neauport-Sautes *et al.*, 1972; Pierres *et al.*, 1975); (*ii*) some public and private H-2D antigens are on separate molecules (Démant *et al.*, 1975); (*iii*) not all the β_2-microglobulin on the cell surface is associated with H antigens (Neauport-Sautes *et al.*, 1974); and (*iv*) Ia antigens are distinct from K,D products (Unanue *et al.*, 1974).

4.2. Solubilization of Cell-Membrane Antigens

Several techniques are available to solubilize membrane antigens. These involve the use of autolytic processes probably depending on endogenous enzymic activity in the starting microsomal material (Sanderson and Davies, 1963), proteolytic enzymes (papain, ficin, and trypsin), phospholipase A, chaotropic agents (for example, 3 M KCl)—which disturbs the ordered water structure of the membrane, sonication, organic solvents, cholate and deoxycholate, and non-ionic detergents (for example, Triton X-100, Triton X-114, and Brij 99).

The use of these techniques is reviewed by Nathenson (1970), Reisfeld and Kahan (1970), Mann and Fahey (1971), Davies (1974), and Davies and Hess (1975). The comparative benefits of the different methods will not be discussed here, but it is worth mentioning that most biological experiments have employed enzymically-derived products. Autolytic processes probably all involve endogenous cathepsin activity, and likewise the use of 3 M KCl, at least in part, involves stimulation of endogenous enzyme activity (Mann, 1972). Enzymic techniques have the disadvantage that they cleave only the exposed part of the antigen from the membrane, and this could have important consequences in biological experiments. Although solubilization of the 'native' molecules is probably achieved using non-ionic detergents the products can only be separated from the detergent under conditions which destroy antigenic activity (8 M urea or 6 M guanidine-hydrochloride). Such products are useless for biological experiments but are suitable for physicochemical analysis. Likewise, antibody-precipitated antigens can only be recovered by similarly harsh techniques.

Once made soluble, either from whole cells or membrane preparations, the purification of H-2 or HLA antigens can be achieved in a variety of ways (summarized in Figure 1), few of which produce homogeneous products. Purification may be followed serologically by the techniques outlined in Section 3. It is estimated that the MHC histocompatibility antigen comprises about $0 \cdot 1$–$0 \cdot 01$ per cent of the total membrane protein, hence a purification of 1000-fold or greater would be needed to obtain homogeneity (Sanderson and Welsh, 1974; Hess and Davies, 1974). For chemical analysis, this is critical and has been approached in several studies (see Davies and Hess, 1975). The problem may be eased by using cultured lymphoid cell lines which carry more than 10 times the amount of HLA protein found on normal cells (Strominger et al., 1974). In biological experiments, the use of homogeneous material is not possible because yields are so small. A minimal requirement is, however, that the material is not aggregated. Most workers accept as operationally soluble any products which resist sedimentation following centrifugation for one to two hours at 100 000 g or more. Such 'crude' soluble preparations contain much material excluded by, for example, Sephadex G-200 which is aggregated and therefore has intrinsic adjuvanticity different from more purified antigens. It seems desirable, therefore, to use H-2 antigens purified by gel filtration at least for biological experiments.

545

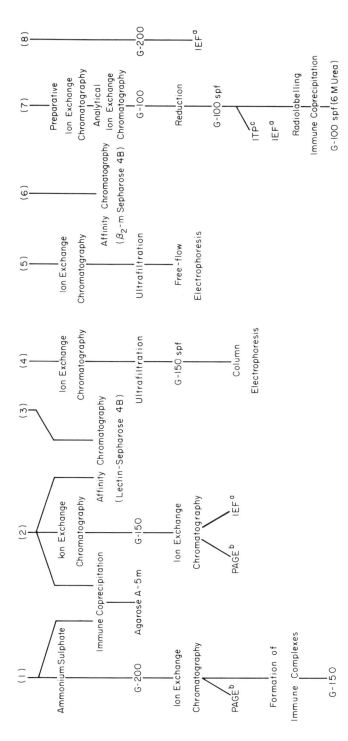

Figure 1 Techniques for the purification of soluble antigens. 1, Shimada and Nathenson (1969), Schwartz et al. (1971); 2, Springer et al. (1974); 3, Snary et al. (1974); 4, Tanigaki and Pressman (1974); 5, Koubek et al. (1973); 6, Cresswell and Dawson (1975); 7, Hess and Davies (1974), Hess and Smith (1974); 8, Bernier et al. (1974). [a]Isoelectric focusing; [b]Polyacrylamide gel electrophoresis; [c]Isotachophoresis

4.3 Chemical Properties of Soluble H-2 and HLA Antigens

Chemical analysis of H-2 and HLA antigens reveals a considerable homology and therefore information on both is presented together. More detailed information is available in reviews cited earlier; see also Mann and Nathenson (1969) and Davies (1970).

Estimates of molecular weight have varied considerably but there is now general agreement that detergent-solubilized H-2 and HLA molecules are composed of two non-covalently linked polypeptide chains with molecular weights of 44 000–45 000 and 11 000–12 000 (Cresswell *et al.*, 1973; Miyakawa *et al.*, 1973; Peterson *et al.*, 1974). Papain solubilization, or cleavage of detergent-solubilized products, releases a molecule containing chains with molecular weights of 34 000 and 12 000, thus leading to the conclusion that a portion of the heavy chain (up to 15 000 molecular weight) is inserted into the lipid membrane matrix (Schwartz *et al.*, 1973). The low molecular weight component is β_2-microglobulin, which is also found in the serum and urine as well as on cell surfaces not associated with H-2 or HLA antigens. Amino acid sequence data of β_2-microglobulin reveal homology with human IgG constant domains and homology between species. This component appears to carry no allotypic variants and to be free of carbohydrate.* These facts have led several authors to propose the existence of dimeric forms of the antigen on the cell surface and to propose a degree of homology between H-2 and IgG (Nathenson and Cullen, 1974; Strominger *et al.*, 1974). The existence in nature of dimeric forms, consisting of two heavy and two light chains, is not proved conclusively; cross-linking agents produce light–heavy combinations but never heavy–heavy pairings. However, detergent-solubilized (HLA) molecules may contain two extra sulphydryl groups absent from papain-solubilized molecules, thus heavy chains may be linked only in the region inserted into the membrane (Strominger, 1975). In the rat, Ag-B antigens of a single polypeptide chain of 30 000–34 000 molecular weight have been solubilized using 3 M KCl; a procedure which would be expected to cleave a portion of the molecule inserted into the membrane and to dissociate any non-covalently linked β_2-microglobulin (Callahan and DeWitt, 1975). This further supports interspecies homology between MHC products.

Preliminary amino acid sequence data from Silver and Hood (personal communication) on one K region and two D region antigens of different haplotypes reveal constant amino acid residues at three out of nine positions so far identified in the first 22 residues. Homology of K,D is as great as D,D homology so far. However, until extensive data are available the homology to IgG and the structure of MHC antigens cannot be established.

Studies of peptides show that genetic polymorphism in the H-2 system is mirrored at the structural level. Brown *et al.* (1974) compared the elution of D and K peptides (prepared by tryptic cleavage) on ion-exchange chromatography

---

* Individual authors are not quoted here, instead the reader is referred to *Transplantation Reviews*, 1974, **21** which contains articles from the major laboratories researching into this aspect.

and found only three out of 12 peptides behaved identically. Furthermore, in two-dimensional peptide mapping, Hess and coworkers (Davies and Hess, 1975; Hess, 1975), found that not all public H-2D.28 determinants were on the same molecule as the private H-2D.4 determinant.

H-2 and HLA antigens are glycoproteins and pronase digestion yields glyco-peptides with molecular weights of 4000–5000, representing 10–20 per cent of the intact molecule. H-2 and HLA contain about 3–6 per cent natural sugars, 2–5 per cent N-acetylglucosamine, and 1 per cent sialic acid. H-2 molecules also contain about 1 per cent N-acetylgalactosamine (Muramatsu and Nathenson, 1970; Sanderson et al., 1971; Nathenson and Cullen, 1974). These glycopeptides possess very little, if any, antigenic activity, and removal of the carbohydrate from intact molecules does not affect antigenicity. Therefore, H-2 and HLA specificities are determined by peptide and not by carbohydrate structure.

Slight differences in the molecular weights of D and K antigens in the mouse (Schwartz et al., 1973), and A and B antigens in man (Snary et al., 1974) have been found. Also, different specificities of both H-2 and HLA antigens are separable by ion-exchange chromatography, electrophoresis, and isoelectric focusing, indicating overall charge differences (Davies, 1969; Mann et al., 1969; Shimada and Nathenson, 1969; Thieme et al., 1974) which may, however, be a function partly of sialic acid residues rather than heterogeneity in the peptide chains (Parham et al., 1974).

It is of considerable importance genetically (and for biological experimentation) to know whether public and private H-2 specificities reside on the same molecule. Separation of specificities by ion-exchange chromatography (Davies, 1969), peptide mapping, and capping data (Démant et al., 1975; Hess, 1975), and comparative serological reactions of public and private antisera (Staines and Archer, 1975) suggest that public and private specificities are not always found on the same molecules.

4.4 Chemical Properties of Soluble Ia Antigens

Ia antigens, like K and D antigens, can be solubilized by detergents and enzymes. They are glycoproteins, their antigenicity being determined by the polypeptide and not by the carbohydrate (Cullen et al., 1975). The molecular weights of NP-40 detergent-solubilized antigens are 25 000–35 000 in SDS gels (Cullen et al., 1974) and of Brij.98-solubilized antigens are about 35 000 (Hess, 1976; Hess and Davies, 1975). Controlled papain digestion produces molecules of about 26 000 molecular weight (Hess, 1975). As with H-2 antigens, enzymic solubilization cleaves a portion of the molecule (with a molecule weight of about 12 000), which is presumably inserted in the cell membrane. As Hess (1976) pointed out, the molecular weight of 26 000 corresponds closely to that of highly purified papain-solubilized H-2 molecules, and although there appears to be no association between Ia and β_2-microglobulin the molecular weight data emphasize the homology between H-2 and Ia antigens supporting the notion that the MHC arose by gene duplication. Some H-2 and Ia molecules thus are not readily separable by gel filtration but they do differ in overall charge and pI, which can be exploited in analytical procedures (see for example Hess and Davies, 1975).

The stability, measured as antigenicity, of Ia and K,D antigens appears to be different in the soluble state, the Ia being more resistant to heat or acid but less resistant to papain than the latter (Hess, 1975; Hess and Davies, 1975). Similarly, Ia^k antigens in the membrane retain antigenicity after heating at 56° for two hours (with 67 per cent of the activity remaining) and treatment in 7 M urea overnight (77 per cent activity remaining), but are unaffected by treatment at pH 3 overnight. These procedures totally destroy H-2 activity.

Ia antigens in strain 2 and 13 guinea-pigs comprise a single polypeptide chain of approximately 25 000 molecular weight (determined using sodium dodecyl sulphate polyacrylamide gel) which distinguishes them from the B alloantigen. The latter is a product of a linked focus, homologous with K,D in the mouse (Sato and DeWeck, 1972), and which consists of two non-covalently linked polypeptide components with molecular weights of 45 000 and 12 000 (Finkelman et al., 1975). It appears that strains 2 and 13 are incompatible for only Ia and not any K,D homologues.

Ia antisera also react with factors produced by T cells, for example with an antigen-specific factor which can arm B cells in T-deficient mice to respond to a T-dependent antigen (Taussig et al., 1975). Further chemical analysis of such factors, however, is required before it is possible to tell whether they are identical with Ia antigens on lymphocyte membranes.

5 BIOLOGICAL PROPERTIES OF SOLUBILIZED ANTIGENS

5.1 Relationship of Antigenicity and Immunogenicity

The potential use of soluble antigens as immunogens for raising defined antisera and as tolerogens for generating DSI was one of the main motives behind solubilizing and studying membrane components. Study of soluble antigens (mainly H-2) has revealed consistently that highly antigenic materials do not always produce the anticipated effects. The relationship of antigenicity to immunogenicity is not simple and has been discussed elsewhere (see for example Reisfeld and Kahan, 1970; Hilgert, 1974). Some factors of importance are outlined below.

5.1.1 Antigen Identity

Immunogenetic studies (see Section 2) reveal that two categories of antigens, H and I, are involved in graft rejection. Serological monitoring of purification (using H-2 antisera) selects H antigens. Thus, it appears that many preparations are deficient in I antigens.

5.1.2 Physicochemical Properties

Solubilization techniques are severe, and it is likely that membrane antigens are altered during solubilization—for example the molecular weight of H-2 antigens is related to the amount of papain used. If the polypeptide is disturbed by solubilization this could affect the precise structure of the epitopes. Serological inhibition assays do not measure binding affinity specifically so changes in epitope structure have not been assessed.

Sialic acid present in H antigens could have profound effects upon immunogenicity (Apffel and Peters, 1969, 1970), even though its presence or absence has no detectable influence upon antigenicity (Nathenson and Muramatsu, 1971; Shimada and Nathenson, 1971). The carbohydrate of soluble molecules may be unaltered but its influence on immunogenicity of soluble products may be different because of other changes.

5.1.3 Adjuvanticity

As a result of solubilization, the intrinsic adjuvanticity (Dresser, 1968) of membrane antigens is decreased. Membrane fragments are probably as immunogenic as whole cells. Soluble antigens are much less immunogenic, and this could be explained by the loss of repeating determinants and a lipid matrix which may possess extrinsic adjuvanticity for the protein antigens associated with it. Soluble protein antigens are tolerogenic if administered intravenously without any extrinsic adjuvant (see review by Dresser and Mitchison, 1968). This fact derives from classical experiments on tolerance to soluble proteins where a depression, but not a complete abrogation, of a humoral response was observed. Its relevance to cellular tolerance—which presumably is required for antigen-induced DSI—can only be guessed at, but the work of Parish (1971) clearly shows a mutually exclusive relationship between humoral and cellular immunogenicity for soluble antigens. Accordingly, a humoral tolerogen may be precisely the wrong molecule to induce cellular tolerance.

5.1.4 Carrier Determinants

The humoral response to H-2 antigens is T-cell dependent (Klein et al., 1974). In practical terms, I antigens may be carriers for H haptens. Precedents for cell-surface antigens acting as carriers or haptens under different conditions exist with chicken blood-group antigens, which are also transplantation antigens (McBride and Schierman, 1970). Soluble membrane antigen are deprived, therefore, of their carrier determinants, and this is borne out by the allogeneic and xenogeneic humoral responses to H-2 antigens (described below) where the latter is greater because of the presence of more recognized epitopes.

5.1.5 Antigen Handling In Vivo

This topic has not been investigated for soluble membrane antigens, but it is likely that they are processed differently from whole membranes or cells. Transplantation antigens normally exist in association with living cell membranes. In a soluble state, they may be processed as effete autochthonous material regardless of their allotypic markers because they display 'self' components normally obscured in the membrane. The clearance of erythrocytes could depend upon the appearance of effete cell antigens on ageing red cells (Rabinovitch, 1967). Measurement of antigen clearance from the circulation is very difficult. Antigenic activity in serum is obscured rapidly by the inhibitory effects of normal serum components and the fate of radioiodinated antigens has been difficult to follow because of the difficulty of labelling the antigens heavily enough without destroying their activity (Staines and Rowland, unpublished results).

5.1.6 Summary

Immunogenicity is thus a function of many variables. Purely practical problems of an adequate source of material and the stability of soluble antigens makes their analysis very difficult.

The following sections will review some of the biological experiments reported in recent years and will concentrate mainly upon the activity of soluble antigens, although reference will be made to insoluble or crude membrane preparations where appropriate. Soluble antigens are, in theory at least, the most suitable for clinical use because of their defined properties, and their freedom from contaminating extraneous antigenic material and adventitious agents.

5.2 Xenogeneic Antibody Response to Soluble Antigens

The immunogenicity of soluble antigen preparations is greater between than within species. This increased immunogenicity appears to be a function of the recognition of a greater number of antigenic determinants in xenoimmunization. Whether determinants not recognized in alloimmunization are strictly invariable within a species is not absolutely clear. In xenoimmunization, allotypes *are* recognized and a proportion of the response is also directed against species-specific antigens.

The xenogeneic recognition of allotypes was the basis upon which Gorer (1936) first identified the H-2 system. Although some workers failed subsequently to confirm this (for example Metzgar *et al.*, 1965; Batchelor and Sanderson, 1968; Batchelor, 1969; DeWitt, 1970), there is ample evidence that allotypes are recognized by xenoantisera. Identification of allotypic specificity in xenoantisera depends upon absorption of the serum with cells from another individual of the immunizing species. An inevitable consequence of absorption is the formation of antigen–antibody complexes which are anti-complementary in lymphocytotoxicity testing and therefore create problems in demonstrating allotypic specificity in absorbed xenoantisera. These problems often can be overcome by ultracentrifugation (Staines *et al.*, 1973), or by using a two-stage lymphocytotoxicity assay (Sachs *et al.*, 1971; Staines *et al.*, 1973, 1976). The xenogeneic recognition of allotypic specificity also can be inferred from the fact that some anti-lymphocyte sera have differential immunosuppressive effects in different strains *in vivo* (Brent *et al.*, 1967; Ogburn *et al.*, 1969; Shorter and Elveback, 1970) and that xenogeneic antisera can passively enhance tumour (Takasugi and Hildeman, 1971), skin (Staines and Guy, unpublished results), and heart or kidney allografts (Hutchinson, personal communication).

Greater genetic disparity between donor and recipient species tends to lead to less recognition of allotypes (Staines *et al.*, 1973; Chen *et al.*, 1974). However, the physical state of the immunizing antigen and its freedom from extraneous material also influence recognition of allotypes. The proportion of allotype-specific antibody appears to increase with solubilization and progressive purification of antigens (Sanderson and Welsh, 1973).

It is worth recalling that most antigenic preparations solubilized by techniques other than those involving detergents are probably the products of enzymic degradation (see Section 4.1). Enzymically solubilized H-2 or HLA antigens lack a lipophilic portion of the molecule, and subsequent processing under acid conditions may remove the lower molecular weight peptide chain associated with them. Such molecular changes could have important consequences for immunogenicity.

5.2.1 Recognition of Human Antigens

Viza (1972) reported that sera raised in rabbits against purified HLA antigens had some allospecificity. Einstein *et al.* (1971*a*,*b*) were also able to produce apparently specific HLA reagents in rabbits against extensively purified HLA antigen derived from human cultured lymphoblast cell lines. In these studies, the rabbits were immunized with papain-solubilized antigen in electrophoretic gel slices emulsified in Freund-type adjuvants, and the xenoantisera were absorbed with other cell lines of different HLA type. Sanderson and Welsh (1973) confirmed these results using purified papain-solubilized antigens to immunize rabbits and human spleen cells for absorption.

The proportion of allotypic HLA antibody produced was higher when similarly purified materials were used to immunize primates (Metzgar and Miller, 1972; Sanderson and Welsh, 1973). Responses of individual animals were variable and in the latter study were found to depend upon the absence of HLA serological reaction in cells of the recipient animals with alloantisera detecting the specificities of the immunizing antigen. Reactive animals did not produce allotypic or xenotypic antibodies. The amount of absorption required to reveal HLA specificity was considerably less with primate sera than with rabbit sera and in the extreme case some sera required no absorption whatsoever. Cross-reactions between human and primate antigens have been recorded many times. At the molecular level, solubilized rhesus monkey antigen can inhibit the reaction of rabbit anti-human lymphoblast serum with human target lymphocytes (Einstein *et al.*, 1971*a*).

5.2.2 Recognition of Mouse Antigens

McKenzie and Painter (1972) immunized rabbits with unpurified ammonium sulphate-precipitated H-2 antigens solubilized ultrasonically from L1210 leukaemia cells. After absorption with allogeneic lymphoid or tumour cells, the sera possessed strain specificity, and in some cases apparent monospecificity for public and private H-2 antigens with a suggestion that the response was stronger against K than against D-end determinants. This has been ascribed to the association of Ia with K rather than D-end specificities in the combinations used. Indeed, McKenzie and Painter (1972) did record a specific reaction against H-2K.34, which is now known to be an Ia antigen of the I-A region (Staines *et al.*, 1976).

Similar results have been obtained by immunizing rabbits with membrane preparations or papain-solubilized spleen or liver H-2 antigens partly purified by gel filtration and ion-exchange chromatography (Staines *et al.*, 1973; Staines, unpublished results). Relatively high proportions (25 per cent) of strain-specific (allotypic) antibodies were produced, and although the reactions of the absorbed sera against different haplotypes was proportional to the number of individual H-2 specificities reacting, there was no clear evidence for the precise recognition of individual specificities. By immunizing with intact lymphoid cells across a closer phylogenetic relationship, Sachs *et al.* (1971) found that rats produced antibodies with good specificity for individual H-2 antigens.

5.2.3 Recognition of Non-MHC Antigens

The immunogenicity of truly soluble rat antigens in xenoimmunization has not been examined. However, two studies have been reported using high molecular weight aggregated solubilized antigens. Neither Gozzo and Rule (1972) using autolytically derived material nor Eshhar (1973) using partially desubstituted citraconylated preparations to immunize rabbits found any evidence for Ag-B specificity. However, in the latter, specificity for thymocyte antigens (in rats and mice) and, in the former, some strain specificity for lymphocyte antigens was found. Sauser *et al.* (1974) raised sera in rabbits against SDS-solubilized mouse antigens (molecular weight 35 000–40 000) which were specific for T cells. Using these antisera and anti-Thy-1 sera, reciprocal blocking on lymphocyte membranes occurred. These results show that non-MHC allotypes retain immunogenicity after solubilization and are recognizable in xenoimmunization.

5.2.4 Allotypic and Xenotypic Specificity in Xenoantisera

A large proportion of the antibodies in xenoantisera appears to have no allotypic specificity. In sera raised against cells, membranes, or purified H-2 or HLA substances, these antibodies are directed against determinants (species-specific xenotypes) on the MHC antigen molecules. Evidence for this has been found in studies on: (*i*) reactions of solubilized, chromatographically fractionated membrane antigens with xenoantisera (Einstein *et al.*, 1971*a*; Staines *et al.*, 1973); (*ii*) competitive binding of soluble H-2 antigens by allo and xenoantibodies (Staines and Davies, 1973; Staines, 1974); (*iii*) Cytotoxicity inhibition (reciprocal) of allo and xenoantisera with F(ab')$_2$ fragments (Chard, 1968; Batchelor, 1969; Staines and Davies, 1973); and (*iv*) competitive absorption of rat Ag-B and non-Ag-B allo and xenoantibodies by cells (DeWitt *et al.*, 1971).

These observations show that most of the anti-species antibody in xenoantisera is directed against molecules carrying MHC allotypes. The molecular relationship of the recognized allotypes and xenotypes has been studied extensively by Pressman and his colleagues (reviewed by Tanigaki and Pressman, 1974). They found that papain-solubilized HLA molecules (molecular weight 48 000) can be acid dissociated into a 33 000 molecular weight fragment carrying HLA (and primate cross-reacting) allotypes and an 11 000 molecular weight fragment (β_2-microglobulin) devoid of allotypic determinants. The bulk of the species activity of the whole molecule is carried by the 11 000 molecular weight fragment. Immunization with the higher molecular weight fragment reveals common species antigens that are absent from the smaller fragment and not easily detectable upon the undegraded whole molecule, and that are probably the result of conformational change during dissociation.

Therefore, rabbits, at least, recognize three types of determinant on MHC gene products—the allotype, a xenotype on the small β_2-microglobulin fragment, and a xenotype on the allotype-carrying (large) fragment. The high xenoimmunogenicity of MHC antigens may result from the xenotypes acting as carrier determinants for the allotypes.

It is remarkable that MHC antigens are immunodominant in xenoimmunization. Non-MHC antigens may not induce antibody formation easily when presented on whole cells. However, when papain-solubilized membrane proteins are fractionated by ion-exchange chromatography on DEAE–A50, the individual fractions (which do not all have H-2 activity) induce high titre sera in rabbits. A range of sera produced in this way was found to react with molecules that can be separated chromatographically from H-2, although the specificity of the antisera was not determined (Staines, 1974). These results are consistent with the interpretation that H-2 molecules operate as haptens and non-H-2 molecules act as carriers on the intact membrane, but in the free state, both classes of molecules have functional hapten and carrier determinants. Why some determinants convert from carriers to haptens is not known.

The polypeptide portion of the H-2 molecule determines allotypic specificity, and it may be assumed that this is also true of the allotype and the β_2-microglobulin-associated xenotype recognized in xenoimmunization. However, xenoantigenic activity tends to be more stable than alloantigenic activity. For example, heating at 83° for 30 minutes destroys all H-2 activity but leaves up to 43 per cent xenoantigenic activity intact in the same preparations (Staines and Davies, 1973). Xenoantigenic activity in C3H and BALB/c mice spleen membrane preparations is also more resistant to treatment with acid (pH 5) or urea (5–8 M at neutral pH) overnight (Staines, unpublished observations). Some xenotypes may be determined, therefore, by a carbohydrate/glycopeptide configuration.

5.3 Allogeneic Antibody Response to Soluble Antigens

The allogeneic humoral response to soluble antigens is very weak. Crude soluble antigens, which inevitably contain aggregated material, may be weakly immunogenic on their own but are usually less effective than whole cells or cell membranes at eliciting antibodies. Purified soluble antigen preparations free of aggregates do not generally induce antibody formation on their own.

Nathenson and Davies (1966a) found that autolytically derived H-2 antigens partly purified on DEAE–A50 induced cytotoxic antibody in allogeneic mice (C3H → BALB/c) when injected subcutaneously alone or intraperitoneally in Freund's complete adjuvant. Similar findings were reported subsequently by Vladimirskii and Govallo (1970). This type of preparation, however, contains aggregated material. The ability of purified H-2 antigens to induce cytotoxic antibodies in allogeneic mice has been examined further (Staines, unpublished results), H-2 antigens were prepared by autolysis (Nathenson and Davies, 1966a,b) or papain solubilization (Shimada and Nathenson, 1969), and were recovered from the included volume of G-200 Sephadex. Some antigens were also subjected to prior ion-exchange chromatography on DEAE–A50. These preparations contain only very small amounts of spontaneously aggregated material as judged by exclusion from G-200.

Repeated intraperitoneal or subcutaneous injection of purified H-2 antigens (50–500 μg/dose) did not induce antibody formation (cytotoxins or haemagglutinins). Incorporation of the antigen in Freund's complete adjuvant or the concurrent administration of *Bordetella pertussis* (10^9 cells) was, in the majority of cases, an effective adjuvant treatment and induced the formation of H-2 and non-H-2 cytotoxic antibodies. This technique would also prime mice to produce higher titres of H-2 antibody upon challenge with spleen cells. On the assumption that aggregated material could be immunogenic, antigen was precipitated by treatment with either ethylchloroformate or glutaraldehyde. Repeated weekly injections of the aggregated materials with *B. pertussis* for nine weeks did not induce antibody formation, although the non-aggregated material did under these conditions.

Although aggregation of antigen decreased its immunogenicity (and antigenicity), material coupled by toluene diisocyanate to bovine serum albumin had increased immunogenicity upon repeated injection in Freund's complete adjuvant. Similarly, H-2 antigen substituted (probably on serine and threonine residues) with 2-phenyl-4-ethoxymethylene-5-oxazolone (at a molar ratio of 1:10) was more immunogenic in Freund's complete adjuvant.

In all these experiments, effective antigen dosage was in excess of 100 μg purified material per injection, and when tested, haemagglutinin formation paralleled cytotoxin formation. Cytotoxic antibody titres were never high (less than 256) and frequently did not induce a maximal release of radiolabel from target lymphocytes even upon two-stage testing. Much of the antibody may be directed, therefore, against Ia antigens, which, when solubilized by hypertonic KCl can induce cytotoxic antibodies in allogeneic mice (Götze et al., 1973). The antigenic preparations used by the author would be expected to contain Ia activity, although this was not investigated.

H-2 antigens solubilized from L1210 (H-2^d) leukaemia cells can in crude form, which contains aggregates, induce the production of H-2 cytotoxic and haemagglutinating antibody in allogeneic mice. The response was found to be dose-dependant and was improved by the use of Freund's complete adjuvant in C57BL/10 (Ranney *et al.*, 1973) and B10.BR mice (Götze and Reisfeld, 1974). In B10.A mice the response is only seen when poly A:U is used as an adjuvant (Götze and Reisfeld, 1974). CBA mice have been reported also to make Thy-1 antibodies against SDS-solubilized allogeneic thymus antigens (Sauser *et al.*, 1974).

Humoral tolerance has never been demonstrated in adult mice in response to repeated injection with soluble histocompatibility antigens. However, in an elegant series of experiments in which papain-solubilized (Sephadex G-150 filtered) H-2 antigens were injected daily for four weeks in newborn mice, Law and colleagues (1972) found that the subsequent haemagglutinin, cytotoxin, and tumour-enhancing antibody responses to a skin allograft (placed at four weeks of age) were abrogated completely, although graft survival was not prolonged. The humoral tolerance was broken down only gradually by repeated injections of allogeneic spleen cells. The antigenic preparations presumably contained both K,D, and Ia activity, but the reasons why split tolerance was generated are not clear. If humoral tolerance involves K,D antigens, and cellular tolerance necessarily involves both types of antigens, then presumably the requirements for tolerance induction in the appropriate responder-cell populations are different.

5.4 Allograft Rejection and Cellular Immunity in Animals Treated with Soluble Antigens

Before it was known that classical low zone tolerance to foreign proteins was inducible by antibody–antigen mixtures (Diener and Feldman, 1970), it was assumed that enhancement and tolerance were distinct phenomena. The prospect of inducing low zone transplantation tolerance led many workers to solubilize cell-membrane antigens for this purpose. The technical problems involved are such that few have tackled the problem comprehensively, and permanent tolerance has never been demonstrated in adult animals. Treatment of adults with live cells or crude membrane preparations tends to induce hastened graft rejection upon subsequent transplantation. In situations where prolonged survival has been recorded, this may be accounted for by active enhancement.

5.4.1 Grafts of Normal Tissues

Many early reports demonstrated hastened graft rejection following immunization with (H-2) antigens solubilized by papain, autolysis, butanol, cholate, triton-X, or phospholipase A. Antigen administered four to five days before the graft was the most effective; adjuvant was generally required and the subcutaneous or intraperitoneal were superior to the intravenous route (see Wilson, 1966; Hutchin, 1968). Contrary to expectation, even repeated intravenous administration did not produce more than a transient delay in graft rejection generally (see for example, Manson and Palm, 1968; Graff and Kandutsch, 1969; Hilgert and Snell, 1969; Graff et al., 1970; Strober et al., 1970). Most of these studies did not employ extensively purified antigen. In many, the material was clearly aggregated or of very high molecular weight. However, the assumed importance of using aggregate-free material to generate donor-specific immunosuppression can be questioned following the results of Halle-Pannenko et al. (1971a, b). They found that a single intraperitoneal or subcutaneous injection of unpurified autosolubilized H-2 antigen (derived from BP8 tumour cells) could immunize C57BL/6 recipient mice for hastened rejection of C3H skin grafts. However, prolonged survival was seen following low or high doses of the antigen (less than 0·1 or greater than 8 mg, respectively), and the prolongation was improved if the dose was divided over several injections. Synergism between antigen and cyclophosphamide was also seen in delaying rejection. However, in no case was rejection delayed by more than a week and therefore genuine tolerance was not induced. Rather, the effect was quantitatively similar to that seen in passive enhancement in which case skin-graft survival is never permanent (McKenzie and Snell, 1973; Staines et al., 1975b).

Graff and Nathenson (1971) followed the immunogenic and antigenic properties of papain solubilized H-2 and non-H-2 antigens through successive states of purification using ammonium sulphate precipitation, G-150 and CM50. The most purified material tested retained immunogenicity, when administered in Freund's complete adjuvant. However, this did not increase in proportion to the antigenic activity suggesting either that the in vivo assay is not very sensitive or that an important active component is lost during purification.

Daily administration of papain-solubilized antigen (recovered from the included volume of G-150) to newborn mice for the first four weeks of life was not effective in producing tolerance to a skin graft, although humoral immunity was considerably suppressed (Law et al., 1972). Concomitantly, other cell-mediated functions were either unaffected (MLR and cell-mediated cytotoxicity) or even amplified (graft-versus-host reaction) by this treatment (Law et al., 1973). Repeated injection of adult animals with potassium chloride-solubilized H-2 antigens (unpurified) has been shown to prolong graft survival and concurrently to elevate antibody levels (Ranney et al., 1973). Using gel-filtered, papain-solubilized H-2 antigen administered daily for two months to adult animals, the author was unable to find any effect on subsequent skin-graft survival over extensive dose ranges of antigen arranged to give circulating H-2 levels of 10^{-13} to 10^{-8} M (Davies and Staines, unpublished results). In rats, papain-solubilized Ag-B antigen administered repeatedly following grafting had no effect on survival of heart allografts. However, permanent graft survival was found if the antigen is complexed (at equivalence) with enhancing antiserum, which on its own has only a small graft-protective effect (Marquet *et al.*, 1975). These studies are not directly comparable in detail but they do indicate that donor-specific immunosuppression in the adult animal may necessarily involve the production of enhancing antibody. Mice treated with allogeneic liver extracts, *B. pertussis*, and ALS retain skin grafts without showing impaired mixed lymphocyte culture, cell-mediated lympholysis or graft-*versus*-host reactivity. The unresponsive state appears to involve suppressor T cells, but even in this case, enhancing antibody may contribute to it and cannot be totally excluded (Kilshaw *et al.*, 1975).

The type of graft used also influences the response to soluble antigens. For example, foetal heart grafts transplanted in the ear pinna may show extended electrical activity whereas skin-graft survival is foreshortened in recipients treated with antigens solubilized with Tris or tris-2-hydroxy-3,5-diiodobenzoate (TIS). Heart survival is extended further by additional treatment with enhancing antibodies, again emphasizing the role of enhancement in the adult (Alspaugh and Davis, 1973).

5.4.2 Growth of Transplanted Tumours

Soluble antigen pretreatment also influences the growth of transplanted tumours. The development of tumour immunity can be seen clearly in mice and guinea-pigs treated with crude soluble antigen preparations (Oettgen *et al.*, 1968; Young and Gyenes, 1973; Pellis *et al.*, 1974). In other cases, tumour growth is favoured and this appears to be correlated with the production of enhancing antibody or serum-blocking factors rather than the development of classical tolerance (Ruszkiewicz, 1971; Rosenberg *et al.*, 1973). The mechanism of control of tumour growth in these situations is outside the scope of this article, but it is worth noting that immunization with potassium chloride-solubilized antigens may grossly suppress cell-mediated immunity (killer-cell activity measured *in vitro*) without influencing either tumour growth or antibody production in any significant way (Bonavida and Zighelboim, 1974). Thus this illustrates the danger of measuring only one parameter of immunity and then extrapolating to define the total immune status of a treated animal.

5.4.3. Graft-versus-Host Reactions

Cellular immunity as measured by graft-*versus*-host reaction can also be increased by immunizing mice with crude membraneous antigens (Marcus, 1969) or with potassium chloride-solubilized H-2 antigens (Götze and Reisfeld, 1974), which are administered once to the cell donors before transplantation. On the other hand, multiple immunization with potassium chloride (Ranney *et al.*, 1973) or autolytically solubilized antigens (Halle-Pannenko *et al.*, 1971*b*) suppresses the graft-*versus*-host reactivity of cells transferred into immature or irradiated adult recipients, respectively. In the latter case, evidence for high and low-dose suppressive effects can be seen which correspond to the donor specific immunosuppression of skin-graft rejection recorded by the same group (Halle-Pannenko *et al.*, 1971*a*).

5.4.4 Non-MHC Incompatibilities

The genetic disparity between donor and recipient profoundly influences the tolerogenic or immunogenic effects of soluble antigen. MHC-Compatible grafts generally are rejected less quickly than MHC-incompatible grafts. Non-H-2 antigen immunization has been recorded in many studies cited above and also has been studied in detail by Hilgert (1974). As far as donor-specific immunosuppression is concerned, this may appear readily in H-2-compatible combinations whereas similar treatment in H-2-incompatible combinations is ineffective (for example, see Judd and Trentin, 1973). From the clinical point of view, donor-specific immunosuppression for non-HLA loci may be relatively unimportant. The good survival of kidneys in HLA-identical siblings indicates that non-HLA incompatibilities are controlled easily by conventional immunosuppressive drug therapy.

5.4.5 Tissue Source of Antigen

Antigens used in these studies were derived from spleen, lymph nodes, thymus, and tumour cells. Liver-derived antigens frequently do not immunize, in fact, they may cause prolonged survival of grafts under certain conditions, and moreover, may destroy the immunizing effect of spleen-derived antigens when administered simultaneously (see for references Hilgert, 1974). In the extreme case in the pig, liver-derived antigens will promote indefinite survival of kidney allografts (Calne *et al.*, 1970). The basis of the peculiar behaviour of liver extracts is not clear, but it is possible that an enzyme present in liver can cleave H-2 molecules, thereby converting them to a more tolerogenic form (Nimelstein *et al.*, 1973).

5.5 Immunogeneicity of Soluble Antigens and MHC Genetics

Several conclusions can be drawn from the *in vivo* experiments described above. Antigens solubilized by a variety of agents retain antigenic and immunogenic properties of their cells of origin. They can induce humoral immunity (haemagglutinin, cytotoxin, and enhancing antibody production) and cellular immunity. The latter is measured by rejection of normal and neoplastic grafts, graft-*versus*-host reactions, mixed lymphocyte culture reactions, and cell-mediated immunity *in vitro*, and also by cell-transfer reactions (Kahan *et al.*, 1967) and delayed hypersensitivity-type skin testing (Oettgen *et al.*, 1968; Ranney *et al.*, 1973). Their immunogenicity is amplified greatly by adjuvants of various types, and subcutaneous administration is preferred. Some degree of so-called cellular tolerance can be induced following repeated intravenous injection, as measured by prolonged graft survival or suppression of graft-*versus*-host reactivity. The involvement of enhancing antibodies is strongly implicated in systems claimed to demonstrate tolerance. If antibody production is necessary for tolerance induction, this would explain the success of unpurified, soluble antigen preparations containing aggregated material; antibody production would be favoured. Indeed, repeated injection with insoluble membrane preparations slightly improves skin-graft survival in mice (Wheeler *et al.*, 1970).

The outcome of administering soluble antigens to graft recipients cannot be predicted. However, with new knowledge of MHC genetics the problems of inducing donor-specific immunosuppression with soluble antigens in adult animals could and should be re-evaluated.

In the mouse, I region antigenic differences are responsible for strong graft-*versus*-host (Klein and Park, 1973) and mixed lymphocyte culture reactivity (Bach *et al.*, 1972). In addition, such differences increase the intensity of graft rejection and humoral responses due to K,D region antigens (Klein, 1972; McKenzie and Snell, 1973).

As antibody (with specificity for the graft) is implicated in generating donor-specific immunosuppression by antigen treatment, an analysis of the mechanism of passive enhancement is pertinent (see reviews by Hutchin, 1968; Hellström and Hellström, 1970, Snell, 1970; Stuart, 1973; Winn, 1974). A considerable effort has been invested in trying to prove that enhancement is a function of a particular class or subclass of immunoglobulin but no success has been achieved (Fuller and Winn, 1973; Rubinstein *et al.*, 1974; Jansen *et al.*, 1975a, b). More important is the specificity of the antiserum; Ia antibodies are the most effective enhancing agents. Experiments in the author's laboratories clearly show that the removal of conventional Ag-B or H-2 antibody from enhancing antisera by absorption with erythrocytes or platelets does not impair the enhancing capacity of such sera for rat heart grafts (Davies and Alkins, 1974) or mouse skin grafts (Archer *et al.*, 1974; Staines *et al.*, 1974), respectively. The absorbed antisera retain residual cytotoxic antibody against Ia antigens on B cells (Staines *et al.*, 1975b, c, 1976). Conventional anti-H-2.K antibodies have at best a trivial graft-prolonging effect.

The mechanism of enhancement is not elucidated totally but the effect involves interference with some early recognition event, which by analogy with mixed lymphocyte culture inhibition by anti-stimulator cell Ia antibody (Meo *et al.*, 1975; Staines *et al.*, 1975b; Fish *et al.*, 1976) appears to prevent the sensitization of T cells to I-region antigens. In the normal course of events, recognition of I-region antigens leads to the subsequent recognition of, and killer-cell production against, K and D region (private) H-2 antigens (Bach *et al.*, 1973; Forman and Möller, 1974). Pretreatment with Ia-antigen preparations therefore should be effective at generating enhancing antibody to prolong graft survival. Indeed, prolonged survival of B10.D2 skin grafts on B10.A(4R) mice, which previously received a B10.A(2R) graft, has been demonstrated. In this system, the two donors share only Ia and not K,D antigen specificity, showing that Ia immunization promotes rather than shortens graft survival. In other systems, where the Ia preimmunizing donor (B10.M) differs from the recipient (B10.A) by K,D as well as Ia, then a subsequent graft (B10.D2) which shares only Ia with the primary donor but differs by Ia and K from the recipient is rejected rapidly, thus suggesting that not all Ia antigens have the same function *in vivo*.

Total coverage of the Ia antigens of the graft by enhancing serum is not necessary to generate donor-specific immunosuppression. On the contrary, sera with limited cross-reactivity promote significant graft prolongation (Fabre and Morris, 1974; Staines *et al.*, 1975*b*, *c*; Staines, 1975). One might expect, therefore, to generate donor-specific immunosuppression by antigen treatment with preparations that do not necessarily carry all the Ia specificities defined in a particular incompatibility.

There is considerable circumstantial evidence from clinical studies (Opelz *et al.*, 1973; Caves *et al.*, 1973; Murray *et al.*, 1974; Van Rood *et al.*, 1975*b*) which has been reviewed elsewhere (Staines and Davies, 1975; Davies and Staines, 1976), that pre-exposure to human I-region antigen analogues in the absence of conventional HLA antigens considerably favours the survival of skin, kidney, and heart transplants. These results are entirely consistent with rodent studies carried out by the author and offer some hope that donor-specific immunosuppression can be generated by active or passive immunization against Ia-type antigens. Exposure to H-2.K and D (or HLA) antigens leads to hastened rejection and also the production of graft-damaging antibodies. On the other hand, Ia antibodies do not cause antibody-mediated hyperacute rejection (Jansen *et al.*, 1975*b*).

Many of the antigen preparations used in *in vivo* experiments would have contained both K,D and Ia antigens, even following gel filtration and ion-exchange chromatography. The variable proportions of these antigens in the preparations could account for the inconsistency and unpredictability of experiments on donor-specific immunosuppression induction. It would, therefore, be profitable to separate K,D and Ia soluble antigens from each other and use them individually in attempts to induce such immunosuppression. Experiments of this kind have not been carried out, but Hilgert has reported (1974) that allogeneic liver extracts have differential immunogenic and tolerogenic effects in systems involving different combinations of K, I, and D incompatibilities. Liver extract may, however, not be the antigen of choice for such experiments since liver tissue does not carry Ia antigens (Davies, 1975).

5.6 Reactions between Cells and Solubilized Membrane Antigens *In Vitro*

The immunogenicity of soluble H-2 antigens, for example, *in vivo* is beyond doubt, but evidence that they are immunogenically active *in vitro* is hard to find. Viza *et al.* (1968) recorded stimulation by allogeneic HLA soluble antigen preparations of human lymphocytes in one-way mixed lymphocyte reaction-type cultures. The level of stimulation was high (10–20 per cent blast cell formation), but in subsequent studies on the stimulation of mouse cells by papain or potassium chloride-solubilized H-2 antigen preparations, the stimulation index never rose above 2·5 (Adler *et al.*, 1970; Ranney *et al.*, 1973). The possibility that the high stimulation first recorded reflects a secondary response in preimmunized humans is substantiated by subsequent findings that papain-solubilized H-2 antigens only effectively stimulate preimmunized allogeneic cells *in vitro* (Leventhal *et al.*, 1971). The failure of soluble antigens to stimulate a significant primary response *in vitro* (Gordon and Rode, 1975) may be due to the inability of dispersed antigens to redistribute receptors on the responder cell surface. Also the affinity of the soluble antigen for the surface receptor may be reduced by the solubilization process. These factors would explain the difficulty experienced by the author in attempts to inhibit target cell lysis specifically by sensitized killer cells, *in vitro* (Cerottini *et al.*, 1971) using soluble H-2 antigens. However, other reports (Bonavida, 1974; Gordon and Rode, 1975) show this can be demonstrated effectively.

The macrophage migration inhibition technique (George and Vaughan, 1962), which is supposed to reflect events involved in delayed hypersensitivity reactions, has been adapted to demonstrate allograft sensitivity. The migration of peritoneal exudate cells is inhibited by the presence of allogeneic cells of donor strain (Al-Askari *et al.*, 1965; Ferraresi *et al.*, 1970; Staines, 1970), or by tumour cells if the sensitized cells are from tumour-immunized animals (Kronman *et al.*, 1969). In similar systems, migration also can be inhibited by crude membraneous preparations (Haskova *et al.*, 1967; Falk *et al.*, 1970a, b; Steiner and Watne, 1970) and antigens solubilized from them (Bloom *et al.*, 1969; Halliday, 1971; Kyriazis *et al.*, 1971). The mechanism of inhibition by soluble antigens has not been elucidated in most cases, but Bloom *et al.* (1969) did find that sensitized lymphocytes incubated with specific autolytically solubilized sarcoma antigen produced the lymphokine macrophage migration inhibition factor. Similarly, the lymphocytes from six out of 14 human subjects suffering from glomerulonephritis, when incubated with a collagenase-solubilized glomerular basement membrane antigen preparation, also produced this factor (Rocklin *et al.*, 1970).

This type of culture system is sensitive to non-specific inhibitory factors, which may act directly upon the migrating macrophages. In most studies, a degree of non-specific inhibition was caused by irrelevant or third party antigens. In attempts to establish the specificity of migration inhibition of peritoneal cells from allografted mice with papain-solubilized H-2 antigens, it was found that syngeneic and allogeneic antigen preparations were inhibitory for normal and sensitized cells (Staines, 1970). Among many possibilities that could account for this, the most attractive is that there is some identity between the migration inhibition factor and the H-2 antigen preparations used which inhibit cell movement in purified macrophage cultures. The precedent for this lies in the reaction of antigen-specific T-lymphocyte factors with Ia antisera (Taussig *et al.*, 1975). Such factors, like lymphokines, are elaborated by sensitized T-lymphocytes when they are confronted by specific antigens *in vitro*. It clearly would be profitable to determine the relationship between cell-surface antigens and lymphokines.

One suspects from these *in vitro* experiments that solubilized antigens are able to bind non-specifically to cell membranes. Specificity has not always been clearly demonstrable. Evidence that skin tissue can incorporate and retain foreign

562

antigens in its fabric is found in experiments where autografts of mouse (Hellman and Duke, 1967) or human skin (Seigler *et al.*, 1970) are rejected as allografts after they have been incubated *in vitro* with allogeneic skin or solubilized HLA antigens respectively. Soluble H-2 antigen preparations non-specifically induce the formation of rosettes between lymphocytes or thymocytes and allogeneic or syngeneic erythrocytes (Micklem and Staines, unpublished results). Is it possible that cell-surface antigens are not always synthesized by the cells on which they are detected?

ACKNOWLEDGEMENTS

The author would like to express his gratitude to many colleagues who have collaborated in work quoted here. In particular to Keith Guy for his long-standing technical collaboration, and to D. Allen L. Davies and Maxime Hess for their discussion and advice. To those many other workers who have not been quoted here through lack of space apologies are expressed.

REFERENCES

Adler, W. H., Takiguchi, T., Marsh, B., and Smith, R. T. (1970). *J. Immunol.*, **105**, 984.

Al-Askari, S., David, J. R., Lawrence, H. S., and Thomas, L. (1965). *Nature (Lond.)*, **205**, 916.

Albert, W. H. W., and Davies, D. A. L. (1973). *Immunology*, **24**, 841.

Alspaugh, M. A., and Davis, W. C. (1973). *Transplantation*, **15**, 270.

Apffel, C. A., and Peters, J. H. (1969). *Prog. Exp. Tumour Res.*, **12**, 1.

Apffel, C. A., and Peters, J. H. (1970). *J. Theoret. Biol.*, **26**, 47.

Archer, J. R., and Davies, D. A. L. (1974). *J. Immunogenet.*, **1**, 113.

Archer, J. R., Smith, D. A., Davies, D. A. L., and Staines, N. A. (1974). *J. Immunogenet.*, **1**, 337.

Bach, F. H., Segall, M., Zier, K. S., Sondel, P. M., Alter, B. J., and Bach, M. L. (1973). *Science, N.Y.*, **180**, 403.

Bach, F. H., Widmer, M. B., Bach, M. L., and Klein, J. (1972). *J. Exp. Med.*, **136**, 1430.

Batchelor, J. R. (1969). *Transplantation*, **7**, 554.

Batchelor, J. R., and Sanderson, A. R. (1968). *Transplant. Proc.*, **1**, 489.

Bernier, I., Dautigny, A., Colombani, J., and Jollés, P. (1974). *Biochim. Biophys. Acta*, **356**, 82.

Bernoco, D., Cullen, S., Scudeller, S., Trinchieri, G., and Cepellini, R. (1972). In *Histocompatibility Testing 1972* (Dausset, J., and Colombani, J., eds.), Munksgaard, Copenhagen, p. 527.

Bloom, B. R., Bennett, B., Oettgen, H. F., McLean, E. P., and Old, L. J. (1969). *Proc. Nat. Acad. Sci., U.S.A.*, **64**, 1176.

Bodmer, W. F. (1972). *Nature (Lond.)*, **237**, 139.

Bodmer, W. F., Tripp, M., and Bodmer, J. (1967). In *Histocompatibility Testing 1967*, (Curtoni, E. S., Mattiuz, P. L., and Tosi, R. M., eds.), Munksgaard, Copenhagen, p. 341.

Bonavida, B. (1974). *J. Immunol.*, **112**, 926.

Bonavida, B., and Zighelboim, J. (1974). *Cell. Immunol.*, **13**, 52.

Brent, L., Courtenay, T., and Gowland, G. (1967), *Nature, (Lond.)*, **215**, 1461.

Brown, J. L., Kato, K., Silver, J., and Nathenson, S. G. (1974). *Biochemistry*, **13**, 3174.

Callahan, G. N., and DeWitt, C. W. (1975). *J. Immunol.*, **114**, 776.
Calne, R. Y., Davis, D. R., Hadjiyannakis, E., Sells, R. A., White, D., Herbertson, B. M., Millard, P. R., Joysey, V. C., Davies, D. A. L., Binns, R. M., and Festenstein, H. (1970). *Nature (Lond.)*, **227**, 903.
Caves, P. K., Stinson, E. B., Griepp, R. B., Rider, A. K., Dong, E., and Shumway, N. E. (1973). *Surgery*, **74**, 307.
Cerottini, J. C., Nordin, A. A., and Brunner, K. T. (1971). *J. Exp. Med.*, **134**, 553.
Chard, T. (1968), *Nature (Lond.)*, **218**, 378.
Chen, C. H., Sabbadini, E., and Sehon, A. H. (1974). *Transplantation*, **17**, 22.
Cooper, S., and Lance, E. M. (1971). *Transplantation*, **11**, 108.
Cresswell, P., and Dawson, J. R. (1975). *J. Immunol.*, **114**, 523.
Cresswell, P., Turner, M. J., and Strominger, J. L. (1973). *Proc. Nat. Acad. Sci., U.S.A.*, **70**, 1603.
Cullen, S. E., David, C. S., Shreffler, D. C., and Nathenson, S. G. (1974). *Proc. Nat. Acad. Sci., U.S.A.*, **71**, 648.
Cullen, S. E., Freed, J. H., Atkinson, P. H., and Nathenson, S. G. (1975). *Transplant. Proc.*, **7**, 237.
Cullen, S. E., and Nathenson, S. G. (1971). *J. Immunol.*, **107**, 563.
Cullen, S. E., Schwartz, B. D., Nathenson, S. G., and Cherry, M. (1972). *Proc. Nat. Acad. Sci., U.S.A.*, **69**, 1394.

Dausset, J., Colin, M., and Colombani, J. (1960). *Vox Sang.*, **5**, 4.
Dausset, J., and Rapaport, F. T. (1966). *Ann. N.Y. Acad. Sci.*, **129**, 408.
David, C. S., Frelinger, J. A., and Shreffler, D. C. (1974). *Transplantation*, **17**, 122.
David, C. S., and Shreffler, D. C. (1974). *Transplantation*, **18**, 313.
David, C. S., Shreffler, D. C., and Frelinger, J. A. (1973). *Proc. Nat. Acad. Sci., U.S.A.*, **70**, 2509.
David, C. S., Stimpfling, J. H., and Shreffler, D. C. (1975). *Immunogenetics*, **2**, 131.
Davies, D. A. L. (1967). *Transplantation*, **5**, 31.
Davies, D. A. L. (1969). *Transplantation*, **8**, 51.
Davies, D. A. L. (1970). In *Blood and Tissue Antigens* (Aminoff, D , ed.), Academic Press, New York and London, p. 101.
Davies, D. A. L. (1974). In *Handbook of Experimental Immunology* (Weir, D. M., ed.), 2nd edn., Blackwell, Oxford, Chapter 4.
Davies, D. A. L. (1975). *Transplant. Proc.*, **7**, 443.
Davies, D. A. L., and Alkins, B. J. (1974). *Nature (Lond.)*, **247**, 294.
Davies, D. A. L., and Hess, M. (1974). *Nature (Lond.)*, **250**, 228.
Davies, D. A. L., and Hess, M. (1977). In *Handbuch der Allgemeinen Pathologie*, Vol. VI/8 (Masshof, W. *et al.*, eds.), Springer Verlag, Berlin, Chapter 2, p. 39.
Davies, D. A. L., and Staines, N. A. (1976). In *Immune Reactivity of Lymphocytes*, (Feldman, M., and Globerson, A., eds.), Plenum Publishing Corporation, New York, p. 381.
Démant, P. (1973). *Transplant. Rev.*, **15**, 162.
Démant, P., Capkova, J., Hinzova, E., and Voracova, B. (1973). *Proc. Nat. Acad. Sci., U.S.A.*, **70**, 863.
Démant, P., Snell, G. D., Hess, M., Lemonnier, F., Neauport-Sautes, C., and Kourilsky, F. M. (1975). *J. Immunogenet.*, **2**, 263.
DeWitt, C. W. (1970). *Transplant. Proc.*, **2**, 468.
DeWitt, C. W., McDonald, J. H., and Miller, C. (1971). *Transplant. Proc.*, **3**, 198.
Diener, E., and Feldman, M. (1970). *J. Exp. Med.*, **132**, 31.
Dresser, D. W. (1968). *Clin. Exp. Immunol.*, **3**, 877.
Dresser, D. W., and Mitchison, N.A. (1968). *Adv. Immunol.*, **8**, 129.

Eijsvoogel, V. P., Dubois, M. J. G. J., Melief, C. J. M., DeGroot-Kooy, M. L., Konong, C. Van Rood., J. J., Van Leeuwen, A., Dutoit, E., and Schellekens, P. Th.A. (1972). In *Histocompatibility Testing 1972*, (Dausset, J., and Colombani, J., eds.), Munksgaard, Copenhagen, p. 501.

Einstein, A. B., Mann, D. L., Gordon, H. G., and Fahey, J. L. (1971*a*). *Tissue Antigens*, **1**, 209.

Einstein, A. B., Mann, D. L., Gordon, H. G., Trappani, R. J., and Fahey, J. L. (1971*b*). *Transplantation*, **12**, 299.

Eshhar, Z. (1973). *Eur. J. Immunol.*, **3**, 668.

Fabre, J. W., and Morris, P. J. (1974). *Transplantation*, **18**, 436.

Falk, R. E., Collste, L., and Möller, G. (1970*a*). *J. Immunol.*, **104**, 1287.

Falk, R. G., Thorsby, E., Möller, E., and Möller, G. (1970*b*). *Clin. Exp. Immunol.*, **6**, 445.

Ferraresi, R. W., Goihmanyahr, M., and Raffel, S. (1970). *Transplantation*, **10**, 237.

Finkelman, F. D., Shevach, E. M., Vitetta, E. S., Green, I., and Paul, W. E. (1975). *J. Exp. Med.*, **141**, 27.

Fish, F., Staines, N. A., Slvorn, J. L., and Davies, D. A. L. (1976). *Transplantation*, **22**, 551.

Flaherty, L., and Bennett, D. (1973*a*). *Transplantation*, **16**, 505.

Flaherty, L., and Bennett, D. (1973*b*). *Transplantation*, **16**, 682.

Forman, J., and Möller, G. (1975). *Immunogenetics*, **3**, 211.

Foschi, G. V., and Manson, L. A. (1970. *Nature (Lond.)*, **225**, 853.

Fox, M. (1962). *Nature (Lond.)*, **195**, 1024.

Frelinger, J. A., Niederhuber, J. E., David, C. S., and Shreffler, D. C. (1974). *J. Exp. Med.*, **140**, 1273.

Fuller, T. C., and Winn, H. J. (1973). *Transplant. Proc.*, **5**, 585.

Gebhardt, B. M., Nakao, Y., and Smith, R. T. (1974). *J. Exp. Med.*, **140**, 370.

George, M., and Vaughan, J. H. (1962). *Proc. Soc. Exp. Biol. Med.*, **111**, 514.

Gordon, J., and Rode, H. N. (1975). *Transplant. Proc.*, **7**, 61.

Gorer, P. A. (1936). *Brit. J. Exp. Path.*, **17**, 42.

Gorer, P. A., and Mikulska, Z. B. (1954). *Cancer Res.*, **14**, 651.

Gorer, P. A., and O'Gorman, P. (1956). *Transplant. Bull.*, **3**, 142.

Götze, D., and Reisfeld, R. A. (1974). *ImmunForsch. Exp. Klin. Immunol.*, **148**, 45.

Götze, D., Reisfeld, R. A., and Klein, J. (1973). *Naturwissenshaften*, **60**, 355.

Gozzo, J. J., and Rule, A. H. (1972). *J. Reticuloendoth. Soc.*, **11**, 175.

Graff, R. J., Hildemann, W. H., and Snell, G. D. (1966). *Transplantation*, **4**, 425.

Graff, R. J., and Kandutsch, A. A. (1969). *Transplantation*, **8**, 162.

Graff, R. J., Mann, D. L., and Nathenson, S. G. (1970). *Transplantation*, **10**, 59.

Graff, R. J., and Nathenson, S. G. (1971). *Transplant. Proc.*, **3**, 249.

Halle-Pannenko, O., Martyre, M. C., and Jolles, P. (1971*a*). *Transplant. Proc.*, **3**, 257.

Halle-Pannenko, O., Martyre, M. C., and Mathe, G. (1971*b*). *Transplantation*, **11**, 414.

Halliday, W. J. (1971). *J. Immunol.*, **106**, 855.

Hämmerling, G. J., Deak, B. D., Mauve, G., Hämmerling, U., and McDevitt, H. O. (1974*a*). *Immunogenetics*, **1**, 68.

Hämmerling, G. J., Mauve, G., Goldberg, E., and McDevitt, H. O. (1974). *Immunogenetics*, **1**, 428.

Haskova, V., Svejcar, J., Pekarek, J., Johanovsky, J., and Hilgert, I. (1967). *Folia Biol. (Praha)*, **13**, 293.

Haughton, G. (1966). *Transplantation*, **4**, 238.

Hauptfeld, V., Klein, D., and Klein, J. (1973). *Science, N.Y.*, **181**, 167.

Hellman, K., and Duke, D. I. (1967). *Transplantation*, **5**, 184.

Hellström, E. K., and Hellström, I. (1970). *Ann. Rev. Microbiol.*, **24**, 373.

Hess, M. (1975). *Folia Biologica*, Prague, **21**, 48.

Hess, M. (1976). *Transplant. Revs.*, **30**, 40.

Hess, M., and Davies, D. A. L. (1974). *Eur. J. Biochem.*, **41**, 1.

Hess, M., and Davies, D. A. L. (1975). *Transplant. Proc.*, **7**, 209.

Hess, M., and Smith, W. (1974). *Eur. J. Biochem.*, **43**, 471.

Hilgert, I. (1974). *Immunogenet.*, **1**, 153.

Hilgert, I., and Snell, G. D. (1969). *Transplantation*, **7**, 401.

Hutchin, P., *Surg. Gynecol. Obst.* (1968), **126**, 1331.

Jansen, J. J., Koene, R. P., van Kamp, G. J., Hagemann, J. F. H. M., and Wijdeveld, P. G. A. B. (1975a). *J. Immunol.*, **115**, 392.

Jansen, J. J., Koene, R. P., van Kamp, G. J., Tamboer, W. P. M., and Wijdeveld, P. G. A. B. (1975b). *J. Immunol.*, **115**, 387.

John, M., Carswell, E., Boyse, E. A., and Alexander, G. (1972). *Nature, New Biol.*, **238**, 57.

Joysey, V. C., Roger, J. H., Evans, D. B., and Herbertson, B. M. (1973). *Nature (Lond.)*, **246**, 163.

Judd, K. P., and Trentin, J. J. (1973). *Transplantation*, **16**, 351.

Kahan, B. D., Reisfeld, R. A., Epstein, L. B., and Southworth, J. G. (1967). In *Histocompatibility Testing 1967* (Curtoni, E. S., Mattiuz, P. L., and Tosi, R. M., eds.), Munksgaard, Copenhagen, p. 295.

Kilshaw, P. J., Brent, L., and Pinto, M. (1975). *Nature (Lond.)*, **255**, 489

Klein, J. (1972). *Tissue Antigens*, **2**, 262.

Klein, J. (1974). *Ann. Rev. Genetics*, **8**, 63.

Klein, J. (1975). *Biology of the Mouse Histocompatibility-2 Complex*, Springer Verlag, New York.

Klein, J., Livnat, S., Hauptfeld, V., Jerabek, L., and Weissman, I. (1974). *Eur. J. Immunol.*, **4**, 44.

Klein, J., and Murphy, D. B. (1973). *Transplant. Proc.*, **5**, 261.

Klein, J., and Park, J. M. (1973). *J. Exp. Med.*, **137**, 1213.

Klein, J., and Shreffler, D. C. (1971). *Transplant. Rev.*, **6**, 3.

Koubek, K., Hilgert, I., and Kristofova, H. (1973). *Folia Biol. (Praha)*, **19**, 397.

Kronman, B. S., Wepsic, H. T., Churchill, W. H., Zbar, B., Borsos, T., and Rapp, H. J. (1969). *Science, N.Y.*, **165**, 296.

Kyriazis, A. P., Wissler, R. W., and Dzoga, K. (1971). *Proc. Soc. Exp. Biol. Med.*, **136**, 75.

Law, L. W., Appella, E., Cohen, J., and Dean, J. H. (1973). *Nature, New Biol.*, **246**, 174.

Law, L. W., Appella, E., Strober, S., Wright, P., and Fischetti, T. (1972). *Proc. Nat. Acad. Sci., U.S.A.*, **69**, 1858.

Leventhal, B. G., Mann, D. L., and Rogentine, G. N. (1971), *Transplant. Proc.*, **3**, 243.

Livnat, S., Klein, J., and Bach, F. H. (1973). *Nature, New Biol.*, **243**, 42.

Lonai, P., and McDevitt, H. O. (1974). *J. Exp. Med.*, **140**, 1317.

Lucas, Z. J. (1970). *Transplantation*, **10**, 512.

McBride, R. A., and Schierman, L. W. (1970). *J. Exp. Med.*, **131**, 377.

McDevitt, H. O., Deak, B. D., Shreffler, D. C., Klein, J., Stimpfling, J. H., and Snell, G. D. (1972). *J. Exp. Med.*, **135**, 1259.

McKenzie, I. F. C., and Painter, M. E. (1972). *J. Immunol.*, **108**, 352.

McKenzie, I. F., and Snell, G. D. (1973). *J. Exp. Med.*, **138**, 259.

Mann, D. L. (1972). *Transplantation*, **14**, 398.

Mann, D. L., and Fahey, J. L. (1971). *Ann. Rev. Microbiol.*, **25**, 679.

566

Mann, D. L., and Nathenson, S. G. (1969). *Proc. Nat. Acad. Sci., U.S.A.*, **64**, 1380.

Mann, D. L., Rogentine, G. N., and Fahey, J. L. (1969). *Science, N.Y.*, **163**, 1460.

Manson, L. A., and Palm, J. (1968). In *Advance in Transplantation*, (Dausset, J., Hamburger, J., and Mathe, G., eds.), Williams and Wilkins, Baltimore, p. 301.

Marcus, Z. (1969). *Transplantation*, **8**, 80.

Marquet, R. L., Heystek, G. A., Tank, B., and VanEs, A. A. (1975). *Transplantation*, **21**, 454.

Meo, T., David, C. S., Rijnbeek, A. N., Nabholz, M., Miggiano, V. C., and Shreffler, D. C. (1975). *Transplant. Proc.*, **7**, 127.

Meo, T., Vives, J., Miggiano, V., and Shreffler, D. C. (1973). *Transplant. Proc.*, **5**, 377.

Metzgar, R. S., and Miller, J. L. (1972). *Transplantation*, **13**, 467.

Metzgar, R. S., Zmijewski, C. M., and Amos, D. B. (1965). In *Histocompatibility Testing* (Russell, P. S., and Winn, H. J., eds.), NAS-NRC, Washington, p. 45.

Miyakawa, Y., Tanigaki, N., Kreter, V. P., Moore, G. E., and Pressman, D. (1973). *Transplantation*, **15**, 312.

Muramatsu, T., and Nathenson, S. G. (1970). *Biochemistry*, **9**, 4875.

Murray, S., Dewar, P. J., Uldall, P. R., Wilkinson, R., Kerr, D. N. S , Taylor, R. M. R., and Swinney, J. (1974). *Tissue Antigens*, **4**, 548.

Nabholz, M., Vives, J., Young, H. M., Meo, T., Miggiano, V., Rijnbeek, A., and Shreffler, D. C. (1974). *Eur. J. Immunol.*, **4**, 378.

Nathenson, S. G. (1970). *Ann. Rev. Genet.*, **4**, 69.

Nathenson, S. G., and Cullen, S. (1974). *Biochim. Biophys. Acta*, **344**, 1.

Nathenson, S. G., and Davies, D. A. L. (1966a). *Proc. Nat. Acad. Sci., U.S.A.*, **56**, 476.

Nathenson, S. G., and Davies, D. A. L. (1966b). *Ann. N.Y. Acad. Sci.*, **129**, 6.

Nathenson, S. G., and Muramatsu, T. (1971). In *Glycoproteins of Blood Cells and Plasma*, (Jamieson, G. A., and Greenwalt, T. J., eds.), Lippincot, Philadelphia, p. 245.

Nathenson, S. G., Schwartz, B. D., and Cullen, S. E. (1972). In *Membranes and Viruses in Immunopathology* (Day, S. B., and Good, R A., eds.), Academic Press, New York and London, p. 117.

Neauport-Sautes, C., Bismuth, A., Kourilsky, F. M., and Manuel, Y. (1974). *J. Exp. Med.*, **139**, 957.

Neauport-Sautes, C., Silvestre, D., Kourilsky, F. M., and Dausset, J. (1972). In *Histocompatibility Testing 1972*, (Dausset, J., and Colombani, J., eds.), Munksgaard, Copenhagen, p. 539.

Nimelstein, S. H., Hotti, A. R., and Holman, H. R. (1973). *J. Exp. Med.*, **138**, 723.

Oettgen, H. F., Old, L. J., McLean, E. P., and Carswell, E. A. (1968). *Nature (Lond.)*, **220**, 295.

Ogburn, C. A., Harris, T. N., and Harris, S. (1969). *Transplantation*, **7**, 112.

Opelz, G., Sengar, D. P. S., Mickey, M. R., and Terasaki, P. I. (1973). *Transplant. Proc.*, **5**, 253.

Parham, P., Humphreys, R. E., Turner, M. J., and Strominger, J. L. (1974). *Proc. Nat. Acad. Sci., U.S.A.*, **71**, 3998.

Parish, C. R. (1971). *Ann. N.Y. Acad. Sci.*, **181**, 108.

Pellis, N. R., Tom, B. H., and Kahan, B. D. (1974). *J. Immunol.*, **113**, 708.

Peterson, P. A., Rask, L., and Lindbolm, J. B. (1974). *Proc. Nat. Acad. Sci., U.S.A.*, **71**, 35.

Pierres, M., Fradelizi, D., Neauport-Sautes, C., and Dausset, J. (1975). *Tissue Antigens*, **5**, 266.

Rabinovitch, M. (1967). *Proc. Soc. Exp. Biol. Med.*, **124**, 396.

Ranney, D. F., Gordon, R. O., Pincus, J. H., and Oppenheim, J. J. (1973). *Transplantation*, **16**, 558.

Ray, J. G., Hare, D. B., Pedersen, P. D., and Kayhoe, D. E. (1974). In *Manual of Tissue Typing Techniques*, (Pedersen, P. D., and Kayhoe, D. E., eds.), National Institute of Health, Bethesda.

Reisfeld, R. A., and Kahan, B. D. (1970). *Adv. Immunol.*, **12**, 117.

Rocklin, R., Lewis, E. J., and David, J. R. (1970). *New Eng. J. Med.*, **283**, 497.

Rosenberg, E. B., Hill, J., Ferrarri, A., Herberman, R. B., Ting, C. C., Mann, D. L., and Fahey, J. (1973). *J. Nat. Cancer Inst.*, **50**, 1453.

Rubinstein, P., Decary, F., and Streun, E. W. (1974). *J. Exp. Med.*, **140**, 591.

Ruszkiewicz, M. (1971). In *Immunogenetics of the H-2 System* (Lengerova, A., and Vojtiskova, M., eds.), Karger, Basel, p. 224.

Rychlikova, M., Demant, P., and Ivanyi, P. (1970). *Folia Biol.* (*Praha*), **16**, 218.

Sachs, D. H., David, C. S., Shreffler, D. C., Nathenson, S. G., and McDevitt, H. O. (1975). *Immunogenetics*, **2**, 301.

Sachs, D. H., Winn, H. J., and Russell, P. S. (1971). *J. Immunol.*, **107**, 481.

Sanderson, A. R. (1965). *Immunology*, **9**, 287.

Sanderson, A. R., Cresswell, P., and Welsh, K. I. (1971). *Nature, New Biol.*, **230**, 8.

Sanderson, A. R., and Davies, D. A. L (1963). *Nature* (*Lond.*), **200**, 32.

Sanderson, A. R., and Welsh, K. I. (1973). *Transplantation*, **16**, 304.

Sanderson, A. R., and Welsh, K. I. (1974). *Transplantation*, **17**, 281.

Sato, W., and DeWeck, A. L. (1972). *ImmunForsch. Allerg. Klin. Immunol.*, **144**, 49.

Sauser, D., Anckers, C., and Bron, C. (1974). *J. Immunol.*, **113**, 617.

Scheid, M., Boyse, E. A., Carswell, E. A., and Old, L. J. (1972). *J. Exp. Med.*, **135**, 938.

Schendel, D. J., and Bach, F. H. (1974). *J. Exp. Med.*, **140**, 1534.

Schwartz, B. D., Kato, K., Cullen, S. E., and Nathenson, S. G. (1973). *Biochemistry*, **12**, 2157.

Seigler, H. F., Mendes, N. F., and Metzgar, R. S. (1970). *Surgery*, **67**, 261.

Severson, C. D., Greazel, N. A., and Thompson, J. S. (1974). *J. Immunol. Meth.*, **4**, 369.

Severson, C. D., and Thompson, J. S. (1968). *Transplantation*, **6**, 549.

Shimada, A., and Nathenson, S. G. (1969). *Biochemistry*, **8**, 4048.

Shimada, A., and Nathenson, S. G. (1971). *J. Immunol.*, **107**, 1197.

Shorter, R. G., and Elveback, L. R. (1970). *Transplantation*, **9**, 253.

Shreffler, D. C., and David, C. S. (1975). *Adv. Immunol.*, **20**, 125.

Shreffler, D. C., David, C. S., Götze, D., Klein, J., McDevitt, H. O., and Sachs, D. H. (1974). *Immunogenetics*, **2**, 11.

Shreffler, D. C., David, C. S., Passmore, H. C., and Klein, J. (1971). *Transplant. Proc.*, **3**, 176.

Shreffler, D. C., and Passmore, H. C. (1971). In *Immunogenetics of the H-2 System* (Lengerova, A., and Vojtiskova, M., eds.), Karger, Basel, p. 58.

Singer, S. J., and Nicholson, G. L. (1972). *Science, N.Y.*, **175**, 720.

Snary, D., Goodfellow, P., Hayman, M. J., Bodmer, W. F., and Crumpton, M. J. (1974). *Nature* (*Lond.*), **247**, 457.

Snell, G. D. (1970). *Surg. Gynecol. Obstet.*, **130**, 1109.

Snell, G. D., Cherry, M., and Demant, P. (1973). *Transplant. Rev.*, **15**, 3.

Snell, G. D., and Stimpfling, J. H. (1966). In *Biology of the Laboratory Mouse* (Green, E. L., ed.), McGraw Hill Book Co., New York, p. 457.

Springer, T. A., Strominger, J. L., and Mann, D. (1974). *Proc. Nat. Acad. Sci., U.S.A.*, **71**, 1539.

Staines, N. A. (1970). Ph.D. Thesis, University of Edinburgh.

Staines, N. A. (1974). *Transplantation*, **17**, 470.

Staines, N. A. (1975). *Behring Inst. Mitt.*, **57**, 122.

Staines, N. A., and Archer, J. R. (1975). *Israel J. Med. Sci.*, **11**, 1319.

Staines, N. A., Ashton, L. J., Cuthbertson, J. L., and Davies, D. A. L. (1976). *Tissue Antigens*, 7, 1.

Staines, N. A., and Davies, D. A. L. (1973). *Transplantation*, 15, 410.

Staines, N. A., and Davies, D. A. L. (1975). In *Histocompatibility Testing 1975* (Kissmeyer-Nielsen, F., ed.), Munksgaard, Copenhagen, p. 625.

Staines, N. A., Guy, K., and Cuthbertson, J. L. (1975b). *J. Immunogenetics*, 2, 317.

Staines, N. A., Guy, K., and Davies, D. A. L. (1974). *Transplantation*, 18, 192.

Staines, N. A., Guy, K., and Davies, D. A. L. (1975c). *Europ. J. Immunol.*, 5, 782.

Staines, N. A., and O'Neill, G. J. (1975). *J. Immunogenet.*, 2, 207.

Staines, N. A., O'Neill, G. J., Guy, K., and Davies, D. A. L. (1973). *Tissue Antigens*, 3, 1.

Steiner, T., and Watne, A. L. (1970). *Cancer Res.*, 30, 2265.

Stimpfling, J. H. (1961). *Transplant. Bull.*, 27, 109.

Strober, S., Appella, E., and Law, L. W. (1970). *Proc. Nat. Acad. Sci., U.S.A.*, 67, 765.

Strominger, J. L. (1975). In *Histocompatibility Testing 1975* (Kissmeyer-Nielsen, F., ed.), Munksgaard, Copenhagen, p. 719.

Strominger, J. L., Cresswell, P., Grey, H., Humphreys, R. E., Mann, D., McCune, J., Papham, P., Robb, R., Sanderson, A. R., Springer, T. A., Terhorst, C., and Turner, M. J. (1974). *Transplant. Rev.*, 21, 126.

Stuart, F. P. (1973). In *Immunological Aspects of Transplantation Surgery* (Calne, R., ed.), MTP, Lancaster, p. 191.

Svejgaard, A., Staub Nielsen, L., Ryder, L. P., Kissmeyer-Nielsen, F., Sandberg, L., Lindholm, A., and Thorsby, E. (1972). In *Histocompatibility Testing 1972* (Dausset, J., and Colombani, J., eds.), Munksgaard, Copenhagen, p. 465.

Takasugi, M., and Hildemann, W. H. (1971). *Israel J. Med. Sci.*, 7, 221.

Tanigaki, N., Miyakawa, Y., Yagi, Y., Kreiter, V. P., and Pressman, D. (1973). *J. Immunol. Meth.*, 3, 109.

Tanigaki, N., and Pressman, D. (1974). *Transplant. Rev.*, 21, 15.

Taussig, M. J., Munro, A. J., Campbell, R., David, C. S., and Staines, N. A. (1975). *J. Exp. Med.*, 142, 694.

Thieme, T. R., Raley, R. A., and Fahey, H. L. (1974). *J. Immunol.*, 113, 323.

Thorsby, E. (1974). *Transplant. Rev.*, 18, 51.

Unanue, E. B., Dorf, M. E., David, C. S., and Benacerraf, B. (1974). *Proc. Nat. Acad. Sci., U.S.A.*, 71, 5014.

Van Rood, J. J., and Van Leeuwen, A. (1963). *J. Clin. Invest.*, 42, 1382.

Van Rood, J. J., Van Leeuwen, A., Parlevliet, J., Termijtelen, A., and Keuning, J. J. (1975a). Submitted for publication.

Van Rood, J. J., Van Oud Alblas, A. E., Keuning, J. J., Frederiks, E., Termijtelen, A., Van Hooff, J. P., Pena, A. S., and Van Leeuwen, A. (1975b). *Transplant. Proc.*, 7, 25.

Viza, D. C. (1972). *Brit. Pat. 1 291 134*.

Viza, D. C., Degani, O., Dausset, J., and Davies, D. A. L. (1968). *Nature (Lond.)*, 219, 704.

Vladimirskii, M. A., and Govallo, V. I. (1970). *Biull. Exp. Biol., Russia*, 70, 1411.

Welsh, K. I., and Cresswell, P. (1971). *Transplantation*, 12, 234.

Wheeler, H. B., DeFronzo, A., and Corson, J. M. (1970). *Transplantation*, 9, 78.

Widmer, M. B., Omodei-Zorini, C., Bach, M. L., Bach, F. H., and Klein, J. (1973). *Tissue Antigens*, 3, 309.

Wigzell, H. (1965). *Transplantation*, 3, 423.

Wilson, L. A., and Amos, D. B. (1972). *Tissue Antigens*, 2, 105.

Wilson, L. A., and Boyle, W. (1972). *J. Immunol.*, 108, 460.

Wilson, R. E. (1966). *Adv. Surg.*, **2**, 109.

Winn, H. J. (1974). In *Progress in Immunology II*, Vol. 3 (Brent, L., and Holborow, J., eds.), North Holland Publishing Co., Amsterdam, p. 207.

Young, J. M., and Gyenes, L. (1973). *Cell. Immunol.*, **6**, 231.

CHAPTER 16

The Chemical Nature of Adjuvants

M. W. Whitehouse

with an appendix by

D. W. Dresser

1 INTRODUCTION

Every immunologist uses adjuvants at some time, usually following time-hallowed practises in preparing them, blending them with the immunogen, and inoculating the resulting 'mixture' into the test animal. This chapter is not a practical guide to this art (some even would call it witchcraft); this has been described adequately elsewhere (Chase, 1967; Herbert, 1973). Rather, attempts will be made to provide a brief review of the materials used to constitute the more commonly used adjuvants, primarily emphasizing their physical and chemical properties, where these might shed light on their biological activities.

It must be recognized that immunobiologists in the past have not concerned themselves excessively with the precise chemical composition or purity of their adjuvant preparations—it was sufficient that they worked. Undoubtedly some of the difficulties in reproducing data obtained by one laboratory in another, or even within the same laboratory on different occasions, have stemmed partly from the introduction of non-biological variables by the use of very impure, often chemically undefined, reagents to prepare the adjuvants. Even a stock bottle of an oily vehicle may change in composition with time (due to acidification and ester hydrolysis, for example), so that adjuvants prepared with supposedly the same constituents may differ in chemical composition, especially if there has been a comparatively large time interval (or increase in the ambient temperature) between separate preparations. It is hoped that with a greater appreciation of the essential chemical components and with the greater availability of relatively cheap pure chemicals with adjuvant activity, it will be feasible for most experimental immunobiologists to use more reproducible adjuvant formulations in the future.

A basic difficulty in any attempt to survey adjuvants is that this deceptively simple term has various meanings. To some it is merely a device to enhance a humoral or a cell-mediated response, while to others, it is a means to arm the body in order to overcome a tumour burden. Some regard adjuvants as the agents that stimulate select populations of cells, such as T or B lymphocytes, and reticuloendothelial system components, but others think of them in terms of enhancing the whole host-defence capability. The latter concept is not necessarily synonymous with the former, as for example tumour rejection may be stimulated by coating the tumour cells to raise their antigenic profile with consequent enhancement of an anti-tumour immunological response. Another view of an adjuvant is as an agent that promotes, rather than prevents or eradicates, a disease. Examples of this situation are initiation of chronic polyarthritis in rats (Pearson, 1972) or the autoallergic monoarticular arthritis in rabbits (Glynn, 1968, 1974).

An attempt has been made to accommodate all these views in selecting material for inclusion in this chapter. It is not proposed, however, to provide an exhaustive catalogue of the range of materials for which adjuvant activity has been claimed. In the interests of brevity, material that is well described elsewhere and that is readily accessible is not reproduced extensively here. The survey of the literature to mid-1975 (see Addendum) provides a point of entry into the more recent literature. A short summary of a review by Phillips and Dresser, which considers the biological properties of adjuvants, has been appended to this chapter. The following reviews are recommended for other background reading on the general subject of immunological adjuvants, including their history (Freund, 1947, 1956; White, 1967, 1972; Asherson and Allwood, 1969; Jollés and Paraf, 1973; Paterson, 1973; Johnson, 1974; Myrvik, 1974). A review by Haas and Thomssen (1961), written in German, has a particularly valuable bibliography.

The subsequent sections are restricted to discussing only adjuvants of known chemical composition.* Poorly characterized mixtures of biological origin, including whole cell preparations, for example *Bordetella pertussis*, have been disregarded generally except in the discussion of Freund's adjuvants.

2 OUTLINE OF METHODS FOR DETERMINING ADJUVANTICITY

2.1 Measurement of Antibody Levels

The titre of serum antibody may be assessed, or *in vitro* antibody production by lymphoid cells (harvested, for example, from spleen) may be measured after removal from animals a few days after establishing a primary immune response. The adjuvant usually is given intraperitoneally or intravenously and the immunogen is administered frequently by the same route, the mouse being commonly used for these studies. Adjuvant effects on a secondary immune response have been investigated much less intensively. A few reports have been concerned with the *in vitro* effects of adjuvants on antibody synthesis by antigen-primed spleen cells cultured in a medium fortified with the agent under study. It is often difficult to determine from these reports if these are truly immune-specific effects or general nutritional effects on cells which may be the case in a partially insufficient or even toxic medium containing for example metals. These assays are used frequently because the effect of the adjuvant is quantified objectively.

* An adjuvant material indexed under a chemical identity in *Chemical Abstracts* was considered to meet this criterion.

2.2 Determination of a Cell-Mediated Hypersensitivity/Autoallergic Response

This approach is carried out in rodents usually. Here the route of immunization is particularly critical as both the immunogen and the adjuvant must pass to or through a chain of lymph nodes, rather than just being presented to the spleen. Various topical, subdermal, intracutaneous or intranodal routes of inoculation have been prescribed to attain this end. Intravenous and intraperitoneal routes of immunization have been generally unsatisfactory, although some exceptions have been recorded. When oily adjuvants are used, there is often a difference in adjuvanticity between presenting oil-in-water and water-in-oil emulsions. Also, the nature and quantity of the emulsifying agent used may be very critical.

2.3 Immunoprophylaxis of Murine or Human Tumours

Here the object is to use the adjuvant to obtain active immunotherapy either specifically against tumour antigens inoculated together with the adjuvant, or non-specifically against other tumours or immunogens (for example, those that are presented before or after giving the adjuvant). A variety of routes of application must be investigated in small animals before any human trials can be contemplated. Experience has shown that while immunoprophylaxis against experimental leukaemias often may be attained successfully, the progression of solid tumours in the same host sometimes may not be affected at all or even may be stimulated (Mathé et al., 1973). Even living micro-organisms, such as *Bacillus Calmette-Guérin* (BCG), may be used as the adjuvant, being given intravenously in doses of the order of 1 mg/mouse. Adjuvant efficacy usually is determined by the extension of the survival time after inoculating a lethal burden of tumour cells. Alternatively, select cell populations, including macrophages or 'killer' lymphocytes, are withdrawn from the adjuvant-treated animal and their properties compared *in vitro* with those of similar cells from control animals.

2.4 Pathogenesis of Disease Promoted by the Adjuvant

A very restricted assay, relating exclusively to Freund's adjuvant and only applicable in rats, is to determine the severity of the arthritis induced by an arthritogen present in the cell walls of highly adjuvant-active bacteria (*Mycobacterium, Corynebacterium, Nocardia*). By varying the composition of the vehicle in which the bacterial arthritogen is administered, then noting the incidence and severity of the ensuing arthritis, some information may be gained about the 'co-arthritogenicity' of the vehicle concerned. This usually parallels its adjuvanticity as determined by other assays (Whitehouse et al., 1974).

The rat is also peculiar in that it is susceptible to cell-mediated immunopathies, especially allergic encephalomyelitis, which can be induced with oily vehicle and autoallergen only. No bacterial component need be added for this purpose. This is discussed further in the section devoted to Freund's adjuvants (see Section 9).

2.5 Summary

It is essential to quantify the adjuvant-induced response *versus* the normal background where this is feasible. Thus, the numerical factor by which the adjuvant has promoted the immune response can be determined, for comparison with the same factor obtained with other adjuvants, or the same adjuvant applied *via* a different route.

Two further comments on drug/adjuvant studies may be appropriate here, since the aim of many experiments using adjuvant-dependent animal diseases as models is to evaluate both new and old compounds for potential immuno-regulatory activity.

(*i*) Where gross inflammation accompanies inoculation of an adjuvant (for example into a footpad), drug metabolism also may be retarded in these animals especially in the case of rats. This can be avoided largely by inoculating the adjuvant (and immunogen) directly into a node (Newbould, 1965) or a less inflammatory focus, such as the tail or ear (Beck and Whitehouse, 1974*a*).

(*ii*) Most experimental studies of adjuvant-like agents employ small animals for their evaluation. These animals usually have high rates of metabolism and drug detoxification. It is important to remember that many adjuvants, like many drugs, have longer half lives and higher toxicities in larger animals. Extrapolation of effective (but safe) doses from smaller to larger species, including primates, can be just as difficult and uncertain in the case of adjuvants, as for other drugs which are intrinsically toxic.

3 IMMUNOPOTENTIATION BY COMPOUNDS OF LOW MOLECULAR WEIGHT

This is currently the subject of considerable research both in the laboratory and the clinic, with a few compounds, such as levamisole and tilorone, being studied in man for antitumour activity and possible efficacy in rheumatoid arthritis. It would be rather premature, therefore, to attempt a detailed review. However, some general principles are beginning to emerge and certainly deserve to be mentioned here.

3.1 Discovery or Rediscovery of Immunopotentiating Agents

The drugs concerned have been investigated primarily for other purposes and the immune competence of the experimental animals or patients has not been noted. Tetramisole (R-8299) was introduced originally as an antihelminthic drug (Thienpont *et al.*, 1966); its *laevo* isomer is the active drug and is now generally known as levamisole. Tilorone was studied first as a broad-spectrum orally active antiviral agent (Krueger and Mayer, 1970), while bromhexine was introduced originally as an expectorant (Engelhorn and Puschmann, 1963). Organic gold compounds were developed initially from Koch's observation, at the end of the

576

last century, of their bactericidal activity for use as tuberculostatic drugs (1910–1930), then they were discovered to have antiarthritic activity in the late 1920s and only examined recently for immunopotentiating activity (Measel, 1975). During this time attempts were made to classify them—inappropriately it now transpires—as anti-inflammatory or immunodepressant agents (Sofia and Douglas, 1973; Walz et al., 1974), to conform with other anti-arthritic drugs. Even this immunopotentiating activity is now disputed, thus indicating the difficulties in reproducing data in different laboratories, even when relatively well-defined chemical entities are used as an adjuvant.

3.2 Chemical Composition

The wide variety of structures featured in Figure 1 clearly shows that adjuvanticity/immunopotentiation is not a property unique to a particular class

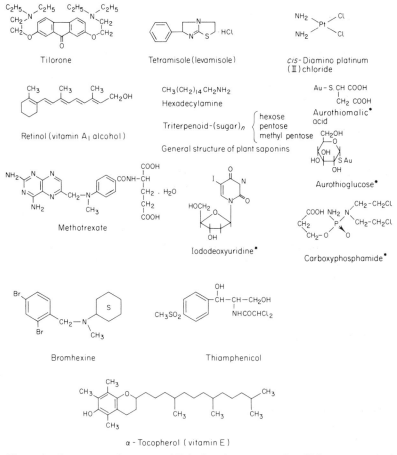

Figure 1 Structures of some established and some putative (*) immunopotentiating agents

of chemical compounds. Furthermore, adjuvanticity is not associated with a narrow range of physical properties, such as detergent activity, hydrophilicity, and pK.

3.3 Essential Physical and Chemical Determinants

It is surprising to find how few investigations of the structure–activity relationship for immunopotentiating activity have been recorded. The lack of activity shown by the *d*-isomer of tetramisole hydrochloride is noteworthy (Renoux and Renoux, 1974), nevertheless the racemic salt is considered to be more effective than the *l*-isomer, levamisole. Some useful structure–activity data have been recorded for analogues of vitamin A (Charabati and McLaren, 1973), tilorone (Munson *et al.*, 1972), and many alkylamines with detergent activity (Gall, 1966).

3.4 Toxicity

Surprisingly few therapeutic indices have been recorded to date, and it is almost impossible to establish the toxicity of some of these compounds, even in the test animal from reports published. The simplest estimation of toxicity, which is to record changes in body weight over a short period (post-adjuvant) compared with untreated animals, is reported rarely. Unfortunately this information cannot be established readily from published LD_{50} data (where they exist), as almost invariably other routes of administration or conditions of stress have been employed to determine the lethal dose. In this respect, some East European authors have much to teach their Western colleagues (see, for example, Zimakov and Zimakova, 1973; Rethy *et al.*, 1968*a*, *b*); their reports eliminate much of this needless guesswork concerning the safety of a proposed adjuvant. The nature of the animal species studied is very important in this context. For example, only the hamster can tolerate the dose of colchicine (100 mg/kg) required to establish an adjuvant effect (Merritt, 1971).

3.5 Multiplicity of Systems/Experimental Conditions for Testing Adjuvants

Table 1 illustrates the variety of systems which has been used; it does not attempt to summarize the nebulous literature describing these compounds in various bioassays. Some of the assays cited here, such as preventing the establishment of tolerance (with actinomycin) or potentiating the activity of an immunogen given orally, presumably be retarding degradation within the gastrointestinal tract (with copper), serve to indicate the breadth of the interpretations that different workers have applied to the idea of an immunological adjuvant. Sometimes the method of administering the test agent, as in the case of vitamin A with oil or emulsifiers, is open to criticism on the grounds that such vehicles are known to function as adjuvants themselves in other test systems.

Table 1 Some immunological test systems used to detect low molecular weight immunopotentiating agents (other than oligonucleotides)

Compound	Species	Quantification immune response	Reference
Metal compounds			
Oral copper	Sheep	Serum antitoxins	Kalic et al. (1965)
Sodium selenite	Mouse	Ab (SRBC)	Spallhoz et al. (1975)
Calcium chloride	Horse	Antitetanus toxin	Schuetzler (1965)
Lanthanum propionate	Mouse	Spleen PFC (SRBC)	Zimakov and Zimakova (1973)
Manganous sulphate	G.P.	Diphtheria antitoxin	Kuleshova (1971)
Gold–sulphur compounds	Mouse	Spleen PFC, RFC (SIII), serum Ab.	Measel (1975)
Platinum II compounds	Mouse/Man	Tumour rejection	Aggarwal et al. (1975)
Beryllium sulphate	Mouse	Ab (haemocyanin)	Unanue et al. (1969)
Nitrogenous bases			
Alkylamines $\geqslant C_{12}$	G.P.	Diphtheria/tetanus antitoxin	Gall (1966)
	Rats	IgG (ovalbumin)	Shier et al. (1974)
Quaternary aliphatic compounds	G.P.	Tetanus antitoxin	Gall (1966), Rethy et al. (1968a, b)
Tetramisole/Levamisole	Mouse	Immunity to Brucella, Spleen PFC (SRBC)	Renoux and Renoux (1972, 1974)
	Chickens	Ab (virus)	Kulkarni et al. (1973)
Tilorone	Mouse	Spleen RFC (SRBC), 'Ig-like' Ab	Munson et al. (1972), Mergel et al. (1974)
Bromhexine	Rabbit	Ab (HSA)	Götz (1975)
Other surface active agents			
Saponin(s)	Cattle	Immunity to rabies	Petermann et al. (1970)
	G.P.	Immunity (Ab) to virus	Dalsgaard (1974)
Sodium dodecyl sulphate	G.P./Man	Skin sensitization to drugs	Marzulli et al. (1968)
Tween 80/Span 80 (mono-oleate esters)	G.P.	Diphtheria antitoxin	Gall (1966)
Other membrane-active agents			
Vitamin A alcohol/ esters	Mouse	Ab rejection of skin grafts	Dresser (1968), Spitnagel and Allison (1970), Jurin and Tannock (1972)
	Rat	Ab	Charabati and McLaren (1973)
Vitamin E (α-tocopherol)	Mouse	Ab in vitro (spleen) cells	Campbell et al. (1974)
		? not in vivo	Spallholz et al. (1975)
	Rat	EAE	Whitehouse et al. (1974)
Vitamin K_1	Rat	EAE	Whitehouse et al. (1974)
Nystatin/amphotericin B	Mouse	Spleen PFC (SRBC) in vitro	Ishikawa et al. (1975)
Other antibiotics			
Thiamphenicol glycinate	Rabbit	Ab (Salmonella typhi)	Barba et al. (1971)
5-Iodo-2'-deoxyuridine (IUdR)	Mouse	Spleen PFC (haemolysin)	Griswold et al. (1975)

Compound	Species	Quantification immune response	Reference
Cytotoxic drugs			
Actinomycin D	Mouse	Prevent tolerance to BGG	Claman and Bronsky (1965)
Colchicine	Hamster	Ab (SRBC)	Merritt (1971)
Methotrexate	Rat	GvHR	Levy and Whitehouse (1974)
Other carcinolytic agents (enhance tumour recognition)			
Platinum (II) complexes	Mice/Man	Tumour rejection	Aggarwal *et al.* (1975)
(Hydrophilic) cyclophosphamide metabolites	Rats	Depress GvHR after application *in vitro*	Whitehouse (1975)

Ab = antibody titre to immunogen shown in parenthesis
BGG = bovine IgG
EAE = induction/severity of allergic encephalomyelitis
G.P. = guinea pig
GvHR = establishment of a graft-*versus*-host reaction
HSA = human serum albumin
PFC = enumeration of plaque-forming cells
RFC = enumeration of rosette-forming cells
SRBC = sheep erythrocytes

3.6 Overlap of Immunodepressant and Immunostimulating Activities

This overlap is often a matter of the timing of the drug regimen relative to the presentation of the immunogen to the animal. For example, methotrexate, a powerful cytostatic and immunosuppressant folate antagonist, stimulates a graft-*versus*-host reaction when given prior to the graft but inhibits the same reaction when given after (Levy and Whitehouse, 1974). Similarly, levamisole both stimulates and inhibits a humoral response, depending on the dose and the time of administration (Renoux and Renoux, 1974). A drug may even generate both immunosuppressant/cytotoxic and immunopotentiating molecular species after biotransformation *in vivo*. An example is cyclophosphamide, a precursor drug which is metabolized to aldophosphamide and phosphoramide mustard— metabolites with powerful carcinostatic/leucopenic activity. Metabolism of cyclophosphamide also yields carboxyphosphamide (and perhaps chloracetaldehyde) which can alkylate the surface of some cells to raise their immunogenic profile and thereby can assist an immunological response. This will be discussed further in Section 3.10.

3.7 Restricted Adjuvant Activity of Small Molecules

Some agents show one activity in affecting a humoral response and another against a cell-mediated response. Thus, Tilorone stimulates antibody synthesis in mice but suppresses the development of cell-mediated immunopathies in rats (Megel *et al.*, 1974). Likewise, octadecylamine only stimulates the humoral response in rats (Shier *et al.*, 1974).

3.8 Enhancement of Host-Defence Reactions in Addition to the Classical Immune Responses

Host-defence reactions include direct activation of macrophages, induction of antiviral activity (usually, but not always, by interferon production), and non-immunological tumour suppression (see Jordan and Merigan, 1975). In some of these activities, these novel immunopotentiating agents are in fact mimicking many of the classical macromolecular adjuvants. Description of these agents as host stimulants or reticuloendothelial-stimulants often would seem to be more appropriate than describing them as immunological adjuvants/immuno-potentiating agents.

3.9 Irritant Properties

The more lipophilic compounds, such as vitamin A, may accumulate rapidly in cell membranes, damaging the plasma, lysosomal, and perhaps even the nuclear, membrane functions due to a membrane-spreading action. Many detergent-like neutral materials or bases, including saponins and long-chain alkylamines, have another type of membrane-disrupting action but still show adjuvant activity. Such agents may cause considerable local tissue injury. Consequently the coadministered immunogen is likely to be exposed to increased blood and/or lymph flow in a highly leucotactic environment, thus facilitating its recognition by circulating lymphocytes and/or transport to the draining lymph node.

3.10 Extralymphoid Stimulants

This special group of immunopotentiating agents has been recognized recently. These compounds, see Table 1 for two examples, may have little effect on the immune system itself in terms of any direct action upon the lymphoid and phagocytic cells that together mount an immune response. Rather, they appear to enhance the immunogenicity of non-self/tumour/viral antigens expressed at the cell surface by combining with these low profile immunogens, such as DNA, to bring them under more effective immunological surveillance.

It is probable that a whole range of drugs of this type will be recognized eventually. They probably will be able to seek out and bind to abnormal cell-surface constituents, but *not* to enter normal lymphoid cells leading to immunosuppression. However, such agents may be able to combine with leukaemic cells, and only be able to associate with the normal cells in such small quantities so that their membrane functions are largely unimpaired. This may sound remarkably like a description of immunoreactants, that is sensitized cells or antibody, but in fact it describes low molecular weight compounds such as platinum (II) complexes which have proved their worth already in clinical trials for cancer treatment (Gale, 1974). A concept that may prove more difficult to appreciate is the proposal that immunoenhancing agents such as platinum (II) or carboxyphosphamide may combine with DNA present at the cell surface (Whitehouse, 1975). A recent development is the rediscovery of reagents such as the platinum blues (Pt(II)-pyrimidine complexes) which can be used both to stain cells carrying DNA selectively at their surface and to control experimental leukaemia. The electron density of these platinum derivatives permits their direct visualization on electron micrographs after cell sorption (Aggarwal *et al.*, 1975).

4 MINERAL ADSORBENTS

This discussion is confined to those minerals that are used in medicine or encountered as occupational hazards.

4.1 Aluminium Salts

The review by Haas and Thomssen (1961) gives a detailed account of these materials, which include the insoluble oxide, hydroxide, and phosphate, and the very soluble sulphates (alums), which also contain a monovalent ion (NH_4^+, Na^+, or K^+). Aluminium salts have been used particularly to raise the immunogenicity of toxoids in the development of antitoxic antisera. Soluble aluminium salts precipitate many proteins or cause them to form large globular aggregates (Joly and Barbu, 1950). The less soluble aluminium adjuvants probably have a twofold action by (*i*) providing a large sorptive area to adsorb fairly soluble (freely diffusable) proteins and limit their biodiffusion; and (*ii*) providing a particulate attraction to immunogen-processing (phagocytic) cells *in vivo* by virtue of their low solubility (hydroxide) or the rather insoluble Al^3–protein salt formed with alums.

Another important property of the aluminium salt is that they are not very toxic to cells mounting the immune response, unlike many other metal ions, such as Cu^2 which also aggregate or precipitate protein antigens. Some evidence has been obtained that the Al^{3+} may have a systemic effect on the immune response over and above its effect in maintaining a depot of immunogen (Kolter *et al.*, 1966).

The suitability of different colloidal forms of aluminium phosphate, hydroxide, and oxide for immunization against bacterial toxins and viral pathogens is discussed further by Knight (1969) and by Grafe (1971). Some reports are difficult to interpret as adsorption properties of various Al^{3+} compounds have been described often in terms of their binding of organic dyestuffs (see Schmidt *et al.*, 1966) rather than binding of proteins or nucleic acids.

Alums are still used as astringents, in styptic agents and mild escharotics, and aluminium hydroxide gels are included in many antacid formulations, including some newer dosage forms of aspirin. Aluminium compounds must, therefore, still be considered as possible accidental adjuvants in man.

4.2 Silicon-Containing Materials

Unlike the aluminium oxides or salts, these materials cannot pass readily into solution either *in vitro* or *in vivo*. Their adjuvant activity depends primarily on their adsorptive and/or macrophage-stimulating properties. Silica particles (usually comprising polymerized, normally hydrated silicon dioxide) carry a negative charge at their surface and can be considered as insoluble polyanions. They may show more adjuvant activity (humoral response) than aluminium gels (Mancino and Bresciano, 1972).

A whole range of mineral silicates abounds in the earth's crust as clays which have been exploited for some time by pharmacists as sorptive agents, laxatives, and in many dermatological formulations, including calamine lotion and poultices. These silicates contain aluminium, magnesium and calcium, some of which may be removed by treatment with dilute acids to enhance the sorptive capacity of the material. Materials related to montmorillonite such as bentonite and fuller's earth have been found to show adjuvant activity in stimulating cell-mediated, as well as humoral responses, in the gunea-pig (Wilkinson and White, 1966; Chase, 1967).

4.3 Thorium Dioxide

This material was used as an X-ray contrast medium and has been employed extensively to 'blockade' the reticuloendothelial system in experimental animals. Nonetheless, it shows antiviral adjuvant activity in mice (Monath and Borden, 1971). Since it has the highest melting point (3390°C) of any known oxide, it is one of the few adjuvant-active materials that can be obtained free of endotoxin contamination. It is prepared routinely by calcination of thorium oxalate at temperatures above 800°.

5 OTHER INSOLUBILIZING AGENTS

These are included here merely for the sake of giving a complete discussion. Non-mineral agents, especially polyelectrolytes that adsorb or form complexes with the immunogen may act as adjuvants, in this respect mimicking aluminium compounds. The complexes formed may be soluble or insoluble. Examples are antigen–IgG complexes used to promote the formation of anti-IgG antibodies such as a rheumatoid factor or methylated albumin to increase the immunogenicity of polyanions, including DNA or polynucleotides (Chase, 1967). Albumin is a highly amphoteric molecule but after esterification of a considerable proportion of the free carboxyl groups using methanol and an acid catalyst, the methylated product behaves as a polycation since the amino and guanidino groups of the albumin molecule are unaffected by the esterification process. A number of other polycations, including histones and polylysine, with molecular weights of greater than 15 000, shows similar adjuvant activity in eliciting antitoxin formation in guinea-pigs and mice (Gall *et al.*, 1972).

There are problems in using macromolecular complexing agents because occasionally they act as competing immunogens. On the other hand, many precipitating or aggregating agents can inhibit an immune response by directly masking the immunogenic determinants (Youmans and Youmans, 1972). It is also possible that a complexing agent may act as an immunosuppressant after being solubilized *in vivo* (by, for example, albumin) or directly engulfed by lymphoid cells and macrophages.

Since so many organic polyanions have been described as adjuvants and many are naturally occurring materials within higher animals, it will be necessary to consider them separately in Section 6.

6 POLYANIONS

6.1 Synthetic Polymers

Acidic and neutral peptides appear to have a low or even negligible adjuvant activity (Gall *et al.*, 1972) in contrast to the polybasic peptides discussed in Section 5. This may be a problem of insufficient size.

The following materials all enhance the humoral response to sheep erythrocytes or diphtheria toxoid in mice: polyacrylic acid (molecular weight) 20 000 (Diamantstein *et al.*, 1971*b*); an immunogenic polyanion formed by copolymerizing styrene with maleic anhydride (Wieczorek *et al.*, 1975); the 'pyran copolymer' (NSC 46015) formed from divinylether and maleic anhydride (Braun *et al.*, 1970); and some polycarboxylates, including Primafloc A-10 and Versicol E-11 (Gall *et al.*, 1972). Polystyrene sulphonic acid, potassium metaphosphate, and onuphic acid (a phosphorylated polysaccharide) showed humoral adjuvant activity in guinea-pigs (Gall *et al.*, 1972).

6.2 Carbohydrate Sulphates

Carrageenan is a mixture of polysaccharides extracted with hot water from the red alga, *Chondrus crispus* (Irish moss). It is used as a stabilizer and homogenizer in toothpaste, cosmetics, and many foodstuff preparations, especially ice cream. The two principal polysaccharides are κ-carrageenan, precipitated as a gel by the addition of K^+, and λ-carrageenan which is isolated subsequently by adding ethanol. These components have similar molecular weights (3×10^5). κ-Carrageenan is a sulphated branched polymer of D-galactose and 3,6-anhydro-D-galactose, and λ-carrageenan has a simpler structure, consisting of a relatively unbranched polygalactose sulphate. The latter is usually present in greater quantity (approximately 60 per cent).

Carrageenan preparations exhibit a variety of biological activities (Di Rosa, 1972) and have been used to treat peptic ulcers. Humoral adjuvant activity has been demonstrated in rabbits (Richou *et al.*, 1968). Even when applied in mineral oil, the Ca^{2+} salt fails to enhance delayed hypersensitivity in guinea-pigs (Salvaggio and Kundur, 1970). However, a comparative study of several carrageenan samples has shown that they differ in their polypeptide content (0·3–4·3 per cent), and in their ability to elicit hypersensitivity in guinea-pigs to both the carrageenan itself (probably determined by the peptide component) and to incorporated protein antigens (Mizushima *et al.*, 1974). Since it is usually the least refined preparations that are used in foods, pharmaceuticals, and cosmetics, the human body may be exposed to possible adjuvanticity from all these sources.

High molecular weight materials such as sulphated dextrans (molecular weight 5×10^5) given intravenously or intraperitoneally stimulate antibody formation in mice (Diamantstein *et al.*, 1971c; Bradfield *et al.*, 1974), but there are conflicting reports about the efficacy of low molecular weight materials—for example pentosan sulphate with a molecular weight of 2000 (Diamantstein *et al.*, 1973; Bradfield *et al.*, 1974). Part of the adjuvant activity of dextran sulphate in mice is believed to be due to diversion of immunogenic sheep erythrocytes from the liver to the spleen, after the Kupffer cells in the liver have become saturated with protein–polysulphate complexes. These complexes are formed when dextran sulphate is given to the animal prior to an immunizing dose of sheep erythrocytes. Heparin and lower molecular weight dextran sulphates do not exhibit this effect (Bradfield *et al.*, 1974). Polysulphates may inhibit antibody formation by spleen cells *in vitro* (Wacker *et al.*, 1970).

6.3 Polyuronides

These are carbohydrate polymers containing hexuronic acid units, which are found abundantly in plants and are present in certain bacteria. They form gel-like viscous materials, especially with certain counter ions such as Ca^{2+}.

Pectin is a material widely distributed in fruits, root vegetables, and wood. Its principal constituent is pectic acid, poly-α-D-galacturonic acid, but arabinose and galactose polymers (araban and galactan, respectively) also are present in most preparations. The humoral adjuvant activity of pectin in rabbits and guinea-pigs has been described by Lallouette *et al.* (1968). It should be noted that the source of the pectin may be important, since pectic acids have been described ranging in size from an average molecular weight of greater than 2×10^5 (found in apples and citrus fruit) to only 2×10^4 (present in pears and plums). It is general experience with other adjuvants, that an increase in molecular size is paralleled usually by an increase in adjuvanticity.

Alginic acid is the main structural carbohydrate of brown seaweeds (*Phaeophyceae*). Very large amounts are used in the food industry as thickeners, emulsifiers, and in preparing edible sausage casings. Alginic acid is very resistant to hydrolysis and forms an insoluble salt with Ca^{2+}. It is composed mainly of D-mannuronic acid with some variable amounts of L-guluronic acid. Originally, alginates were used as absorbable haemostatic dressings, with a solution of sodium alginate being applied to a bleeding area and immediately being converted to a firm gel by the addition of a solution of calcium chloride. This principle was extended to introducing an antigen in a solution of sodium alginate which then was rendered insoluble *in vivo* (within the injection site) by endogenous Ca^{2+}. Satisfactory antitoxin titres have been obtained by this procedure (Amies, 1959). Subsequent experience has shown that it may be necessary, or even essential, to gelify this immunogen–alginate inoculum by first adding Ca^{2+} to ensure an adequate vaccination (Kohn *et al.*, 1969).

Alginates may stimulate antibody synthesis *in vivo* (Wacker *et al.*, 1970). For *in vivo* activity, alginates do not need to be given simultaneously with an immunogen such as sheep erythrocytes (Diamantstein *et al.*, 1971a).

The type III pneumococcal polysaccharide (polycello-biuronic acid) has been shown to stimulate B cells in mice (Mitchell, 1975).

6.4 Polynucleotides and Nucleic Acids

Much of the earlier literature on this subject has been reviewed in two books (Plescia and Braun, 1968; Beets and Braun, 1971). Originally, interest was aroused in these polyphosphates, which contain the common purines and pyrimidines, since it was believed that endogenous oligonucleotides—formed in some quantity after X-irradiation, or treatment with cytostatic drugs or cell-necrotic agents such as endotoxins—were responsible for the heightened (humoral) immune responsiveness observed in all these conditions. Concurrent discoveries that these same materials also induced antiviral or antitumour activity under certain conditions considerably increased the interest in them.

RNase-sensitive ribonucleoprotein from *Mycobacterium tuberculosis* induces immunity to tuberculous infection but does not induce general hypersensitivity in guinea-pigs or mice (Youmans and Youmans, 1969). Double-strand RNA (dsRNA) has been studied intensively, not only for its interferon-inducing (antiviral) activity, but also for its humoral adjuvant activity. This is dependent upon the time of administration relative to antigen, and prior treatment with dsRNA will suppress a subsequent immune response (Cunnington and Naysmith, 1975).

With the discovery of polynucleotide phosphorylase in 1955, which permitted the facile enzymic synthesis of polynucleotides and the development of techniques for the chemical synthesis of large oligonucleotides, interest became centred on the biological properties of these materials. Polynucleotides are most effective when presented as dsRNA usually polyuridylic acid complexed to polyadenylic acid (poly U:A) or polyinosinic acid complexed to polycytidylic acid (poly I:C). A corresponding series of homodeoxyribopolymers (DNA analogues) has also been investigated.

A shortcoming in many reports describing the biological properties of these materials is a lack of any clear indication of their molecular size and the nature of the counter ions present (since these compounds are in fact polyphosphoric acids). Their immunogenicity has been discussed by Lacour and colleagues

(1973). This material is considerably less toxic than poly I:C in mice. The (humoral) adjuvant activity of the ribose-containing polymers, poly A:U has been reviewed by Johnson (1973).

In guinea-pigs, both mycobacterial RNA and synthetic poly A:U applied in an oily vehicle with the encephalitogen act as adjuvants to induce the autoallergic disease allergic encephalomyelitis (Gumbiner *et al.*, 1973). Cytoplasmic RNA from Group A *Streptococcus* was found to be a much stronger adjuvant than the cytoplasmic DNA from the same source in stimulating the appearance of haemolysin-forming spleen cells (Bueltmann *et al.*, 1975).

7 NEUTRAL MATERIALS

Some macromolecules which are not polyelectrolytes, but which seem to offer considerable promise for future studies, will be discussed in this section.

7.1 Lentinan and Related Glucans

Lentinan is a high molecular weight linear $(1 \rightarrow 3)$linked polymer of D-glucose isolated from the edible Japanese mushroom *Lentinus edodes* by hot-water extraction, followed by precipitation with cetyl trimethyl ammonium hydroxide at pH 11 (Chihara *et al.*, 1970). In mice, the LD_{50} is greater than 2 g/kg when given intraperitoneally. It has excited considerable interest not only because of its antitumour activity but also because it is a potent stimulant of T-helper cells in mice (Maeda and Chihara, 1971; Dennert and Tucker, 1973). It is insoluble in most solvents, including water, but is brought into solution with aqueous alkali, in which it decomposes easily at an elevated temperature. Since it contains no nitrogen, phosphorous, or sulphur and yields no minerals on incineration, it must be presumed to be non-acidic despite its bizarre solubility properties, which are, however, similar to those of other known $\beta(1 \rightarrow 3)$glucans. Some related $\beta(1 \rightarrow 3)$glucans (pachymaran and schizophyllan) also show dramatic anti-tumour activity in mice (Hamiro *et al.*, 1971), presumably through a similar immunopotentiating mechanism.

A $\beta(1 \rightarrow 3)$glucan isolated from the cell walls of *Saccharomyces cerevisiae* and from fungal wall materials shows adjuvanticity in guinea-pigs for humoral and cell-mediated responses (Kotani *et al.*, 1975a).

7.2 Polyvinyl Alcohol

This soluble material stimulates and extends antibody production after administering a plague vaccine to rabbits and pigs (Dokukin *et al.*, 1972). This polymer would seem to merit further study.

7.3 Carbonyl Iron

Carbonyl iron is used as a suspension and induces allergic encephalomyelitis in rat strains resistant to complete Freund's adjuvants (Levine and Sowinski, 1975).

8 BACTERIAL ENDOTOXINS

These are toxic principles, usually designated lipopolysaccharides, produced by gram-negative bacteria. They are bound firmly to the bacterial cell wall in a complex with protein, from which they are shed when the cell undergoes lysis. The term 'endotoxin' is therefore a misnomer since these substances originate from outside the cells, nor are they always toxic, having the property of increasing resistance to infection. They exhibit a range of biological activities at quite remarkably low doses in some instances; 1 ng/kg given intravenously will raise the body temperature of many sensitive mammals, including man, horse, and rabbit. They also stimulate nerve regeneration, activate the fibrinolytic, complement, and reticuloendothelial systems, induce the production of interferon, and are mitogens for B lymphocytes. By virtue of their strong binding to cell membranes, they also promote platelet aggregation, release of histamine and catecholamines from the appropriate storage cells, and will induce tumour necrosis directly (besides stepping up the host's immunosurveillance). In addition to stimulating the humoral response, by acting as classic adjuvants at doses of less than 1 μg given intravenously to rabbits, but not in guinea-pigs (Johnson et al., 1956), also they suppress delayed hypersensitivity in guinea-pigs (Floersheim and Szeszak, 1971). Adjuvant activity is demonstrable in vitro with cultured mouse spleen cells (Ortiz-Ortiz and Jaroslow, 1970). Neter (1969) has provided a valuable review of both the adjuvant and immunosuppressive properties of endotoxins.

For all these diverse activities, including adjuvant/immunodepressant effects, there is a relationship between pyrogenicity or general toxicity and the magnitude of the response obtained. Thus, rabbits are very susceptible, while some mouse strains and primates (especially baboons) are very resistant.

After extraction of *Enterobacteriaceae* and other endotoxin-producing organisms with hot aqueous phenol, protein-free lipopolysaccharide complexes are obtained containing 60–85 per cent polysaccharide. It is the lipid component that primarily determines the toxicity and the adjuvant activity. The polysaccharide components from these lipopolysaccharides may differ in different bacterial strains and contain many unusual sugars including a family of 3,6-dideoxy-hexoses (paratose, abequose, tyvelose, and colitose) which, themselves or as their 2-O-acetyl derivatives, contribute to the serological specificity.

The structure of the lipid component known as lipid A, isolated from *Salmonella* mutants, is shown in Figure 2. It contains a repeating disaccharide unit composed of two molecules of D-glucosamine linked through a $\beta(1 \rightarrow 6)$-glycosidic bond, each unit being bound to another disaccharide unit *via* an $\alpha(1 \rightarrow 4)$phosphate diester linkage. In most other bioconstituents, the amino group of glucosamine is acylated with short-chain fatty acids (formyl, acetyl, and glycolyl), but in lipid A it is acylated with the C_{14} hydroxyacid, β-hydroxymyristic acid. Three of the four available hydroxyl groups of the disaccharide are esterified with 2-myrystyloxy-myristyl, lauryl (C_{12}), and palmityl (G_{16}) moieties with the fourth hydroxyl group being the site of

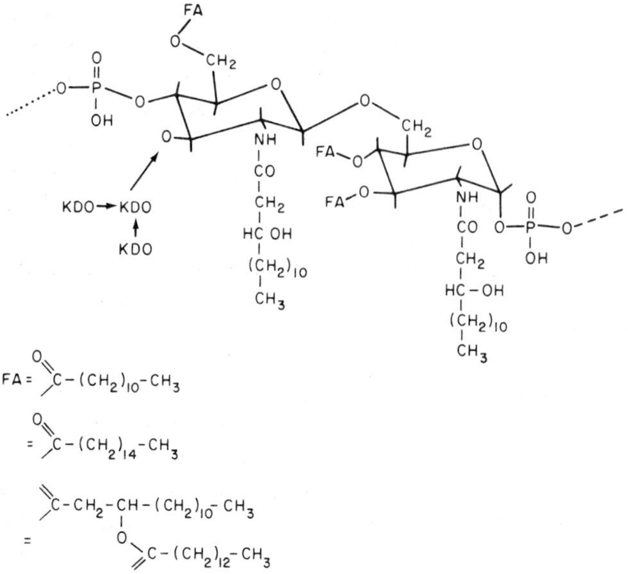

FA
O
CH₂

O
..........O—P—O
OH

O

KDO→KDO
↑
KDO

NH
CO
CH₂
HC OH
(CH₂)₁₀
CH₃

FA—O
FA—O

O
CH₂

O

NH
CO
CH₂
HC—OH
(CH₂)₁₀
CH₃

O—P—O——
OH

$$FA = \overset{O}{\underset{}{C}} - (CH_2)_{10} - CH_3$$

$$= \overset{O}{\underset{}{C}} - (CH_2)_{14} - CH_3$$

$$= C - CH_2 - CH - (CH_2)_{10} - CH_3$$
$$\underset{}{O} \overset{}{C} - (CH_2)_{12} - CH_3$$

Structure of lipid A

(a)

O-Specific Chains (Region I)

```
[2-Ac-Abep                    o-Glcp      ]        2-Ac-Abep
    1│α                        1│α                     1│α
    │3        α            │4      α          │3                α                    α                  β
  D-Manp(I→4) L-Rhap(I→3)D-Galp(I→2)  =7   D-Manp(I→4) L-Rhap(I→3) D-Galp(I→4)
```

Core Polysaccharide (Region II)

```
D-GlcNAcp      Glc       D-Galp         Hep            ℗-OCH₂-CH₂NH₂            7
    1│α         1│        1│α            1│℗              ℗              KDO-℗-OCH₂-CH₂NH₂
    │2   α      │6  α     │6             │7               │4               2│   │?
  D-Glcp(I→2)D-Galp(I→3)D-Glc(I→3) L-α-D-Hepp(I→3) L-α-D-Hepp(I→5)KDO(2→?)KDO(2→3)
```

```
        ℗                          ℗            S.typhimurium LPS
        │4                         │1                 (4,5,12)
    D-GlcNp-(FA)(I→6)D-GlcN-(FA)
```

Lipid A (Region III)

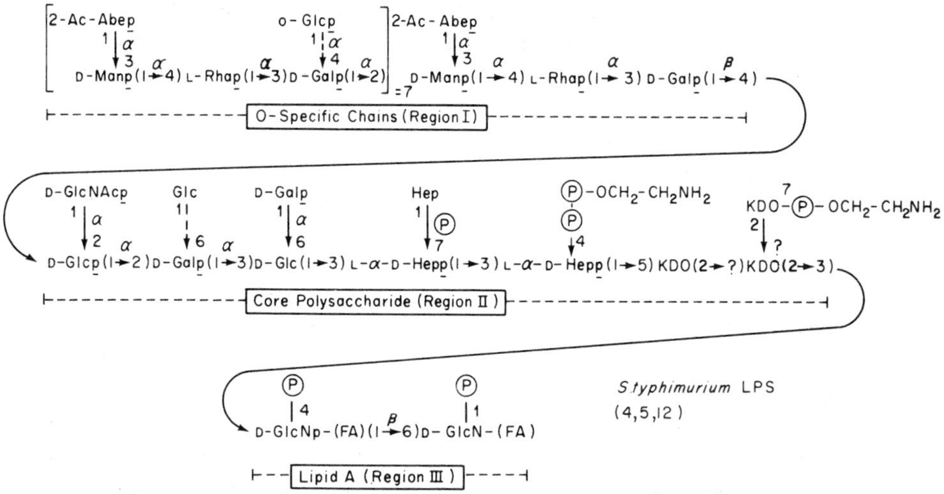

(b)

Figure 2 (After Westphal, 1975)

glycosidic linkage to a ketodeoxyoctonoic acid moiety, the first carbohydrate unit of the so-called 'core' polysaccharide (see Figure 2b).

The history of the long, painstaking, sometimes tortuous and ever misleading trail of research which resulted in the elucidation of the structure of lipid A has been recounted by Westphal (1975). Lipid A, solubilized with serum albumin, has been shown to exhibit nearly all of the biological activities associated with whole endotoxins, including adjuvanticity (see Westphal, 1975).

Treatment of the whole lipopolysaccharide with succinic or phthalic anhydrides has yielded more water-soluble, anionic acyl-lipopolysaccharide preparations with adjuvant activity but considerably diminished toxicity (McIntire, 1970). Further studies of derivatives of lipopolysaccharide along these lines and/or the synthesis of lipid A analogues may provide more suitable materials for development as adjuvants for humoral immunity.

9 FREUND'S ADJUVANTS

9.1 General Observations

Freund's adjuvants induce powerful cell-mediated responses, humoral immunity, break tolerance, and potentiate tumour rejection. Their nomenclature honours the work of Jules Freund and his coworkers, who established the conditions required to obtain reproducible activity despite relying on materials of uncertain composition and of varying physical and chemical properties.

The history of these adjuvants is briefly outlined (also see Freund, 1947, 1956). Dienes and Schoenheit (1930) found that an antigen injected into a tuberculous 'focus' gave heightened antibody titres and elicited a greater degree of delayed hypersensitivity in guinea-pigs than when it was injected at other (non-tuberculous) sites. Furthermore, they showed that heat-killed tubercle bacilli gave a marked tissue reaction, and antigens injected into this area of inflammation also elicited hypersensitivity. The same antigens injected into acute inflammatory foci produced with non-bacterial irritants, including silica, tapioca, or turpentine, however did not elicit any greater immune response than when injected into non-inflammatory tissue. This finding led Freund and McDermott (1942) to develop adjuvants containing mycobacteria. A key constituent of their adjuvant formulation was a lanolin-like substance contained in Aquaphor, which is derived from wool fat and which contains added petrolatum hydrocarbons.

Further research has shown that adjuvant activity for induction of cell-mediated immunity can be obtained also with variations from the classical (complete) Freund's adjuvants which consists of dead *Mycobacterium* suspended in mineral oil, usually with added emulsifier. Such variations can be achieved by (*i*) using either live or dead bacteria without an oily vehicle, or (*ii*) using an oily vehicle without a bacterial component.

This first variant has been studied with a view to using adjuvant (immuno) therapy to treat cancer, with viable *Bacillus Calmette-Guérin* (BCG), a strain of

Mycobacterium bovis (Mackaness *et al.*, 1973), or formalin-treated *Corynebacterium parvum* (Wolmark *et al.*, 1974) given in saline as the sole adjuvant material.

The second variant seems to apply only to the immunization of rats, particularly in the context of sensitizing an animal to develop autointolerance to its own myelinated nervous tissue (allergic encephalomyelitis). For this purpose, the animal is usually challenged with a crude extract of spinal cord as the encephalitogen, a material which may contain natural emulsifiers, considerable lipid, and other intrinsic pro-adjuvant components. As an extrinsic adjuvant, it is only necessary to use an oily vehicle, which need not be a mineral oil (Whitehouse *et al.*, 1974). This phenomenon clearly contradicts the generally accepted view that it was the bacterial component which provided the essential adjuvanticity for cell-mediated immunity.

This second variant has been evaluated at some length for it has not always been appreciated that the vehicle may be of prime importance in determining the ultimate magnitude of an autoallergic response. It has long been known that mineral oil (with or without an emulsifying agent) is a sufficient adjuvant to stimulate a humoral response to a simultaneously applied immunogen, and when used for this purpose it is commonly described as a Freund's incomplete adjuvant. In order to avoid ambiguity it is suggested that the terminology be revised, and the following recommendations are proposed.

(*i*) Adjuvants containing an oily vehicle should be continued to be described as Freund's adjuvants, referring to them by the prefix Fd, rather than Fr, (*a*) to distinguish Freund from Fr = fraction as used in the biochemical literature and (*b*) in accordance with the general practice of designating items by first and last letters.

(*ii*) Every adjuvant should be designated by its composition encoded as bacterial component, emulsifier, oil—abbreviated to BEO. Thus, the traditional Freund's complete adjuvant would be designated Fd/BEO. The gain in clarity more than compensates for the need to use three extra ciphers. An incomplete adjuvant would be Fd/EO if it contained an emulsifier, and Fd/O if it did not.

(*iii*) Wherever possible, B and E (and O) should be identified once in the experimental section of any report describing the use of Freund's adjuvants (Whitehouse, 1973).

Herbert (1973) has given a detailed guide to the art of preparing mineral oil adjuvants and using them to immunize laboratory animals. For initiating adjuvant disease in rats, with its characteristic polyarthritis (Swingle, 1974), some Fd/BO adjuvants are available commercially which contain various bacterial materials and oily vehicles (see Whitehouse and Beck, 1974). Other commercial adjuvants have proved unsatisfactory for initiating the arthritis, presumably because they contain insufficient arthritogenic material.

9.2 Nature of the Bacterial Component

A great deal of effort is being devoted currently to 'refining' the activity of the whole crude *Mycobacterium*, *Corynebacterium* or *Nocardia* species, in order to isolate and identify the actual material with adjuvant properties.

Inoculation of the whole dead micro-organism causes considerable local injury—granuloma formation—and some systemic disturbances—for example, altered drug metabolism (Beck and Whitehouse, 1973)—which restrict the utility of Freund's adjuvants in cancer immunotherapy. Purification of the adjuvant to the point where a low molecular weight material with less irritancy/toxicity can be substituted for the original whole organism constitutes one advance; the elimination of competing immunogens from within the same organism constitutes another. There seem to be two schools of thought as to how this might be achieved: (*i*) by starting with the cell wall of the micro-organism and chemically degrading it, removing extraneous lipid and protein, etc.; and (*ii*) by isolating polyanions that are not part of the cell envelope, but are known to have adjuvant-like activity.

The former approach has been used in France and in Japan in recent years. With the recent flood of publications from both these countries, it seems impossible to provide in this review little more than a very dated progress report (see Addendum). The second approach, focusing on mycobacterial RNA, is currently receiving far less attention (see, for example, Gumbiner *et al.*, 1973).

The work by Jollés and Paraf (1973) gives an account of the earlier investigations to determine the chemistry of the wax material extracted from whole cells of *M. tuberculosis* (or their cell walls) and to obtain from this wax fraction a water-soluble adjuvant-active material, after removing the bulk of the fatty acids by saponification with alkali. The resultant water-soluble material is a mixture of peptidoglycans and polysaccharides. Similar destructive fractionation procedures have been carried out starting from cell-wall materials from *Mycobacterium* (including BCG), *Corynebacterium* (especially *C. parvum*), and *Nocardia* species (Azuma *et al.*, 1974*a*, *b*). Some of these chemical isolation methods are so vigorous that it is a problem to know whether the products obtained are artefacts, or whether the real adjuvant principle is not being lost (see Stewart-Tull *et al.*, 1975). Alternative modes of degradation using enzymes such as lysozyme, fungal and bacterial peptidases, and carbohydrases under much milder conditions are therefore particularly valuable and receiving due attention in various Japanese and French laboratories.

The following reports describe materials of identified composition, which are claimed to have adjuvant activity (Azuma *et al.*, 1974*b*; Ellouz *et al.*, 1974; Fleck *et al.*, 1974; Migliore-Samour *et al.*, 1974; Kotani *et al.*, 1975*b*). These small molecular weight products, some of which are indicated in Figure 3, do not seem to be able to induce arthritis in rats, at least not without the addition of some further (adjuvant-like) factors. Thus, a distinction must be made between isolating low molecular weight adjuvants and isolating an arthritogen from the same micro-organism. Materials of similar composition and adjuvant activity

– Acetyl Muramyl– L – Ala –D – Isoglutamine –

Figure 3 Structures with adjuvant activity (for CMI) from microbial cell walls

also have been obtained from cell walls of *Micrococcus* (Ellouz *et al.*, 1974), *Staphylococcus*, and *Lactobacillus* (Kotani *et al.*, 1975c), and various other gram-positive bacteria (Kotani *et al.*, 1975d), from culture filtrates of *M. tuberculosis* (Stewart-Tull *et al.*, 1975), and from the nucleotide precursors of cell-wall peptidoglycan synthesis which accumulate in various micro-organisms poisoned with D-cycloserine (Ellouz *et al.*, 1974). Simple peptide or oligosaccharide degradation products are apparently devoid of activity (see Fleck *et al.*, 1974). Instead, the adjuvant activity is associated with the hybrid molecular species, a glycopeptide. Muramic acid (the 3-*O*-lactic acid ether of D-glucosamine) is an essential constituent but it may be either *N*-glycolated (as in material derived from some BCG strains) or *N*-acetylated. The presence of D-isoglutamine in this minimal molecular weight adjuvant deserves comment. Not only is this a D-amino acid but the amide group is adjacent to the amino group (position 1), whereas in glutamine it is at position 3. Isoglutamine therefore can be considered as a γ-amino acid.

Some of these low molecular weight adjuvants have relatively low activity in suppressing murine tumours, although they will induce hypersensitivity in guinea-pigs. It will be necessary therefore to establish another structure–action relationship for other molecular fragments isolated from these immunopotentiating organisms, which show antitumour activity. Yet another structure–activity relationship may emerge eventually for the mitogenic activity of the water-soluble fragments obtained from this range of micro-organisms. Of some interest is the suggestion that the antihumour activity of bacterial peptidoglycans is due to antibodies directed against a polysaccharide portion of the peptidoglycan which cross-reacts with a tumour cell-surface carbohydrate moiety present at the tumour cell surface (Anon, 1975).

At the time of writing a glycodipeptide has been shown to be the smallest molecule of natural origin, with true adjuvant activity. Other portions of the original cell-wall peptidoglycan probably bear the antitumour and the arthritogenic (for the rat) activities. A common structural feature of the cell walls from adjuvant-active/arthritogenic strains of *Mycobacterium*, *Corynebacterium*, and *Nocardia* species is the presence of a heteropolysaccharide containing arabinose and galactose (arabinogalactan) (Azuma *et al.*, 1974a), and possibly also mannose (Stewart-Tull *et al.*, 1975), which may have some significance for the arthritogenic activity. Some progress has been made towards characterizing the arthritogen from *M. tuberculosis* (Koga and Pearson, 1973; Koga *et al.*, 1976). Arthritogenic activity also has been located in cell-wall materials of many other bacteria, for example, *Staphylococcus*, *Streptomyces*, and *Lactobacillus* species, and these may provide a better source of arthritogen(s) for eventual chemical characterization.

9.3 Nature of the Oily Vehicle

Early work with Freund's adjuvants tended to emphasize the use of paraffin wax or liquid paraffin (see Turk, 1975), and since these proved adequate vehicles for most immunizations there was little incentive to alter the vehicle component.

However, this was not always the case when inducing adjuvant disease in rats; different mineral oils sometimes gave a varied incidence of disease. Mineral oils refined for medicinal use as emollients and laxatives, are available under a bewildering variety of names—vaseline oil, liquid petrolatum, white mineral oil, liquid paraffin, and seneca oil They are characterized by their physical properties (viscosity, density, insolubility in alcohol, resistance to concentrated sulphuric acid, and high boiling range) rather than by chemical composition. The latter can be extremely complex and can vary quite considerably according to the source of the material. Occasionally, there have been problems due to bacterial contamination at source, and since these oils usually have a high boiling range and considerable viscosity, it is not always feasible to carry out small scale purifications by distillation or filtration.

Some detailed structure–activity relationships have been assessed for vehicles that can be used instead of mineral oil, in conjunction with (i) arthritogenic bacteria to induce polyarthritis and drug metabolism deficits in rats, and (ii) encephalitogens, with or without a bacterial adjuvant, to induce allergic encephalomyelitis in rats and guinea-pigs (Shaw et $al.$, 1964; Whitehouse et $al.$, 1974). These relationships can be summarized as follows:

(i) Linear alkanes with a chain length C_{12} or more and linear 1-alkenes with a chain length C_{14} or more are very suitable, except that they are only liquids at room temperature up to hexadecane (melting point = 18°) and 1-octadecene (melting point = 17°). Bigger, branched-chain hydrocarbons with suitably low melting points, for example phytane (C_{19}) and squalene (C_{30}) are also satisfactory substitutes for mineral oil.

(ii) Coadjuvanticity is reduced by cyclization of the hydrocarbon, or by the presence of double bonds or oxygen functions.

(iii) Many esters and triglycerides of fatty acids with chain length of C_{12} or more are suitable substitutes, especially those containing oleic (octadec-9-enoic) acid, also vitamins E and K, and vitamin A acetate (but not palmitate).

(iv) Plant oils and fats show very variable activity as substitutes for mineral oil, and with certain exceptions (olive oil), cannot be recommended generally for adjuvant formulation (Whitehouse et $al.$, 1974).

Alternative oily vehicles such as squalene or butyl oleate, which, in contrast to most mineral oil constituents, can be metabolized readily, seem to offer considerable promise—being less likely to load macrophages permanently or to facilitate chronic granuloma reactions. Preliminary studies have shown that they offer the further advantage that the experimental arthritis or allergic encephalomyelitis in rats induced by adjuvants containing alternative oily vehicles are usually more drug-sensitive than those (granulomatous) diseases engendered with mineral oil adjuvants (Beck and Whitehouse, 1974b, 1975).

9.4 Nature of the Emulsifier

The emulsifier serves at least two purposes. Firstly, it blends the oily vehicle with the lipid-rich mycobacterial adjuvant component which is usually enmeshed in lipophobic materials (protein, nucleates) in the whole killed micro-organism. Secondly, the emulsifier blends the whole dispersate of bacterial material in oil with an immunogen which is dissolved or suspended in an aqueous phase. Paradoxically, after removing much of the readily extractable lipid from the dried bacteria with ethanol and ether, the defatted residue often blends more readily with an oily vehicle and an emulsifier may not be required to obtain a dispersion of bacterial matter in oil. This Fd/BO dispersion is usually sufficient to initiate arthritogenesis in the rat.

Not much information has been published in recent years concerning variations in adjuvanticity produced by altering the emulsifier of a Freund's adjuvant formulation. The early investigations were carried out using crude commercial, usually liquid, emulsifiers of uncertain composition. Their reproducibility and stability were often much below acceptable standards. Thus, Arlacel-A which has been recommended repeatedly for the preparation of Freund's adjuvants (Herbert, 1973), may contain 30 or more components, only half of which are carbohydrate esters (e.g. mannide mono-oleate) with the desired detergent characteristics (Bollinger, 1970). Anionic, cationic and even neutral detergents such as alkyl sulphates, alkylamine derivatives and carbohydrate alkanoate esters, respectively, of greater than 95 per cent purity are now available and should be studied further in this context.

Another problem deserving further consideration is the fact that most detergents have shorter biological half lives than the conventional oily vehicles so they are likely to be removed first from an adjuvant depot *in vivo*. This may not always be desirable, as this may promote coalescence of the oil droplets *in situ*, perhaps retarding access to the immunogen or its processing by macrophages.

10 TOXIC PROTEINS

There are many adjuvant materials which might be included under this heading. However, only two examples will be discussed here, one being drawn from the plant kingdom, the other from a micro-organism.

10.1 Ricin D

This is the principal toxic principle of the castor bean, *Ricinus communis*. It should not be confused with a lectin from the same source. In mice the LD_{50} is $0.2 \mu g$/mouse but at one-tenth this dose, it acts as a humoral adjuvant (Koga *et al.*, 1971). It is a glycoprotein, with a molecular weight of 55 000, containing approximately 5 per cent carbohydrate. The toxicity is reduced 80-fold by cleaving the single disulphide bridge which holds together the two constituent polypeptide chains (Funatsu *et al.*, 1971). It would be of value to know if the adjuvanticity is diminished correspondingly by this manipulation.

10.2 Endotoxin from *Pseudomonas aeruginosa*

The lipopolysaccharide endotoxins have been discussed in general previously (see Section 8). This particular endotoxin comprises more than 85 per cent protein and was more commonly known as original endotoxin protein (OEP). It occurs, together with a lipopolysaccharide with endotoxin activity, in the cell wall of this gram-negative bacterium. OEP is apparently superior to the autologous lipopolysaccharide in inducing non-specific resistance to infection and implanted tumours in mice, and in stimulating interferon production by lymphoid cells (Homma and Abe, 1972). Since this bacillus resists conventional chemotherapy using, for example, penicillin, it causes frequent adventitious infection after burns, tissue grafting, intensive radiation, or steroid therapy, often with serious morbidity. OEP is now of further interest being an antigen common to very many *Pseudomonas* species (Homma, 1974) so that, under the name of 'common antigen', it is now being investigated quite intensively as a means of establishing effective immunity and therapy in *Pseudomonas* infections when conventional chemotherapy is inadequate. This has two consequences that must be of interest to the immunologist. Firstly, OEP is becoming increasingly more readily available, and secondly considerable experience is being accumulated about its safety and spectrum of side effects in man.

11 POSSIBLE HAZARDS OF ADJUVANTS

While the aetiology of many autoallergic disorders still remains unknown, it may be of some value to enquire if the average man is not unduly exposed to adjuvant-like immunostimulation from his everyday environment. One such stimulus is a biological one, in the form of persistent viral infection (Paterson, 1973).

Throughout this chapter it has been stressed how many materials with adjuvant activity are brought into contact with the body's surfaces or the gastrointestinal tract, not only in processed foodstuffs and cosmetics, but also during clinical treatment by the use of poultices, laxatives, suppositories, anti-diarrhoreal sorptive agents and massive vitamin supplementation. Normal human sebum and wool fat contain a number of lipids which will replace mineral oil in constituting Freund's adjuvants for inducing hypersensitivity disease in laboratory animals (Whitehouse *et al.*, 1974). Furthermore, the increasing burden of petroleum products in the environment such as greases or oil droplets (in insecticidal sprays) also should be considered, since these also must accumulate on the skin. In combination with many bacterial and fungal cell walls, they may become potential adjuvants, for either boosting non-specific host resistance on the one hand or triggering an autoallergy on the other, if they should happen to penetrate the external integument.

The safety of some Fd/EO adjuvants used with viral vaccines has been carefully evaluated (Hilleman, 1966, 1972). There is a real need for further reports on the long-term safety/toxicity of other adjuvants and immunopotentiating drugs.

ACKNOWLEDGEMENT

The author is indebted to Mrs M. Lee (Canberra) and Drs P. Y. Paterson (Chicago), O. Kohashi (Fukuoka), and D. W. Dresser (London) for their help at various stages in the preparation of this manuscript.

REFERENCES

Aggarwal, S. K., Wagner, R. W., McAllister, P., and Rosenberg, B. (1975). *Proc. Nat. Acad. Sci., U.S.A.*, **72**, 928.
Amies, C. R. (1959). *J. Pathol. Bacteriol.*, **77**, 435.
Anon. (1975). *Nature (Lond.)*, **254**, 18.
Asherson, G. L., and Allwood, G. G. (1969). In *The Biological Basis of Medicine*, Vol. 4, (Bittar, E. E., and Bittar, N., eds.), Academic Press, New York and London, p. 327.
Azuma, I., Kanetsuna, F., Taniyama, T., Yamamura, Y., Hori, M., and Tanaka, Y. (1975). *Bikens J.*, **18**, 1.
Azuma, I., Ribi, E. E., Meyer, T. J., and Zbar, B. (1974a). *J. Nat. Cancer Inst.*, **52**, 95.
Azuma, I., Yamamura, Y., and Ribi, E. (1974b). *Jap. J. Microbiol.*, **18**, 327.

Barba, G., Merlo, N., and Valguarnera, G. (1971). *Boll. Soc. Ital. Biol. Sper.*, **47**, 292.
Beck, F. J., and Whitehouse, M. W. (1973). *Biochem. Pharmacol.*, **22**, 2453.
Beck, F. W. J., and Whitehouse, M. W. (1974a). *Proc. Soc. Exp. Biol. Med.*, **145**, 135.
Beck, F. W. J., and Whitehouse, M. W. (1974b). *Proc. Soc. Exp. Biol. Med.*, **146**, 665.
Beck, F. W. J., and Whitehouse, M. W. (1975). *Proc. W. Pharmacol. Soc.*, **18**, 136.
Beets, R. F., and Braun, W., eds. (1971). *Biological Effects of Polynucleotides*, Springer Verlag, New York.
Bollinger, J. N. (1970). *J. Pharm. Sci.*, **59**, 1088.
Bradfield, J. W., Southami, R. L., and Addison, I. E. (1974). *Immunology*, **26**, 383.
Braun, W., Regelson, W., Yajima, Y., and Ishizuka, M. (1970). *Proc. Soc. Exp. Biol. Med.*, **133**, 171.
Bueltmann, B., Finger, H., Heymer, B., Schachenmayer, W., Hof, H., and Haferkamp, O. (1975). *Z. ImmunForsch. Exp. Klin. Immunol.*, **148** 425.

Campbell, P. A., Cooper, H. R., Heinzerling, R. H., and Tengerdy, R. P. (1974). *Proc. Soc. Exp. Biol. Med.*, **146**, 465.
Charabati, M. F., and McLaren, D. S. (1973). *Experientia*, **29**, 343.
Chase, M. W. (1976). In *Methods in Immunology and Immunochemistry* (Williams, C. A., and Chase, M. W., eds.), Vol. 1, Academic Press, New York and London, p. 197.
Chihara, G., Hamuro, J., Maeda, Y. Y., Arai, Y., and Fukuoka, F. (1970). *Cancer Res.*, **30**, 2776.
Claman, H. N., and Bronsky, E. A. (1965). *J. Immunol.*, **95**, 718.
Cunnington, P. G., and Naysmith, J. D. (1975). *Immunology*, **28**, 451.

Dalsgaard, K. (1974). *Archs ges. VirusForsch.*, **44**, 243.
Dennert, G., and Tucker, D. (1973). *J. Nat. Cancer Inst.*, **51**, 1727.
Diamantstein, T., Odenwald, G., and Odenwald, D. (1971a). *Experientia*, **27**, 953.

Diamantstein, T., Stork, C., and Malenus, R. (1973). *Experientia*, **29**, 214.

Diamantstein, T., Wagner, B., Beyse, I., Odenwald, M. V., and Schulz, G. (1971*b*). *Eur. J. Immunol.*, **1**, 335.

Diamantstein, T., Wagner, B., Beyse, I., Odenwald, M. V., and Schulz, G. (1971*c*). *Eur. J. Immunol.*, **1**, 340.

Dienes, L., and Schoenheit, E. W. (1930). *J. Immunol.*, **19**, 41.

Di Rosa, M. (1972). *J. Pharm. Pharmacol.*, **24**, 89.

Dokukin, I. S., Samoilova, A. I., and Yamashev, S. G. (1972). *Chem. Abstr.*, **104**, 145.

Dresser, D. W. (1968). *Nature (Lond.)*, **217**, 527.

Ellouz, F., Adam, A., Ciorbaru, R., and Lederer, E. (1974). *Biochem. Biophys. Res. Commun.*, **59**, 1317.

Engelhorn, R., and Püschmann (1963). *ArzneimittelForsch.*, **13**, 474.

Fleck, J., Mock, M., Tytgat, F., Nauciel, C., and Minck, R. (1974). *Nature (Lond.)*, **250**, 517.

Floersheim, G. K., and Szeszak, J. J. (1971). *Ag. Act.*, **2**, 150.

Freund, J. (1947). *Ann. Rev. Microbiol.*, **1**, 295.

Freund, J. (1956). *Adv. Tubercul. Res.*, **7**, 130.

Freund, J., and McDermott, K. (1942). *Proc. Soc. Exp. Biol. Med.*, **49**, 548.

Funatsu, M., Funatsu, G., Masatsune, I., and Kenji, H. (1971). *Proc. Japan Acad.*, **47**, 786.

Gale, G. R. (1975). In *Handbook of Experimental Pharmacology*, Vol. 38/2 (Sartorelli, A. C., and Johns, D. G., eds.), Springer Verlag, Heidelberg, p. 829.

Gall, D. (1966). *Immunology*, **11**, 369.

Gall, D., Knight, P. A., and Hampson, F. (1972). *Immunology*, **23**, 569.

Glynn, L. E. (1968). *Ann. Rheumat. Dis.*, **27**, 113.

Glynn, L. E. (1974). In *Proceedings of the International Symposium on Rheumatology* (Ballabio, C. B., Weissmann, G., Willoughby, D. A., and Ziff, M., eds.), Carlo Elba Foundation, Milan, p. 28.

Götz, H. (1975). *ArzneimittelForsch.*, **25**, 607.

Grafe, A. (1971). *Arzneimittel-Forsch.*, **21**, 903.

Griswold, D. E., Heppner, G. H., and Calabresi, P. (1975). *Cancer Res.*, **35**, 88.

Gumbiner, C., Paterson, P. Y., Youmans, G. P., and Youmans, A. S. (1973). *J. Immunol.*, **110**, 309.

Haas, R., and Thomssen, R. (1961). *Ergebn. Mikrobiol. ImmunForsch. Exp. Therap.*, **34**, 27.

Hamiro, J., Maeda, Y. Y., Arai, Y., Fukuoka, F., and Chihara, G. (1971). *Chem. Biol. Interactions*, **3**, 69.

Herbert, W. J. (1973). In *Handbook of Experimental Immunology* (Weir, D. M., ed.), 2nd edn., Blackwell, Oxford, Appendix 2.

Hilleman, M. R. (1966). *Prog. Med. Virol.*, **8**, 131.

Hilleman, M. R. (1972). *Ann. Allergy*, **30**, 477.

Homma, J. Y. (1974). *Jap. J. Exp. Med.*, **44**, 1.

Homma, J. Y., and Abe, C. (1972). *Jap. J. Exp. Med.*, **42**, 23.

Ishikawa, H., Narimatsu, H., and Saito, K. (1975). *Cell. Immunol.*, **17**, 300.

Johnson, A. G. (1973). *J. Reticuloendoth. Soc.*, **14**, 441.

Johnson, A. G. (1974). *Ann. Reports. Med. Chem.*, **9**, 244.

Johnson, A. G., Gaines, S., and Landy, M. (1956). *J. Exp. Med.*, **103**, 225.

Jollés, P., and Paraf, A. (1973). *Chemical and Biological Basis of Adjuvants*, Chapman and Hall, London.

598

Joly, M., and Barbu, E. (1950). *Bull. Soc. Chim. Biol.*, **32**, 908.

Jordan, G. W., and Merigan, T. C. (1975). *Ann. Rev. Pharmacol.*, **15**, 157.

Jurin, M., and Tannock, I. F. (1972). *Immunology*, **23**, 283.

Kalic, R. V., Batty, I., and Vukicevic, Z. (1965). *Bull. Acad. Vet. France*, **38**, 453; *Chem. Abstr.*, *1965*, **65**, 4428f.

Knight, P. A. (1969). *Prog. Immunbiol. Stand.*, **3**, 252; *Chem. Abstr.*, *1971*, **75**, 25291.

Koga, T., and Pearson, C. M. (1973). *J. Immunol.*, **111**, 599.

Koga, T., Sugiyama, K., and Tanaka, K. (1971). *Experientia*, **27**, 323.

Koga, T., Tanaka, A., and Pearson, C. M. (1976). *Int. Archs Allergy Appl. Immunol.*, **51**, 583.

Kohn, A., Helering, I., and Ben Efraim, S. (1969). *Int. Archs Allergy Appl. Immunol.*, **36**, 156.

Kolter, L., Herrmann, C., Ring, C., and Corsico, G. (1966). *Zentbl. VetMed. (Reihe B)*, **13**, 613; *Chem. Abstr.*, *1966*, **66**, 115035.

Kotani, S. *et al.* (1975*a*). *Biken J.*, **18**, 135.

Kotani, S. *et al.* (1975*b*). *Biken J.*, **18**, 105.

Kotani, S. *et al.* (1975*c*). *Biken J.*, **18**, 93.

Kotani, S. *et al.* (1975*d*). *Z. ImmunForsch.*, **149**, 302.

Krueger, R. F., and Mayer, G. D. (1970). *Science, N.Y.*, **169**, 1213.

Kuleshova, O. V., and Preger, S. M. (1971). *Chem. Abstr.*, **75**, 107608.

Kulkarni, V. B., Mulbagal, A. N., Paranjape, V. L., Khot, J. B., and Manda, A. V. (1973). *Ind. Vet. J.*, **50**, 225; *Chem. Abstr.*, *1973*, **79**, 27141.

Lacour, F., Nahon-Merlin, E., and Michelson, M. (1973). *Curr. Top. Microbiol. Immunol.*, **62**, 1.

Lallouette, P., Richou, R., Legger, H., and Schwartz, A. (1968). *C.r. Acad. Sci., Ser. D*, **267**, 2391.

Levine, S., and Sowinski, R. (1975). *J. Immunol.*, **114**, 597.

Levy, L., and Whitehouse, M. W. (1974). *Ag. Act.*, **4**, 113.

Mackaness, G. B., Auclair, D. J., and Lagrange, P. H. (1973). *J. Nat. Cancer Inst.*, **51**, 1655.

Maeda, Y. Y., and Chiahara, G. (1971). *Nature*, **229**, 634.

Mancino, D., and Bresciano, E. (1972). *Atti Accad. Naz. Lincei*, **53**, 612; *Chem. Abstr.*, *1974*, **81**, 2239.

Marzulli, F. N., Carson, T. R., and Maibach, H. I. (1968). *Proc. Joint Conf. Cosmet. Sci.*, p. 107; *Chem. Abstr.*, *1969*, **70**, 104684.

Mathé, G., Kamel, M., Dezfulian, M., Halle-Pannenko, O., and Bourut, C. (1973). *Cancer Res.*, **33**, 1987.

McIntire, F. C. (1970). *Chem. Abstr.*, **73**, 91233.

Measel, J. W., Jr. (1975). *Infect. Immunol.*, **11**, 350.

Megel, H., Raychaudhuri, A., Goldstein, S., Kinsolving, C. R., Shemano, T., and Michael, J. G. (1974). *Proc. Soc. Exp. Biol. Med.*, **145**, 513.

Merritt, K. (1971). *Infect. Immunol.*, **4**, 393.

Migliore-Samour, D., Korontzis, M., Jollés, P., Maral, R., Floch, F., and Werner, G. H. (1974). *Immunol. Commun.*, **3**, 593.

Mitchell, G. F. (1975). *Immunology*, **29**, 39.

Mizushima, Y., Wada, Y., and Yasumira, K. (1974). *Int. Archs Allergy Appl. Immunol.*, **46**, 731.

Monath, T. P. C., and Borden, E. C. (1971). *J. Infect. Dis.*, **123**, 297.

Munson, A. E., Munson, J. A., Regelson, W., and Wampler, G. L. (1972). *Cancer Res.*, **32**, 1397.

Myrvick, Q. N. (1974). *Ann. N.Y. Acad. Sci.*, **1974**, 221, 324.

Neter, E. (1969). *Curr. Top. Microbiol. Immunol.*, **47**, 82.
Newbould (1965). *Immunology*, **9**, 613.

Ortiz-Ortiz, L., and Jaraslow, B. N. (1970). *Immunology*, **19**, 387.

Paterson, P. Y. (1973). *J. Reticulo-endoth. Soc.*, **14**, 426.
Pearson, C. M. (1972). In *Arthritis and Allied Conditions*, 8th edn. (Hollander, J. L., and McCarty, D. J., Jr., eds.), Lea and Febiger, Philadelphia, p. 195.
Petermann, H. G., Soulebot, J. P., Lang, R., and Branche, R. (1970). *C.r. Acad. Sci., Ser. D*, **270**, 234.
Plescia, O. J., and Braun, W., eds. (1968). *Nucleic Acids in Immunology*, Springer Verlag, New York.

Renoux, G., and Renoux, M. (1972). *J. Immunol.*, **109**, 761.
Renoux, G., and Renoux, M. (1974). *J. Immunol.*, **113**, 779.
Rethy, L., Hegedus, V. P., Juhasz, V. P., and Bacskai, L. (1968). *Ann. Immunol. Hung.*, **11**, 87; *Chem. Abstr.*, *1970*, **72**, 98533.
Richou, R., Lallouette, P., and Hugues, L. (1968). *C.r. Acad. Sci., Series D*, **267**, 257.

Salvaggio, J., and Kundur, V. (1970). *Proc. Soc. Exp. Biol. Med.*, **134**, 1116.
Schmidt, G., Hennessen, W., and Schlosser, G. (1966). *Z. Med. Mikrobiol. Immunol.*, **152**, 73.
Schuetzler, H. (1965). *Archs Exp. VetMed.*, **19**, 331; *Chem. Abstr.*, **64**, 20395b.
Shaw, C. M., Alvord, E. C., Jr., and Kies, M. W. (1964). *J. Immunol.*, **92**, 24.
Shier, W. T., Trotter, J. T., III, Reading, C. L., and Lennon, V. A. (1974). *Int. Archs Allergy Appl. Immunol.*, **47**, 688.
Sofia, R. D., and Douglas, J. F. (1973). *Ag. Act.*, **3**, 335.
Spallholz, J. E., Martin, J. L., Gerlach, M. L., and Heinzerling, R. H. (1975). *Proc. Soc. Exp. Biol. Med.*, **148**, 37.
Spitznagel, J. K., and Allison, A. C. (1970). *J. Immunol.*, **104**, 119.
Stewart-Tull, D. E. S., Shimono, T., Kotani, S., Kato, M., Ogawa, Y., Yamamura, Y., Koga, T., and Pearson, C. M. (1975). *Immunology*, **29**, 1.
Swingle, K. F. (1974). In *Anti-inflammatory Agents*, Vol. II (Scherrer, R. A., and Whitehouse, M. W., eds.), Academic Press, New York and London, p. 92.

Thienpont, D. *et al.* (1966) *Nature (Lond.)*, **209**, 1084.
Turk, J. L. (1975). In *Delayed Hypersensitivity*, 2nd edn., North Holland Publishing Co., Amsterdam, p. 16.

Unanue, E. R., Askonas, B. A., and Allison, A. C. (1969). *J. Immunol.*, **103**, 71.

Wacker, A., Chandra, P., Haenzel, I., and Gericke, D. (1970). *Z. Phys. Chem.*, **351**, 1273.
Walz, D. T., Di Martino, M. J., and Sutton, B. M. (1974). In *Anti-inflammatory Agents*, Vol. I (Scherrer, R. A., and Whitehouse, M. W., eds.), Academic Press, New York and London, p. 209.
Westphal, O. (1975). *Int. Archs Allergy Appl. Immunol.*, **49**, 1.
White, R. G. (1967). *Brit. Med. Bull.*, **23**, 39.
White, R. G. (1972). In *Immunogenicity* (Borek, F., ed.), North Holland Publishing Co., Amsterdam, p. 112.
Whitehouse, M. W. (1973). *Ag. Act.*, **3**, 221.
Whitehouse, M. W. (1975). *Ag. Act.*, **5**, 508.

600

Whitehouse, M. W., and Beck, F. W. J. (1974). *Ag. Act.*, **4**, 227.
Whitehouse, M. W., Orr, K. J., Beck, F. W. J., and Pearson, C. M. (1974). *Immunology*, **27**, 311.
Wieczorek, Z., Staroscik, K., Lisowski, J., and Zimecki, M. (1975). *Eur. J. Immunol.*, **5**, 157.
Wilkinson, P. C., and White, R. G. (1966), *Immunology*, **11**, 229.
Wolmark, N., Levine, M., and Fisher, B. (1974). *J. Reticulo-endoth. Soc.*, **16**, 252.

Youmans, G. P., and Youmans, A. S. (1969). *Curr. Top. Microbiol. Immunol.*, **48**, 129.
Youmans, A. S., and Youmans, G. P. (1972). *Infect. Immunity*, **6**, 798.

Zimakov, Y. A., and Zimakova, I. E. (1973). *Chem. Abstr.*, **79**, 51706.

ADDENDUM (mid-1977)

The World Health Organization has issued a valuable 40-page pamphlet discussing immunological adjuvants (WHO, 1976). Other recent reviews discuss the adjuvant effects of microbial products (Jolles, 1976; White, 1976).

Bacterial glycolipids (Azuma *et al.*, 1976; Kumazawa *et al.*, 1976; Saito *et al.*, 1976), dextran sulphate (McCarthy *et al.*, 1977), DEAE-dextran (Houston *et al.*, 1976), polymethylmethylacrylate (Kreuter *et al.*, 1976), amorphous silica (Mancino and Bevilacqua, 1977), double-stranded RNA (Butlin and Cunnington, 1976), alkylated (i.e. detoxified) endotoxins (Chedid *et al.*, 1975), and OEP (Sasaki *et al.*, 1976) all continue to attract attention as alternatives to Freund's adjuvants.

Synthetic (glyco)lipids may be important adjuvants in the future. Significant prototypes are analogues of lysolecithin containing an ether linkage *in lieu* of lipase-sensitive ester linkages (Weltzien, 1975; Strannegärd and Roupe, 1976) and *N*-alkanoyl-D.glucosamines which mimic lipid A (see p. 587) with less toxicity (Behling *et al.*, 1976).

Synthetic muramyldipeptide (Figure 3, p. 591) is now commercially available (e.g. from Bachem Inc., Torrance, Calif. 90505) and the subject of many reports including structure–activity surveys (Adam *et al.*, 1976; Azuma *et al.*, 1976; Chedid *et al.*, 1977; Tanaka *et al.*, 1977). Remarkably, it is orally active (Chedid *et al.*, 1977). It is not arthritogenic in rats (Kohashi *et al.*, 1976) and apparently activates T-lymphocytes rather than macrophages (Löwy *et al.*, 1977).

Experiments with liposomes, to entrap immunogen and conserve it from rapid biodegradation, suggest that a new adjuvant technology is being rapidly developed (Allison and Gregoriadis, 1974; Uemara *et al.*, 1974; Heath *et al.*, 1976).

The complications of using mineral oils to prepare Freund's adjuvants has been noted again with some oils giving a toxic immunosuppressive effect, rather than the desired adjuvanticity (Stewart-Tull *et al.*, 1976). These authors conclude: 'It would seem timely in adjuvant research to re-examine the oil component of Freund-type adjuvants in order to obtain a well-defined, non-toxic, non-biodegradable mixture (sic) of hydrocarbons suitable for use in vaccine preparations'.

REFERENCES

Adam, A., Devys, M., Souvannavong, V., Lefrancier, P., Choay, J., and Lederer, E. (1976). *Biochem. Biophys. Res. Comm.*, **72**, 339.
Allison, A. C., and Gregoriadis, G. (1974). *Nature*, **252**, 252.
Azuma, I., Sugimura, K., Itoh, S., and Yamamura, Y. (1976a). *Jap. J. Microbiol.*, **20**, 465.
Azuma, I., Sugimura, K., Taniyama, T., Yamawaki, M., Yamamura, Y., Kusumoto, S., Okada, S., and Shiba, T. (1976b). *Inf. Immun.*, **14**, 18.

Behling, U. H., Campbell, B., Chang, C-M., Rumpf, C., and Nowotny, A. (1976). *J. Immunol.*, **117**, 847.
Butlin, P. M., and Cunnington, P. G. (1976). *Eu. J. Immunol.*, **6**, 607.

Chedid, L., Audibert, F., Bona, C., Damais, C., Parant, F., and Parant, M. (1975). *Inf. Immun.*, **12**, 714.
Chedid, L., Parant, M., Parant, F., Lefrancier, P., Choay, J., and Lederer, E. (1977). *Proc. Natl. Acad. Sci. USA*, **74**, 2089.

Heath, T. D., Edwards, D. C., and Ryman, B. E. (1976). *Biochem. Soc. Trans.*, **4**, 129.
Houston, W. E., Crabbs, C. L., Kremer, R. J., and Springer, J. W. (1976). *Infect. Immun.*, **13**, 1559.

Jolles, P. (1976). *Experientia*, **32**, 677.

Kohashi, O., Pearson, C. M., Watanabe, Y., Kotani, S., and Koga, T. (1976). *J. Immunol.*, **116**, 1635.
Kreuter, J., Mauler, R., Gruschkau, H., and Speiser, P. P. (1976). *Exp. Cell Biol.*, **44**, 12.
Kumazawa, Y., Shibusawa, A., and Suzuki, T. (1976). *Immunochem.*, **13**, 173.

Löwy, I., Bona, C., and Chedid, L. (1977). *Cell Immunol.*, **29**, 195.

Mancino, D., and Bevilacqua, N. (1977). *Int. Arch. Allergy appl. Immun.*, **53**, 97.
McCarthy, R. E., Arnold, L. W., and Babcock, G. F. (1977). *Immunology*, **32**, 963.

Saito, R., Tanaka, A., Sugitama, K., Azuma, I., Yamamura, Y., Kato, M., and Goren, M. B. (1976). *Infect. Immun.*, **13**, 776.
Sasaki, M., Ito, M., and Komma, J. Y. (1976). *Jap. J. Exp. Med.*, **45**, 335.
Stewart-Tull, D. E. S., Shimono, T., Kotani, S., and Knights, B. A. (1976). *Int. Arch. Allergy appl. Immun.*, **52**, 118.
Strannegärd, O., and Roupe, G. (1976). *Int. Arch. Allergy appl. Immun.*, **51**, 198.

Tanaka, A., Nagao, S., Saito, R., Kotani, S., Kusumoto, S., and Shiba, T. (1977). *Biochem. Biophys. Res. Comm.*, **77**, 621.

Uemura, K-I., Nicolotti, R. A., Six, H. R., and Kinsky, S. C. (1974). *Biochemistry*, **13**, 1572.

Weltzien, H. U. (1975). *Exp. Cell. Res.*, **92**, 111.
White, R. G. (1976). *Ann. Rev. Microbiol.*, **30**, 579.
WHO Scientific Group (1976). *WHO Tech. Rep.*, Ser. No. **595**, pp. 40.

Notes on the Cellular Basis of the Immuno-potentiating Action of Adjuvants

D. W. Dresser

1 CELLULAR ORIENTATION

There are three major cellular compartments concerned in the humoral immune response; these are the T and B-lymphocytes and macrophages (Miller and Mitchell, 1969). *Bordetella pertussis* vaccine has been shown to be an adjuvant affecting all three compartments. (*i*) It can have an effect on antigen processing and on the production of lymphocyte-activating factors by macrophages (Unanue *et al.*, 1969). (*ii*) It can stimulate T cells at low doses of antigen. (*iii*) It can have preferential effects on B cells at high-dose of antigen (Dresser, 1972). In contrast, lipopolysaccharide, a well-known B cell mitogen (Andersson *et al.*, 1972), is an adjuvant oriented towards B cells, and lentinan is an adjuvant which is oriented towards T cells (Dresser and Phillips, 1973; Maeda *et al.*, 1973).

2 CELLULAR BASIS OF IMMUNOPOTENTIATION

Examination of plaque sizes shows that increased antibody production per cell cannot account for the potentiating effect of adjuvants on serum antibody levels. Potentiation is the result of an increase in the number of cells producing antibody. In terms of the clonal selection theory of acquired immunity, adjuvants may be seen to act on the response of mice to sheep erythrocytes in two ways. Firstly, they increase the number of stem cells induced to proliferate into clones of antibody cells. The result of this is an increase in the heterogeneity of the response as measured by the isoelectric focusing–overlay assay (Phillips and Dresser, 1973). Secondly, they increase the amount of proliferation taking place in each clone. The increase in burst-size is reflected by larger amounts of antibody in each spectrotype (clonal product) detected by the isoelectric focusing-overlay assay (Dresser *et al.*, 1975).

3 THE TOLERANCE–IMMUNITY SWITCH

Non-immunogenic antigens induce a specific state of tolerance unless there is a concomitant administration of an adjuvant. An antigen-sensitive cell receiving a 'pure' antigenic stimulus is induced to enter a process of tolerant induction— suicide. If, however, the antigen-sensitive cell receives an adjuvant stimulus in addition to, and concomitantly with, the antigenic stimulus, a process of immune induction will be initiated. Early experiments leading to a two-stimulus model of the immune response (Dresser, 1962) have been modified recently and extended considerably by Bretscher and Cohn (1970) in the form of the 'two-signal model'. In this model, antigen provides signal one, and carrier determinants (in combination with an associative antibody derived from a third party cellular source) provide signal two, which gives an antigen-sensitive cell a mitotic stimulus. Failure to receive the mitotic signal two, after receiving an antigenic signal one, is interpreted as a tolerance-inducing signal.

4 CELL DIFFERENTIATION AND THE ACTION OF ADJUVANTS IN BLOCKING TOLERANCE INDUCTION

It seems reasonable to postulate that antibody production is an extension of a basic mechanism of cell differentiation. Some inducers of cell differentiation are likely to be generated within the cell (Jacob and Monod, 1961). Others may pass from one cell to another, as is envisaged for 'embryonic inducers' or hormones (see Tiedmann, 1971). In immunodifferentiation, the system has evolved to cope with two apparently conflicting demands. These are the need, for reasons of spacial and thermodynamic economy, to be able to respond specifically to a wide range of environmental inducers, and also a means of preventing an immune response to self-determinants (Burnet and Fenner, 1949). Many authors have pointed out that not only is differentiation obviously a function of cell division, but also that it is likely that the decision-making mechanism is itself an integral part of the cell cycle (see Holtzer *et al.*, 1973).

Thomas and Lingwood (1975) have shown that a tumour cell line (P815Y) is sensitive to external inducers during a short switch point in early G_1 phase. Cells which have already received a mitotic (transformation) stimulus can be switched at this critical point from a pathway of continued cycling to a pathway where, after completion of the cycle, the two daughter cells enter a null state perhaps equivalent to G_0, despite culture conditions being excellent. The model has been extended to account for the tolerance–immunity switch (Dresser and Phillips, 1975; Dresser, 1976). In this model, antigen-sensitive cells receive a mitotic stimulus from antigen, and pass into the critical transition point of early G_1 where they become susceptible to adjuvant-like inducers (switch-point stimuli). If they fail to receive a switch stimulus the daughter cells enter G_0 and become null (or dead), whereas receipt of a switch (adjuvant-like) stimulus results in the commencement of differentiation towards the formation of a 'clone' of antibody-forming cells. In this model of the tolerance–immunity switch, an antigen is the trigger stimulus for mitosis and the adjuvant is a permissive stimulus operating a differentiational gate.

5 MECHANISM OF IMMUNOPOTENTIATION

It is proposed that adjuvants may potentiate the immune response in at least one of several ways.

(i) By acting as an additional switch-point stimulus, operating the differentiational gate so that immune induction is favoured at the expense of tolerance induction. This effect is particularly significant with antigens of low immunogenicity.

(ii) By supplying a permissive switch-point stimulus which allows prolonged post-antigen proliferation and hence a greater number of producing cells in each clone derived from a successfully 'hit' antigen-sensitive cell. This is of greater significance for immunogenic antigens, such as with sheep erythrocytes in mice (Dresser *et al.*, 1975).

(iii) By increasing the probability of successful contact between T and B cells, macrophages, and antigens through activation of the lymphocyte-trapping mechanism (Taub *et al.*, 1970; Frost and Lance, 1973).

(iv) By increasing the number of helper T cells in relation to the number of suppressor T cells (Dresser and Tao, 1974).

(v) By a depot effect in which antigen is released over a prolonged period (Freund, 1953).

(vi) By increasing the sensitivity of the detector systems, such as in the increased histamine sensitivity seeen after the administration of *B. pertussis* vaccine (Malkiel, 1953).

REFERENCES

Andersson, J., Sjöberg, O., and Möller, G. (1972). *Transplant. Rev.*, **11**, 131.

Bretscher, P., and Cohn, M. (1970). *Science, N.Y.*, **169**, 1042.
Burnet, F. M., and Fenner, F. (1949). *The Production of Antibodies*, Macmillan, Melbourne.

Dresser, D. W. (1962). *Immunology*, **5**, 378.
Dresser, D. W. (1972). *Eur. J. Immunol.*, **2**, 50.
Dresser, D. W. (1976). *Brit. Med. Bull.*, **32** (2), 147.
Dresser, D. W., and Phillips, J. M. (1973). *Ciba Symp.*, **18**, 3.

Dresser, D. W., and Phillips, J. M. (1975). *Modulation of host immune resistance in the prevention or control of induced neoplasia*, Vol. **28**, Foggarty International Center Proceedings, U.S. Govt. Printing Office, Washington, p. 303.

Dresser, D. W., and Tao, T. W. (1974). *Immunology*, **28**, 443.

Dresser, D. W., Phillips, J. M., and Pryjma, J. (1975). *Proc. 4th Convoc. Immunol.*, **194**, p. 191.

Freund, J. (1953). In *Nature and significance of the antibody response* (Pappenheimer, A. M., ed.), Columbia University Press, Colombia.

Frost, P., and Lance, E. M. (1973). *Ciba Symp.*, **18**, 29, p. 46.

Holtzer, H., Weintraub, H., Mayne, R., and Mochan, B. (1973). *Contemp. Top. Dev. Biol.*, **7**, 229.

Jacob, F., and Monod, J. (1961). *Cold Spring Harbor Symp. Quant. Biol.*, **26**, 193.

Maeda, Y. Y. *et al.* (1973). *Ciba Symp.*, **18**, 257.

Malkiel, S. (1953). *Att. 6th Congr. Int. Microbiol.*, **2**, 265.

Miller, J. F. A. P., and Mitchell, G. F. (1969). *Transplant. Rev.*, **1**, 3.

Phillips, J. M., and Dresser, D. W. (1973). *Eur. J. Immunol.*, **3**, 524.

Taub, R. N., Krantz, A. R., and Dresser, D. W. (1970). *Immunology*, **18**, 171.

Thomas, D. B., and Lingwood, C. A. (1975). *Cell*, **5**, 37.

Tiedmann, H. (1971). *Symp. Soc. Exp. Biol.*, **25**, 223.

Unanue, E. R., Askonas, B. A., and Allison, A. C. (1969). *J. Immunol.*, **103**, 71.

INDEX

628